MEMORY DISORDERS

Neurological Disease and Therapy

Series Editor
William C. Koller
Department of Neurology
University of Kansas Medical Center
Kansas City, Kansas

Volume 1   Handbook of Parkinson's Disease
Edited by William C. Koller

Volume 2   Medical Therapy of Acute Stroke
Edited by Mark Fisher

Volume 3   Familial Alzheimer's Disease: Molecular Genetics and Clinical
Perspectives
*Edited by Gary D. Miner, Ralph W. Richter, John P. Blass,
Jimmie L. Valentine, and Linda A. Winters-Miner*

Volume 4   Alzheimer's Disease: Treatment and Long-Term Management
Edited by Jeffrey L. Cummings and Bruce L. Miller

Volume 5   Therapy of Parkinson's Disease
Edited by William C. Koller and George Paulson

Volume 6   Handbook of Sleep Disorders
Edited by Michael J. Thorpy

Volume 7   Epilepsy and Sudden Death
Edited by Claire M. Lathers and Paul L. Schraeder

Volume 8   Handbook of Multiple Sclerosis
Edited by Stuart D. Cook

Volume 9   Memory Disorders: Research and Clinical Practice
Edited by Takehiko Yanagihara and Ronald C. Petersen

Additional Volumes in Preparation

MEMORY DISORDERS
Research and Clinical Practice

Edited by

Takehiko Yanagihara

Ronald C. Petersen

Mayo Clinic and Mayo Foundation
Rochester, Minnesota

MARCEL DEKKER, INC.   **New York · Basel · Hong Kong**

Library of Congress Cataloging-in-Publication Data

Memory disorders : research and clinical practice/ edited by Takehiko
   Yanagihara and Ronald C. Petersen.
       p.   cm. -- (Neurological disease and therapy ; v. 9)
   Includes bibliographical references.
   Includes index.
   ISBN 0-8247-8489-8 (alk. paper)
   1. Memory disorders.   I. Yanagihara, Takehiko
II.   Petersen, Ronald C.   III. Series.
   [DNLM: 1. Memory. 2. Memory Disorders. W1 NE33LD v. 9 / WM
173.7 M5327]
   RC394.M46M49 1991
   616.8'4--dc20
   DLC   91-9454
   for Library of Congress   CIP

This book is printed on acid-free paper

MARCEL DEKKER, INC.
270 Madison Avenue, New York, New York 10016

Current printing (last digit):
10 9 8 7 6 5 4 3 2 1

PRINTED IN THE UNITED STATES OF AMERICA

Preface

Memory function is not unique to human beings. However, it is one of the most important cognitive functions and essential to independent human life. Accordingly, both normal memory functions and memory disorders have been investigated intensely by clinicians and cognitive neuroscientists in recent decades. Thanks to these investigators, a great deal of information has been accumulated in the literature regarding memory functions and memory disorders, and we now have fair understanding of many of the anatomical, biochemical, pharmacological and psychological aspects of memory functions. Obviously, there is much more to be learned. It appears, however, that clinicians and cognitive neuroscientists often address the issues regarding memory functions and memory disorders from different perspectives. Normal memory function has been the main focus of cognitive neuroscientists who have used a variety of theoretical models and experimental paradigms, while much of the work on memory disorders has been the focus of clinical investigators who have relied on a variety of clinical and neuropsychological assessment techniques. One of our goals was to make a large volume of literature from these two different approaches comprehensible to both clinicians and cognitive neuroscientists. In this volume, an attempt has been made by the cognitive neuroscientists to prepare their material for the clinicians, and by the clinical investigators to prepare their material for the cognitive neuroscientists. We hope that this large volume of work related to memory disorders has been presented in a readable fashion for practicing clinicians, psychologists, and cognitive neuroscientists and that this monograph will serve as a reference book for them as well as for students studying neuropsychology and cognitive neurosciences.

We are grateful to Mr. Paul Dolgert, Executive Editor of Marcel Dekker, Inc. Medical Division, for providing us this opportunity and Ms. Della McEneaney, Senior Production Editor, for her excellent editorial assistance. We also express our appreciation to Mrs. Gail Sim and Ms. Ellen Ptacek of the Mayo Clinic for their assistance for preparation of this monograph.

Takehiko Yanagihara
Ronald C. Petersen

Contributors

John P. Aggleton, Ph.D.   Department of Psychology, University of Durham, Durham, England

Marilyn S. Albert, Ph.D.   Departments of Psychiatry and Neurology, Massachusetts General Hospital, Harvard Medical School, Boston, Massachusetts

Warren T. Blume, M.D.   Epilepsy Unit, University Hospital, University of Western Ontario, London, Ontario, Canada

Nelson Butters, Ph.D.   Psychology Service, San Diego Veterans Administration Medical Center, La Jolla; Departments of Psychiatry and Neurosciences, University of California School of Medicine at San Diego, San Diego, California

Richard J. Caselli, M.D.   Department of Neurology, Mayo Clinic and Mayo Foundation, Rochester, Minnesota

Fergus I. M. Craik, Ph.D.   Department of Psychology, University of Toronto, Toronto, Ontario, Canada

Felicia C. Goldstein, Ph.D.   Department of Neurology, Emory University, Atlanta, Georgia

William C. Heindel, Ph.D.   Psychology Service, San Diego Veterans Administration Medical Center, La Jolla; Departments of Psychiatry and Neuroscience, University of California School of Medicine at San Diego, San Diego, California

Robert J. Ivnik, Ph.D.   Department of Psychiatry and Psychology, Mayo Clinic and Mayo Foundation, Rochester, Minnesota

Alfred W. Kaszniak, Ph.D.   Department of Psychology, University of Arizona, Tucson, Arizona

John F. Kihlstrom, Ph.D.   Department of Psychology, University of Arizona, Tucson, Arizona

Ginette Lafleche, Ph.D.   Departments of Psychiatry and Neurology, Massachusetts General Hospital, Harvard Medical School, Boston, Massachusetts

Brian A. Lawlor, M.D.   Division of Psychogeriatrics, Mount Sinai School of Medicine, New York, New York

Harvey S. Levin, Ph.D.   Division of Neurosurgery, University of Texas Medical Branch, Galveston, Texas

Christopher J. Mace, M.R.C. Psych.   Department of Neuropsychiatry, The National Hospital for Neurology and Neurosurgery, London, England

Rick A. Martinez, M.D.   Unit on Geriatric Psychopharmacology, Section on Clinical Neuropharmacology, Laboratory of Clinical Science, National Institute of Mental Health, National Institutes of Health, Bethesda, Maryland

M.-Marsel Mesulam, M.D.   Division of Neuroscience and Behavioral Neurology, Department of Neurology, Dana Research Institute and Beth Israel Hospital, Harvard Medical School, Boston, Massachusetts

John W. Miller, M.D., Ph.D.   Department of Neurology and Neurological Surgery (Neurology), Washington University School of Medicine, St. Louis, Missouri

Richard C. Mohs, Ph.D.   Department of Psychiatry, Mount Sinai School of Medicine, New York, New York

Susan E. Molchan, M.D.   Unit on Geriatric Psychopharmacology, Section on Clinical Neuropharmacology, Laboratory of Clinical Science, National Institute of Mental Health, National Institutes of Health, Bethesda, Maryland

Ronald C. Petersen, Ph.D., M.D.   Department of Neurology, Mayo Clinic and Mayo Foundation, Rochester, Minnesota

David P. Salmon, Ph.D.   Psychology Service, San Diego Veterans Administration Medical Center, La Jolla; Departments of Psychiatry and Neurosciences, University of California School of Medicine at San Diego, San Diego, California

Daniel L. Schacter, Ph.D. Department of Psychology, University of Arizona, Tucson, Arizona

Mary Lou Smith, Ph.D. Department of Psychology, Erindale College, University of Toronto, Mississauga, Ontario, Canada

Trey Sunderland, M.D. Unit on Geriatric Psychopharmacology, Section on Clinical Neuropharmacology, Laboratory of Clinical Science, National Institute of Mental Health, National Institutes of Health, Bethesda, Maryland

Michael R. Trimble, FRCP, FRCPsych. Department of Neuropsychiatry, The National Hospital for Neurology and Neurosurgery, London, England

Herbert Weingartner, Ph.D. Unit on Geriatric Psychopharmacology, Section on Clinical Neuropharmacology, Laboratory of Clinical Science, National Institute of Mental Health, National Institutes of Health, Bethesda, Maryland

Takehiko Yanagihara, M.D. Department of Neurology, Mayo Clinic and Mayo Foundation, Rochester, Minnesota

Contents

Preface   iii

Contributors   v

Part I   Introduction

1. **Memory Disorders: An Overview**   3
   Takehiko Yanagihara and Ronald C. Petersen

2. **Memory Nomenclature**   9
   Ronald C. Petersen and Herbert Weingartner

Part II   Memory Structure and Function

3. **Anatomy of Memory**   23
   John P. Aggleton

4. **Central Cholinergic Pathways: Neuroanatomy and Some Behavioral Implications**   63
   M.-Marsel Mesulam

5. **Drugs and Memory**   97
   *Brian A. Lawlor, Trey Sunderland, Rick A. Martinez,
   Susan E. Molchan, and Herbert Weingartner*

6.   Models of Memory and the Understanding of Memory Disorders   111
     Daniel L. Schacter, Alfred W. Kaszniak, and John F. Kihlstrom

Part III   Evaluation of Memory Function

7.   Memory Assessment at the Bedside   137
     Ronald C. Petersen

8.   Memory Testing   153
     Robert J. Ivnik

9.   Neuropsychological Testing of Memory Disorders   165
     Marilyn S. Albert and Ginette Lafleche

Part IV   Memory Dysfunction in Neuropsychiatric Disorders

10. Memory Disorders in Cerebral Vascular Diseases   197
     Takehiko Yanagihara

11. Alcoholic Korsakoff's Syndrome   227
     William C. Heindel, David P. Salmon, and Nelson Butters

12. Memory Disorders After Closed Head Injury   255
     Felicia C. Goldstein and Harvey S. Levin

13. Transient Global Amnesia   279
     John W. Miller, Ronald C. Petersen, and Takehiko Yanagihara

14. Memory Function and Epilepsy   299
     Warren T. Blume

15. Amnesia Associated with Temporal Lobectomy   321
     Mary Lou Smith

16. Memory Functions in Normal Aging   347
     Fergus I. M. Craik

17. Memory Disorders in Degenerative Neurological Diseases   369
     Richard J. Caselli and Takehiko Yanagihara

18. Memory Disorders in Encephalitides, Encephalopathies, and
     Demyelinating Diseases   397
     Takehiko Yanagihara

19. Memory Disorders Associated with Brain Tumors,
     Hydrocephalus, and Neurosurgical Procedures   413
     Takehiko Yanagihara

20. Psychogenic Amnesias   **429**
Christopher J. Mace and Michael R. Trimble

Part V   Treatment

21. Treatment of Memory Disorders   **457**
Ronald C. Petersen, Takehiko Yanagihara, Richard C. Mohs,
Harvey S. Levin, and Felicia C. Goldstein

Index   **505**

MEMORY DISORDERS

Part I

INTRODUCTION

1

Memory Disorders: An Overview

Takehiko Yanagihara
and
Ronald C. Petersen

Mayo Clinic and Mayo Foundation
Rochester, Minnesota

Memory is one of the most important cerebral functions for human beings and essential to independent life. Even a relatively mild impairment may interfere with aspects of one's professional or personal life. Consequently, patients with memory impairments frequently seek medical attention for a specific diagnosis and treatment. Since the description over 100 years ago of what is now known as Korsakoff's syndrome, a great deal of knowledge has accumulated on normal and abnormal memory function, and memory disorders remain a major focus of interest among neurologists, psychiatrists, psychologists, cognitive neuroscientists, and computer scientists. Undoubtedly, much more remains to be learned.

This volume is designed to address basic structural and functional aspects of normal and abnormal memory function and apply this knowledge to a variety of clinical conditions associated with memory impairments. A problem encountered frequently by clinicians who care for patients with memory impairments is the disparity between the information derived from cognitive neuroscientists using a variety of theoretical models and the information compiled by clinicians using a variety of clinical and neuropsychological assessment techniques. In this volume, an attempt has been made to interrelate these two investigative approaches and make currently available information more comprehensive to readers ranging from practicing clinicians to cognitive neuroscientists. In this chapter, we review the material which will be covered in greater detail in succeeding chapters.

BASIC RESEARCH ON MEMORY DISORDERS

There has been considerable progress in basic research on memory disorders in the anatomical, biochemical, pharmacological, and psychological fields which has enhanced our understanding of the pathophysiologic mechanisms involved in a variety of memory disorders.

ANATOMICAL BASIS OF MEMORY AND MEMORY DISORDERS

Our interest and understanding of the anatomical basis of memory and memory disorders were stimulated in 1957 by Scoville and Milner who observed a patient (HM) who suffered a profound anterograde amnesia following a bilateral temporal lobectomy for control of seizures [see The Anatomy of Memory (Chap. 3) and Amnesia Associated with Temporal Lobectomy (Chap. 16)]. Clinical cases which have accumulated since that time have clearly demonstrated that the hippocampal formation plays a key role in encoding new information and that the CA1 region of the hippocampus is particularly important in this regard. Animal experimentation using primates have demonstrated cortical and subcortical structures crucial to memory encoding and have established a memory circuit from the hippocampus to the mamillary bodies through the fornix, to the anterior nucleus of the thalamus through the mamillothalamic tract, to the cingulate gyrus and back to the hippocampus (see Chap. 3). Destruction of these structures and pathways in patients by various pathologic processes have resulted in varying degrees of amnesia.

In 1971, Victor, Adams, and Collins observed degeneration of the dorsomedial nucleus of the thalamus in patients with alcoholic Korsakoff's syndrome and a second memory circuit has been recognized which originates in the amygdala and sends efferent pathways to the dorsomedial nucleus of the thalamus and subsequently to the prefrontal cortex (see Chap. 3). The prefrontal cortex sends efferent pathways to the ventral striatum and forms a "cognitive loop" with the dorsomedial nucleus of the thalamus as well as the amygdala [see the Memory Disorders in Degenerative Neurologic Diseases (Chap. 17)]. The role of this frontostriatal cognitive loop in human memory has not been studied as extensively as the previously mentioned memory circuits, but it appears to be important in certain disorders involving the basal forebrain.

PHARMACOLOGY OF MEMORY AND MEMORY DISORDERS

Several neurotransmitters play an important role in memory function. Acetylcholine has a key role in memory and learning, and several central cholinergic pathways originating from the basal forebrain have been well established [see Central Cholinergic Pathways. Neuroanatomy and Some Behavioral Implications (Chap. 4)]. The cholinergic system is affected in Alzheimer's disease with a loss of cholinergic cells in the basal forebrain and a reduction of choline acetyltransferase [see Chap. 4 and Treatment of Memory Disorders (Chap. 21)]. Noradrenaline has also been implicated in memory and learning and this system is also affected in Alzheimer's disease with neuronal loss in the locus coeruleus (see Chap. 21). The role of the frontostriatal dopaminergic cognitive loop has not been demonstrated in Alzheimer's disease, although this system is affected in many subcortical degenerative diseases (see Chap. 17). Finally, a variety of drugs have been used to investigate memory functions (see Drugs and Memory (Chap. 5)], and these pharmacological agents have aided in the delineation of various processes involved in memory acquisition and retrieval.

EXPERIMENTAL PSYCHOLOGY AND MEMORY DISORDERS

One of the primary problems in reading the literature of different investigators on memory disorders involves terminology. It is often difficult for the clinician to translate the terminology used in a model of memory to a particular clinical condition. Consequently, the chapters on Memory Nomenclature (Chap. 2) and Models of Memory and the Understanding of Memory Disorders (Chap. 6) address this issue and attempt to correlate the various sets of theoretical terminology with normal and abnormal memory function in the clinical setting. In the succeeding chapters, terms such as "episodic," "semantic," "declarative," "procedural," "explicit," and "implicit," memories will be applied to various disorders including Korsakoff's syndrome, Alzheimer's disease, and Huntington's disease.

MEMORY DISORDERS IN CLINICAL PRACTICE

Complaints of failing memories by patients and family members are common in clinical practice. Clinicians have to identify whether their complaints are based on the impairments of sensory processing and attention or are based on primary impairments of acquisition, retention, and retrieval of information (see Chaps. 2 and 5). Several bedside memory assessment techniques may be helpful in further defining the nature of the problem [see Memory Assessment at the Bedside (Chap. 7)]. Once a memory impairment has been identified, neuropsychological testing can delineate the cognitive processes underlying the learning and recall dysfunction, and compare memory function with other cognitive capacities [see Psychometric Memory Tests (Chap. 8)].

Memory Dysfunction in Neuropsychiatric Disorders (Part IV) describes a multitude of conditions with memory dysfunction as a prominent feature. An attempt has been made to correlate the memory dysfunction in these disorders with anatomical and pharmacological knowledge as well as with concepts derived from theoretical models of normal and abnormal memory. In addition to the primary disorders of memory, memory dysfunction may be secondary to an impairment of attention and concentration, or part of a more generalized cognitive impairment such as that seen in dementia. Finally, some memory impairments may be psychogenic in origin.

IMPAIRMENT OF ATTENTION AND CONCENTRATION

The classical condition in this group of disorders is the acute confusional state [see Memory Disorders in Encephalitides, Encephalopathies and Demyelinating Diseases (Chap. 18)], but more sustained impairments of attention and concentration can be associated with other disorders such as brain tumors, hydrocephalus and closed head injury [see Memory Disorders Associated with Brain Tumors, Hydrocephalus and Neurosurgical Procedures (Chap. 19) and Memory Disorders after Closed Head Injury (Chap. 12)]. Subtle impairments of attention and concentration may occur in patients taking certain central nervous system depressants (see Chap. 5) and impairments of attention and concentration can also occur in the setting of more widespread cognitive disorders such as in degenerative diseases of the central nervous system (see Chap. 17).

AMNESIA AS THE PRIMARY
NEUROLOGIC DYSFUNCTION

In this group of disorders, memory dysfunction is not only the prominent feature but perhaps the sole cognitive dysfunction. Case illustrations of major neurologic disorders with amnesia as the primary manifestation are presented in Neuropsychological Testing of Memory Disorders (Chap. 9). This group of disorders has been called the amnesic syndrome in the past but probably represents several disorders all affecting common anatomical structures and memory circuits. Characteristically, patients learn new information but cannot retain it for a sustained period. Historically, the prototype of this group of disorders is Korsakoff's syndrome [see Alcoholic Korsakoff's Syndrome (Chap. 11)]. However, there are several other disorders which produce fairly pure amnesias as the result of temporal lobe dysfunction such as those seen in some patients with seizure disorders and following temporal lobectomies [see Memory Function and Epilepsy (Chap. 14) and Amnesia Associated with Temporal Lobectomy (Chap. 15)]. Relatively pure memory disorders can arise from a variety of other neurological disorders such as herpes simplex encephalitis (see Chap. 18), cerebral infarction in the posterior cerebral artery distribution, infarcts or hemorrhage in the paramedian thalamic region and ruptured aneurysms arising from the anterior communicating artery [see Memory Disorders in Cerebral Vascular Diseases (Chap. 10)]. In addition, strategically located brain tumors can cause a relatively pure amnesia (see Chap. 19) and amnesia may be the most significant residual dysfunction in head injury (see Chap. 12). One of the most intriguing pure amnesias is transient global amnesia [see Transient Global Amnesia (Chap. 13)]. While several hypotheses have been offered for its etiology, no clear explanation for this transient memory dysfunction has arisen in the majority of patients. Finally, a decline of memory function can occur in normal aging and the distinction between these changes and early dementia can be difficult [see Memory Functions in Normal Aging (Chap. 16)] and may be necessary to retain (Chap. 6).

MEMORY DYSFUNCTION IN DEMENTIAS

In patients with dementia, memory dysfunction is a primary feature but it is embedded in a more widespread pattern of cognitive dysfunction. Case illustrations of major neurologic disorders with dementias are presented in Chapter 9. In most dementias, memory dysfunction is the earliest sign and often the hallmark of the disorder. This is certainly true with the most common dementia, Alzheimer's disease, but is often characteristic of other dementias such as Pick's disease, Huntington's disease, Parkinson's disease, and progressive supranuclear palsy (Chap. 17). Recently, a distinction has been drawn between cortical and subcortical dementias. While this characterization is probably too simplistic, it does highlight some differences in the characteristics of the dementias, particularly with respect to the nature of the memory dysfunction in these two classes of dementias (see Chap. 17).

PSYCHOGENIC AMNESIAS

Amnesias can occur without apparent neurological basis and are typically labelled as "psychogenic amnesias" [see Psychogenic Amnesias (Chap. 20)]. Dissociation and repression have been the traditional psychological explanations offered for this type of disorder. Depending on the acuteness of the traumatic events, they can be divided into situational amnesia, posttraumatic stress syndrome, and psychogenic fugue. Psychogenic amnesia should be distinguished from transient global amnesia, epileptic/postictal amnesia, and drug-induced amnesia, where clinical features of the history and examination are essential for the differential diagnosis.

TREATMENT OF MEMORY DISORDERS

Some neuropsychiatric disorders involving memory impairments are amenable to treatment. However, memory disorders are difficult to treat in general, and research in this field is still in its infancy. Therapy for memory disorders can be broadly classified into two main categories: pharmacological and behavioral (see Chap. 21). Current pharmacological research and drug trials are concentrated on the treatment of dementia, particularly Alzheimer's disease, partly because of its prevalence and serious socioeconomic implications. A major effort has been directed to cholinergic drugs, including precursors of acetylcholine, inhibitors of acetylcholinesterase, and cholinergic agonists. Neuropeptides including vasopressin, have been investigated as well as nootropic drugs, vasodilators, and metabolic enhancers. While no single drug has emerged as universally effective, this area of investigation is being pursued actively.

The behavioral approach or cognitive rehabilitation of memory disorders is a controversial area, but its proponents have made considerable progress in recent years. Because of the age of patients and the nature of memory impairments, most studies have involved patients with head injuries. As a part of this approach, computer technology has been introduced to enhance memory rehabilitation. While complete remediation of memory impairments may not be possible even with pharmacological and behavioral intervention, partial improvement may have a significant impact on the daily lives of patients with memory disorders.

SUMMARY

Since Korsakoff observed prominent memory impairments in alcoholic patients more than 100 years ago, various forms of memory disorders have been identified and considerable progress has been made to delineate the anatomical, biochemical, pharmacological, and psychological mechanisms for memory impairments. The chapters of this volume deal with these issues and attempt to bring these principles together to characterize different types of memory disorders. Toward this goal, the contributors have attempted to make their work relevant for a wide range of readers from clinicians who take care of patients with memory disorders to cognitive neuroscientists who deal with the theoretical aspects of memory and memory disorders.

2

Memory Nomenclature

Ronald C. Petersen
Mayo Clinic and Mayo Foundation
Rochester, Minnesota

Herbert Weingartner
National Institute òf Mental Health
National Institutes of Health
Bethesda, Maryland

INTRODUCTION

Memory functions are not unitary and can be quite complex. Many different types of models and schemes are used to describe learning and recall functions. It is not surprising therefore that the clinician encounters a problem in making sense of the contrasting terms used to describe various memory processes. The clinician can encounter a mixture of terminology derived from different models found in the clinical, experimental psychology, and neuropsychology literatures. Unfortunately, often no attempt is made to draw correlations among the various concepts. For example, if a memory study on a group of normal elderly individuals or demented patients has been performed by an experimental psychologist, we may find terms such as effortful versus automatic processing or implicit versus explicit learning; yet the relationship of these terms to memory tasks with which the clinician may be familiar, such as the Wechsler Memory Scale, the Wechsler Memory Scale-Revised, or the Rey Auditory Verbal Learning Test, is not clear. Similarly, the neuropsychologist may use a variety of memory tests to assess patients; yet the relationship of these tests to theoretical memory descriptions such as those espoused by the experimental psychologist is lacking. In fact, most of these tests were not derived from any particular theoretical model of memory. Finally, when the neurologist, psychiatrist, or internist without any psychological background attempts to read this literature, he/she often becomes discouraged because of the jargon and lack of correspondence between the experimental psychologists' terminology and that of the neuropsychologist.

While the authors make no attempt in this chapter to solve this dilemma, we will present an overall framework for thinking about and assessing memory disorders. It is therefore helpful to include a compendium of definitions of some of the theoretical terms to be encountered in other chapters of this volume.

CONCEPTUAL FRAMEWORK

In a general fashion, learning and memory functions can be assessed in terms of input and output processes. The general scheme is shown in Figure 1. This model emphasizes how, in a set of sequential and sometimes parallel steps, the input is processed, stored, and later retrieved (output). A specific example of this scheme is also presented in the chapter on Drugs and Memory. On the input side, there are a variety of functions which are active in processing the information to be remembered. The model presented serves primarily to order these events but not to define specific determinants or mechanisms that account for the components of memory. Initially, the material is received through our sensory organs and retained there for a brief period of time until the information is further encoded. Attentional processes are oper-

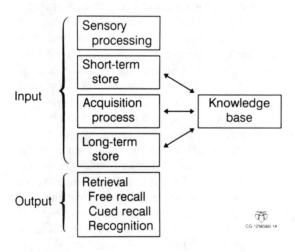

Figure 1

ating at this stage to maintain the information in our consciousness, keeping in mind the fact that material can be learned in spite of our apparent lack of awareness. During the acquisition phase, the material is encoded into a type of brief processing store for further analysis and elaboration. Attentional processes are operating here as well, and various terms have been used to describe this storage process such as short-term memory and primary memory. In a simplistic sense, material is then encoded depending upon its relevance/importance/salience/familiarity to the learner, and contact is made with previously learned information.

Next, there is a retention phase where a "plastic" reconstruction of the true experience is consolidated and made into a permanent record. During this phase, the material is revised and modified depending on other knowledge and on the basis of new experiences. Some of the information is transformed and perhaps some is lost.

Finally, the material must be retrieved. Either the material is spontaneously recalled by the person, or cues or prompts are used to aid in the recall process. Certain methodological problems arise at this point since our assessment of memory is dependent upon the means by which we test recall. That is, if a person does not spontaneously recall a name, does that mean that the name has been forgotten or is just not retrievable? If we use cues, prompts, or provide additional context and the name is still not recalled, is it indeed forgotten? This is probably an unanswerable question, but raises the issue of how memory assessment techniques influence our interpretation of theoretical concepts.

A variety of terms come into play at this phase concerning the nature of the retrieval processes. For example, as will be discussed below, terms such as implicit and explicit and the priming effect refer to inferences drawn about the learning/remembering process based on the specific testing procedures used. It will also become apparent that various terms can be used to describe the same phenomena depending on one's theoretical position.

CLINICAL TERMS

A variety of terms are used in the clinical description of memory and memory disorders, and several of the more commonly used descriptions are reviewed below.

ANTEROGRADE AMNESIA

This term refers to the inability to learn or remember new contemporary experiences. This form of amnesia is quite common and, for example, is seen in head trauma, seizures, or drug exposures. Anterograde amnesia is manifested when subjects, having just experienced something, fail to remember that particular experience a short time later (minutes, hours). The anterograde feature refers to the timing of the amnesia (i.e., from the ictal event forward). This concept is similar to an impairment in new learning and may be complete or incomplete. Anterograde amnesia typically occurs with damage to medial temporal or diencephalic structures such as seen in herpes simplex encephalitis, Korsakoff's syndrome, temporal lobectomy, head trauma, or Alzheimer's disease.

RETROGRADE AMNESIA

This term refers to the inability to recall material learned *prior* to a particular point in time (e.g., head trauma, seizure, or drug exposure). The two main features of the type of difficulty are its retrograde nature (i.e., an inability to recall information prior to the ictal event), and a time-dependent gradient. Again, it may be incomplete and often has a temporal gradient with events occurring immediately prior to the ictus being more difficult to remember. Retrograde amnesia is usually less severe than anterograde amnesia and may occur in head trauma, Korsakoff's syndrome, and Alzheimer's disease.

POSTTRAUMATIC AMNESIA

This term has been defined in various fashions by different authors. Some call posttraumatic amnesia the period of both dense retrograde amnesia and anterograde amnesia surrounding a head injury (1). Recovery from posttraumatic amnesia must include return to full orientation, not just recovery of consciousness. Other authors refer to posttraumatic amnesia as that period between the head injury and the resumption of normal continuous memory (2). The latter definition is the more common usage.

LEARNING/ACQUISITION

This term refers to the process of acquiring an experience or entering new information into memory stores. The process of learning or acquisition refers to the actual laying down of memory traces or the establishment of an engram (the term used in the older literature). A distinction should be drawn between simple conditioning and higher order learning. Conditioning refers to the establishment of stimulus-response bonds, and various conditioning paradigms have been well studied (3). However, the neuroanatomical structures which mediate conditioning may be quite different from those involved in higher order learning.

FREE RECALL

The process of retrieving information from memory without any external cues or prompts is referred to as free recall. This is typical of the memory assessment used in many laboratory and clinical memory tests. For example, when we ask patients, "Do you remember the words I presented to you five minutes ago?," we are testing for free recall. Free recall is often the most difficult type of memory retrieval task and is impaired in many forms of amnesia including Karsokoff's syndrome, herpes simplex encephalitis, head trauma, and Alzheimer's disease.

CUED RECALL

This term refers to the task used for assessing memory with the assistance of cues or prompts. For example, the instructions might read, "Remember the list of vegetables I gave you. . . ." In this instance, "vegetable" is the cue to assist the person in remembering the specific items. This is commonly used when free recall fails and is the next most difficult memory retrieval task.

RECOGNITION

In this form of memory test the to-be-remembered items are presented to the person along with distractor items (foils), and the person is asked to identify the correct items. A multiple choice test is a recognition test. This is generally the least difficult memory retrieval task and is often spared in mild forms of amnesia.

RETRIEVAL FAILURE

This term describes the difference in performance between what someone can remember on demand at a given point in time compared with what is available in memory. For example, when a person forgets someone's name but is able to select it from a list of names, the person has a retrieval failure. Alternatively, in a clinical laboratory setting, patients are typically asked to recall a list of words. They may not be able to recall all of the words but are subsequently able to select additional words from a larger list when given several choices. This is also an example of free recall failure with successful subsequent recognition constitutes a retrieval failure.

TERMINOLOGY IN TEXT

A variety of terms have been used to describe the various aspects of acquisition/learning/retention and retrieval. The terms are often not mutually exclusive but rather refer to different theoretical formulations of memory function. Recent reviews on memory function discuss this terminology in more detail (4,5).

SHORT-TERM MEMORY

This is an imprecise term in clinical practice and there is little consensus on the specific meaning of the term. As originally defined in the experimental psychology literature, short-term memory referred to a limited capacity storage buffer held for a brief period of time (seconds to a minute) without the opportunity to think about or rehearse the items (6,7). Its function was to hold information for further processing. However, in clinical practice it is used loosely to refer to material held in memory for minutes to hours or perhaps days without a more precise definition. Consequently, it may be best to avoid this term clinically. Short-term memory is relatively spared in many memory disorders until perhaps the later stages of the disease process. Short-term memory relies heavily on attentional processes and consequently, when it is impaired markedly, one needs to consider conditions that primarily affect attention.

LONG-TERM MEMORY

Long-term memory refers to material held over 60 seconds as defined originally in experimental psychology (6,7). Again, in clinical use this term is defined in various fashions. Typically, the clinical literature uses the term "recent memory" to refer to memories of hours to days in duration. The term "remote memory" is used to refer to memories of may years' duration. The precise temporal delineation of these terms is lacking. Long-term memory is the type of memory impaired in most forms of amnesia and as such refers to the functions most people consider as "memory."

PRIMARY MEMORY

This term is similar in temporal domain to short-term memory but refers more to the processing nature of this type of memory than to an actual store. It also de-emphasizes a precise temporal gradient. Primary memory refers to the continued processing or activation of a memory trace for further encoding. This is similar to the notion of "attending to" material in consciousness (8,9). The term "working memory" belongs to this category of memory. When primary memory is affected out of proportion to other cognitive functions, one needs to consider primary disorders of attention.

SECONDARY MEMORY

In the primary-secondary memory distinction, secondary memory refers to processes that support retention across long retention intervals. The emphasis is once again on the process rather than the storage concept. In general, secondary memory refers to material retained over long periods and relates to processes involved in storage and retrieval (8,9). As in long-term memory, secondary memory comprises the bulk of what most people refer to as "memory."

EPISODIC MEMORY

Episodic memory refers to memory for events which are related to specific spatial or temporal contexts (10-14). This is a type of autobiographical memory whereby the person not only remembers the event or information but remembers when and where he learned it. There is no temporal dimension which necessarily underlies this type of memory. Episodic memory is severely affected in processes involving the medial temporal lobes and diencephalic structures in a fashion similar to alterations of anterograde memory.

SEMANTIC MEMORY

In contrast to episodic memory, semantic memory refers to general knowledge of the world independent of the particular learning circumstances (10-14). That is, a person may have knowledge of an event but is uncertain as to when and where he learned that information. Semantic memory can be relatively resistant to disruption in many memory disorders until later in the disease process, as in, for example, Alzheimer's disease.

EXPLICIT MEMORY

This term refers to the conscious recollection of recent events such as that found in typical laboratory learning exercises when a person is instructed to learn a list of words (15,16). This is similar to the term "intentional memory" whereby people are instructed to learn a body of material and they are aware of the intent. This term is used to refer to processes operating at the time of retrieval. When a person is asked to remember "what occurred," the person is asked to use explicit memory processes to recall the information. This is a type of memory of which the person is aware and can process in consciousness.

IMPLICIT MEMORY

In contradistinction to explicit memory, implicit memory refers to the demonstration of learning having taken place in spite of the person being unaware of actually learning the information (15,16). This is similar to the concept of "incidental memory" whereby a person recalls more about a learning situation than is apparent to him. Implicit memory is inferred to have taken place when performance is facilitated in spite of no conscious or intentional recollection of learning. Again, this refers primarily to a retrieval process, since someone can intentionally learn material but nonetheless years later be unable to remember the material unless given an implicit test of memory. That is, in spite of the intentionality at the time of learning, the memory may only be manifest through an appropriately structured implicit memory task.

DECLARATIVE MEMORY

This refers to memory that is directly accessible to consciousness; in this sense, one can declare this memory (17,18). This type of memory deals with facts and data and is typically impaired in amnesia caused by damage to medial temporal and diencephalic structures.

PROCEDURAL MEMORY

In contrast to declarative memory, this form of memory refers to learned skills or modifiable cognitive operations (17,18). This type of memory is often spared in amnesia, implying that structures other than medial temporal and diencephalic regions mediate this type of memory. Both declarative and procedural memory refer to how material is represented in long-term memory.

PRIMING

Priming refers to subsequent facilitation of memory of material after having been exposed to the material earlier in spite of a lack of awareness of the priming exposure (19). This facilitation can occur despite impaired recall and recognition of the material.

METACOGNITIVE PROCESSES

This term refers to one's ability to monitor and make judgments about his own performance and includes the ability to plan and allocate cognitive resources (20-22). In addition to remembering information, we also are able to assess how accurately we are remembering; that is, we are able to judge our own performance. This type of judgment is differentially affected in various disease processes. For example, depressed patients typically underestimate their ability to remember, while patients who have consumed alcohol or benzodiazepines may overestimate their ability to recall.

EFFORT-DEMANDING PROCESSING

Some tasks require extensive cognitive effort and concentration to accomplish, while others are relatively effortless (23-26). These tasks can be useful in differentiating patients with certain types of disorders. For example, patients with depression or Parkinson's disease may have more difficulty with effortful processes implying diminished concentration or attention. They may perform well, however, on automatic tasks.

AUTOMATIC (NONEFFORTFUL) PROCESSING

In contrast to effort-demanding tasks, these tasks are relatively automatic and do not require extensive conscious attention (23-26). Automatic task performance is not altered by changing the intention or set of the subject. Automatic operations can be performed at the same time as effort-demanding cognitive processes. For example, driving an automobile or reciting multiplication tables which are overlearned are automatic tasks. These tasks are preserved in depression but may be impaired in dementia, and consequently can be useful in distinguishing between these two disorders.

OVERALL SCHEME OF INFORMATION PROCESSING

Figure 2 demonstrates the general relation between the conceptual framework involving input and output processes outlined earlier and the theoretical terminology discussed above. This figure shows that the input processes involved in registration of the material correspond to the conceptual terms of "attention, short-term memory and primary memory" discussed above. When discussing the other theoretical issues, this is the primary locus of effortful processes. Insofar as effortful processes are attention demanding, the initial registration and input processes would be affected by disorders of attention.

In the next phase of the input processing of the material, Figure 2 shows the acquisition process whereby input information is related, compared, and

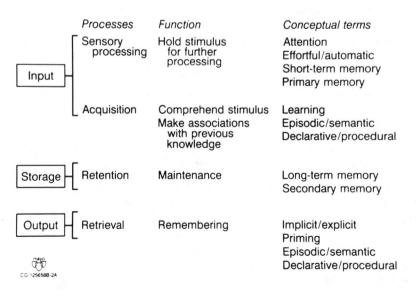

Figure 2

evaluated in the context of prior learning. This is necessary for comprehending and encoding new information. In memory theory terms, we are dealing with learning and elaboration. Elaboration refers to the investment of meaning in the material to-be-remembered or trying to embellish or enhance the meaningfulness of the material to the learner. Generally we are speaking of transferring material to long-term memory or secondary memory in this phase. Terms such as episodic and semantic memory and declarative versus procedural learning are relevant here. These terms refer to different characterizations of the way in which material is learned, stored, or represented in long-term memory.

On the output side, a variety of memory recall procedures have been employed. Initially, patients are often asked to free recall the material, i.e., "Do you remember . . . ?." If they are unsuccessful at free recall, they are then given cues or prompts such as "Do you remember the vegetables . . .," or "Do you remember the name of the city?." If still unsuccessful, they are then given a recognition test and asked to identify the items they were to remember from a list of correct items and foils.

From the conceptual point of view, factors such as implicit and explicit memory are relevant here since recall may, in part, be dependent upon the patient's awareness of remembering the material. Alternatively, certain testing procedures can be designed to demonstrate that the patient actually learned material in spite of his/her own lack of awareness (implicit learning). Similarly, concepts such as episodic and semantic memory and declarative and procedural memory are relevant here since they may be variably influenced by disease processes and testing procedures must be designed to elicit each type of memory. The effects of priming are best assessed during the retrieval phase as well, since, as with implicit learning, the patient is not aware of the influence of these processes.

Finally, metacognition pervades the entire process of learning and retrieving since it involves one's assessment of his own performance. This allows the person to form judgments on his own ability to function and may be affected by some disease processes.

CONCLUSION

One can see in this highly simplified schematic that many of these conceptual issues are not mutually exclusive. That is, several of these processes are operating at a given time in the input/output schema, but one set of terms may be more appropriate for describing the psychological processes operating than another. For example, if one were describing recall failures in amnesia in contrast to preserved motor skill retention, the declarative/procedural distinction would be most relevant. That is not to say that one could not discuss the performance in terms of episodic and semantic processes; however, it might be less appropriate.

There are many ways to describe the same phenomena based on one's theoretical predisposition. Consequently, the seeming myriad of terminology can be confusing. This chapter was designed to help organize this confusing body of literature to assist the reader in comprehending subsequent chapters.

REFERENCES

1. Strub, R. L., and Black, R. L. (1988). *Neurobehavioral Disorders.* Philadelphia, F. A. Davis Co., pp. 313-348.
2. Alexander, M. P. (1982). Traumatic brain injury. In *Psychiatric Aspects of Neurologic Disease*, Vol. II. Edited by D. F. Benson and D. Blumer. New York, Grune and Stratton, Inc., pp. 219-249.
3. Woodruff-Pak, D. S., and Thompson, R. F. (1985). Classical conditioning of the eyelid response in rabbits as a model system for the study of brain mechanisms of learning and memory in aging. *Exp. Aging Res. 11*:109-112.
4. Richardson-Klavehn, A., and Bjork, R. A. (1988). Measures of memory. *Ann. Rev. Psychol. 39*:475-543.
5. Johnson, M. K., and Hasher, L. (1987). Human learning and memory. *Ann. Rev. Psychol. 38*:631-668.
6. Brown, J. (1958). Some tests of the decay theory of immediate memory. *Q. J. Exp. Psychol. 10*:12-21.
7. Peterson, L. R., and Peterson, M. J. (1959). Short-term retention of individual verbal items. *J. Exp. Psychol. 58*:193-198.
8. Craik, F. I. M., and Levy, B. A. (1976). The concept of primary memory. In *Handbook of Learning and Cognitive Processes*, Vol. IV. Edited by W. K. Estes. New York, Academic Press, pp. 133-175.
9. Waugh, N. C., and Norman, D. A. (1965). Primary memory. *Psychol. Rev. 72*:89-104.
10. Tulving, E. (1972). Episodic and semantic memory. In *Organization of Memory.* Edited by E. Tulving and W. Donaldson. New York, Academic Press.
11. Tulving, E. (1983). *Elements of Episodic Memory.* Oxford, Clarendon Press.
12. McKoon, G., and Ratcliff, R. (1986). A critical evaluation of the semantic/episodic distinction. *J. Exp. Psychol. 12*:295-306.
13. Tulving, E. (1984). Multiple learning and memory systems. In *Psychology in the 1990s.* Edited by K. M. J. Lagerspetz and P. Niemi. North-Holland, Elsevier Science Publishers, pp. 163-184.
14. Tulving, E. (1989). Remembering and knowing the past. *Am. Sci. 77*:361-367.
15. Graf, P., and Schacter, D. L. (1985). Implicit and explicit memory for new associations in normal subjects and amnesic patients. *J. Exp. Psychol. 11*:502-518.
16. Schacter, D. L. (1987). Implicit memory: History and current status. *J. Exp. Psychol. 13*:501-518.
17. Squire, L. R. (1987). *Memory and Brain.* New York, Oxford University Press.

18. Cohen, N. J. (1984). Preserved learning capacity in amnesia: Evidence for multiple memory systems. In *Neuropsychology of Memory*. Edited by L. R. Squire and N. Butters. New York, Guilford Press, pp. 83-103.

19. Tulving, E., Schacter, D. L., and Stark, H. (1982). Priming effects in word-fragment completion are independent of recognition memory. *J. Exp. Psychol. Learn. Mem. Cog. 8*:336-342.

20. Jacoby, L. L. (1984). Incidental versus intentional retrieval: Remembering and awareness as separate issues. In *Neuropsychology of Memory*. Edited by L. R. Squire and N. Butters. New York, Guildford Press, pp. 145-156.

21. Jacoby, L. L., and Witherspoon, D. (1982). Remembering without awareness. *Can. J. Psychol. 36*:300-324.

22. Johnson, M. K., Kahan, T. L., and Raye, C. L. (1984). Dreams and reality monitoring. *J. Exp. Psychol. 113*:329-344.

23. Hasher, L., and Zacks, R. T. (1979). Automatic and effortful processes in memory. *J. Exp. Psychol. 108*:356-388.

24. Hasher, L., and Zacks, R. T. (1984). Automatic processing of fundamental information: The case of frequency of occurrence. *Am. Psychol. 39*:1372-1388.

25. Weingartner, H., Burns, S., Diebel, R., and LeWitt, P. A. (1984). Cognitive impairments in Parkinson's disease: Distinguishing between effort-demanding and automatic cognitive processes. *Psychiatry Res. 11*:223-235.

26. Weingartner, H., Chen, R. M., Sunderland, T., Tariot, P. N., and Thompson, K. (1987). Diagnosis and assessment of cognitive dysfunction in the elderly. In *Psychopharmacology: The Third Generation of Progress*. Edited by H. Meltzer. New York, Raven Press, pp. 909-919.

Part II

MEMORY STRUCTURE AND FUNCTION

3

Anatomy of Memory

John P. Aggleton
University of Durham
Durham, England

However presumptious it may appear to describe an anatomy of memory, there is abundant evidence that such an anatomy does exist and there is considerable agreement over many of its component parts. In fact, it is also agreed that one anatomy will not suffice; there must be multiple anatomies reflecting multiple classes of learning and memory. Some of these 'systems' are well established while the existence of others has emerged only recently and our suggestions as to their anatomical basis remain merely speculative.

Probably the best understood 'system' underlies our ability to learn new everyday information and events, this understanding coming primarily from studies of anterograde amnesia. Nevertheless, while we know an increasing amount concerning those structures involved in this process, we know far less as to how this involvement results in memory storage and retrieval.

ANTEROGRADE AMNESIA

Anterograde amnesia refers to the inability to learn new information such as events, people's names, and places. It has been repeatedly shown that certain patterns of brain damage can produce a dramatic anterograde amnesia and yet leave intact a wide range of other cognitive abilities. This important finding leads to one inescapable conclusion; that certain brain structures are necessary for the formation or retrieval of new memories and yet are not necessary for a wide range of other cognitive abilities. Thus there must be a specific anatomy of memory mechanisms and an obvious starting point will be to define those regions responsible for anterograde amnesia. A second important feature of some anterograde amnesic syndromes is that memories prior to the onset of the impairment may be left intact. This, in turn, indicates that while those brain regions damaged may be crucial for normal memory function they are unlikely to represent actual sites of memory storage.

Neuropathological studies have repeatedly shown that anterograde amnesias can be broadly defined as having either a temporal lobe or diencephalic origin. These two regions will initially be considered separately although, as will become apparent, they are almost certainly different components of the same system or systems.

CLINICAL STUDIES

TEMPORAL LOBE AMNESIA

Patient HM is surely the best known single case in clinical psychology. In 1953, at the age of 27, he received a bilateral resection of approximately the most rostral 8 cm of the medial temporal lobe in an attempt to control major epileptic seizures (1). The full extent of the surgery remains unknown as HM is still alive, but it is thought that all of the grey and white matter medial to the temporal horns of the lateral ventricles was removed. As a consequence, it has always been assumed that the surgery involved the prepiriform cortex, uncus, amygdala, hippocampus, entorhinal cortex, and parahippocampal gyrus (Fig. 1).

Postoperatively HM showed no obvious deficits in perception, abstract thinking, reasoning, or immediate short-term memory, and indeed on re-testing his Wechsler-Bellevue Intelligence Scale had increased from 104 to 112 (1). In dramatic constrast, he suffered a most profound global antero-grade amnesia which remains to this day. He does not know where he now lives, who cares for him, what he ate for his last meal, or even his age. This dense amnesia has been confirmed by many formal psychometric tests (2). Initial estimates of HM's premorbid memories suggested a retrograde amnesia which was restricted to about 2 years before the operation (3). Recently more objective tests indicate retrograde deficits back to the age of 16, an age which coincides with the first onset of major seizures (2).

HM was only one of a group of patients who received bilateral medial temporal surgery (1) and it was the results of HM's case combined with those of other patients which particularly directed attention to the hippocampal formation. Thus Scoville and Milner (1) reported that the most severe memory impairments were found in those cases in which the surgery extended most caudally; in other words, the greater the hippocampal involvement the more profound the amnesia. In contrast, a patient who underwent bilateral removal

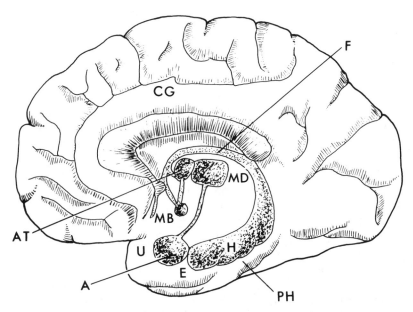

Figure 1 Lateral view of the medial surface of the human brain showing brain regions implicated in the formulation of long-term memories. A, amygdala; AT, anterior thalamic nuclei; CG; cingulate gyrus; E, entorhinal cortex; F, fornix; H, hippocampus; MB, mammillary bodies; MD, nucleus medialis dorsalis; PH, parahippocampal gyrus; U, uncus.

of the rostal 4 cm of the temporal lobe, involving the amygdala, uncus, and temporal pole, and presumably sparing the hippocampus, displayed no obvious memory deficit. Although Scoville and Milner were not the first to link the hippocampus to amnesia (4-6), their study has had by far the greatest impact.

More evidence for the role of the hippocampal formation came from two patients who unexpectedly displayed severe memory deficits immediately after unilateral temporal lobectomies (7). In one of these cases the surgery had been performed in two stages and the amnesia appeared only after removal of the amygdala and hippocampus. It was supposed that these amnesias reflected abnormalities in the intact temporal lobe, and in one case, this was later confirmed by autopsy which revealed a severely shrunken, necrotic hippocampus in the remaining temporal lobe. The amygdala appeared normal (7).

These findings, which clearly strengthened the notion that the hippocampus is involved in temporal lobe amnesia do not, however, imply that unilateral damage has no effect on memory. Indeed, many studies have shown that unilateral damage can disrupt memory, although there appear to be clear differences between the effects of right and left hemispheric damage. Right temporal lobe damage can disrupt tactile and visual maze learning, spatial position, facial recognition, and spatial memory (8-10), while left temporal lobe damage can impair the recall of word lists, stories, nonsense syllables, digit span plus one (11).

It is no surprise that other pathologies which affect the medial temporal lobes can also produce amnesia. Following encephalitis due to herpes simplex virus, both anterograde and retrograde amnesia may often be a prominent, persistent symptom. This disease primarily affects limbic structures and related cortical regions in the temporal and frontal lobes, most consistently damaging the amygdala, the hippocampal formation including the subiculum, the parahippocampal gyrus, the perirhinal cortex, the anterior insula cortex, the posterior orbitofrontal cortex, and the anterior cingulate cortex (12,13).

A more restricted temporal pathology was described in the case of a woman who suffered a bilateral embolic stroke which produced a severe generalized amnesia (14). Postmortem examination revealed extensive damage to the medial temporal-occipital region in the left hemisphere, but only selective damage restricted to the posterior two thirds of the hippocampus and subiculum in the right hemisphere. If bilateral lesions are necessary for the production of permanent amnesia then the hippocampus would appear to be a crucial structure.

The key role of the hippocampus in temporal lobe amnesia is further underlined by two recent cases in which highly selective pathological changes were reported. In one of these cases, a 36-year-old-man, who displayed a relatively pure and severe anterograde amnesia of unknown origin, suffered bilateral lesions restricted to the amygdala and hippocampus (15). While nearly all of the pyramidal cells in hippocampal fields CA1, CA2, and CA3 (Fig. 2) had disappeared the dentate gyrus, subiculum, and all of the parahippocampal gyrus were unaffected. The amygdaloid damage was mainly centered in the basolaterial nuclei.

In the second case, a 52-year-old man RB suffered a sudden ischemic episode which left him with a persistent anterograde amnesia coupled with a relatively mild retrograde amnesia extending back 1 or 2 years (16). The particular value of patient RB is that his amnesia was thoroughly investigated while the pathology was essentially confined to field CA1 of the hippocampus. While minor damage was found elsewhere none of this could reasonably be associated with his amnesia. This case therefore provides the strongest evidence yet that hippocampal damage disrupts new memories.

One other subcortical temporal lobe structure, the amygdala, merits special mention. While amygdaloid damage does not on its own produce a clear cut amnesia the amygdala may still have an important mnemonic function. Evi-

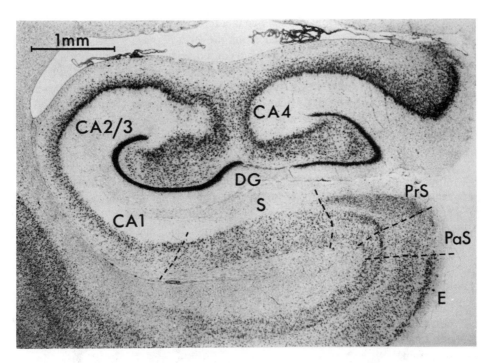

Figure 2 Photomicrograph showing the normal appearance of the hippocampal formation in the monkey (*Macaca fascicularis*). CA, CA fields as described by Lorento de No (61); DG, dentate gyrus; E, entorhinal cortex; PaS, parasubiculum; PrS, prosubiculum; S, subiculum. (Coronal section, Nissl stain.)

dence that selective amygdaloid damage does not produce amnesia comes from the series of patients which included HM (1). Further evidence comes from the hundreds of patients who received psychosurgical lesions of the amygdala. These surgeries, which were typically intended to control aggression and/or epilepsy (17,18) usually produced no apparent memory dysfunctions.

This conclusion must, however, be limited by two considerations. First, the postoperative assessment of the large majority of psychosurgical cases failed to include appropriate psychometric testing, and so mild changes may have gone unobserved. Second, many of the surgeries were unilateral and most, if not all, attempted to produce only partial damage to the structure. Nevertheless, slight impairments in memory have been noted in occasional cases (19, 20). Indeed, the sole thorough study of the cognitive effects of unilateral amygdalotomy (partial amygdaloid lesions) found evidence of a subtle change which was interpreted as a retrieval deficit (21).

While the contribution of the amygdala to temporal lobe amnesia remains uncertain, there is growing evidence that the most pervasive form of anterograde amnesia, Alzheimer's disease, is a consequence of medial temporal lobe damage. This disease produces widespread neuronal loss in a range of structures including the temporal lobe, the prefrontal cortex, and basal forebrain regions such as the basal nucleus of Meynert. While considerable attention has been focused upon the basal nucleus of Meynert (22,23) there are good reasons for supposing that the medial temporal lobes are responsible for the loss of recent memory which is so often the first symptom. First, those structures which suffer the greatest degree of cell loss include the amygdala and hippocampus (24-26). The hippocampal pathology, which is primarily concentrated in the subiculum, field CA1, and entorhinal cortex (24, 25), is of particular interest as it maps onto those regions described in the more circumscribed amnesias (15, 16) and would functionally isolate the hippocampus from nearly all of its afferent and efferent targets (26, 27). Second, longitudinal studies of Down's syndrome, which may be a valid model of Alzheimer's disease, strongly indicate that the plaques which are a characteristic feature of both diseases first form in the amygdala and hippocampus while tangles initially concentrate in the entorhinal cortex (28). Given the early appearance of the memory loss these findings clearly implicate the medial temporal lobe although they do not preclude a contributory effect from the basal forebrain.

In summary, evidence for the involvement of the hippocampus in a wide range of amnesias of different etiologies appears to be incontrovertible. More precise localization within the hippocampal formation remains difficult, and indeed the anatomical organization of the structure makes it almost impossible to isolate one particular subfield. Nevertheless, the present pathological evidence clearly implicates at least field CA1. As the hippocampus has both direct afferent and efferent connections with much of the temporal lobe cortex, it is also most likely that closely related regions such as the parahippocampal or entorhinal cortices will also prove to have mnemonic functions. The status of the amygdala, based on human clinical evidence, remains, however, unproven.

DIENCEPHALIC AMNESIA

It is just over 100 years since S.S. Korsakoff first described the amnesic and confabulatory syndrome to which his name is now attached. Many studies have described the neuropathology of Korsakoff's syndrome and it is accepted that the amnesic state is associated with damage in hypothalamic and thalamic regions adjacent to the third ventricle (29, 30). More specific descriptions have emphasized the invariable damage to the mammillary bodies. This structure typically appears discolored and shrunken, neuronal loss being found most frequently, if not always, in the medial mammillary nucleus (31).

The presumed key role of the mammillary bodies in diencephalic amnesia arose from descriptions of Korsakoff's disease in which the pathology appeared to be limited to the mammillary bodies (30, 32-34). Additional evidence came from reports that colloid cysts and tumors located in the floor and walls of the third ventricle, and hence adjacent to the mammillary bodies, may produce an amnesic state (35). Furthermore, drainage or removal of the cyst has occasionally relieved the amnesia (35-37). The fact that one of the major inputs to the mammillary bodies is from the hippocampus seemed to provide the final confirmation of this structure's key mnemonic role.

The role of the mammillary bodies was not questioned until the extensive neuropathological studies of Victor, Adams, and Collins (31). It had earlier been observed that thalamic, as well as mammillary body, damage was a very frequent occurrence in cases of Korsakoff's disease (31, 38, 39), and it has been suggested that thalamic nuclei may contribute to the amnesic syndrome. Victor and his co-workers went one stage further and argued that thalamic damage may be sufficient to produce anterograde amnesia and that mammillary body damage may not be required. This conclusion arose from a detailed neuropathological study of 43 cases diagnosed with the Wernicke-Korsakoff syndrome. Victor's group (31) noted that the mammillary bodies were always necrotic, a finding in clear accord with other studies. But they also noted that in 38 of these cases there was degeneration in at least the medial part of the dorsomedial nucleus of the thalamus, and it was only these 38 cases that showed obvious memory impairments. They concluded that the critical lesions needed to produce amnesia were in the thalamus and not the mammillary bodies. The failure of some previous studies to report thalamic damage was ascribed to a failure to search the appropriate brain region.

There is now a wealth of supporting evidence that thalamic damage contributes to some amnesias, and the large majority of these studies point to the nucleus medialis dorsalis (40). It has already been noted that tumors in the region of the third ventricle may induce amnesia, and in many of these cases there is direct thalamic damage. Most attention has been focused on those cases in which the thalamus, and in particular the nucleus medialis dorsalis (MD), has suffered damage while the mammillary bodies appear to have been spared (41-43). Such cases cannot, however, rule out indirect mammillary body involvement as a result of either increased intracranial pressure, or damage to the fornix or mammillothalamic tract (the bundle of Vicq d'Azyr) which runs through the rostral thalamus (44, 45).

Further evidence of thalamic amnesia has been provided by the discovery that bilateral or even unilateral paramedian thalamic infarcts may produce memory disturbances (46, 47). Unfortunately in those cases with confirmed pathology the damage involved not only MD but also the mammillothalamic tract (47). Other reports of more selective infarcts restricted to the dorsomedial region of the thalamus have relied on CT scans and must await confirmation (48, 49). The results of such cases may, however, still prove inconclusive as damage outside MD may nevertheless disrupt its connections.

It has been argued that the well-described patient NA provides an example of diencephalic amnesia in which there is thalamic but not mammillary body damage (50). This patient received an accidental stab wound with a miniature fencing foil which penetrated to the dorsomedial thalamic region. There is, however, good reason to believe that the foil inflicted significant damage in the region of the mammillary bodies and therefore this case does not provide incontrovertible evidence for a thalamic contribution to diencephalic amnesia.

While there is considerable circumstantial evidence for the existence of a distinct thalamic amnesia, none of it can be regarded as conclusive. As yet there has not been a single amnesic case with confirmed pathology restricted to MD (40). Furthermore, when selective surgical lesions have been placed within MD only transient declines in memory have been noted (51-53). These stereotaxic lesions were, however, intended to be subtotal and recent evidence suggests that damage of up to 15% MD need not adversely affect memory (54). Taken together these findings suggest that either extensive damage to the whole, or to a particular part, of the nucleus is required or that a combination of damage to MD and another diencephalic structure is required to produce a clear cut amnesia.

Other thalamic nuclei have been implicated in amnesia although their status remains uncertain. In Korsakoff's disease, it has been noted frequently that there is damage in the lateral dorsal nucleus, the anterior nuclei, and the medial pulvinar (30, 31, 55). These regions are of particular interest as they receive direct hippocampal inputs (56) while the anterior thalamic nuclei receive additional dense inputs from the mammillary bodies through the mammillothalamic tract. Furthermore, Hassler (57) described a case in which stereotaxic lesions of the anterior thalamic nuclei resulted in a severe but temporary amnesia. As has already been noted, it is quite possible that many ischemic accidents or tumors involving the thalamus may damage connections to the anterior thalamic nuclei. Indeed, some reports of thalamic amnesia following ischemic lesions attribute the critical pathology to the mammillothalamic tract and not MD (46, 58). Given the close anatomical relationship between the anterior thalamic nuclei, the mammillary bodies and the hippocampus it would, in fact, seem most unlikely that this thalamic region has no contribution to memory mechanisms.

One other thalamic region, the parataenial nucleus, has been implicated in amnesia. Mair, Warrington, and Weiskrantz (59) provided very detailed psychometric and pathological data for two alcoholic Korsakoff patients. They described a very restricted pattern of diencephalic damage which was essentially confined to the mammillary bodies and the parataenial nucleus, which lies just medial to MD, while MD itself appeared normal. The close proximity of this nucleus to MD suggests that some pathological studies may have neglected to distinguish these regions.

From a consideration of the evidence it is clear that a distinct diencephalic amnesia exists. While few would argue that the mammillary bodies or their connections do not contribute to the syndrome, the status of other diencephalic regions remains unclear. The lack of confirmed, near complete lesions confined to particular diencephalic nuclei still continues to hamper any unequivocal statement concerning the anatomical basis of diencephalic amnesia. Indeed, it may well prove that a combination of more than one structure or pathway is required to produce the full amnesic syndrome (59).

ANIMAL STUDIES OF ANTEROGRADE AMNESIA

The rarity of amnesic subjects with confirmed, selective lesions has led many investigators to turn to experimental studies using animals. These studies have not only examined the behavioral effects of specific lesions but have also provided detailed electrophysiological and anatomical information which would be unobtainable from studies on humans.

TEMPORAL LOBE AMNESIA

Following descriptions of the amnesic subject HM a number of studies tried to confirm that hippocampal lesions had a similar catastrophic effect upon recent memory in monkeys. The results of such studies proved disappointing. Monkeys with bilateral hippocampal lesions were found to be able to master a large number of tasks such as object discrimination learning, object reversal learning, nonspatial go/no go tasks, and delayed response (60). While some studies reported minor deficits for some of these tasks it soon became evident that the hippocampal formation was not necessary for a variety of learning tasks. Furthermore, it became apparent that hippocampal lesions had a much greater effect upon spatial rather than nonspatial versions of the same task; for example, spatial delayed alternation versus nonspatial go/no go; spatial reversal learning versus object reversal learning. While human amnesics clearly do display severe spatial deficits they are also impaired on a wide range of nonspatial problems.

This apparent mismatch suggested a number of possible solutions. First, the function of the hippocampus may have undergone a dramatic species change. Second, the hippocampus might not be necessary for normal memory in spite of the apparent clinical evidence. Third, the behavioral tasks used to assess memory dysfunctions in animals may have been in some way inappropriate. Clearly, none of these possibilities are mutually exclusive and a combination of any two, or even all three, may be closer to the truth.

The first possibility, that of a species difference, is in many ways the hardest to disprove. There can be no doubt that the connections, and in particular the cortical connections, of the hippocampal formation will differ between humans and other primates. Indeed, the contribution of language to memory, coupled with the clear evidence that damage to different hemispheres can have different effects upon human memory surely underlines the fact that some changes have occurred. Nevertheless, this must be weighed against the fact that the cytoarchitectonic appearance of the structure and its major connections appear to be remarkably constant across a wide range of mammalian species. Indeed, Lorente de No's (61) classic description of the detailed anatomical structure of the hippocampal formation and entorhinal cortex repeatedly emphasizes these cross-species similarities. For example he states that

> The similarity between the Cornu Ammonis and Fascia Dentata (the two major subdivisions of the hippocampus) in man and monkey is so extreme that the description will be made on the basis of drawings taken from brains of monkeys (p. 147).

Given the belief that structure and function are interdependent it would seem almost inconceivable that a virtually identical hippocampus should play a vital part in human, but not monkey memory mechanisms.

The second possibility is that the hippocampus itself is not a key mnemonic structure. There is, for example, recent behavioral and electrophysiological evidence from studies of monkeys that the entorhinal and perirhinal cortices play a far greater role in recognition memory than has usually been accorded (62, 63). Nevertheless, such evidence must still implicate the hippocampus as it is closely related to both cortical areas. Indeed, the entorhinal cortex is often regarded as part of the hippocampal formation.

A more radical suggestion is that the white matter of the temporal stem and not the hippocampus itself is responsible for temporal lobe amnesia (64). It has been proposed that damage to the temporal stem would disconnect the temporal cortex and so produce an anterograde amnesia. This idea arose from the discovery that such lesions severely impair the acquisition of pattern discriminations by monkeys. It is now, however, possible to rule out this "temporal stem hypothesis" as it has been confirmed that some subjects with temporal lobe amnesia do not suffer temporal stem damage (65). Furthermore, it has been elegantly shown that while temporal stem damage does indeed disrupt simultaneous visual discriminations (66), such lesions do not affect memory tests which have been shown to be sensitive to human anterograde amnesia (Fig. 3; 66-68). The discovery that some behavioral tests appear sensitive to experimental amnesias while other tests of learning and memory, such as pattern discrimination learning, appear insensitive, brings us to the third possibility; inappropriate testing methods.

It is now clear that anterograde amnesia does not affect all types of learning memory. Examples of "preserved learning" by amnesic subjects include

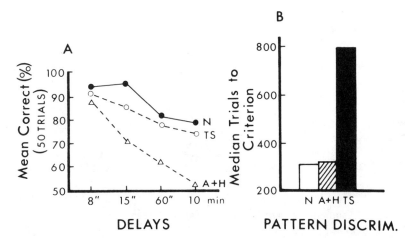

Figure 3 (A) Delayed nonmatching-to-sample. The ability of normal (N) monkeys (*Macaca fascicularis*) and those with temporal stem lesions (TS) or conjoint amygdala-hippocampus lesions (A + H) to recognize a single object after retention delays of 8 seconds to 10 minutes. (B) Acquisition scores for two pattern discrimination tasks learned in succession by N, TS, and A + H monkeys. The TS group was markedly impaired on (B) but not (A), the reverse pattern of results was found for the A + H group. (From Ref. 66.)

classical conditioning, priming, passive avoidance, reading mirror letters, mirror tracing, assembling jigsaws, the Tower of Hanoi problem, and various motor-perception tasks such as the pursuit rotor task. It is becoming increasingly evident that long-term memory should be divided into at least two distinct divisions, one or more of which may be unaffected by anterograde amnesia. From this it is also evident that animal tests of amnesia must tax the appropriate aspects of memory.

With these considerations in mind Zola-Morgan and Squire (69) have suggested that the following four tasks should form part of a standard battery for the assessment of anterograde amnesia in nonhuman primates. The tasks are delayed nonmatching-to-sample, concurrent learning of visual discriminations, delayed retention of object discriminations, and delayed response. Of these, the delayed nonmatching-to-sample task (DNMS) has proved the most influential, and its value has been strengthened by recent studies showing that analogous versions of this task are sensitive to human amnesic syndromes (67, 68).

In the most widely used version of the DNMS task, the animal is shown a novel sample object (Fig. 4). By displacing the object and taking the food reward which lies under the object the animal is forced to attend to this sample

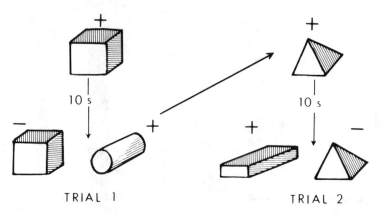

TRIAL 1   TRIAL 2

Figure 4 Diagrammatic representation of the testing procedure used standardly in the delayed nonmatching-to-sample task.

stimulus. After a delay of typically 6 to 10 s, during which the sample object is removed, the initial sample object and a novel alternative object are shown simultaneously to the animal. In "nonmatching" the animal is rewarded for selecting the novel stimulus. New pairs of stimuli are then usually used for each set of trials.

In spite of some initial controversy it has become accepted that hippocampectomy or transection of its major efferent pathway, the fornix, produces only mild impairments upon standard DNMS acquisition in monkeys (70-72). While impairments may also be observed when the retention interval is increased beyond 10 s or when the animal is required to remember lists of more than one sample object at a time, these impairments are often regarded as mild (71-73). The same is true when the amygdala is removed (70). But, in striking contrast, combined removal of both the amygdala and the hippocampus has a catastrophic effect upon task acquisition and subsequent performance over increasing retention intervals (Fig. 5). These findings have been found for both visual and tactile DNMS (66, 70, 74) and there seems no reason to suppose that they would not extend to other modalities such as audition.

These results have led to the intriguing proposal that the full-blown temporal lobe amnesia is a consequence of combined damage to the amygdala and hippocampus (70). This is not meant to imply that the amygdala and hippocampus have interchangeable roles; indeed there is ample evidence that they are quite distinct. Nor does this imply that all cases of amnesia must have complete or near-complete lesions of these two structures. For example, the subject described by Penfield and Mathieson (7) suffered bilateral hippo-

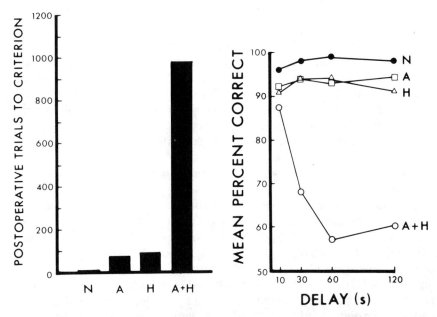

Figure 5 Delayed nonmatching-to-sample performance of normal (N) monkeys (*Macaca mulatta*) and those with lesions in either the amygdala (A), the hippocampus (H), or both (A + H). Left; mean trials to reacquire the preoperative learning criterion. Right; mean trials correct when the retention interval was increased from 10 to 120 s. (From Ref. 70.)

campal damage but only unilateral amygdaloid damage. The amnesia in this case was slightly milder than that in HM's case, suggesting that an increase in total damage to the two structures is paralleled by an increase in the severity of the amnesia. Experimental support comes from a study using monkeys which showed that bilateral amygdala plus unilateral hippocampal lesions, or bilateral hippocampal plus unilateral amygdala lesions, produce similar impairments on the DNMS task which were greater than those seen after lesions confined to just the hippocampus or the amygdala but less than those seen after combined, bilateral lesions to both structures (75).

The proposal that combined amygdala and hippocampal system damage is involved in severe amnesias accounts for the frequent failure of selective hippocampal lesions in monkeys to have severe effects upon memory. It is also consistent with the evidence that both structures are involved in herpes encephalitis and Alzheimer's disease, both of which can lead to exceptionally dense amnesias. This proposal can also account for the apparent failure of damage to the fornix to produce a consistent, severe amnesia in humans (76);

indeed some descriptions of subjects with fornical damage have reported no apparent memory disturbances (37, 77-79). While other cases have noted memory problems (80-83), these are difficult to interpret for a number of reasons. In some, the fornical damage was caused by a ventricular tumor (80, 82), making localization of the dysfunction a problem, while in other cases there was additional damage to other regions which may have contributed to the amnesic state (80, 83). In at least one case, the severity of the amnesia can only be regarded as mild when compared with subjects like HM (82), in another the short survival time of the patient means that it is impossible to tell if the amnesic state was permanent (81), while in a third case the lack of postmortem confirmation limits confidence in the full extent of the damage (80).

A recent challenge to the view that a combination of hippocampal and amygdaloid damage is required to produce full-blown temporal lobe amnesia comes from studies into the perirhinal, prorhinal, and entorhinal cortices. Evidence has been provided that stereotaxic lesions of the amygdala which do not involve these adjacent cortical regions fail to potentiate the effects of hippocampal lesions on the DNMS task (84). Furthermore, removal of the perirhinal and parahippocampal cortices may produce a severe deficit on performance on the same task (85). These findings have been interpreted as showing that it is the hippocampal formation and related cortical regions that form the critical substrate for temporal lobe amnesia and that the amygdala, while important for other cognitive functions, is not involved.

A number of difficulties are, however, raised by this alternative view. First, this key role for the hippocampal formation is inconsistent with the relatively minor contribution of either the fornix or the mammillary bodies in amnesia (76, 86), unless the hippocampal-diencephalic projections via the fornix have little mnemonic function and the critical efferents are those from the hippocampus to the entorhinal cortex (86). While this explanation may deal with the initial problem it raises the far greater problem of how there could be two very similar amnesic syndromes (one temporal, the other diencephalic) from quite independent causes. Second, it has been shown that dorsal amygdaloid lesions, which involve a very restricted portion of the most rostral entorhinal cortex, can markedly potentiate the effects of fornix transsection on DNMS performance in monkeys (87). Lastly, this analysis assumes that the amygdala has no clear mnemonic role and yet studies of its afferents, its electrophysiological properties, and the effects of amygdaloid damage all point to its contribution in the linking of extrinsic stimuli with reward, a role which logically requires an important mnemonic capacity (88).

In summary, while there is every reason to suppose that the perirhinal and parahippocampal cortices will prove to be important components in a temporal lobe 'memory system,' current evidence would require a role for the amygdala. Further support for the view that damage to single brain sites causes only a relatively mild amnesia comes from a comparison of the severity of the memory loss following different degrees of temporal and diencephalic damage in humans. Figure 6 depicts the WAIS-WMS (Wechsler Adult Intelligence Scale, Wechsler Memory Scale) differences for a number of amnesics with increasingly selective medial temporal lobe damage. These cases include one additional subject from the original Scoville and Milner series (89) and a subject (Case 7) who had undergone a frontal lobotomy, with little apparent effect, followed by a bilateral hippocampectomy (90). While the temporal lobe cases refer to individual studies, the data for alcoholic Korsakoff subjects are taken from groups of 9 (91) and 8 (16) subjects.

While the WMS test remains, in many respects, a very blunt instrument for the assessment of anterograde amnesias, its almost universal use does allow such direct comparisons to be made and it can be seen that bilateral damage to multiple temporal sites is associated with the most severe amnesias. As mentioned above, the effects of fornix lesions remain uncertain and as it is only those cases which report clear memory impairments which also provide WAIS and WMS scores it is likely that the typical effects of such damage have been exaggerated.

DIENCEPHALIC AMNESIA

Relatively few experimental studies of memory in nonhuman primates have been directed at diencephalic regions such as the mammillary bodies or the thalamus. Nevertheless, a number of recent studies examining the diencephalon suggest a similar story to that emerging from studies of the temporal lobe.

It has been shown that mammillary body lesions in monkeys impair spatial, but not object, reversal learning (92). Mammillary body lesions also impair spatial alteration when long delays are used (93). These findings bear obvious similarities with those observed following hippocampal ablation (94, 95) and fornical transsection (96, 97) and are clearly consistent with the close anatomical links between these structures. Furthermore, just as fornix transsection has only mild effects upon DNMS (71, 72), so lesions centered on the medial mammillary nuclei (86, 98), that part damaged by Korsakoff's disease, produce only small DNMS acquisition and performance impairments (Fig. 7) impairments which may only be transient (86). Clearer evidence of a memory impairment following mammillary body damage was reported for a yes/no running recognition task by Saunders (99), although once again the magnitude of the deficit matched that seen after fornix transsection. Thus, while there is a clear need to extend these analyses to a much wider range of behavioral tasks, it would appear that mammillary body damage and fornix transsection often have similar effects which, in themselves, do not resemble a severe, global amnesia (Fig. 7).

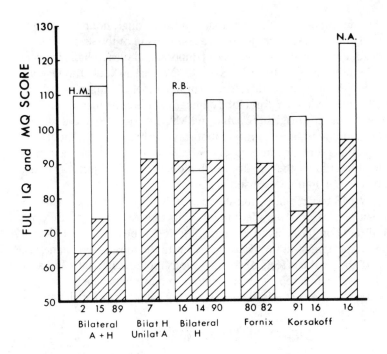

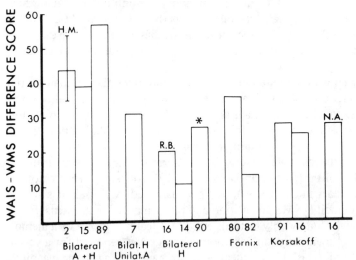

Figure 6 Upper panel shows full scale Wechsler Adult Intelligence Scale (WAIS) and Wechsler memory (WMS) scores for a variety of patients with anterograde amnesia. Lower panel shows the WAIS-WMS difference scores for the same patients. For case H.M. the range of WAIS-WMS differences from repeated assessments (2) is shown, while for one case (asterisk) the drop in WMS score following surgery is depicted (90). The numbers correspond to the appropriate references.

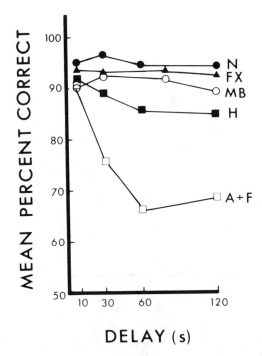

Figure 7   Delayed nonmatching-to-sample: showing performance of normal monkeys (N) and those with lesions in the fornix (Fx), hippocampus (H), mammillary bodies (MB), and the amygdala and fornix combined (A + F). All data refers to *Macaca fascicularis* (data from Refs. 62, 87, 98).

Remarkably little is known about the effects of thalamic damage upon memory in monkeys, and most relevant studies have concentrated upon MD. Early studies emphasized the important anatomical links between MD and the prefrontal cortex and so used tests known to be sensitive to prefrontal damage such as delayed response and delayed alternation. While the results have been inconsistent, it appears that damage to the more caudal parts of MD produces slight impairments in both tasks (100).

More recent studies using the DNMS task have shown that an extensive, medial thalamic lesion (MT, Fig. 8) which removed the midline nuclei, the medial, magnocellular portion of MD, and parts of the anterior thalamic nuclei produces a severe acquisition and performance deficit (101). When this medial thalamic lesion was divided into an anterior (AMT; anterior midline nuclei, medial anterior nuclei and mammillothalamic tract) and a posterior (PMT; posterior midline nuclei and medial MD) portion similar small, but insignificant, DNMS performance deficits (Fig. 8) were found (102). This pattern of results clearly echoes that found after amygdala and hippo-

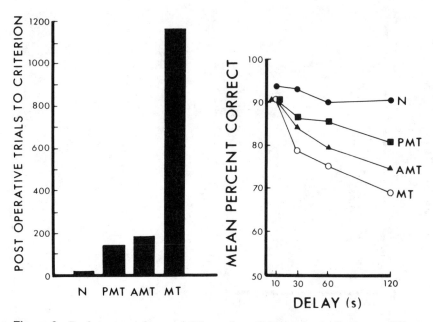

Figure 8   Performance of normal (N) monkeys (*Macaca fascicularis*) over different retention intervals on the delayed nonmatching-to-sample task compared to monkeys with lesions in either the anterior medial thalamus (AMT), the posterior medial thalamus (PMT), or both (MT). (From Ref. 102.)

campal lesions, as ablation of the anterior or posterior medial thalamic tissue produced only mild effects while combined damage produced a severe deficit (102).

Evidence that the MD damage was responsible for the posterior medial thalamic deficit has come from studies showing that lesions more restricted to MD also impair DNMS performance (103) while midline thalamic lesions have no effect (101). It is more difficult to define the critical site in the anterior medial thalamic lesions as the ablation caused retrograde degeneration in the mammillary bodies. Furthermore, transsection of the mammillothalamic tract, which spared the anterior thalamic nuclei but produced marked degeneration in the mammillary bodies, brought about a similar mild, but significant, DNMS deficit (102). This suggests that the mammillary body involvement was sufficient to bring about a mild recognition memory impairment in those animals with anterior medial thalamic lesions. However, given the close anatomical links between the mammillary bodies and the anterior thalamic nuclei, it may prove more appropriate to regard these diencephalic regions as part of a single mnemonic system, especially as they both receive dense inputs from the hippocampus.

In summary, there is evidence to support that, as in the medial temporal lobes, full-blown diencephalic amnesia is a consequence of damage to a combination of structures and that selective damage to only one structure may produce relatively mild memory impairments. This idea is not only consistent with the animal evidence, but it coincides with much of the clinical evidence. For example, the severe amnesia of Korsakoff's disease may reflect combined mammillary body and thalamic damage, while damage restricted to structures such as MD or the mammillary bodies produces relatively mild impairments or even none at all (31, 40). In the next section we will consider how diencephalic and temporal lobe amnesias relate anatomically to one another.

THE ANATOMICAL BASIS OF ANTEROGRADE AMNESIAS

The advent of axonal tracing methods has heralded a dramatic improvement of our understanding of the fine anatomical relationships between those structures thought to be needed for normal memory. This technical advance has, however, meant that there is now an enormous discrepancy between our understanding of human neuroanatomy and that of experimental species such as the rat or monkey. Consequently, this section concentrates on the neural pathways that have been mapped out in monkeys, and in particular the rhesus macaque (*Macaca mulatta*) and the cynomolgus macaque (*Macaca fascicularis*).

While they are structurally different, the amygdala and hippocampus share at least one very important attribute. Both structures receive dense cortical inputs which allow sensory information from a range of modalities to gain access to these limbic structures. This would appear to be a prerequisite feature for structures involved in anterograde amnesia as the memory deficits are polysensory in nature and yet, with the exception of olfaction, there is no specific sensory loss.

In the case of the amygdala, the sensory afferents arise directly from a number of cortical association areas such as the inferotemporal cortex, the superior temporal cortex, the insula, the temporal pole, the orbitofrontal cortex and the superior temporal sulcus (Fig. 9). Some of these cortical regions provide sensory-specific information (inferotemporal cortex, superior temporal cortex, insula) while the other cortical inputs will include polysensory information. As a consequence, highly processed sensory information is allowed to converge upon the amygdala (104).

The organization of inputs to the hippocampus is slightly different (Fig. 10) in that the sensory afferents are first relayed through the parahippocampal, entorhinal, perirhinal, and prorhinal cortices (105). These cortices then project through the perforant pathway to the hippocampus proper, many of the afferents terminating initially in the CA4 region, from whence they pass, in

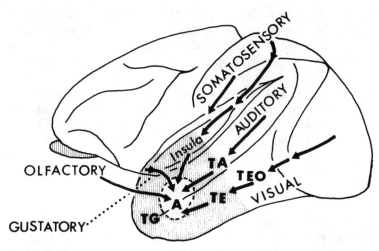

Figure 9 Schematized representation of sensory inputs of the amygdala in the macaque monkey. The lateral fissure is shown opened to expose the insula. The shaded regions designate the various sensory pathways' final cortical stations, which are the
sources of the direct amygdaloid afferents. (From Ref. 104, courtesy of Academic
Press.)

a stepwise fashion, to CA2, CA1, and the subiculum (105, 106). Both the
amygdala and the hippocampus project back upon the neocortex (104-106).
In the case of the hippocampus many of these efferents being relayed via the
entorhinal and parahippocampal cortices (Fig. 10). Of particular interest is
that the projections from the amygdala and from the hippocampus, via the
parahippocampal gyrus, project to very widespread areas of cerebral association cortex (Fig. 10); these reciprocal connections being at least as widespread as the inputs from the cortex to these limbic structures (105, 107).

While the structure and functions of the amygdala and hippocampus are
clearly different, the two regions are reciprocally connected. It is well known
that indirect interconnections may pass through the entorhinal cortex. It is
now also clear that there are direct amygdalohippocampal interconnections
(108). The hippocampal projections run from the subiculum to the lateral basal
and medial basal nuclei of the amygdala, while the amygdaloid projections
run from the basal amygdaloid nuclei to the most rostral portions of hippocampal fields CA1-3 and throughout parts of the subiculum. Clearly, it is
wrong to consider these two limbic structures to be independent of one another.

Examination of the subcortical projections from the amygdala and hippocampus provides a further valuable clue. Both structures project to diencephalic targets which themselves have been implicated by studies of amnesia.

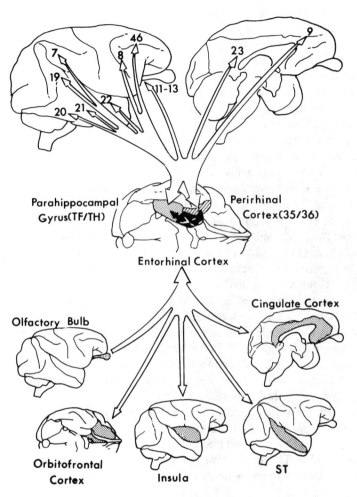

Figure 10 Summary of cortical afferent and efferent connections of entorhinal cortex, which is the major source of projections to the hippocampus. The major cortical input originates in the adjacent parahippocampal gyrus and perirhinal cortex. These regions in turn receive inputs from a variety of sensory association areas. (From Ref. 156, courtesy of Elsevier Publications, Cambridge.)

In this two way parallel limbic-diencephalic systems emerge, one from the hippocampus via the fornix to the mammillary bodies and the anterior thalamic nuclei, the other from the amygdala to the magnocellular portion of MD (Fig. 11). These direct connections between the temporal and diencephalic regions implicated in anterograde amnesia must surely be more than coincidence and indicate that temporal lobe and diencephalic amnesias are different facets of the same underlying amnesic syndrome.

The dense hippocampal projections to the mammillary bodies arise from all cell layers of the subiculum and presubiculum to pass exclusively through the fornix and terminate throughout the medial mammillary nucleus (109, 110), that part most consistently damaged by Korsakoff's disease. Additional projections terminate in the tuberomammillary nucleus. As in the case of MD and the amygdala, so the medial mammillary nucleus does not project back upon the hippocampus. Instead, the mammillary body efferents to the hippocampus arise from the supra- and perimammillary regions to terminate in CA2 and the dentate gyrus (111, 112). Whether there are intramammillary body connections which permit reciprocal connections between this structure and the hippocampus remains an important, but as yet unanswered question, although a detailed analysis of the efferents from the medial mammillary nuclei failed to find appropriate connections (112).

The hippocampus also provides extensive thalamic inputs which may well be involved in mnemonic processes. In particular, dense projections arise from the subicular and entorhinal cortices to pass through the fornix to the anterior thalamic nuclei. In the case of the subiculum these projections terminate most heavily in the anterior medial and anterior ventral nuclei. Other subicular and entorhinal projections terminate in nucleus lateralis dorsalis, the medial pulvinar, and several of the more rostral midline nuclei. Some of the projections to the pulvinar and nucleus lateralis dorsalis appear to use nonfornical routes (113). The anterior medial and anterior ventral nuclei are of particular interest as they receive dense inputs from the hippocampus via

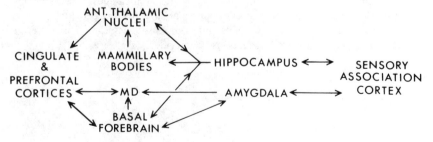

Figure 11 Schematic diagram showing relationships between those structures forming an anatomy of anterograde amnesia.

the fornix and from the medial mammillary bodies via the mammillothalamic tract. These nuclei also project back upon the hippocampus (111) and hence could provide an indirect route from the mammillary bodies to the hippocampus. The lateral dorsal thalamic nucleus, which is regarded as a member of the anterior complex, also has dense reciprocal hippocampal connections and hence should not be ignored in any consideration of diencephalic memory systems.

The amygdalothalamic projections arise primarily from the basal amygdaloid nuclei and terminate in characteristic patches in the rostral half of the medial, magnocellular portion of MD (114, 115). Furthermore, both the entorhinal and perirhinal cortices project to magnocellular MD although there is little overlap with the amygdaloid projections (115). In spite of the substantial input from the amygdala to MD, there are no direct reciprocal projections; in other words, MD cannot influence the amygdala directly. This is clearly of great importance when considering the relationship between temporal lobe and diencephalic amnesias.

The lack of a reciprocal connection from MD to the amygdala or temporal association cortex inevitably directs attention upon the major efferent target of MD, the prefrontal cortex. Particular attention has focused upon the caudal orbital cortex and caudal medial cortex as these adjacent areas receive inputs not only from the medial portion of MD but also from the amygdala (107) and the hippocampus (106). Parts of the rostral cingulate cortex receive inputs from the amygdala and hippocampus as well as the anterior thalamic nuclei, although most of the thalamic inputs terminate in the caudal cingulate cortex (116).

Although the prefrontal cortex may well form an important further component in a medial temporal-medial diencephalic system, there is little evidence that prefrontal damage produces an amnesic syndrome comparable to that seen after damage to either diencephalic or temporal regions. While some descriptions of prefrontal damage report the regular occurrence of anterograde memory problems (117) many others do not. These latter cases include descriptions of the outcomes of prefrontal lobotomies and lobectomies, some of which involve damage to those orbital regions most implicated by their anatomical connections (118). Furthermore, when memory disorders are observed they most often refer to difficulties such as learning the temporal order of events, assessing the relative frequency and recency of stimuli (119), and the learning of conditional associative tasks (120). While it is the case that frontal damage may often be associated with memory problems (117) they are often qualitatively different from those associated with temporal or diencephalic damage (118).

An apparent exception has been the observation that rupture of the anterior cerebral artery or the anterior communicating artery can produce an anterograde amnesic state resembling Korsakoff's disease (23, 121). As such cases frequently involve the orbital cortex they appear to strengthen the case for a prefrontal contribution to amnesia. Unfortunately, these vascular accidents also involve basal forebrain regions and it may be the case that this subcortical damage is a better predictor of amnesia (121).

More direct support for a prefrontal contribution to anterograde amnesic syndromes has come from recent animal studies. It has been shown that combined removal of the ventral and medial prefrontal tissue disrupts DNMS performance in a way similar to that seen after medial temporal or medial thalamic damage (122). It is important to note that these are the same regions of prefrontal cortex which receive the majority of projections from the hippocampus, the amygdala, the anterior thalamic nuclei, and medial MD. In contrast, removal of the dorsolateral prefrontal cortex has little effect upon DNMS performance. These findings indicate that there may be a further station to both the hippocampal and amygdaloid mnemonic systems within the prefrontal cortex, which given its anatomical connections may be reciprocal.

In summary, a complex series of temporal-diencephalic connections has emerged which tightly link the amnesic syndromes observed after damage to the respective areas. This does not, however, mean that temporal lobe and diencephalic amnesias can be regarded as identical syndromes as the different regions will have different functional contributions. Nevertheless, if the critical flow of information is from temporal regions to the diencephalon then the similarities will outweigh the differences. These similarities include comparable performances on standardized neuropsychological tests, difficulty in new learning, intact digit span or immediate memory, and intact general intellectual ability. It has been argued that temporal and diencephalic amnesias may be distinguished by different rates of forgetting (123), but recent studies have cast doubt on this distinction (124), and at present there is no generally agreed qualitative difference between these amnesias. Given the apparent lack of appropriate back projections from some diencephalic regions to the temporal lobe it is tempting to suppose that the major flow of information is on to the prefrontal cortex, although the nature of this step requires further investigation.

With hindsight it is fascinating to read an account published near the beginning of the century of a man who had a pronounced anterograde amnesia following a stroke (125). At autopsy symmetrical areas of infarction were observed in the frontal white matter, immediately anterior to the head of the caudate nucleus. The authors suggested that these lesions would have interrupted long association fibers from the frontal to the temporal and occipital lobes, and indeed the extensive corticocortical projections from the prefrontal cortex would link this region with a wide area of association cortex. A similar disconnection view of amnesia has been proposed much more recently by Warrington and Weiskrantz (126), who argued that amnesias may reflect a disconnection of temporal-diencephalic-frontal structures in which different memory systems are isolated from one another. Whichever proves nearer to the truth, it is becoming clear that the prefrontal cortex cannot be ignored and that a series of interrelated structures (Fig. 11) have been identified which form a complex anatomy of structures necessary for normal recent memory. It is, however, also apparent that this series of structures is most unlikely to represent the sites of memory storage, and this will be considered in the next section.

ANTEROGRADE AMNESIA AND THE STORAGE OF MEMORIES

One of the most striking aspects of the anterograde amnesic syndrome is that premorbid memories may remain essentially intact. This in turn tells us that those regions responsible for anterograde amnesia are not sites of memory storage, nor can they be necessary for the retrieval of old memories. If we take the case of HM, it would appear that his event memory prior to the age of 16 years, when his first seizures occurred, is normal (2). Given that he has lost all of the medial temporal structures and that the presumed initial flow of sensory information is from the temporal cortex to the subcortex, then the storage of his premorbid memories must be 'upstream' from the site of the lesion, namely the cortex. A similar logic dictates that diencephalic structures, which are 'downstream,' cannot be a site of memory storage, and as predicted there are diencephalic amnesic cases with normal retrograde memory (49). Nevertheless, the existence of a diencephalic syndrome shows that a closed reciprocal temporal cortex-hippocampus/amygdala system is insufficient for the encoding, storage and retrieval of memories. This is born out by the recent case RB in whom a circumscribed hippocampal lesion led to severe anterograde but essentially normal retrograde memory (16).

The notion that the cortex, and in particular, sensory association cortex, is the repository of the elusive memory trace or 'engram' is of course not new. The dramatic discovery by Wilder Penfield that direct stimulation of the temporal cortex in conscious patients during neurosurgery could on rare occasions evoke an apparent memory immediately focused attention upon the neocortex. These apparent 'memories' included hearing music, walking into a timber yard, and watching a baseball game (127). Although others have questioned whether the original events ever occurred (128) and have provided evidence that these 'experimental' effects require afterdischarges in the amygdala or hippocampus (129), the involvement of association cortex in these phenomena is not disputed.

Further evidence for a cortical role in storage has come from those diseases which can produce a persistent retrograde amnesia. Although it may be logically impossible to distinguish a retrieval deficit from a storage deficit it is the case that certain diseases which can produce extensive cortical damage, for example, Alzheimer's disease or herpes encephalitis, may be accompanied by a severe, permanent retrograde amnesia. In both cases the cortical damage is typically most severe in the temporal and frontal lobes. Further evidence for the involvement of temporal association cortex has come from anatomical studies on the flow of visual information from the striate cortex to the parietal and temporal cortices and the effects of inferotemporal, area TE, damage upon complex visual learning tasks (130). Such studies strongly suggest that the inferior temporal cortex acts as a storehouse for the central representation of visual stimuli (130, 131).

From a more theoretical viewpoint, it is evident that the sheer number of bits of information required in a lifetime must demand an enormous storage capacity. For example, estimates of the number of bits required to master a language completely, multiplied by the number of languages a single person can master at the same time gives something of the order of 4-5 $\times$ 10^6 bit (132). Given the vast number of neurons in the cortex, its modular organization, and the increasing acceptance that memory depends on synaptic changes in a distributed population of neurons, it is no surprise that many regard the cortex as the prime site of memory storage in humans.

This conclusion allows us to further our anatomy of event memory by assuming that those subcortical systems outlined in the previous section must feed back upon the cortex, either to allow storage or retrieval or both. This does, however, produce a slight paradox, for although we know that the amygdala and hippocampus have extensive direct and indirect projections upon the cortex which would allow just such a function, we have also argued that their diencephalic projections form the next part of the circuit. This in turn lead us to consider the reciprocal diencephalic-limbic projections which are indirect and far less numerous. In contrast, there are extensive projections from the diencephalon to the frontal cortex which may well converge with direct inputs from cortical and subcortical structures in the temporal lobe. While the role of the frontal lobe in memory mechanisms remains enigmatic, its unique set of cortical and subcortical connections denote that this region forms part of our notional memory system.

It is also clear that the widespread back projections from the amygdala and hippocampal formation (Fig. 10) upon association cortex must be considered, but it has already been made clear that these connections on their own are insufficient. It may prove that projections from the medial diencephalon, frontal cortex, or basal forebrain upon these limbic structures, or upon those cortical regions that the amygdala and hippocampus project to, are necessary to permit these limbic-cortical connections to contribute to memory mechanisms. At present these issues remain unanswered and pose

some of the greatest challenges; a challenge made all the more difficult by the widely held view that a particular memory cannot be localized to a particular neuronal site and that memory formation involves changes in many ensembles of neurons.

OTHER MEMORY SYSTEMS

At the outset, it was made clear that there are in fact multiple anatomies of memory, and some of the strongest evidence has come from dissociations between those types of memory disrupted by anterograde amnesia and those that are spared. In this section the possible neuroanatomical bases of those kinds of learning that are spared will be considered.

SHORT-TERM MEMORY

An accepted feature of anterograde amnesia is that it may be accompanied by normal performance on a range of tasks thought to tax short-term memory. Evidence for a qualitative distinction between short-term and long-term memory is made all the stronger by the existence of patients who have a severely limited auditory verbal short-term memory but near-normal long-term memory (133). Patients with damage in the supramarginal and angular gyri of the left hemisphere have been found to perform very poorly on Brown-Petersen tasks and show very reduced immediate memory spans for digits, words, or letters using auditory presentation (133, 134). Similarly, in free recall tasks these cases may show a recency effect of only one item. In contrast, the same subjects can show normal performance in tasks such as paired-associate learning, recall of stories, and the learning of word lists. It has been argued that these deficits reflect a specific loss of a temporary articulatory store which forms a component of the short-term memory store (134).

These patients provide a double dissociation with amnesic subjects who fail tests of long-term memory yet can perform normally on these tests of short-term memory and vice versa (134). While the critical anatomical locus in those cases with reduced auditory verbal short-term memory is poorly understood it does appear to lie close to regions known to be important for auditory verbal reception.

DIVISIONS WITHIN LONG-TERM MEMORY: SEMANTIC/EPISODIC AND PROCEDURAL/DECLARATIVE MEMORY

On talking to an amnesic subject it is impossible not to be struck by his or her impaired learning or recall of new events which is in marked constrast to a normal use of language and naming. This distinction is all the more stark

in occasional postencephalitic cases who have extraordinary dense anterograde and retrograde amnesias and yet still show a highly accurate and sophisticated use of language (135). Such a division is reminiscent of that put forward
by Tulving (136), who proposed that long-term memories could be regarded
as either 'episodic' (autobiographical information concerning events in our
lives) or 'semantic' (language, facts, general concepts, and rules about the
world).

While it is tempting to transpose this distinction directly to the amnesic
syndrome, it is evident that there are shortcomings. It has been shown (137)
that amnesic subjects are impaired in learning both new facts (semantic) (e.g.
geographical locations of places), as well as new specific events (episodic).
As a consequence, amnesic subjects show very clear impairments in semantic
knowledge about the world when that knowledge is linked to events occurring
after the onset of the amnesia. For example, in 1973 the subject HM could
not identify Watergate or John Dean even though he watched the TV news
every night, in 1980 he stated that he thought that a hippie was a type of dancer
(2). These examples illustrate how amnesia does not respect the semantic/
episodic memory distinction and indeed they highlight some of the logical
problems inherent in such a distinction as one could argue that semantic memory is drawn from a number of episodes or examples which help build up
and confirm that 'fact.' One extreme version of this view is that all episodic
memory may eventually become semantic memory (138).

A more promising distinction with regard to amnesia is that between 'procedural' and 'declarative' memory. Declarative memory concerns knowing
that while procedural memory concerns knowing how (139). Declarative
memory can in many ways be seen as an amalgam of episodic and semantic
memory (140), many aspects of which as we have seen are affected by anterograde amnesia. Procedural memory involves the learning of perceptual, motor,
and cognitive skills. These usually require multiple learning trials and often
allow little insight into what it is we have actually learned.

Evidence that procedural abilities rely on a distinct neural system comes
from the finding that subjects with a variety of anterograde amnesias are
able to learn tasks that could be classified as procedural. These include mirror-
tracing, rotary pursuit tasks, mirror reading, solving jigsaw puzzles, mathematical puzzles, and the Tower of Hanoi problem (126, 141, 142). A further
subcategory of procedural memory is classical conditioning which, like the
previous examples, can be preserved in amnesia (143). It is interesting to note
that in all of these cases of preserved learning, the amnesic subject may be
able to master the desired skill but fail to remember where, when, and under
what conditions it was acquired (i.e., the episodic aspects of the task).

While studies of amnesia indicate that procedural memory does not rely
on the medial temporal lobe or medial diencephalon, clinical studies have

told us little more. Animal studies may, however, afford us further insights. The learning of repetitive tasks, such as visual discriminations, which are thought to involve automatic stimulus-response associations or 'habits' (144) can be seen as analogous to procedural memory tasks. In contrast, a task such as DNMS, which requires the recognition of a stimulus seen only once, would be expected to tax declarative memory. Of particular interest therefore is the finding that combined A + H lesions impair DNMS but not visual discrimination learning, while temporal stem lesions spare DNMS but impair the visual discrimination task (66). This double dissociation provides strong evidence for two neurally distinct systems.

It has been proposed that the learning of habits (i.e., procedural memory) depends on cortical inputs from sensory association areas to the striatum or basal ganglia (144). Not only do the two key structures in the striatum, the putamen and caudate nucleus, receive dense cortical inputs, they also project to the globus pallidus and its associated structures within the extrapyramidal system. In this way sensory inputs could become linked with motor outputs. This proposal is also consistent with the limited number of studies on the effects of striatal damage upon discrimination learning; although this must await more critical investigation (144).

One category of procedural learning which has been studied extensively in animals is classical conditioning. In rats and rabbits simple classically conditioned responses such as eyeblink responses are not affected by hippocampal removal. Indeed, neodecorticate rats are capable of classical conditioning providing that the stimuli are not too complex (145). One subcortical site that has been implicated in classical conditioning is the cerebellum, and highly selective lesions have been shown to produce impairments in nictitating membrane responses (146, 147). While this does not mean that cerebellar lesions disrupt all forms of classical conditioning (148), considerable advances have been made in mapping out a possible circuitry involving the interpositus nucleus of the cerebellum, the red nucleus of the midbrain, the inferior olive, and the fibers that interconnect them, in the conditioned nictitating membrane response in rabbits (147).

The final category of preserved learning in amnesia concerns priming effects. Priming refers to the facilitation of performance by the prior exposure of material to be tested. This effect can be found even in the subject who shows impaired recall or recognition of the same material and the effect persists well beyond the span of short-term memory. Tests of priming usually involve showing a subject a set of words or pictures and then at a later stage providing that subject with the first few letters or a fragment of the picture. When amnesic subjects are asked to form the first word or picture that comes into their mind on seeing the fragment they can perform like normal subjects; that is they will often provide the original sample (149, 150). In contrast, the amnesic subject may be impaired when he or she is told to use the fragment to recall a recently presented item (149).

Another example of intact priming in amnesic subjects was reported by Jacoby and Witherspoon (151). In this study, subjects were asked a series of questions (e.g., name a musical instrument that uses a reed). Each sentence contained a critical word which was one part of a homophone pair (reed/read) and the subjects were later asked to spell these critical words. Both the amnesic subjects and the controls showed a tendency to conform to the usage they had previously heard and so would more often spell 'reed' rather than 'read' and so on.

The classification of priming with respect to other possible types of memory poses a problem. While it fits more closely to an episodic/declarative type division, it is unusual in that the subject is unaware of that knowledge. The presence of other characteristics which do not resemble declarative memory (152) coupled with its preservation in amnesia have led some to argue that priming represents a further subcategory of procedural memory which is honored in the brain (153). We have very little information regarding the anatomy of priming effects although a comparison of patients with matched memory problems but different degrees of cortical damage suggests that priming relies on the neocortex (154).

CONCLUDING REMARKS

In this survey of the neural bases of memory particular emphasis was placed on clinical and experimental studies that have examined the consequences of brain damage. There is little doubt that this approach has helped highlight a series of brain regions that hold key roles in memory processes. Furthermore, by attempting to dissociate the effects of different patterns of brain damage, it has been possible to provide some of the strongest evidence for the existence of multiple memory systems. The fact that it may be possible to dissociate different types of memory does not, however, mean that they rely on totally independent neural systems, merely that at some stage or stages in their processing different neural regions are employed.

The reliance on studies of brain injury and amnesia has placed particular emphasis on those regions necessary for a given function. Other regions may be involved, but if the brain can compensate for their loss then their involvement in memory processes may remain obscured. To give a particular example, it may well be the case that the thalamic nucleus lateralis dorsalis has a role in memory mechanisms, yet this may never be disclosed by clinical studies. In other words, a range of other classes of evidence and hence other investigative procedures will be needed to reveal the full involvement of such regions. It is also evident that while the study of human and experimental amnesia can provide a skeletal outline of memory systems it will never on its own provide a satisfactory account of the neural mechanisms involved in memory storage and retrieval. An obvious starting point for a detailed analysis of such mechanisms in the primate brain is the relationship between association cortex and its limbic and diencephalic inputs. Recent evidence from electrophysiological studies of humans (155) and monkeys (63) have indicated that neurons in the parahippocampal and entorhinal cortices, the subiculum, the amygdala, the hippocampus, and the anterior thalamus may all be involved in signaling familiarity, a role consistent with their contribution to anterograde amnesia and its associated recognition deficit. Such studies point to ways in which the role of these temporal and diencephalic regions can profitably be investigated at a neuronal level once the critical regions and their possible roles have been highlighted by clinical methods.

REFERENCES

1. Scoville, W.B., and Milner, B. (1957). Loss of recent memory after bilateral hippocampal lesions. *J. Neurol. Neurosurg. Psychiat. 20*:11-21.
2. Corkin, S. (1984). Lasting consequences of bilateral medial temporal lobectomy: Clinical course and experimental findings in H.M. *Sem. Neurol. 4*:249-259.
3. Milner, B., Corkin, S., and Teuber, H.L. (1968). Further analysis of the hippocampal amnesic syndrome: 14 year follow-up study of H.M. *Neuropsychologia 6*:215-234.
4. Bechterew, W.V. (1900). Demonstration eines Gehirnes mit Zerstorung der vorderen und inneren Theile der Hirnrinde beider Schlafenlappen. *Neurol. Zentbl. 19*:990-991.
5. Grunthal, E. (1947). Uber das klinische Bild nach umschriebenem beiderseitigem Ausfall der Ammonshornrinde. Ein Beitrag zur Kenntnis der Funktion des Ammonshorns. *Mschr. Psychiat. Neurol. 113*:1-16.
6. Glees, P., and Griffith, H.B. (1952). Bilateral destruction of the hippocampus (Cornu ammonis) in a case of dementia. *Monatsschr. Psychiat. Neurol. 123*: 193-204.
7. Penfield, W., and Mathieson, G. (1974). Memory. Autopsy findings and comments on the role of hippocampus in experimental recall. *Arch. Neurol. 31*:145-154.
8. Milner, B. (1965). Visually-guided maze learning in man: Effects of bilateral hippocampal, bilateral frontal, and unilateral cerebral lesions. *Neuropsychologia 3*:317-338.
9. Milner, B. (1968). Visual recognition and recall after right temporal-lobe excision in man. *Neuropsychologia 6*:191-209.
10. Smith, M.L., and Milner, B. (1981). The role of the hippocampus in the recall of spatial location. *Neuropsychologia 19*:781-793.
11. Milner, B. (1967). Brain mechanisms suggested by studies of temporal lobes. In *Brain Mechanisms Underlying Speed and Language*. Edited by F.L. Darley. New York, Grune & Stratton.

12. Hierons, R., Janota, I., and Corsellis, J.A.N. (1978). The late effects of necro-
    tizing encephalitis of the temporal lobes and limbic areas: A clinico-pathological
    study of 10 cases. *Psychol. Med. 8*:21-42.
13. Damasio, A.R., and Van Hoesen, G.W. (1985). The limbic system and the local-
    ization of herpes simplex encephalitis. *J. Neurol. Neurosurg. Psychiat. 48*:297-
    301.
14. Woods, B.T., Schoene, W., and Kneisley, L. (1982). Are hippocampal lesions
    sufficient to cause lasting amnesia? *J. Neurol. Neurol. Neurosurg. Psychiat.
    45*:243-247.
15. Duyckaerts, C., Derouesne, C., Signoret, J.L., Gray, F., Escourolle, R., and
    Castaigne, P. (1985). Bilateral and limited amygdalohippocampal lesions causing
    a pure amnesic syndrome. *Ann. Neurol. 18*:314-319.
16. Zola-Morgan, S., Squire, L.R., and Amaral, D.G. (1986). Human amnesia and
    the medial temporal region: Enduring memory impairment following a bilateral
    lesion limited to field CA1 of the hippocampus. *J. Neurosci. 6*:2950-2967.
17. Balasubramaniam, V., and Kanaka, T.S. (1975). Sedative neurosurgery. *Proc.
    Inst. Neurol. Madras 5*:98-101.
18. Narabayashi, H. (1977). Stereotoxic amygdalatomy for epileptic hyperactivity-
    long range results in children. Topics in Child Neurology. In *M.E. Blaw*. Edited
    by I. Rapin and M. Kinsbourne. New York, Spectrum Publ. Inc. pp. 319-331.
19. Hitchcock, E., and Cairns, V. (1973). Amygdalatomy. *Postgrad. Med. J. 49*:
    894-904.
20. Small, I.F., Heimburger, R.F., Small, J.D.G., Milstein, V., and Moore, D.F.
    (1977). Follow up of stereotaxic amygdalotomy for seizure and behavioral dis-
    orders. *Biol. Psychiatry 12*:401-411.
21. Anderson, R. (1978). Cognitive changes after amygdalectomy. *Neuropsychologia
    16*:439-451.
22. Whitehouse, P.J., Price, D.L., Clark, A.W., Coyle, J.T., and Delong, M.R.
    (1981). Alzheimer's disease: Evidence for selective loss of cholinergic neurons in
    the nucleus basalis. *Ann. Neurol. 10*:122-126.
23. Damasio, A.R., Graff-Radford, N.R., Eslinger, P.J., Damasio, H., and Kassell,
    N. (1985b). Amnesia following basal forebrain lesions. *Arch. Neurol. 42*:263-
    271.
24. Hooper, M.W., and Vogel, F.S. (1976). The limbic system in Alzheimer's dis-
    ease. *Am. J. Pathol. 85*:1-14.
25. Herzog, A.G., and Kemper, T.L. (1980). Amygdaloid changes in aging and
    dementia. *Arch. Neurol. 37*:625-629.
26. Hyman, B.T., Van Hoesen, G.W., Damasio, A.R., and Barnes, C.L. (1984).
    Alzheimer's disease: Cell-specific pathology isolates the hippocampal formation.
    Science 225:1168-1170.
27. Hyman, B.T., Van Hoesen, G.W., Kromer, L.J., and Damasio, A.R. (1986).
    Perforant pathway changes and the memory impairment of Alzheimer's disease.
    Ann. Neurol. 20:472-481.
28. Mann, D.M.A., and Esiri, M.M. (1988). The site of the earliest lesions of Alzhei-
    mer's disease. *N. Engl. J. med. 318*:789-790.

29. Brierley, J.B. (1977). Neuropathology of amnesic states. In *Amnesia*. Edited by C.W.M. Whitty and O.L. Zangwill. London, Butterworths, pp. 199-223.
30. Delay, J., and Brion, S. (1969). *Le syndrome de Korsakoff*. Paris, Masson & Cie.
31. Victor, M., Adams, R.D., and Collins, G.H. (1971). *The Wernicke-Korsakoff Syndrome*. Oxford, Blackwell.
32. Colmant, H.J. (1965). *Enzephalopathien bei chronischem Alkoholismus, insbesondere Thalamusbefunde bei Wernickescher Enzephalopathie*. F. Enke, Stuttgart.
33. Kant, F. (1932). Die Pseudoencephalitis Wernicke der Alkoholiker. (Polioencephalitis haemorrhagica superior acuta.) *Arch. Psychiat. Nervenkrankht. 98*: 702-768.
34. Remy, M. (1942). Contribution a l'etude de la maladie de Korsakow. *Mschr. Psychiat. Neurol. 106*:128-144.
35. Ignelzi, R.J., and Squire, L.R. (1976). Recovery from anterograde and retrograde amnesia after percutaneous drainage of a cystic craniopharyngioma. *J. Neurol. Neurosurg. Psychiat. 39*:1231-1235.
36. Williams, M., and Pennybaker, J. (1954). Memory disturbances in third ventricle tumours. *J. Neurol. Neurosurg. Psychiat. 17*:115-123.
37. Cairns, H., and Mosberg, W.H. (1951). Colloid cyst of the third ventricle. *Surg. Gynec. Obstet. 92*:546-570.
38. Malamud, N., and Skillicorn, S.A. (1956). Relationship between the Wernicke and the Korsakoff syndrome. *Archs. Neurol. Psychiat. 76*:586-596.
39. Rigges, H.E., and Boles, R.S. (1944). Wernicke's encepholopathy: clinical and pathological studies of 42 cases. *Q. J. Stud. Alcohol. 5*:361-370.
40. Markowitsch, H.J. (1982). Thalamic mediodorsal nucleus and memory: A critical evaluation of studies in animals and man. *Neurosci. Biobehav. Rev. 6*:351-380.
41. McEntee, W.J., Biber, M.P., Perl, D.P., and Benson, D.F. (1976). Diencephalic amnesia: a reappraisal. *J. Neurol. Neurosurg. Psychiat. 39*:436-441.
42. Smythe, G.E., and Stern, K. (1938). Tumours of the thalamus—a clinico-pathological study. *Brain 61*:339-374.
43. Mills, R.P., and Swanson, P.D. (1978). Vertical oculomotor apraxia and memory loss. *Ann. Neurol. 4*:149-153.
44. Sprofkin, B.E., and Sciarra, D. (1952). Korsakoff's psychosis associated with cerebral tumours. *Neurology 2*:427-434.
45. Ziegler, D.K., Kaufman, A., and Marshall, H.E. (1977). Abrupt memory loss associated with thalamic tumor. *Arch. Neurol. 34*:545-548.
46. Barbizet, J., Degos, J.D., Louarn, F., Nguyen, J.P., and Mas, J.L. (1981). Amnesia from bilateral ischemic lesions of the thalamus. *Rev. Neurol. 137*:415-424.
47. Casaigne, P., Lhermitte, F., Buge, A., Escourolle, R., Hauw, J.J., and Lyon-Caen, O. (1981). Paramedian thalamic and midbrain infarcts: Clinical and neuropathological study. *Ann. Neurol. 10*:127-148.
48. Speedie, L.J., and Heilman, K.M. (1982). Amnestic disturbance following infarction of the left dorsomedial nucleus of the thalamus. *Neuropsychologia 20*: 597-604.

49. Winocur, G., Oxbury, S., Roberts, R., Agnetti, V., and Davis, C. (1984). Amnesia in a patient with bilateral lesions to the thalamus. *Neuropsychologia 22*:123-143.
50. Squire, L.R., and Moore, R.Y. (1979). Dorsal thalamic lesions in a noted case of human memory pathology. *Ann. Neurol. 6*:503-506.
51. Spiegel, E.A., Wycis, H.T., Orchinik, C., and Freed, H. (1956). Thalamic chronotaraxis. *Am. J. Psychiat. 113*:97-105.
52. Orchinik, C.W. (1960). Some psychological aspects of circumscribed lesions in the diencephalon. *Confin. Neurol. 20*:292-310.
53. Hassler, R., and Dieckmann, G. (1973). Relief of obsessive-compulsive disorders, phobias and tics by stereotaxic coagulation of the rostral intralaminar and medial-thalamic nuclei. In: *Surgical Approaches to Psychiatry*. Edited by L.V. Laitinen and K. Livingstone. Lancaster, Medical and Technical Press, pp. 206-212.
54. Kritchevsky, M., Graff-Radford, N.R., and Damasio, A.R. (1987). Normal memory after damage to medial thalamus. *Arch. Neurol. 44*:959-964.
55. Brion, S., and Mikol, J. (1978). Atteinte du noyou lateral dorsal du thalamus et syndrome de Korsakoff alcoolique. *J. Neurol. Sci. 38*:249-261.
56. Aggleton, J.P., Desimone, R., and Mishkin, M. (1986). The origin, course, and termination of the hippocampo-thalamic projections in thge macaque. *J. Comp. Neurol. 243*:409-421.
57. Hassler, F. (1962). New aspects of brain functions revealed in brain diseases. In *Frontiers in Brain Research*. Edited by J.D. French. New York, Columbia University Press, pp. 242-285.
58. Cramon, D.Y., Von, Hebel, N., and Schuri, U. (1985). A contribution to the anatomical basis of thalamic amnesia. *Brain 108*:993-1008.
59. Mair, W.G.P., Warrington, E.K., and Weiskrantz, L. (1979). Memory disorder in Korsakoff psychosis. A neuropathological and neuropsychological investigation of two cases. *Brain. 102*:749-783.
60. Squire, L.R., and Zola-Morgan, S. (1983). The neurology of memory: The case for correspondence between the findings for man and non-human primate. In *The Physiological Basis of Memory*, 2nd ed. Edited by J.A. Deutsch. New York, Academic Press, pp. 199-268.
61. Lorente de No, R. (1934). Studies of the structure of the cerebral cortex. II contamination of the study of the ammonic system. *J. Psychol. Neurol. (Leipsig). 46*:113-177.
62. Murray, E.A., and Mishkin, M. (1986). Visual recognition in monkeys following rhinal cortical ablations combined with either amygdalectomy or hippocampectomy. *J. Neurosci. 6*:1991-2003.
63. Brown, M.W., Wilson, F.A.W., and Riches, P. (1987). Neuronal evidence that inferomedial temporal cortex is more important than hippocampus in certain processes underlying recognition memory. *Brain Res. 409*:158-162.
64. Horel, J.A. (1978). The neuroanatomy of amnesia. A critique of the hippocampal memory hypothesis. *Brain 101*:403-445.
65. Cummings, J.L., Tomiyasu, K., Read, S., and Benson, F. (1984). Amnesia with hippocampal lesions after cardiopulmonary arrest. *Neurology 34*:671-681.

66. Zola-Morgan, S., Squire, L.R., and Mishkin, M. (1982). The neuroanatomy of amnesia: Amygdala-hippocampus versus temporal stem. *Science 218*:1337-1339.
67. Aggleton, J.P., Nicol, R.M., Huston, A.E., and Fairbairn, A.F. (1988). The performance of amnesic subjects on tests of experimental amnesia in animals: Delayed matching-to-sample and concurrent learning. *Neuropsychologia 26*: 265-272.
68. Squire, L.R., Zola-Morgan, S., and Chen, K.S. (1988). Human amnesia and animal models of amnesia: Performance of amnesic patients on tests designed for the monkey. *Behav. Neurosci. 102*:210-221.
69. Zola-Morgan, S., and Squire, L.R. (1985). Medial temporal lesions in monkeys impair memory on a variety of tasks sensitive to human amnesia. *Behav. Neurosci. 99*:22-34.
70. Mishkin, M. (1978). Memory in monkeys severely impaired by combined, but not by separate removal of amygdala and hippocampus. *Nature 273*:297-298.
71. Bachevalier, J., Saunders, R.C., and Mishkin, M. (1985). Visual recognition in monkeys: Effects of transection of fornix. *Exp. Brain. Res. 57*:547-553.
72. Gaffan, D., Gaffan, E.A., and Harrison, S. (1984). Effects of fornix transection on spontaneous and trained non-matching by monkeys. *Q.J. Exp. Psychol. 36B*: 285-303.
73. Ringo, J.L. (1988). Seemingly discrepant data from hippocampectomized macaques are reconcited by detectability analysis. *Behav. Neurosci. 102*:173-177.
74. Murray, E.A., and Mishkin, M. (1984). Severe tactual as well as visual memory deficits follow combined removal of the amygdala and hippocampus in monkeys. *J. Neurosci. 4*:2565-2580.
75. Mishkin, M., Speigler, B.J., Saunders, R.C., and Malamut, B.L. (1982). An animal model of global amnesia. In *Alzheimer's Disease: A report of Progress*, Vol. 19. *Aging*. Edited by S. Corkin, K.L. Davis, J.H. Growden, E. Usdin and R.J. Wurtman. New York, Raven Press, pp. 235-247.
76. Parkin, A.J. (1984). Amnesic syndrome: A lesion-specific disorder. *Cortex. 20*: 479-508.
77. Jarho, L. (1973). Korsakoff-like amnesic syndrome in penetrating brain injury. A study of English war veterans. *Acta Neurol. Scand. 49 Suppl. 54*:1-156.
78. Woolsey, R.M., and Nelson, J.S. (1975). Asymptomatic destruction of the fornix in man. *Archs. Neurol. 32*:566-568.
79. Bengochea, F.G., Torre, O. de la, Esquivel, O., Vieta, R., and Fernandez, C. (1954). The section of the fornix in the surgical treatment of certain epilepsies. *Transact. Am. Neurol. Assoc. 39*:176-178.
80. Heilman, K.M., and Sypert, G.W. (1977). Korsakoff's syndrome resulting from bilateral fornix lesions. *Neurology 27*:490-493.
81. Hassler, R., and Riechert, T. (1957). Uber einen Fall von doppelseitiger Fornicotomie bei sogenannter temporaler Epilepsie. *Acta Neurochirurg. 5*:330-340.
82. Sweet, W.H., Talland, G.A., and Ervin, F.R. (1959). Loss of recent memory following section of fornix. *Transact. Am. Neurol. Assoc. 84*:76-82.
83. Laplane, D., Degos, J.D., Baulac, M., and Gray, F. (1981). Bilateral infarction of the anterior cingulate gyri and of the fornices. *J. Neurol. Sci. 51*:289-300.

84. Zola-Morgan, S., Squire, L.R., and Amaral, D.G. (1989). Lesions of the amygdala that apare adjacent cortical regions do not impair memory or exacerbate the impairment following lesions of the hippocampal formation. *J. Neurosci. 9*: 1922-1936.

85. Zola-Morgan, S., Squire, L.R., and Amaral, D.G. (1988).Amnesia following medial temporal lobe damage in monkeys: The importance of the hippocampus and adjacent cortical regions. *Soc. Neurosci. Abst. 14*:1043.

86. Zola-Morgan, S., Squire, L.R., and Amaral, D.G. (1989). Lesions of the hippocampal formation but not lesions of the fornix or the mammillary nuclei produce long-lasting memory impairment in monkeys. *J. Neurosci. 9*:898-913.

87. Bachevalier, J., Parkinson, J.K., and Mishkin, M. (1985). Visual recognition in monkeys: effects of separate vs. combined transection of fornix and amygdalofugal pathways. *Exp. Brain Res. 57*:554-561.

88. Kentridge, R.W., and Aggleton, J.P. (1990). Emotion: Sensory representation, reinforcement and the temporal lobe. *Cognit. Emot.* In press.

89. Drachman, D.A., and Arbit, J. (1966). Memory and the hippocampal complex. *Arch. Neurol. 15*:52-61.

90. Gol, A., and Faibish, G.M. (1967). Effects of human hippocampal ablation. *J. Neurosurg. 26*:390-398.

91. Butters, N., and Cermak, L.S. (1980). *Alcoholic Korsakoff's Syndrome.* New York, Academic Press, pp. 8-9.

92. Holmes, E.J., Butters, N., Jacobson, S., and Stein, B.M. (1983). An examination of the effects of mammillary-body lesions on reversal learning sets in monkeys. *Physiol. Psych. 11*:159-165.

93. Holmes, E.J., Jacobson, S., Stein, B.M., and Butters, N. (1983). Ablations of the mammillary nuclei in monkeys: Effects on postoperative memory. *Exp. Neurol. 81*:97-113.

94. Mahut, H. (1971). Spatial and object reversal learning in monkeys with partial temporal lobe ablations. *Neuropsychologia 9*:409-424.

95. Jones, B., and Mishkin, M. (1972). Limbic lesions and the problem of stimulus-reinforcement associations. *Exp. Neurol. 36*:362-377.

96. Mahut, H. (1972). A selective spatial deficit in monkeys after transection of the fornix. *Neuropsychologia 10*:65-74.

97. Mahut, H., and Zola, S.M. (1973). A non-modality specific impairment in spatial learning after fornix lesions in monkeys. *Neuropsychologia 11*:255-269.

98. Aggleton, J.P., and Mishkin, M. (1985). Mammillary-body lesions and visual recognition in monkeys. *Exp. Brain. Res. 58*:190-197.

99. Saunders, R.C. (1983). Impairment in recognition memory after mammillary body lesions in monkeys. *Soc. Neurosci. Abst. 9*:12.9.

100. Isseroff, A., Rosvold, H.E., Galkin, T.W., and Goldman-Rakic, P.S. (1982). Spatial memory impairment following damage to the mediodorsal nucleus in the thalamus of rhesus monkeys. *Brain Res. 232*:97-113.

101. Aggleton, J.P., and Mishkin, M. (1983). Visual recognition impairment following medial thalamic lesions in monkeys. *Neuropsychologia 21*:189-197.

102. Aggleton, J.P., and Mishkin, M. (1983). Memory impairments following restricted medial thalamic lesions in monkeys. *Exp. Brain Res. 52*:199-209.

103. Zola-Morgan, S., and Squire, L.R. (1985). Amnesia in monkeys after lesions of the mediodorsal nucleus of the thalamus. *Ann. Neurol. 17*:558-564.
104. Aggleton, J.P., and Mishkin, M. (1986). The amygdala: sensory gateway to the emotions. In *Biological Foundations of Emotion*. Edited by R. Plutchik and H. Kellerman. New York, Academic Press, pp. 281-300.
105. Van Hoesen, G.W. (1982). The parahippocampal gyrus. New observations regarding its cortical connections in the monkey. *Trends Neurosci. 5*:345-350.
106. Rosene, D.L., and Van Hoesen, G.W. (1977). Hippocampal efferents reach widespread areas of cerebral cortex and amygdala in the rhesus monkey. *Science 198*:315-317.
107. Amaral, D.G., and Price, J.L. (1985). Amygdalo-cortical projections in the monkey (Macaca fascicularis). *J. Comp. Neurol. 230*:465-497.
108. Aggleton, J.P. (1986). A description of the amygdalo-hippocampal interconnections in the macaque monkey. *Exp. Brain Res. 64*:515-526.
109. Poletti, C.E., and Creswell, G. (1977). Fornix system efferent projections in the squirrel monkey: An experimental degeneration study. *J. Comp. Neurol. 175*:101-128.
110. Krayniak, P.F., Siegel, A., Meibach, R.C., Fruchtman, D., and Scrimenti, M. (1979). Origin of the fornix system in the squirrel monkey. *Brain Res. 160*: 401-411.
111. Amaral, D.G., and Cowan, W.M. (1980). Subcortical efferents to the hippocampal formation in the monkey. *J. Comp. Neurol. 189*:573-591.
112. Veazey, R.B., Amaral, D.G., and Cowan, W.M. (1982). The morphology and connections of the posterior hypothalamus in the cynomolgus monkey (*Macaca fascicularis*). II Efferent connections. *J. Comp. Neurol. 207*:135-156.
113. Aggleton, J.P., Desimone, R., and Mishkin, M. (1986). The origin, course and termination of the hippocampothalamic projections in the macaque. *J. Comp. Neurol. 243*:409-421.
114. Aggleton, J.P., and Mishkin, M. (1984). Projections of the amygdala to the thalamus in the cynomolgus monkey. *J. Comp. Neurol. 222*:56-68.
115. Russchen, F.T., Amaral, D.G., and Price, J.L. (1987). The afferent input to the magnocellular division of the mediodorsal thalamic nucleus in the monkey. *Macaca fascicularis. J. Comp. Neurol. 256*:175-210.
116. Vogt, B.A., Pandya, D.N., and Rosene, D.L. (1987). Cingulate cortex of the rhesus monkey: I cytoarchitecture and thalamic afferents. *J. Comp. Neurol. 262*:256-270.
117. Angelergues, R. (1969). Memory disorders in neurological disease. In *Handbook of Clinical Neurology*, Vol. 3, *Disorders of Higher Nervous Activity*. Edited by P.J. Vinken and G.W. Bruyn. New York, American Elsevier, pp. 268-292.
118. Stuss, D.T., Kaplan, E.F., Benson, D.F., Weir, W.S., Chiulli, S., and Sarazin, F.F. (1982). Evidence for the involvement of orbitofrontal cortex in memory functions: An interference effect. *J. Comp. Physiol. Psychol. 96*:913-925.
119. Milner, B., Petrides, M., and Smith, M. (1985). Frontal lobes and temporal organisation of memory. *Human Neurobiol. 4*:137-142.
120. Milner, B. (1982). Some cognitive effects of frontal-lobe lesions in man. *Phil. Tran. R. Soc. Lond. B. 298*:211-226.

121. Vilkki, J. (1985). Amnesic syndromes after surgery of anterior communicating artery aneurysms. *Cortex 21*:431-444.
122. Bachevalier, J., and Mishkin, M. (1986). Visual recognition impairment follows ventromedial but not dorsolateral prefrontal lesions in monkeys. *Behav. Brain Res. 20*:249-261.
123. Huppert, F.A., and Piercy, M. (1979). Normal and abnormal forgetting in organic amnesia: Effect of locus of lesion. *Cortex 15*:385-390.
124. Freed, D.M., Corkin, S., and Cohen, N.J. (1987). Forgetting in H.M.—A second look. *Neuropsycholgia 25*:461-472.
125. Mabille, E., and Pitres, A. (1913). Sur un cas d'Amnesie de fixation post-apoplectique ayant persiste vingt trois ans. *Rev. Med. 33*:257-279.
126. Warrington, E.K., and Weiskrantz, L. (1982). Amnesia: A disconnection syndrome? *Neuropsychologia 20*:233-248.
127. Penfield, W., and Perot, P. (1963). The brain's record of auditory and visual experience. *Brain 86*:595-696.
128. Loftus, E.F., and Loftus, G.R. (1980). On the permanence of stored information in the human brain. *Am. Psychol. 35*:409-420.
129. Halgren, E., Walter, R.D., Cherlon, D.G., and Crandall, P.H. (1978). Mental phenomena evoked by electrical stimulation of the human hippocampal formation and amygdala. *Brain 101*:83-117.
130. Mishkin, M., and Petri, H.L. (1984). Memories and habits: some implications for the analysis of learning and retention. In *Neuropsychology of Memory*. Edited by L.R. Squire and N. Butters. New York, Guilford Press, pp. 287-296.
131. Weiskrantz, L., and Saunders, R.C. (1984). Impairments of visual object transforms in monkeys rhesus. *Brain 107*:1033-1072.
132. Kornhuber, H.H. (1973). Neural control of input into long-term memory: Limbic system and amnestic syndrome in man. In *Memory and Transfer of Information.* Edited by H.P. Zippel. New York, Plenum Press, pp. 1-22.
133. Warrington, E.K., Logue, V., and Pratt, R.T.C. (1971). The anatomical localisation of selective impairment of auditory verbal short-term memory. *Neuropsychologia 9*:377-387.
134. Baddeley, A. (1988). Cognitive psychology and human memory. *Trends Neurosci. 11*:176-181.
135. Parkin, A.J. (1987). *Memory and Amnesia. An Introduction.* Oxford, Basil Blackwell Ltd.
136. Tulving, E. (1972). Episodic and semantic memory. In *Organization of Memory*. Edited by E. Tulving and W. Donaldson. New York, Academic Press, pp. 381-403.
137. Shimamura, A.P., and Squire, L.R. (1987). A neuropsychological study of fact memory and source amnesia. *J. Exp. Psychol. (Learn. Mem. Cog.). 13*:464-473.
138. Cermak, L.S. (1984). The episodic-semantic distinction in amnesia. In *Neuropsychology of Memory*. Edited by L.R. Squire and N. Butters. New York, Guildford Press, pp. 55-62.
139. Ryle, G. (1949). *The Concept of Mind*. London, Hutchinson.

140. Tulving, E. (1983). *Elements of Episodic Memory.* Oxford, Clarendon Press.
141. Corkin, S. (1968). Acquisition of motor skill after bilateral medial temporal-lobe excision. *Neuropsychologia 6*:255-265.
142. Cohen, N.J., and Squire, L.R. (1980). Preserved learning and retention of pattern-analyzing skill in amnesia: dissociation of knowing how and knowing that. *Science 210*:207-210.
143. Weiskrantz, L., and Warrington, E.K. (1979). Conditioning in amnesic patients. *Neuropsychologia 17*:187-194.
144. Mishkin, M., Malamut, B., and Bachevalier, J. (1984). Memories and habits: two neural systems. In *The Neurobiology of Learning and Memory.* Edited by G. Lynch, J.L. McGaugh and N.M. Weinberger. New York, Guildford Press, pp. 65-77.
145. Oakley, D.A., and Russell, I.S. (1972). Neocortical lesions and classical conditioning. *Physiol. Behav. 8*:915-926.
146. Thompson, R. (1983). Neuronal substrates of simple associative learning: classical conditioning. *Trends Neurosci. 6*:270-274.
147. Yeo, C.H., Hardiman, M.J., and Glickstein, M. (1984). Discrete lesions of the cerebellar cortex abolish the classically conditioned nicitating membrane response of the rabbit. *Behav. Brain Res. 13*:261-266.
148. Lavond, D.G., Lincoln, J.C., McCormick, D.A., and Thompson, R.F. (1983). Effect of bilateral cerebellar lesions in heart rate and nicitating membrane/eyelid conditioning in the rabbit. *Neurosci. Abst. 189*:1.
149. Graf, P., Squire, L.R., and Mandler, G. (1984). The information that amnesic patients do not forget. *J. Exp. Psychol. (Learn. Mem. Cog.). 10*:164-178.
150. Warrington, E.K., and Weiskrantz, L. (1968). A new method of testing long-term retention with special reference to amnesic patients. *Nature 217*:972-974.
151. Jacoby, L.L., and Witherspoon. (1982). Remembering without awareness. *Can. J. Psychol. 36*:300-324.
152. Graf, P., Shimamura, A.P., and Squire, L.R. (1985). Priming across modalities and across category levels: extending the domain of preserved function in amnesia. *J. Exp. Psychol. (Learn. Mem. Cog.) 11*:386-396.
153. Squire, L.R. (1987). *Memory and Brain.* Oxford, University Press.
154. Shimamura, A.P., Salmon, D., Squire, L.R., and Butters, N. (1987). Memory dysfunction and word priming in dementia and amnesia. *Behav. Neurosci. 101*: 347-351.
155. Heit, G., Smith, M.E., and Halgren, E. (1988). Neural encoding of individual words and faces by the human hippocampus and amygdala. *Science 333*:773-775.
156. Squire, L.R., and Zola-Morgan, S. (1988). Memory: brain systems and behavior. *Trends Neurosci. 11*:170-175.

4

Central Cholinergic Pathways: Neuroanatomy and Some Behavioral Implications

M.-Marsel Mesulam

*Dana Research Institute and
Beth Israel Hospital, Harvard Medical School
Boston, Massachusetts*

Neurons which synthesize and secrete acetylcholine (ACh) for the purpose of neurotransmission are designated as cholinergic. The pioneering work of Otto Loewi established ACh as a neurotransmitter in the peripheral nervous system (Loewi, 1921). Soon thereafter, the suggestion was made that ACh could also serve a similar purpose in central nervous structures (Dale, 1938). Partial support for this possibility was obtained by pharmacological and physiological investigations which showed that ACh, acetylcholinesterase (AChE), choline acetyltransferase (ChAT), and cholinergic receptor sites were widely distributed throughout the neuraxis and that many central neurons were responsive to ACh (for review see Silver, 1974; Fibiger, 1982; Mesulam et al., 1983b). Observations based on AChE histochemistry provided additional information on the anatomical arrangement of cholinergic pathways in the brain stem, diencephalon, limbic system, and neocortex (Krnjević and Silver, 1965; Shute and Lewis, 1967). However, uncertainty has always been associated with conclusions based on AChE histochemistry since this enzyme is also present in many noncholinergic neurons. The production of monoclonal and monospecific antibodies to ChAT by several research groups has now provided new and much more reliable information on the distribu-

Reprinted from M. Avoli, T. Reader, R. Dykes, and P. Gloor (eds.) *Neurotransmitters and Cortical Function*, Plenum Press, New York, 1988, pp. 237-260, with permission of the author and publishers.

tion of cholinergic neurons and on the organization of their connections (Rossier, 1984; Wainer et al., 1984). Since the presence of ChAT is necessary and probably also sufficient for the synthesis of ACh, the immunohistochemical demonstration of ChAT currently constitutes the most specific anatomical marker for putative cholinergic·neurons and their processes. Although it is not yet known if all neurons that contain ChAT also secrete ACh, this seems like a reasonable assumption to make, but will ultimately need definitive confirmation through a combination of anatomical and physiological approaches.

The contemporary literature on the anatomy of cholinergic neurons is vast and varied. The purpose of this chapter is not to provide a critical review of these developments but to summarize some observations on central cholinergic pathways that my colleagues and I have made in the past 10 years. The papers cited provide additional references to the rich literature on this subject.

CHOLINERGIC INNERVATION OF THE STRIATAL COMPLEX

The striatal complex has four major components: the *caudate* and *putamen*, collectively designated as the neostriatum, and the *olfactory tubercle* and *nucleus accumbens* also known as the limbic striatum. All four components contain cholinergic neurons. In the rhesus monkey, ChAT-positive cholinergic neurons in the caudate and putamen are larger but less densely packed than those in the olfactory tubercle and nucleus accumbens (Mesulam et al., 1984a). The concentration of cholinergic neurons in the limbic striatum is particularly high around the islands of Calleja (Fig. 1). The density of other cholinergic markers (e.g., AChE, muscarinic receptors) also displays patchy variations in the striatum. These patches have been designated as striosomes (Nastuk and Graybiel, 1985).

The striatal complex contains populations of large and small neurons. The cholinergic cells of the striatum belong to the class of large aspiny neurons seen in Golgi preparations (Wainer et al., 1984). Only 1-2% of the striatal perikarya are cholinergic. These neurons do not see to have projections outside the striatum (Woolf and Butcher, 1981). In fact, the striatal complex provides the best known example of a telencephalic structure which receives almost all of its cholinergic input from local circuit interneurons. In addition to these local projections, the striatum also receives what is probably a relatively minor cholinergic innervation from the ChAT-positive neurons of the basal forebrain (Arikuni and Kubota, 1984).

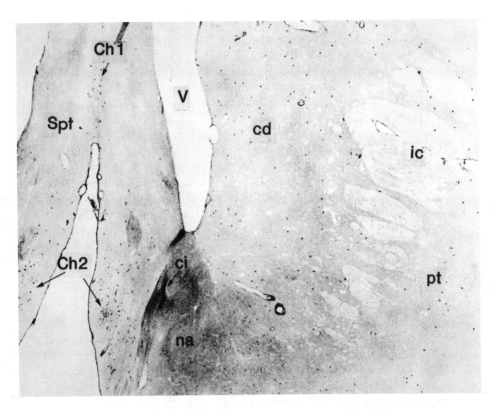

Figure 1 ChAT immunohistochemical staining in the macaque brain. Curved arrow-heads point to interstitial elements of Ch4. Magnification is 24×. The photomicrograph is taken from coronal sections that are from progressively more posterior levels of the brain. (From Mesulam et al., 1984a.)

SOURCE OF CHOLINERGIC INNERVATION FOR THE HIPPOCAMPUS, OLFACTORY BULB, AMYGDALA, AND CEREBRAL CORTEX—THE Ch1—Ch2 CELL GROUPS

In contrast to the striatum, the great majority of the cholinergic innervation for the hippocampus, olfactory bulb, amygdala, and neocortex comes from extrinsic sources located in the basal forebrain. The adult rodent neocortex and hippocampus contain intrinsic ChAT-positive cell bodies which may provide approximately 30% of their cholinergic innervation (Johnston et al.,

1981; Eckenstein and Thoenen, 1983; Houser et al., 1983; Levey et al., 1984). Immunohistochemical observations suggest that such neurons are either less conspicuous or perhaps absent in the adult brain of other species including reptiles, carnivores, and primates (Kimura et al., 1981; Mesulam et al., 1984a; Mufson et al., 1984). Extrinsic sources therefore account for as much as 70% of the cortical cholinergic input in the rodent brain and this proportion may be even higher in the adult primate.

The cholinergic innervation of olfactory, limbic, and neocortical regions arises from basal forebrain nuclei which contain cholinergic as well as non-cholinergic cells. In order to focus attention on the cholinergic component of these nuclei, we have designated the ChAT-positive cell groups in these regions as Ch1-Ch4 (Mesulam et al., 1983a,b, 1984a). The Ch1-Ch4 nomenclature is based not only on the location of the neurons but also on their connectivity patterns. The following discussion will concentrate on observations in the primate even though comparative information from the rodent brain will also be included.

CH1-CH2

The Ch1 and Ch2 cell groups collectively provide (by way of the fornix, fimbria, and perhaps supracallosal fibers) the major cholinergic innervation of the hippocampal formation. In the rhesus monkey as well as in the rat, Ch1 consists of the ChAT-positive neurons within the traditional boundaries of the medial septal nucleus (Fig. 1). These are the smallest of the basal forebrain cholinergic neurons. The proportion of medial septal cells that are ChAT-positive varies from about 50% in the rat brain to even less in the monkey. The boundary between the Ch1 and Ch2 groups is not sharp. In both rat and monkey, approximately 70% of the cell bodies within the vertical nucleus of the diagonal band of Broca are cholinergic and make up the Ch2 cell group (Fig. 1).

Experiments based on the concurrent demonstration of retrogradely transported horseradish peroxidase (HRP) and perikaryal cholinergic markers have shown that only about half of the projections from the septal area to the hippocampal formation arise from cholinergic Ch1-Ch2 neurons (Mesulam et al., 1977, 1983b; Baisden et al., 1984; Wainer et al., 1985). The septohippocampal pathway is therefore not uniformly cholinergic. The transmitter(s) for the other components of the septohippocampal pathway remain unknown. This anatomical arrangement is consistent with physiological observations on hippocampal theta, a rhythm which is dependent on the integrity of the septohippocampal projections. According to these observations, the hippocampal theta rhythm has at least two components only one of which can be abolished by cholinergic antagonists (Rawlins et al., 1979; Vanderwolf, 1983).

Ch3

The Ch3 cell group provides the principal source of cholinergic innervation for the olfactory bulb. In the rhesus monkey, approximately 2% of the cell bodies in the horizontal limb nucleus of the diagonal band of Broca are ChAT-positive. This cell group makes up the major aggregate of cholinergic cells projecting to the olfactory bulb and is designated as Ch3 (Figs. 2 and 3). In the rat, the Ch3 designation fits most appropriately the cholinergic neurons only in the *lateral* portion of the horizontal limb nucleus since this is the component from which the principal connection to the olfactory bulb arises. Approximately 20% of the cell bodies in this lateral portion of the rodent's horizontal limb nucleus are ChAT-positive. The great majority of projections from the horizontal nucleus of the diagonal band to the olfactory bulb in the rodent as well as in the monkey arise from noncholinergic neurons (Mesulam et al., 1977, 1983b).

Ch4

The Ch4 neurons provide the major cholinergic innervation for the amygdala and all neocortical regions. In keeping with the highly developed cerebral cortex of the primate brain, the Ch4 group is very extensive in monkeys and humans (Fig. 2-6). In the primate brain, the Ch4 complex contains the cholinergic neurons within the nucleus basalis (NB) of the substantia innominata (Mesulam and Van Hoesen, 1976; Parent et al., 1977; Mesulam et al., 1983a). At least 90% of the neurons in the NB are cholinergic and belong to Ch4. For practical purposes, therefore, the NB and Ch4 are coextensive and share an identical topography in the primate brain (Mesulam et al., 1986b). In the rat, however, the Ch4 group (defined as the collection of ChAT-positive forebrain cells which provide the major cholinergic innervation of cortex and amygdala) is more modest in size and less easily confined to any specific nuclear formation (Mesulam et al., 1983b). Studies based on the concurrent demonstration of perikaryal cholinergic markers and retrogradely transported HRP suggest that the Ch4 of the rodent includes ChAT-positive neurons in the *medial* part of the horizontal limb nucleus of the diagonal band and also in a location just medial and ventral to the globus pallidus. It is this latter region that is usually designated as the nucleus basalis in the rat brain. Many ChAT-positive neurons in the lateral portion of the vertical limb nucleus of the rat also project to neocortex and probably belong to the Ch4 group.

The Ch4-NB complex of the primate brain extends from the level of the olfactory tubercle anteriorly to that of the lateral geniculate body posteriorly. In the human, this complex contains approximately 200,000 neurons in each hemisphere (Arendt et al., 1985). This extensive nuclear complex comes into intimate contact with many other cell groups including those of the ventral

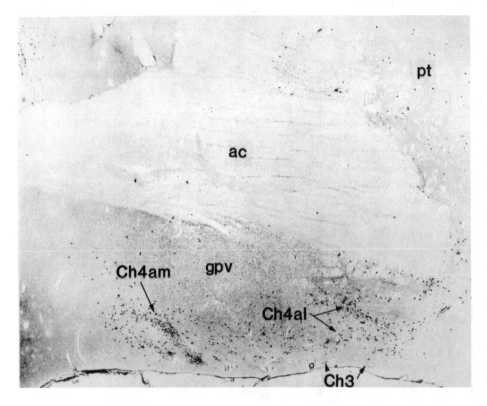

Figure 2 ChAT immunohistochemical staining in the macaque brain. Curved arrowheads point to interstitial elements of Ch4. Magnification is 24×. (From Mesulam et al., 1984a.)

striatum, the septal area, the ventral globus pallidus, the amygdaloid complex, the preoptic region, and the lateral hypothalamus. In addition to the compact cell group which is coextensive with the NB, Ch4 also contains interstitial elements embedded among the fibers of the diagonal band of Broca, the anterior commissure, the stria terminalis, the ansa peduncularis, the ansa lenticularis, the inferior thalamic peduncle, and the medullary laminae of the globus pallidus. The Ch4 complex can be subdivided into several sectors. The anterior sector of Ch4 is located at the level of the decussation of the anterior commissure. A vascular marking or a rarefaction in cell density divides this into anteromedial (Ch4am) and anterolateral (Ch4al) subsectors (Fig. 2). The passage of the ansa peduncularis through the basal forebrain

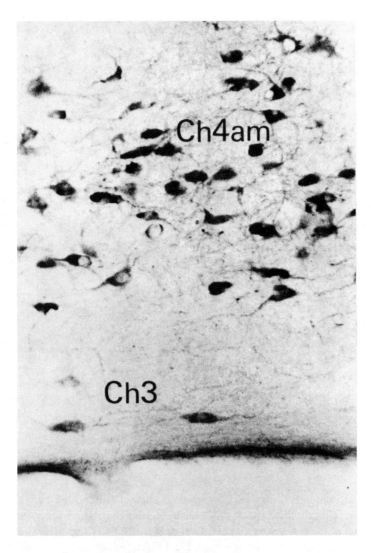

Figure 3 ChAT immunohistochemical staining in the macaque brain. Curved arrowheads point to interstitial elements of Ch4. Magnification is 150×. (From Mesulam et al., 1984a.)

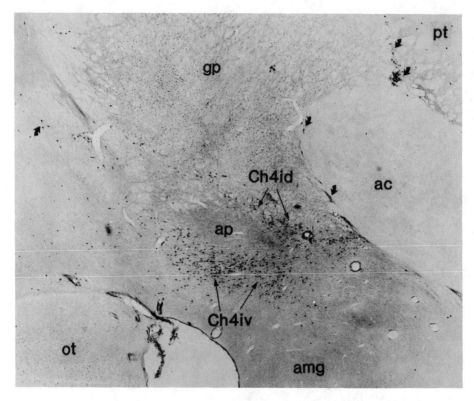

Figure 4 ChAT immunohistochemical staining in the macaque brain. Curved arrowheads point to interstitial elements of Ch4. Magnification is 24 ×. (From Mesulam et al., 1984a.)

identifies the intermediate sector of Ch4 which is further subdivided by the ansa into dorsal (Ch4id) and ventral (Ch4iv) subsectors (Fig. 4). Behind the ansa peduncularis lies the extensive posterior sector of Ch4 (Ch4p) (Figs. 5 and 6). If the few noncholinergic neurons of the NB are also taken into account, these topographical subdivisions could be designated as NBam, NBal, NBiv, and NBp. A similar arrangement is present in the human brain (Mesulam et al., 1983a; Arendt et al., 1985).

The three-dimensional reconstruction of the Ch4-NB cell group, even without including its interstitial elements, shows a remarkable structural com-

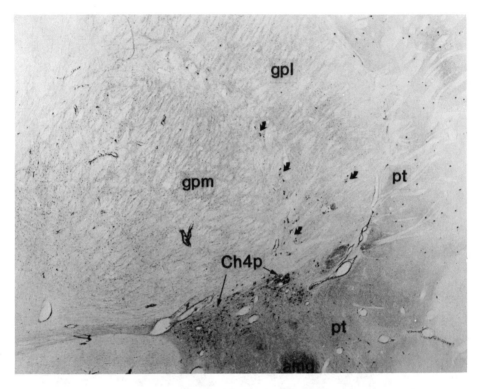

Figure 5 ChAT immunohistochemical staining in the macaque brain. Curved arrowheads point to interstitial elements of Ch4. Magnification is 24×. (From Mesulam et al., 1984a.)

plexity (Fig. 7A). In the absence of specific cholinotoxins, attempts at destroying Ch4-NB would lead to extensive damage in a large number of additional noncholinergic structures.

TOPOGRAPHY OF PROJECTIONS FROM Ch4 TO THE AMYGDALA AND CORTEX

Observations based on 36 rhesus monkeys, each with an HRP injection within a specific brain region, and each prepared for the concurrent visualization of retrogradely transported HRP and perikaryal cholinergic markers, indicated

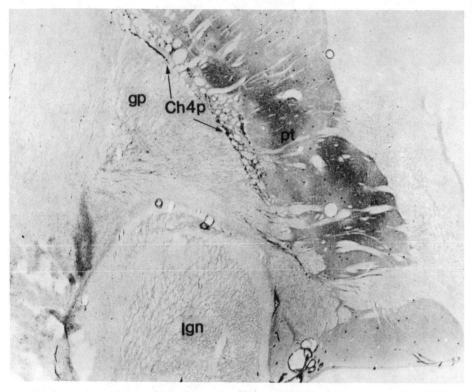

Figure 6 ChAT immunohistochemical staining in the macaque brain. Curved arrowheads point to interstitial elements of Ch4. Magnification is 24×. (From Mesulam et al., 1984a.)

that different cortical regions receive their principal cholinergic innervation from different Ch4 subsectors (Mesulam et al., 1983a, 1986b). Thus, Ch4am is the major source of projections for the dorsomedial surface of the cerebral hemispheres including medial parietal, medial frontal, and cingulate cortex; Ch4al is the major source of cholinergic projections for the frontoparietal operculum and the amygdaloid complex; the Ch4i sector provides the major cholinergic input for lateral prefrontal, parietal, peristriate, midtemporal, and inferotemporal cortex; Ch4p provides the major cholinergic innervation for the superior temporal gyrus and the adjacent temporal pole (Figs. 7B and 8, Table 1). Although this topography is not as specific as the arrangement of thalamocortical connections, there is anatomical organization in that each cortical region receives its primary cholinergic input from a circumscribed

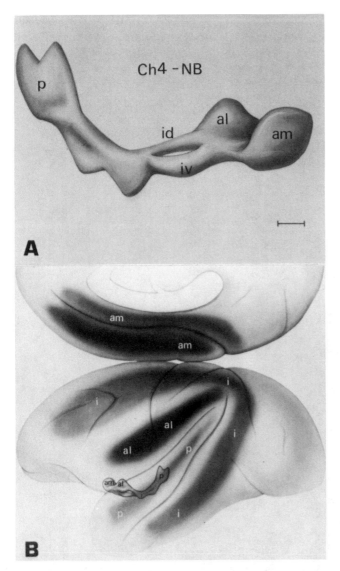

Figure 7 (A)Three-dimensional drawing of the left NB-Ch4 in the macaque brain showing its anteromedial (am), anterolateral (al), intermediodorsal (id), intermedioventral (iv), and posterior (p) sectors. The ansa peduncularis passes through the space between id and iv. Bar ~ 1.3 mm. Dorsal is toward the top. In the primate brain and at the macroscopic level of analysis, Ch4 is coextensive with what is now commonly designated as the nucleus basalis. Therefore, this three-dimensional representation applies equally well to NB as well as to Ch4. (B) A schematic diagram showing the distribution of cortical areas that receive their major cholinergic input from am, al, intermediate (i), and p sectors of Ch4. Definitive information is not yet available for the occipital lobe. (From Mesulam et al., 1986b.)

Table 1   Percentage of Retrograde Labeling and Number of Retrogradely Labeled Neurons in the Ch Sectors of Two Macaque Hemispheres[a,b]

Percent of total labeling:	Case I—HRP in frontoparietal operculum								Case II—HRP in superior temporal gyrus							
	Ch1	Ch2	Ch3	Ch4am	Ch4al	Ch4id	Ch4iv	Ch4p	Ch1	Ch2	Ch3	Ch4am	Ch4al	Ch4id	Ch4iv	Ch4p
	0%	1%	0%	11%	52%	12%	12%	11%	4%	2%	0%	3%	0%	1%	1%	89%
Level[b]																
1	1	3							3	3						
2	0	2	1	6	25				0	2	1	0	0			
3	0	0	0	9	66				1	0	0	1	0			
4			0	12	83						0	2	0			
5			0	9	18	5	11				0	0	0	0		
6						18	19							1	1	
7						23	14							0	0	
8								15								16
9								16								5
10								9								12
11								1								28
12								0								8
13								0								9
14								0								4

[a]From Mesulam et al. (1986b).
[b]Level 1 is most anterior, level 14 most posterior. The distance between each level is approximately 1 mm. The numbers at each level represent the counts of retrogradely labeled Ch4 neurons. Observations based on 36 macaque cerebra show that these topographical patterns are quite reliable.

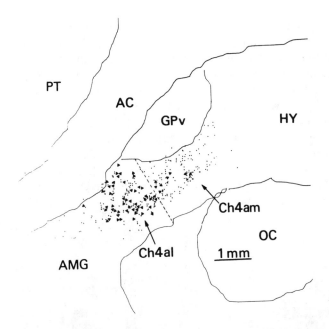

Figure 8 Tracing obtained from an X-Y plotter electronically coupled to the microscope stage. Triangles indicate retrogradely labeled Ch4 neurons after a large HRP injection in frontoparietal opercular cortex of a macaque brain. The dots represent Ch4 neurons not labeled with the retrogradely transported HRP. The dashed line provides an approximate demarcation between Ch4am and Ch4al. (From Mesulam et al., 1986b.)

portion of Ch4. Approximately 96% of the projections from the NB to cortex arise from ChAT-positive cell bodies (Mesulam et al., 1986b). The transmitter for the noncholinergic NB neurons remains unknown. Extremely few (less than 2%) Ch4 neurons have contralateral projections (Mesulam et al., 1983a). Observations in the rat suggest that each Ch4 neuron innervates a small cortical area, approximately 1 mm in diameter, without sending additional collaterals to other cortical regions (Price and Stern, 1983). This question deserves more attention, especially in the monkey brain where the total number of Ch4 neurons appears to be too low if each cell is to innervate such a small area of cortex.

SOURCES OF CHOLINERGIC PROJECTIONS FOR THE THALAMUS AND SOME MESENCEPHALIC STRUCTURES—THE Ch5-Ch8 GROUPS

Ch5-Ch6

No ChAT-positive thalamic neurons have yet been reported in any animal species. Although this does not prove the absence of such neurons, it raises the possibility that the cholinergic innervation for this region of the brain may be predominantly, if not entirely, extrinsic. Approximately 80% of all cholinergic neurons that project to the thalamus are located within two pontomesencephalic cholinergic cell groups that we have designated as Ch5 and Ch6 (Figs. 9 and 10). The rest of the cholinergic neurons that project to the thalamus are located primarily within the Ch1-Ch4 groups (Mesulam et al., 1983b). The Ch5-Ch6 groups also contain about 10% of cholinergic cell bodies projecting to limbic and cortical regions (Mufson et al., 1982; Mesulam et al., 1983b). Therefore, cortical and limbic regions are under three types of cholinergic influence: (1) a major direct input from Ch1-Ch4; (2) a minor direct input from Ch5-Ch6; (3) an indirect input with a cholinergic relay from Ch5-Ch6 to the thalamus and a noncholinergic relay from the thalamus to cortex.

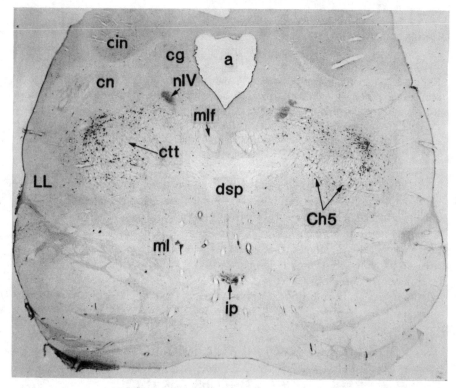

Figure 9 ChAT immunohistochemical staining in the macaque brain stem at the pontomesencephalic level. Magnification 10×. (From Mesulam et al., 1984a.)

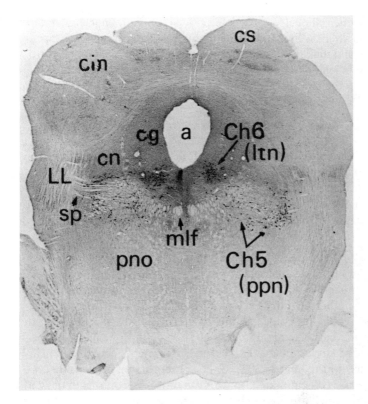

Figure 10 ChAT immunohistochemical staining in the rat brain stem at the ponto-mesencephalic level. Magnification 17×. (From Mesulam et al., 1983b.)

The Ch5 group is made up of large (75-80 by 40-45 μm in the monkey) ChAT-positive neurons which are aggregated mostly in the pedunculopontine nucleus but which also extend into the nucleus cuneiformis and the parabrachial region (Fig. 9 and 10). In the pedunculopontine region Ch5 has a compact lateral portion which abuts upon the lateral lemniscus and a more diffuse medial component which is largely embedded within the central tegmental tract and the superior cerebellar penduncle (Figs. 9 and 10). Large and small cells are intermingled with each other in the pedunculopontine nucleus. About 75% of the large neurons in the lateral part of this nucleus and 25% of those in the medial part belong to Ch5. The remainder of the neurons in these regions do not stain positively for ChAT.

The Ch6 sector consists of relatively smaller (40-45 by 50-55 μm in the monkey) cholinergic neurons which are located within the boundaries of the laterodorsal tegmental nucleus. The laterodorsal tegmental nucleus contains both large and small cells. Approximately 90% of the larger neurons are ChAT-positive and make up the Ch6 group. The majority of projections from the laterodorsal tegmental nucleus and pedunculopontine nuclei to the thalamus arise from the cholinergic Ch5-Ch6 component of neurons (Mesulam et al., 1983b; Isaacson and Tanaka, 1986).

Ch7

The medial habenular nucleus contains oval, lightly ChAT-positive neurons (30 by 35 μm in the monkey). Although we have not checked this directly by combined transport and immunohistochemical methods, it is reasonable to assume that these neurons send cholinergic projections to the interpeduncular nucleus via the habenulo-interpeduncular tract (Kataoka et al., 1974).

Ch8

Studies in the mouse show that most of the cholinergic cell bodies which project to the superior colliculus are located in the parabigeminal nucleus (Mufson et al., 1986). Another but smaller contingent of cholinergic cells projecting to the superior colliculus is located in Ch5 and Ch6. About 80-90% of the cell bodies in the parabigeminal nucleus are ChAT-positive and have been designated as Ch8. In keeping with the proportion of cholinergic to noncholinergic neurons, approximately 80% of the parabigeminal neurons that project to the superior colliculus are also ChAT-positive. In contrast to the Ch1-Ch6 projections which are predominantly, if not exclusively, ipsilateral, the projection from Ch8 to the superior colliculus is mostly crossed.

FEEDBACK CONTROL OF THE Ch4-NB IN THE MONKEY BRAIN

The Ch4 cell group provides the cholinergic innervation for the entire cortical surface and the amygdala. It had been known that the Ch4 region receives neural input from limbic structures such as the amygdala, septal nuclei, and hypothalamus (Saper et al., 1979; Price and Amaral, 1981). As evidence accumulated for an extensive net of projections from Ch4 to the cortical surface, it became important to determine if these cortical regions also sent reciprocal projections back into Ch4. This question was addressed in a study based on 35 rhesus monkeys, each with an injection of tritiated amino acids within a specific cerebral area (Mesulam and Mufson, 1984). These studies showed that virtually none of the primary sensory-motor and association areas in the frontal, parietal, occipital, and temporal lobes projected back to Ch4-NB. The only cortical areas with substantial projections to Ch4-NB were located in the orbitofrontal, anterior insular, temporopolar, and parahippocampal, and probably cingulate regions (Fig. 11). Almost all of these regions

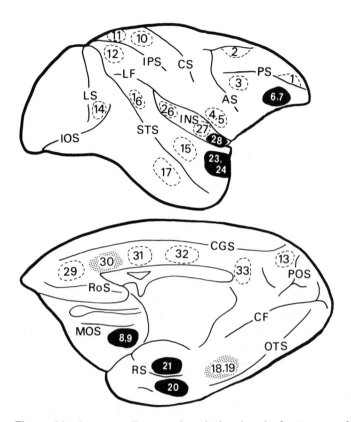

Figure 11 Summary diagram of cortical regions in the macaque that project to the Ch4-NB complex. Each animal involved in this study received a tracer injection in only one of the regions shown in this summary diagram. The dashed circles indicate regions where tritiated amino acid injections did not result in anterograde transport to Ch4-NB. Lightly stippled regions indicate areas that send fibers through the substantia innominata and perhaps also a relatively minor projection to Ch4-NB. Tracer injections within the blackened regions resulted in definite projections to the Ch4-NB complex. The diagram on top shows the lateral surface of the cerebral hemisphere and the one at the bottom, the medial and basal surfaces. The descriptive location of the regions are as follows: 1-3: dorsolateral prefrontal association cortex, 4-5: frontal operculum, 6-7: lateral orbitofrontal cortex, 8-9: caudal orbitofrontal cortex, 10: somatosensory cortex, 11: somatosensory association cortex, 12-13: caudal parietal association cortex, 14: peristriate visual association cortex, 15-16: auditory association cortex, 17: inferotemporal visual association cortex, 18-19: parahippocampal cortex, 20: medial inferotemporal and parahippocampal areas, 21: entorhinal cortex, 23-24: temporopolar cortex, 26: posterior insula, 27: middle insula, 28: anterior insula, 29-30: anterior cingulate gyrus, 31: middle cingulate gyrus, 32: posterior cingulate gyrus, 33: retrosplenial area. Injections 22 and 25 (within the hippocampus and piriform olfactory cortex, respectively) are not shown. Of these two, only the piriform injection showed anterograde transport to Ch4-NB. (From Mesulam and Mufson, 1984.)

that project to Ch4-NB belong to the paralimbic group of cortical regions. These anatomical conclusions have been confirmed by subsequent studies based on HRP injections within the Ch4-NB region (Russchen et al., 1985). This remarkable selectivity of corticofugal projections into Ch4-NB indicates that primary and association areas have little or no direct feedback upon the cholinergic input that they receive whereas a handful of limbic and paralimbic areas can regulate not only the cholinergic input that they receive but also the cholinergic innervation directed to the rest of the cortical surface. This anatomical arrangement suggests that the Ch4-NB region is in a position to act as a cholinergic relay for modulating the activity of the entire cortical surface according to the prevailing motivational state as encoded by limbic and paralimbic regions (Mesulam and Mufson, 1984).

THE CORTICAL DISTRIBUTION OF CHOLINERGIC INNERVATION

Cortical fibers form a dense and intricate plexus in almost all cortical areas. Observations based on the distribution of ChAT and AChE in the monkey show that these cholinergic markers display marked and statistically significant regional variations (Mesulam et al., 1984b, 1986a; Lehmann et al., 1984).

The hippocampus and amygdala contain high levels of the presynaptic cholinergic marker ChAT. This confirms the well-accepted notion that these two limbic structures receive a rich cholinergic input. In addition, we found that the paralimbic (mesocortical) areas of the brain (e.g., parahippocampal, insular, caudal orbitofrontal, temporopolar, and parolfactory cortex) also contain high levels of cholinergic input. In contrast, the concentration of ChAT was much lower (by as much as sevenfold) within all frontal and temporoparietal association areas. As a group, the primary sensory and motor regions contained an intermediate level of ChAT activity. The cingulate gyrus was the only major paralimbic area with a relatively low level of ChAT. Within each paralimbic area, the more primitive nonisocortical sectors tended to have higher levels of cholinergic innervation than the immediately adjacent isocortical regions (Fig. 12, Table 2).

As mentioned above, several lines of observation suggest that regional ChAT activity in the adult primate cortex is likely to reflect primarily the density of cholinergic fibers which arise from extrinsic sources located within the Ch4 sectors (Mesulam et al., 1986a). The observations on regional ChAT activities therefore suggest that the projections from Ch4 to the cerebral cortex are not uniformly distributed and that the variations in these projections respect architectonic and functional boundaries. Our preliminary observations on the distribution of cortical AChE axons suggest that a similar pattern of regional variations may be present in the human cerebral cortex (Green et

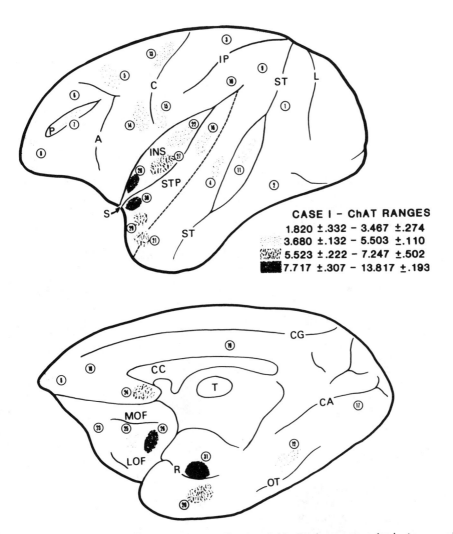

Figure 12 Regional distribution of ChAT activities in the macaque brain (expressed as nanomoles of ACh produced per 15 min per milligram protein). The ChAT activities are divided into four nonoverlapping ranges. The sample numbers correspond to those in Table 2 which can be consulted for specific values and anatomical descriptions. All assays were performed in triplicate. (From Mesulam et al., 1986a.)

Table 2 ChAT Enzymatic Activities and Standard Errors[a,b]

Sample number	Area	ChAT (nmoles/15 min per mg protein)	
		Case I	Case II
	Association areas	**3.465 ± 0.278**	**7.202 ± 0.790**
1	(OA,OB) Peristriate visual association	3.467 ± 0.274	3.938 ± 0.186
2	(TE) Temporal visual association	1.820 ± 0.332	5.560 ± 0.077
3	(PE) Somatosensory association	3.213 ± 0.162	4.327 ± 0.043
4	(TA) Auditory association	4.357 ± 0.047	9.081 ± 0.520
5	(FB) Dorsal premotor association	3.990 ± 0.336	9.708 ± 0.466
6	(FD) Dorsolateral prefrontal	2.740 ± 0.075	6.096 ± 0.208
7	(FD) Principalis cortex (prefrontal)	3.680 ± 0.132	6.758 ± 0.014
8	(FD) Frontopolar cortex	4.157 ± 0.162	5.827 ± 0.290
9	(PG) Caudal inferior parietal lobule	2.070 ± 0.123	4.092 ± 0.225
10	(PF) Rostral inferior parietal lobule	2.867 ± 0.132	11.320 ± 0.144
11	Banks of superior temporal sulcus	4.157 ± 0.113	11.707 ± 0.470
12	(TF) Caudal inferotemporal cortex	5.047 ± 0.283	8.002 ± 0.039
	Primary sensory-motor	**4.394 ± 0.576**	**9.820 ± 3.068**
13	(FA) Dorsal primary motor	4.013 ± 0.084	6.335 ± 0.255
14	(FBA-FA) Ventral primary motor	5.443 ± 0.154	7.191 ± 0.070
15	(PC(3b))Primary somatosensory	5.503 ± 0.110	10.511 ± 0.480
16	(TC) Primary auditory	4.653 ± 0.177	21.307 ± 1.213
17	(OC) Primary visual	2.367 ± 0.124	3.762 ± 0.078
	Cingulate gyrus	**3.170 ± 0.130**	**7.600 ± 1.440**
18	(LA) Anterior cingulate	3.040 ± 0.310	9.043 ± 0.507
19	(LC) Caudal cingulate	3.300 ± 0.134	6.158 ± 0.126
	Isocortical paralimbic areas	**5.405 ± 0.775**	**14.358 ± 3.166**
20	(TE$_m$) Medial inferotemporal visual association	5.523 ± 0.222	11.268 ± 0.564
21	(STPg-anterior TA) Temporopolar auditory association	7.247 ± 0.502	23.366 ± 0.182
22	(Ig) Granular insula	5.387 ± 0.122	13.870 ± 0.533
23	(OFg) Granular anterior orbitofrontal	3.457 ± 0.156	8.933 ± 0.142
	Nonisocortical paralimbic	**8.686 ± 1.280**	**17.282 ± 2.162**
24	(FL) Paralfactory area	6.670 ± 0.326	9.574 ± 0.311
25	(OFdg) Dysgranular mid-orbitofrontal	5.147 ± 0.135	14.282 ± 0.395
26	(OFap) Agranular caudal orbitofrontal	13.733 ± 1.025	28.754 ± 1.133
27	(Idg) Dysgranular insula	5.703 ± 0.136	15.358 ± 0.683
28	(Iap) Agranular insula	7.717 ± 0.307	22.827 ± 0.675
29	(TPdg) Dysgranular temporopolar	5.767 ± 0.350	18.418 ± 0.233
30	(TPap) Agranular temporopolar	13.817 ± 0.193	16.850 ± 0.442
31	Entorhinal-prorhinal	10.927 ± 0.513	12.206 ± 0.281

Table 2

Sample number	Area	ChAT (nmoles/15 min per mg protein)	
		Case I	Case II
	Limbic areas	**21.675 ± 12.795**	**39.730 ± 11.850**
32	Midhippocampus	8.883 ± 0.613	27.878 ± 0.340
33	Amygdala	34.470 ± 2.023	51.582 ± 1.128
	Comparison areas		
	Nucleus basalis	37.527 ± 1.292	41.050 ± 2.555
	Putamen	45.380 ± 1.300	46.477 ± 1.200
	Corpus callosum	1.670 ± 0.071	3.578 ± 0.092
	Cerebellum	0.210 ± 0.150	1.012 ± 0.017

[a]From Mesulam et al. (1986a).
[b]The anatomical location of samples 1-31 are shown in Fig. 2. Values in bold type indicate group means. Letters in parentheses indicate the architectonics designation of Mesulam and Mufson (1982) and von Bonin and Bailey (1947).

al., 1986). It is not yet known if cortical regions with a more intense cholinergic input receive projections from a larger number of Ch4 neurons or if the input from an individual Ch4 neuron in these regions has more ramifications and a greater ChAT content.

The cholinergic receptors in cortex and hippocampus are mostly muscarinic. Although most of these receptors are postsynaptic, some presynaptic receptor sites may also exist and may participate in the autoregulation of ACh secretion. In cortical slices, the effect of ACh upon pyramidal neurons consists of a short-latency inhibition followed by a prolonged increase in excitability (McCormick and Prince, 1985). The inhibitory effect seems to be mediated by GABAergic interneurons whereas the excitatory effect reflects a direct action of ACh upon pyramidal neurons. The increase of excitability in response to ACh appears to be caused by a reduction of membrane K^+ conductance (Krnjević, 1981). Since this effect lasts for a relatively long time, ACh is considered to act, at least in part, as an excitatory neuromodulator upon pyramidal neurons.

Recent observations indicate the existence of more than one type of muscarinic receptor in the CNS (Mash et al., 1985). We examined the regional distribution of cholinergic receptor subtypes within the cortex of the monkey brain (Mash and Mesulam, 1986). The pirenzepine-sensitive M1 subtype (which is also the dominant species of cortical muscarinic receptor) was distributed according to a pattern that approximated the variations of ChAT activity. Thus, both M1 receptor density and ChAT enzyme activity displayed peaks mostly within limbic and paralimbic regions such as the amygdala, hippocampal complex, parahippocampal cortex, orbitofrontal cortex, and the temporopolar region. However, there were also discrepancies. For example, peak M1 receptor densities were seen in posterior cingulate cortex and in some patches of association cortex even though these areas contain relatively low levels of ChAT activity. Furthermore, the insula and the baso-lateral nucleus of the amygdala contain very high levels of ChAT and AChE but did not display M1 density peaks.

The primate cortex contains substantially fewer M2 than M1 receptor sites. The cortical distribution of M2 receptors displayed a rather unexpected pat-tern characterized by distinct peaks in the primary areas of all five sensory modalities and in parts of the primary motor cortex. We speculated that these receptors may be associated with cholinergic reticulocortical projec-tions (perhaps emanating from Ch5-Ch6), thus providing a physiological mechanism through which all primary sensory and motor areas can be acti-vated in concert according to the prevailing state of arousal (Mash and Mesu-lam, 1986).

A closer analysis of muscarinic and nicotinic receptors in the hippocampal complex revealed marked regional variations that reflected cytoarchitectonic subdivisions. Thus, the M1 receptor showed regional density peaks in the dentate gyrus (molecular layer), the CA3, and CA4 hippocampal sectors and in some parahippocampal regions. The M2 receptor sites showed the highest density in the subiculum, parasubiculum, ventral entorhinal cortex, and the prorhinal region. Nicotinic receptors, although much less dense than either muscarinic subtype, showed a regional peak within the presubicular component of the hippocampal formation. Thus, selective cholinergic agon-ists could conceivably be used to selectively influence specific sectors of the heterogeneous hippocampal formation (Mash et al., 1987).

The lack of a perfect fit between the distribution of ChAT and that of the M1 and M2 receptor subtypes may initially appear surprising since one might have expected the distribution of postsynaptic receptor sites to mirror the distribution of the incoming presynaptic innervation. One possibility for this discrepancy is that we do not yet possess a ligand which reliably binds to all postsynaptic cholinergic receptors and to nothing but these receptors. Alternatively, a very large number of neural membranes may contain sites that will bind to available receptor ligands but these sites may remain physio-logically inactive unless coupled to the proper presynaptic innervation. Yet a third possibility is that the distribution of active receptor sites simply does not parallel the distribution of presynaptic fibers (Herkenham, 1987). Perhaps some transmitter systems (e.g., cholinergic, dopaminergic) are distributed not only in the form of traditional neural pathways with spatially coupled pre- and postsynaptic junctional complexes but also in the form of more diffuse arrays within the transmitter substance acts as a hormone, at much larger distances. These considerations, while they do not alter the implications based on the differential distribution of cortical ChAT, indicate that the organiza-tion of central cholinergic pathways contains additional complexities that need to be elucidated.

BEHAVIORAL AFFILIATIONS OF
CENTRAL CHOLINERGIC PATHWAYS

In keeping with their widespread anatomical distribution, a number of behavioral affiliations have been attributed to central cholinergic pathways. These can be divided into four major groups: (1) extrapyramidal motor function, (2) sleep and arousal, (3) mood and affect, and (4) memory and learning.

With respect to motor function, many centrally acting cholinergic agonists are known to be tremorogenic. Especially in parkinsonian patients, cholinergic agents intensify the tremor whereas anticholinergic medication provides effective symptomatic relief. It is thought that the motor deficit in parkinsonism results from an impairment in the balance between cholinergic and dopaminergic innervation within the striatum (Calne, 1978). It is not known if the Ch1-Ch8 cell groups also participate in the cholinergic regulation of extrapyramidal motor function. Several studies indicate that the pedunculopontine nucleus (which contains most of the Ch5 neurons) may have some interaction with the mesencephalic locomotor region and that it may participate in extrapyramidal pathways (Moon-Edley and Graybiel, 1983; Skinner et al., 1985; Isaacson and Tanaka, 1986). Recent anatomical studies, however, have shown that the mesencephalic sites with the most extrapyramidal connections are adjacent to but not overlapping with the pedunculopontine nucleus (Rye et al., 1987).

With respect to the regulation of arousal, cholinergic pathways have traditionally been considered as major components of the ascending reticular activating system (Shute and Lewis, 1967). In keeping with this concept, physiological studies show that cholinergic activation in the thalamus is likely to have a net facilitatory effect upon the thalamocortical transmission of neural impulses (McCance et al., 1968; Dingledine and Kelly, 1977). This activating effect is probably mediated predominantly by the Ch5-Ch6 neurons of the pontomesencephalic reticular formation since they supply most of the thalamic cholinergic innervation.

Behavioral arousal as well as electrical stimulation of the brain stem reticular formation are associated with a low-voltage fast-activity pattern in the neocortical EEG. This EEG pattern, which is largely abolished by cholinergic antagonists and enhanced by cholinergic agonists, also shows a positive correlation with the amount of neocortical ACh release (Kanai and Szerb, 1965; Sie et al., 1965; Steward et al., 1984). This cholinergic influence upon neocortical low-voltage fast activity is thought to be mediated by corticopetal projections from the nucleus basalis (Ch4) rather than by thalamocortical projections (Stewart et al., 1984). The extent to which direct cholinergic projections from Ch5-Ch6 to neocortex (and perhaps to Ch4) also contribute to the regulation of this neocortical low-voltage fast activity has not yet been determined specifically. If the influence of septohippocampal projections (arising from Ch1-Ch2) upon the arousal-related hippocampal theta activity is also taken into consideration, it becomes clear that the cholinergic cell groups in the basal forebrain as well as those in the brain stem participate extensively in the electrophysiological regulation of arousal states. These considerations lend further credence to the suggestion that the nuclei containing the Ch1-Ch4 groups represent, at least in part, a telencephalic extension of the brain stem reticular formation (Ramon-Moliner and Nauta, 1966).

The putative role of cholinergic pathways in emotion and memory is entirely consistent with the preferential association of the Ch1-Ch4 cell groups with the limbic system. As shown above, limbic and paralimbic regions receive a heavier cholinergic input than other cortical areas and also play a more important role in the feedback regulation of the Ch1-Ch4 neurons. With respect to emotion, cholinergic agonists such as physostigmine have, in my experience, produced acute dysphoria in individuals with no evidence of prior mood disturbance. Furthermore, this same agent has been advocated as an effective treatment for acute manic episodes. It has also been suggested that the antidepressant effect of tricyclic substances is partly due to their well-known anticholinergic activity. Conceivably, certain emotional states may represent a balance between cholinergic and monoaminergic innervation within the limbic system (Janowsky et al., 1972).

The relationship of central cholinergic pathways to memory and learning has recently attracted a great deal of attention. For example, young experimental animals and human volunteers show an impairment of new learning when given anticholinergic agents such as scopolamine. The similarity of this scopolamine-induced effect to the memory difficulty that emerges in the course of aging has led to the suggestion that the memory decline of senescence could be caused by an age-related depletion of cholinergic innervation within cortex and limbic structures (Drachman and Leavitt, 1974; Bartus et al., 1982; Mesulam et al., 1987). The importance of cholinergic innervation to memory is further shown by experiments where Ch4 ablations which result in a loss of neocortical AChE and ChAT also result in memory deficits (Flicker et al., 1983). An excessive loss of cortical and limbic cholinergic innervation, above and beyond what is expected on the basis of age alone, has been reported in Alzheimer's disease and this could contribute to the emergence of the severe amnesia (and perhaps some of the other clinical features) seen in this dementing condition (Davies and Maloney, 1976). In keeping with the loss of cortical and limbic cholinergic innervation in Alzheimer's disease, the Ch1, Ch2, and Ch4 regions show marked cell loss in patients with this condition (Whitehouse et al., 1981; Arendt et al., 1985).

The pattern of regional variations in ChAT activity has led us to speculate that cortical cholinergic pathways may participate in memory processes by regulating sensory-limbic interactions (Mesulam et al., 1986a). Sensory-limbic interactions are thought to underlie many important behaviors including

the ability to direct drives toward the appropriate object and also the ability
to store and retrieve memory traces. Paralimbic areas provide one important
avenue for sensory-limbic interactions and these regions have among the
highest ChAT activities. It is also known that there are additional multisyn-
aptic pathways for conveying modality-specific information in each of the
major sensory modalities into core limbic structures such as the hippocampus
and the amygdala (Van Hoesen, 1981; Mishkin, 1982; Mesulam, 1985). An
analysis of regional ChAT activities along these pathways shows that this
sensory information is likely to come under progressively more intense cholinergic influence as it approaches the limbic system (Fig. 13). Furthermore,
single-unit studies in awake and behaving rhesus monkeys have shown that
the Ch4-NB neurons which provide this cholinergic influence are particularly
responsive to the delivery of reward and to the motivational relevance of
sensory events (DeLong, 1971; Rolls et al., 1979). Taken together, these observations lead to the speculation that cortical cholinergic pathways could
provide a gating mechanism for channeling motivationally relevant sensory
information into and out of the limbic system. Therefore, a dysfunction of
these pathways (e.g., by ablations of Ch4, scopolamine administration, or

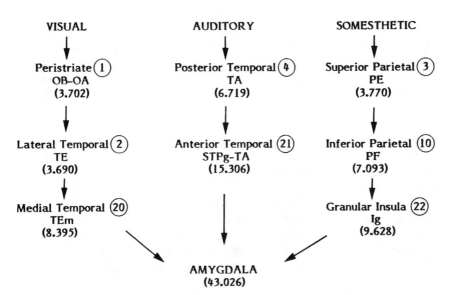

Figure 13   The amygdalopetal flow of sensory information in the three major modalities. The circled numbers and the architectonic designations correspond to those
in Table 2. The numbers in parentheses show the mean ChAT activity in that area as
calculated from values obtained in the two macaque monkeys which were used for
the regional enzymatic assays. (From Mesulam et al., 1986a.)

in the course of Alzheimer's disease) could cause a memory impairment by interfering with crucial sensory-limbic interactions (Mesulam et al., 1986a). In partial support for this hypothesis, it has been shown that procaine or GABA injections into the nucleus basalis of the rat inhibit the response of frontal neurons to a sensory cue that signaled the delivery of reward (Rigdon and Pirch, 1984). Thus, cortical cholinergic innervation could be regulating the neuronal response to motivationally relevant sensory stimuli in a way that determines whether or not the pertinent information gets relayed into the limbic system. This gating hypothesis also explains how cholinergic input within sensory and association areas (not particularly known for their involvement in learning) could participate in the overall process of memory storage and retrieval. The gating function of cholinergic pathways is a hypothesis that lends itself to experimental verification.

SUMMARY

Although ubiquitous, central cholinergic projections also have a specific topographic organization. The cholinergic innervation of the striatal complex is predominantly intrinsic whereas that of thalamic, limbic, and cortical regions is mostly extrinsic. Four groups of neurons in the basal forebrain (Ch1-Ch4) provide the major cholinergic innervation for limbic, olfactory, and cortical structures; two cell groups in the pontomesencephalic reticular formation (Ch5-Ch6) provide the major cholinergic input for thalamic nuclei; neurons in the medial habenula (Ch7) provide the cholinergic input for the interpeduncular nucleus; and the ChAT-positive cells in the parabigeminal nucleus (Ch8) provide the major cholinergic input for the superior colliculus. The most extensive of these cell groups, the Ch4 complex, innervates the amygdala and the entire cortical mantle. There is further internal topography in the projections from Ch4 to the cortical surface so that each cortical region receives its major cholinergic input from one of the Ch4 subsectors. Furthermore, the Ch4 complex sends a more intense cholinergic projection to limbic and paralimbic structures than to the other portions of the cortical surface. In turn, these limbic and paralimbic areas seem to have a greater feedback influence upon the activity of the Ch4 neurons. These details of anatomical organization are consistent with many of the behavioral affiliations that have been attributed to central cholinergic pathways.

ACKNOWLEDGMENTS

The preparation of this chapter was supported in part by a Javits Neuroscience Investigator Award, the McKnight Foundation, and and Alzheimer's Disease Research Center Grant (AG05134). I am grateful to Leah Christie for expert secretarial assistance.

ABBREVIATIONS

A	arcuate sulcus
a	cerebral aqueduct
ac	anterior commissure
al	anterolateral subsector of Ch4
am	anteromedial subsector of Ch4
amg	amygdala
ap	ansa peduncularis
AS	arcuate sulcus
C	central sulcus
CA	calcarine fissure
CC	corpus callosum
cd	caudate nucleus
CF	calcarine fissure
cg	central gray substance
CG(S)	cingulate gyrus
Ch1	first cholinergic cell group
Ch2	second cholinergic cell group
Ch3	third cholinergic cell group
Ch4	fourth cholinergic cell group
Ch5	fifth cholinergic cell group
Ch6	sixth cholinergic cell group
Ch4al	anterolateral subsector of Ch4
Ch4am	anteromedial subsector of Ch4
Ch4id	intermediodorsal subsector of Ch4
Ch4iv	invermedioventral subsector of Ch4
Ch4p	posterior subsector of Ch4
ci	islands of Calleja
cin	inferior colliculus
cn	cuneiform nucleus
CS	central sulcus
cs	superior colliculus
ctt	central tegmental tract
dsp	decussation of the superior cerebellar peduncle
gp	globus pallidus
gpl	lateral globus pallidus
gpm	medial globus pallidus
gpv	ventral globus pallidus
HY	hypothalamus
i	intermediate sector of Ch4
ic	internal capsule
id	intermediodorsal subsector of Ch4

INS   insula
IOS   inferior occipital status
ip   interpeduncular nucleus
IP   intraparietal (sulcus)
iv   intermedioventral subsector of Ch4
L   lunate sulcus
LF   lateral (sylvian) fissure
lgn   lateral geniculate nucleus
LL   lateral lemniscus
LOF   lateral orbitofrontal sulcus
LS   lunate sulcus
ltn   laterodorsal tegmental nucleus
ml   medial lemniscus
mlf   medial longitudinal fasciculus
MOF   medial orbitofrontal sulcus
MOS   medial orbitofrontal sulcus
na   nucleus accumbens
NB   nucleus basalis
nIV   fourth cranial nerve
OC   optic chiasm
ot   optic tract
OT   occipitotemporal (sulcus)
P   principal sulcus
p   posterior sector of Ch4
pno   oral division of the pontine reticular nucleus
POS   parietooccipital sulcus
ppn   pedunculopontine nucleus
PS   principal sulcus
pt   putamen
R   rhinal sulcus
RoS   rostral sulcus
RS   rhinal sulcus
S   sylvian fissure
sp   superior cerebellar peduncle
Spt   septal area
STP   supratemporal plane
ST(S)   superior temporal sulcus
T   thalamus

REFERENCES

Arendt, T., Bigl, V., Tennstedt, A., and Arendt, A. (1985). Neuronal loss in different parts of the nucleus basalis is related to neuritic plaque formation in cortical target areas in Alzheimer's disease. *Neuroscience 14*:1-14.

Arikuni, T., and Kubota, K. (1984). Substantia innominata projection to caudate nucleus in macaque monkeys, *Brain Res. 302*:184-189.

Baisden, R.H., Woodruff, M.L., and Hoover, D.B. (1984). Cholinergic and non-cholinergic septo-hippocampal projections: A double-label horseradish peroxidase-acetylcholinesterase study in the rabbit, *Brain Res. 290*:146-151.

Bartus, R.T., Dean, R.L., III, Beer, B., and Lippa, A.S. (1982). The cholinergic hypothesis of geriatric memory dysfunction. *Science 217*:408-417.

Calne, D.B. (1978). Parkinsonism, clinical and neuropharmacological aspects. *Postgrad. Med. 2*:1457-1459.

Dale, H.H. (1938). Acetylcholine as a chemical transmitter. *J. Mt. Sinai Hosp. 4*: 401-429.

Davies, P., and Maloney, A.J.F. (1976). Selective loss of central cholinergic neurons in Alzheimer's disease. *Lancet 2*:1403.

DeLong, M.R. (1971). Activity of pallidal neurons during movement. *J. Neurophysiol. 34*:414-427.

Dingledine, R., and Kelly, J.S. (1977). Brain stem stimulation and the acetylcholine-evoked inhibition of neurons in the feline nucleus reticularis thalami. *J. Physiol (London) 271*:135-154.

Drachman, D.A., and Leavitt, J. (1974). Human memory and the cholinergic system— A relationship to aging? *Arch. Neurol. Psychiatry 30*:113-121.

Eckenstein, F., and Thoenen, H. (1983). Cholinergic neurons in the rat cerebral cortex demonstrated by immunohistochemical localization of choline acetyltransferase. *Neurosci. Lett. 36*:211-215.

Fibiger, H. (1982). The organization and some projections of cholinergic neurons of the mammalian forebrain. *Brain Res. Rev. 4*:322-388.

Flicker, C., Dean, R.L., Watkins, D.L., Fisher, S.K., and Bartus, R.T. (1983). Behavioral and neurochemical effects following neurotoxic lesions of a major cholinergic input to the cerebral cortex in the rat. *Pharmacol. Biochem. Behav. 18*:973-981.

Green, R.C., Moran, M.A., Martin, T.L., Mash, D.C., Mufson, E.J., and Mesulam, M.-M. (1986). Distribution of acetylcholinesterase fiber staining in the human hippocampus and parahippocampal gyrus. *Soc. Neurosci. Abstr. 12*:356.

Herkenham, M. (1987). Mismatches between receptor and transmitter localizations in the brain: observations and implications. *Neuroscience 23*:1-38.

Houser, C.R., Crawford, G.D., Barber, R.P., Salvaterra, P.M., and Vaughn, J.E. (1983). Organization and morphological characteristics of cholinergic neurons; An immunohistochemical study with a monoclonal antibody to choline acetyltransferase. *Brain Res. 266*:97-119.

Isaacson, L.G., and Tanaka, D., Jr. (1986). Cholinergic and non-cholinergic projections from the canine pontomesencephalic tegmentum (Ch5 area) to the caudal intralaminar thalamic nuclei. *Exp. Brain Res. 62*:179-188.

Janowsky, D.S., Davies, J.M., El-Yousef, M.K., and Sekerke, H.J. (1972). A cholinergic-adrenergic hypothesis of mania and depression. *Lancet 2*:632-635.

Johnston, M.V., McKinney, M., and Coyle, J.T. (1981). Neocortical cholinergic innervation: A description of extrinsic and intrinsic components in the rat. *Exp. Brain Res. 43*:159-172.

Kanai, T., and Szerb, J.C. (1965). The mesencephalic reticular activating system and cortical acetylcholine output. *Nature 205*:80-82.

Kataoka, R., Nakamura, Y., and Hassler, R. (1974). Habenulointerpeduncular tract: A possible cholinergic neuron in the rat brain. *Brain Res. 62*:264-267.

Kimura, H., McGeer, P.L., Peng, J.H., and McGeer, E.G. (1981). The central cholinergic system studied by choline acetyltransferase immunohistochemistry in the cat. *J. Comp. Neurol. 200*:151-201.

Krnjević, K. (1981). Acetylcholine as a modulator of amino-acid-mediated synaptic transmission. In: *The Role of Peptides and Amino Acids as Neurotransmitters.* Liss, New York, pp. 124-141.

Krnjević, K., and Silver, A. (1965). A histochemical study of cholinergic fibers in the cerebral cortex. *J. Anat. 99*:711-759.

Lehmann, J., Struble, R.G., Antuono, P.G., Coyle, J.T., Cork, L.C., and Price, D.L. (1984). Regional heterogeneity of choline acetyltransferase activity in primate neocortex. *Brain Res. 322*:361-364.

Levey, A.I., Rye, D.B., Wainer, B.H., Mufson, E.J., and Mesulam, M.-M. (1984). Choline acetyltransferase-immunoreactive neurons intrinsic to rodent cortex and distinction from acetylcholinesterase-positive neurons. *Neuroscience 13*: 341-353.

Loewi, O. (1921). Uber humorale Ubertragbarkeit der Herznervenwirkung. *Pfluegers Arch. Gesamte Physiol. Menschen Tiere 189*:239-242.

Mash, D.C., White, F., Mufson, E.J., and Mesulam, M.-M. (1987). Muscarinic and nicotinic acetylcholine receptors in the hippocampal formation of the monkey. *Neurology 37*(Suppl. 1):194.

Mash, D.C., and Mesulam, M.-M. (1986). Muscarine receptor distributions within architectonic subregions of the primate cortex. *Soc. Neurosci. Abstr. 12*:809.

Mash, D.C., Flynn, D.D., and Potter, L.T. (1985). Loss of M2 receptors in the cerebral cortex in Alzheimer's disease and experimental cholinergic denervation. *Science 228*:1115-1117.

McCance, I., Phillis, J.W., and Westerman, R.A. (1968). Acetylcholine-sensitivity of thalamic neurons: Its relationship to synaptic transmission. *Br. J. Pharmacol. 32*:635-651.

McCormick, D.A., and Prince, D.A. (1985). Two types of muscarinic responses to acetylcholine in mammalian cortical neurons. *Proc. Natl. Acad. Sci. (USA) 82*: 6344-6348.

Mesulam, M.-M. (1985). Patterns in behavioral neuroanatomy. In: *Principles of Behavioral Neurology.* Edited by M.-M. Mesulam. Davis, Philadelphia, pp. 1-70.

Mesulam, M.-M., and Muson, E.J. (1982). Insula of the Old World monkey. Part I. Architectonics in the insuloorbito-temporal component of the paralimbic brain. *J. Compl Neurol. 212*:1-22.

Mesulam, M.-M., and Mufson, E.J. (1984). Neural inputs into the nucleus basalis of the substantia innominata (Ch4) in the rhesus monkey. *Brain 107*:253-274.

Mesulam, M.-M., and Van Hoesen, G.W. (1976). Acetylcholinesterase-rich projections from the basal forebrain of the rhesus monkey to neocortex. *Brain Res. 109*:152-157.

Mesulam, M.-M., Van Hoesen, G.W., and Rosene, D.L. (1977). Substantia innominata, septal area of nuclei of the diagonal band in the rhesus monkey: Organization of efferents and their acetylcholinesterase histochemistry. *Soc. Neurosci.
Abstr. 3*:202.

Mesulam, M.-M., Mufson, E.J., Levey, A.I., and Wainer, B.H. (1983a). Cholinergic
innervation of cortex by the basal forebrain: Cytochemistry and cortical connections of the septal area, diagonal band nuclei, nucleus basalis (substantia innominata) and hypothalamus in the rhesus monkey. *J. Comp. Neurol. 214*:170-197.

Mesulam, M.-M., Mufson, E.J., Wainer, B.H., and Levey, A.I. (1983b). Central
cholinergic pathways in the rat: An overview based on an alternative nomenclature (Ch1-Ch6). *Neuroscience 10*:1185-1201.

Mesulam, M.-M., Mufson, E.J., Levey, A.I., and Wainer, B.H. (1984a). Atlas of
cholinergic neurons in the forebrain and upper brainstem of the macaque based
on monoclonal choline acetyltransferase immunohistochemistry and acetylcholinesterase histochemistry. *Neuroscience 12*:669-686.

Mesulam, M.-M., Rosen, A.D., and Mufson, E.J. (1984b). Regional variations in
cortical cholinergic innervation: Chemoarchitectonics of acetylcholinesterase-
containing fibers in the macaque brain. *Brain Res. 311*:245-258.

Mesulam, M.-M., Volicer, L., Marquis, J.K., Mufson, E.J., and Green, R.C. (1986a).
Systematic regional differences in the cholinergic innervation of the primate cere-
bral cortex: Distribution of enzyme activities and some behavioral implications.
Ann. Neurol. 19:144-151.

Mesulam, M.-M., Mufson, E.J., and Wainer, B.H. (1986b). Three-dimensional representation and cortical projection topography of the nucleus basalis (Ch4) in
the macaque: Concurrent demonstration of choline acetyltransferase and retrograde transport with a stabilized tetramethylbenzidine method for HRP. *Brain
Res. 367*:301-308.

Mesulam, M.-M., Mufson, E.J., and Rogers, J. (1987). Age-related shrinkage of cortically projecting cholinergic neurons: A selective effect. *Ann. Neurol. 22*:31-36.

Mishkin, M. (1982). A memory system in the monkey. *Phil. Trans. R. Soc. London
Ser. B. 298*:85-92.

Moon-Edley, S., and Graybiel, A.M. (1983). The afferent and efferent connections
of the feline nucleus tegmenti pedunculopontinus, pars compacta. *J. Comp.
Neurol. 217*:187-215.

Mufson, E.J., Levey, A.I., Wainer, B.H., and Mesulam, M.-M. (1982). Cholinergic
projections from the mesencephalic tegmentum to neocortex in rhesus monkey.
Soc. Neurosci. Abstr. 8:135.

Mufson, E.J., Desan, P.H., Mesulam, M.-M., Wainer, B.H., and Levey, A.I. (1984).
Choline acetyltransferase-like immunoreactivity in the forebrain of the red-eared
pond turtle (*Pseudemys Scripta elegans*). *Brain Res. 323*:103-108.

Mufson, E.J., Martin, T.L., Mash, D.C., Wainer, B.H., and Mesulam, M.-M. (1986).
Cholinergic projections from the parabigeminal nucleus (Ch8) to the superior
colliculus in the mouse: A combined analysis of HRP transport and choline acetyltransferase immunohisto-chemistry. *Brain Res. 370*:144-148.

Nastuk, M.A., and Graybiel, A.M. (1985). Patterns of muscarinic cholinergic binding in the striatum and their relation to dopamine islands and striosomes. *J. Comp. Neurol. 237*:176-194.

Parent, A., Poirier, L.J., Boucher, R., and Butcher, L.L. (1977). Morphological characteristics of acetylcholinesterase-containing neurons in the CNS of DEP-treated monkeys. *J. Neurol. Sci. 32*:9-28.

Price, J.L., and Amaral, D.G. (1981). An autoradiographic study of the projections of the central nucleus of the monkey amygdala. *J. Neurosci. 1*:1242-1259.

Price, J.L., and Stern, R. (1983). An autoradiographic study of the projections of the central nucleus of the monkey amygdala. *J. Neurosci. 1*:1242-1259.

Ramon-Moliner, E., and Nauta, W.J.H. (1966). The isodendritic core of the brain stem. *J. Comp. Neurol. 126*:311-335.

Rawlins, J.N.P., Feldon, J., and Gray, J.A. (1979). Septo-hippocampal connections and the hippocampal theta rhythm. *Exp. Brain Res. 37*:49-63.

Rigdon, G.C., and Pirch, J.H. (1984). Microinjection of procaine or GABA into the nucleus basalis magnocellularis affects cue-elicited unit responses in the rat frontal cortex. *Exp. Neurol. 85*:283-296.

Rolls, E.T., Sanghera, M.K., and Roper-Hall, A. (1979). The latency of activation of neurons in the lateral hypothalamus and substantia innominata during feeding in the monkey. *Brain Res. 164*:121-135.

Rossier, J. (1984). On the mapping of the cholinergic neurons by immunocytochemistry. *Neurochem. Int. 6*:183-184.

Russchen, F.T., Amaral, D.G., and Price, J.L. (1985). The afferent connections of the substantia innominata in the monkey. *Macaca fascicularis. J. Comp. Neurol. 24*:1-27.

Rye, D.B., Saper, C.B., Lee, H.J., and Wainer, B.H., Pedunculopontine tegmental nucleus of the rat: Cytoarchitecture, cytochemistry, and some extrapyramidal connections of the mesopontine tegmentum. *J. Comp. Neurol. 259*:483-528.

Saper, C.B., Swanson, L.W., and Cowan, W.M. (1979). Some afferent connections of the rostral hypothalamus in the squirrel monkey (*Saimiri sciureus*) and cat. *J. Comp. Neurol. 184*:5-242.

Shute, C.C.D., and Lewis, P.R. (1967). The ascending cholinergic reticular system: Neocortical, olfactory and subcortical projections. *Brain 90*:497-520.

Sie, G., Jasper, H.H., and Wolfe, I. (1965). Rate of ACh release from cortical surface in encephale and cerveau isole preparations in relation to arousal and epileptic activation of the EEG. *Electroencephalogr. Clin. Neurophysiol. 18*:206.

Silver, A. (1974). *The Biology of Cholinesterases*. Elsevier, Amsterdam.

Skinner, R.D., and Garcia-Rill, D., Conrad, C., and Mosley, C. (1985). The mesencephalic locomotor region. II. Ascending and descending projections in the rat. *Anat. Rec. 211*:180a.

Steward, D.J., and MacFabe, D.F., and Vanderwolf, C.H. (1984). Cholinergic activation of electrocorticogram: Role of the substantia innominata and effects of atropine and quinuclidinyl benzylate. *Brain Res. 322*:219-232.

Vanderwolf, C.H. (1983). The role of the cerebral cortex and ascending activating systems in the control of behavior. In: *Handbook of Behavioral Neurobiology*. Edited by E. Satinoff and P. Teitelbaum. Plenum Press, New York, pp. 67-104.

Van Hoesen, G.W. (1981). The differential distribution, diversity and sprouting of cortical projections to the amygdala in the rhesus monkey. In: *The Amygdaloid Complex*. Edited by Y. Ben-Ari, Elsevier, Amsterdam, pp. 77-90.

von Bonin, G., and Bailey, P. (1947). *The Neocortex of Macaca Mulatta*. University of Illinois Press, Urbana.

Wainer, B.H., Levey, A.I., Mufson, E.J., and Mesulam, M.-M. (1984). Cholinergic systems in mammalian brain identified with antibodies against choline acetyltransferase. *Neurochem. Int. 6*:163-182.

Wainer, B.H., Levey, A.I., Rye, D.B., Mesulam, M.-M., and Mufson, E.J. (1985). Cholinergic and noncholinergic septohippocampal pathways. *Neurosci. Lett. 54*:45-52.

Whitehouse, P.J., Price, D.L., Clark, A.W., Coyle, J.T., and DeLong, M.R. (1981). Alzheimer's disease: Evidence for selective loss of cholinergic neurons in the nucleus basalis. *Ann. Neurol. 10*:122-126.

Woolf, N.J., and Butcher, L.L. (1981). Cholinergic neurons in the caudate-putamen complex proper are intrinsically organized: A combined Evans blue and acetylcholinesterase analysis. *Brain Res. Bull. 7*:487-507.

5

Drugs and Memory

Brian A. Lawlor
Mount Sinai School of Medicine
New York, New York

Trey Sunderland, Rick A. Martinez,
Susan E. Molchan, and Herbert Weingartner
National Institute of Mental Health
National Institutes of Health
Bethesda, Maryland

INTRODUCTION

A great deal of research on cognitive science has been published during the past few decades and has provided us with both tools and theories for considering the features and determinants of cognitive functions (1). Much of this research has focused on uncovering the psychobiological basis of various aspects of cognitive processes (2-6). This work has emerged from clinical studies and from research involving the study of various biological treatments in animals, as well as from studies using drugs as tools to explore cognition. The central theme of all this research is that a cognitive function, such as memory, is determined by several identifiable and psychobiologically distinct component processes. It is this theme of specificity that links these research findings to this chapter describing how drugs alter cognitive functions.

INFORMATION PROCESSING SYSTEMS
AND THEIR FAILURES

The clinician is often faced with the complex clinical problem of understanding why a patient cannot remember some recent events. Specifically, let us consider what it means if a patient cannot remember an event that has occurred earlier in the day. This exercise will allow us to delineate a scheme of information processing systems involved in memory and also will help us establish at what point drugs affect the processing systems that involve memory.

SENSORY PROCESS FAILURE

The patient's recall of an event is likely to be unsuccessful if the patient cannot perceive the incoming stimulus because of perceptual problems. This is often the case in elderly subjects with primary hearing problems. If patients are unable to hear incoming information, they cannot process the event. In the elderly, it is particularly important to determine the hearing status of a patient before diagnosing memory impairment. The same difficulty also applies to patients with primary visual problems. The sedative and behavioral effects of drugs can also interfere with perceptual processes and prevent subjects from accessing incoming stimuli. This type of disruption in memory is referred to as a "sensory processing failure."

ATTENTIONAL PROCESS FAILURE

If a patient cannot focus on the stimulus, or is already concentrating on another stimulus, then the patient will not remember the event very well. This type of memory failure is called an "attentional processing failure" and is a common reason why subjects do not remember events. Similarly, children with an attention deficit disorder are unable to focus on specific stimuli in the environment and, therefore, have difficulty learning and remembering. Drugs such as stimulants can help these children with attentional processing difficulties, allowing them to focus their attention on tasks and, thus, improving behavior and school performance.

KNOWLEDGE MEMORY FAILURE

Patients must be able to access previously acquired knowledge if sensory events are to be meaningfully understood and related to past experience (3). This component of information processing is essential to encoding information in a form that permits it to be stored effectively in memory and remembered later. Access to information is also part of our knowledge base and is crucial to our ability to perceive stimuli in our environment. Perceiving what objects look like is dependent on having access to knowledge that labels stimuli and draws inferences about how any stimulus is related to other stimuli. Tasks as basic as perceiving the constancy of an object depend on efficient access to knowledge memory. Understanding that an object remains the same even though it may change position or look different as a function of lighting conditions depends on efficient access to knowledge memory. Alzheimer's disease is the best clinical example of a disease process that disrupts knowledge memory. This type of cognitive impairment typically involves apraxia and problems in finding words and completing well-learned procedures and routines. In fact, many of the impairments in recent memory that are so obvious in Alzheimer patients are associated with the patient's inability to search quickly and use previously acquired knowledge in decoding, encoding, and elaborating information. For example, these patients may have difficulty adding to a list of fruits or clothing articles. They may also have problems describing the sequence of events in a routine day. This disruption of information processing when patients cannot access and encode what they know is called "knowledge memory failure." It is this serious disruption in memory processes, as well as recent memory loss, that makes the functional impairment of Alzheimer patients so devastating. A similar pattern of memory disruption can be caused by certain drugs (such as the anticholinergic drug, scopolamine), which are useful in the pharmacological modelling of Alzheimer's disease in animals and humans (7).

EPISODIC MEMORY FAILURE

Episodic memory refers to memory for events linked to a unique context and specific time (8). When patients can attend and appreciate an event in terms of past experience, it is still possible that these patients cannot make a permanent record of this experience because they cannot consolidate the memory. For instance, patients may have immediate recall of items on a list, but when asked to recite the list minutes or hours later, they have no recall of ever having learned the list. In this situation, there is a problem between perception and registration of the stimulus, and encoding the stimulus in memory. This type of memory failure commonly occurs in amnestic patients with Korsakoff's disease, who are unable to consolidate or remember recent events (5,9). A similar clinical situation can also exist in patients with bilateral damage to the temporal lobes and hippocampus. Such patients can attend and access what they already know to make sense of the incoming stimuli, but cannot remember recent events because they cannot consolidate memories. A similar condition operates in drug-induced amnestic states such as those following benzodiazepines, which are known to interfere with cognitive functions involved in establishing a permanent record of ongoing experiences. Such patients, like amnestics, can remember events that have just occurred but have difficulty recalling events that have occurred hours earlier. This type of memory dysfunction is called a "failure in recent memory" by clinicians and "episodic memory process failure" by cognitive neuroscientists. Several recent publications have reviewed this complex and multifaceted area of research (5,6).

EFFORT-DEMANDING VERSUS NONEFFORT-DEMANDING PROCESSES

Another useful way of dividing memory into psychobiologically distinct components is to look at effort-demanding versus noneffort-demanding processes

(10-15) since some cognitive operations require more effort and concentration than others. Patients with certain neuropsychiatric illnesses characteristically have difficulty with effort-demanding tasks, while they perform normally on tasks not requiring effort. For example, patients with depression and Parkinson's disease, often have problems with tasks requiring prolonged concentration, while they have no difficulty with less effort-demanding tasks (14). Such patients may not be able to retain information about the news heard from a car radio but still not lose their way or make errors in shifting gears while driving the car. The dementia patient, however, has problems with both effort- and noneffort-demanding tasks. Consequently, this type of memory process failure may be useful in differentiating between patients with a true dementia, and those with the so-called "pseudodementia" or memory loss associated with depression.

SPECIFIC DRUG CLASSES
AND THEIR EFFECTS ON MEMORY

In addition to being useful clinically, the classification of different memory processes and types of memory process failure should be considered when examining the effects of various drugs on memory. In this section, various classes of drugs and their differential effects on memory are discussed. However, it is important to make the following generalization before describing each class of drugs in detail: Differences between effects of different drugs may be caused by several variables such as dose, route of administration, and bioavailability of the drug. For example, a high dose versus a low dose of ethanol may have different effects on cognition. The social and educational background of the patient may also influence the cognitive effects of various drugs. For instance, Alzheimer patients who are well-educated and have had a high degree of success in their professional, interpersonal and social lives, may exhibit a different pattern of cognitive changes from patients who have had little formal education and been socially disadvantaged.

ANTICHOLINERGIC DRUGS

There has been extensive research on the effects of anticholinergic agents on memory. The studies of Deutsch (16) have documented a clear role for cholinergic neurotransmission in memory. Clinical studies with the central muscarinic antagonist, scopolamine, provide evidence for the involvement of the cholinergic system in memory and learning (17). Some of these studies provide the theoretical bases for the cholinergic hypothesis in geriatric memory loss (18). Studies have shown that an antagonist like scopolamine can transiently impair performance on a variety of memory tasks, including episodic memory, and retrieval and access to semantic memory. Scopolamine affects the learning of new information; immediate recall on digit span is not affected but the storage of new memories is disrupted, as shown by testing on "supra-span" sequences (17). There are some conflicting data about the effects of scopolamine on retrieval of previously learned information. Some authors report that scopolamine does not impair the recall of information learned immediately before drug treatment (19,20), while others report that the drug interferes with the retrieval of previously learned information (17). Most studies suggest that scopolamine can interfere with the acquisition and storage of new information (19-22). It also appears that anticholinergic agents can disrupt the retrieval process from knowledge memory (17,23). These deficits in memory can be partially reversed by physostigmine, a cholinesterase inhibitor, suggesting that the effects of scopolamine on memory are specific to the cholinergic system. The effect of scopolamine on memory in younger subjects mimics the changes seen with normal aging (17), and the effect of scopolamine on memory in older normals mimic the changes seen in Alzheimer's disease (7). The effect of scopolamine on attention may be dose related. It has been shown that attention was not affected at a lower dose, but was impaired at a higher dose. This impairment was independent of the sedative and behavioral effects of the drug (22).

Alzheimer's disease is characterized clinically by progressive memory impairment. Neuropathological studies have demonstrated prominent loss of cholinergic cell bodies in the nucleus basalis of Meynert (24) and loss of presynaptic choline acetyltransferase (25), an enzyme involved in the synthesis of acetylcholine. Studies have shown an association between the severity of the cholinergic deficits and the degree of the memory impairment (26). In Alzheimer's disease, there is usually disruption of episodic and knowledge memory processes (3). Patients with Alzheimer's disease have difficulty in accessing what has already been encoded in their knowledge memory. This pattern of cognitive impairment can be seen in elderly normals following administration of scopolamine, suggesting that the cognitive and memory impairments in Alzheimer's disease are closely linked to the widespread derangement in the cholinergic system associated with this illness. Furthermore, short-term treatment with agents such as tetrahydroaminoacridine and physostigmine which enhance the chilinergic system have shown some improvement in the performance of cognitive tasks in patients with Alzheimer's disease (27,28). These data further support the importance of the cholinergic system in human memory.

The pharmacological modelling of Alzheimer's disease with anticholinergic agents, however, may not be specific. Benzodiazepines can produce an "Alzheimer-like" response in normals, although these effects have been seen at higher doses and are therefore potentially less selective than respective doses of anticholinergic agents (29). Furthermore, memory disruption induced in animals by administration of scopolamine can be reversed with serotonin reuptake blockers (30) and nootropic agents (31). Thus, although some evidence for the specificity of the cholinergic system in the memory loss of Alzheimer's disease is available, it is far from conclusive. Other neurotransmitter systems, such as the serotonergic and peptidergic systems, may also be involved.

BENZODIAZEPINES

The cognitive effects of benzodiazepines have been well characterized in humans (32). The best documented cognitive effect of benzodiazepines has been anterograde amnesia (33). The time of onset and duration of this effect varies according to the benzodiazepine used, but the effect can last more than 6 hours. Although they disrupt the encoding and consolidating phase of learning, benzodiazepines have not been found to affect immediate recall and access to previously acquired information. One problem of using benzodiazepines as a model of dementia is the difficulty in separating different components of memory since the amnestic effects of these agents are also accompanied by sedative effects. Therefore, it is difficult to say whether the effects of benzodiazepines on memory are specific, or whether they are secondary to the sedative effect. Memory impairment without sedation, however, has been demonstrated in a number of studies, suggesting that the effect of the benzodiazepines on memory is specific.

The pattern of memory impairment produced by benzodiazepines is different from that produced by anticholinergic agents. In contrast to the anticholinergic agents, benzodiazepines do not interfere with previously learned information (34). Benzodiazepines have more selective disruptive effect on episodic memory, so the encoding of new memories is specially impaired. This type of memory impairment most closely resembles that of the alcoholic amnestic syndrome. In an elaborate experiment supporting the hypothesis that memory has distinct components that can be separated out by specific pharmacologic agents, physostigmine antagonized the effect of scopolamine on memory, but had no effects on the effect of diazepam on memory (21). This finding suggests that the effects of benzodiazepines on memory are pharmacologically distinct from those of anticholinergic agents and cannot be antagonized by cholinergic stimulation. It is well accepted that the effects of benzodiazepines are mediated via specific benzodiazepine receptors in the central nervous system (CNS) (35), which occur with high density in the hippocampus. The fact that the amnestic effect of the benzodiazepines can be reversed by the benzodiazepine antagonist, RO 15-1788, suggests that the benzodiazepine receptor complex is involved in memory (36). The effect of benzodiazepines on memory is probably mediated, at least indirectly, through GABA, since agents that enhance GABAergic transmission impair memory (37,38) and agents that interfere with GABA facilitate memory task performance in animal models (37). The finding that diazepam-induced memory loss is not reversed by physostigmine also suggests that the amnestic effect of benzo-diazepines involves noncholinergic mechanisms.

Benzodiazepines can produce an amnestic syndrome that impairs new memory formation without affecting access to previously learned information. Increasing doses of benzodiazepines produce a marked deficit in episodic memory with knowledge memory remaining completely intact (33,39,40). These studies further support the hypothesis that episodic and knowledge memory functions are psychobiologically distinct. This amnestic syndrome is indistinguishable from the alcohol amnestic syndrome associated with chronic alcohol consumption. Benzodiazepines may provide a human model for this amnestic syndrome and thus be used in experiments designed to modify this cognitive dysfunction.

NEUROPEPTIDES

During the past two decades, there has been an explosion of research concerning the possible role of neuropeptides in CNS functioning. Neuropeptides, such as vasopressin, oxytocin, endorphins, ACTH, CCK, and MSH, have all been implicated in learning, memory, attention, and habituation (41-45). The hypotheses implicating these various neuropeptides have largely come from studies of the behavioral effects of these substances in animals (41). For example, rats lacking antidiurectic hormone (ADH) are impaired in the acquisition and retention of certain learned behaviors and these behaviors are corrected by the administration of ADH. Such treatments also improve learning and memory of normal rats whose memory have been impaired by puromycin, CO_2 treatment, or electroconvulsive shock.

Data on the effects of the neuropeptides on human memory processes are not as compelling (46,47) and studies with head injury patients and alcoholics have produced conflicting results (48-51). Studies in patients with dementia have shown that a single administration of lysine-vasopressin (LVP) improved performance on word retention tasks and semantic memory (52,53). In another study of cognitive performance, LVP affected only the reaction time, leading the authors to conclude that vasopressin had a nonspecific activating effect on memory (49,50). Thus the effect of vasopressin on cognition resembles that of central and peripheral catecholamines and other stimulants (44,45). These substances affect the different aspects of information processing in a way that is entirely consistent with the body's integrated arousal response-enhanced selective attention and with facilitation of effortful processing. These similarities are also consistent with the biochemical and electrophysiological data, which show vasopressin to increase catecholamine activity in the brain (46) and, with animal data, which show the behavioral effects of vasopressin to be dependent of an intact catecholaminergic system (42,54).

ETHANOL

Many studies have documented cognitive impairment in response to the consumption of alcohol-containing beverages (55). Many of these studies suggest that alcohol, when given acutely, primarily affects the acquisition of new information rather than the retrieval of previously learned material (56-59). If information is presented to the subjects while they are in an intoxicated state, their ability to recall a series of events is markedly impaired, regardless of whether retrieval takes place when subjects are sober or intoxicated. While intoxicated subjects have difficulty learning new information, they show little impairment in remembering previously acquired learning. In some instances, subjects even demonstrate some improved retrieval of information learned prior to consumption of ethanol. Therefore, it is unlikely that alcohol impairs retrieval ability (60). Furthermore, ethanol does not appear to impair retention of previously learned material. This finding has been demonstrated in experiments in which subjects acquired and retrieved information in sober states and became intoxicated between these two processes. No memory impairments are found when ethanol is administered between storage and retrieval of new information.

However, subjects may show ethanol-induced impairments in acquisition of new information for several reasons. Intoxicated subjects may not perceive the incoming stimuli as well as sober subjects. Furthermore, intoxicated subjects may not attend to the stimuli, or may not process and encode information efficiently. Ethanol may also produce disruption in attention. Data in support of such a hypothesis comes from the results of recall tasks, in which alcohol caused the greatest impairment on the recall of the first few events. In these studies, recall of events in the middle of a sequence was slightly impaired, whereas recall of the last few events was generally unimpaired. If impaired perception accounts for these learning deficits, then subjects would be expected to show deficits in recalling events from all locations on the list.

Since learning impairment have been associated with decreases in arousal and since ethanol possesses CNS depressant properties, it is possible that the effect of ethanol on cognition could be mediated in part by its sedative effects. The interrelationship between sedative and cognitive effects has yet to be fully understood.

In contrast to the finding that ethanol intoxication impairs learning, there is some evidence that ethanol can improve memory if given after a learning task. It may be that alcohol causes an indirect stimulant effect, or produces some positive cognitive effects by causing a "retrograde facilitation" that reduces interfering stimuli presented after adminstration of ethanol. This "retrograde facilitation" has also been observed with benzodiazepines (39), whose effects on cognition closely resemble those of ethanol.

STIMULANTS

Amphetamine and other stimulants affect cognition by directly releasing the neurotransmitters, dopamine and norepinephrine, and by blocking catecholamine reuptake. In animal studies, psychostimulants have been shown to have consistent effects on learning and memory variables (61,62). Although many studies have examined the cognitive effects of these agents in human populations, there are many contradictory findings. Some studies have shown that prior treatment with amphetamine can accelerate acquisition of a list of word pairs (63), while one study (64) has demonstrated a similar enhancement of persistence and recall of learned material. The most consistent effects of stimulants have been on measures of attention and arousal. Amphetamine usually improves performance on tasks that require sustained attention (65, 66), particularly in subjects who are fatigued (65). Although such studies suggest that stimulants may improve some aspects of cognition, it has yet to be shown whether effects are simply a reversal of some deficit state induced by fatigue and decreased attention. These findings suggest that stimulants have a greater effect on effort-demanding processes than on automatic processes.

CONCLUSION

We have attempted to construct here a clinically and experimentally useful model to evaluate memory by separating it into psychobiologically distinct processes. This model allows us to examine various memory disorders and to begin to characterize how specific components of memory may be differentially affected in each disorder. We have also demonstrated the capacity of certain psychopharmacological agents to disrupt some psychobiologically distinct components of memory, making these drugs useful in pharmacological models of human memory failure.

With the recent progress made in neuroscience, it is now appropriate to apply cognitive science to neuropsychopharmacology. However, simply documenting human responsivity to drugs is not sufficient if we are to understand how drugs alter mental functions. Instead, current knowledge of different types of memory failure provides us with the means to evaluate with some precision the specific ways that drugs alter cognitive function. This knowledge, in turn, provides a rational scheme for developing a neurochemical taxonomy of distinct cognitive processes.

   This convergence of fields has several implications for future research and clinical applications. First, drug strategies are being used increasingly to explore the psychobiological bases of cognitive functions. Drug studies in neuropsychiatric populations have important advantages over studies of patients with lesions because drug challenges with neuropharmacological probes allow us to use subjects as their own controls. Second, information on how different classes and doses of psychoactive drugs alter cognition can be used to classify and define groups of patients for diagnostic purposes. With this information, we can use drugs to highlight existing changes in CNS function by further disrupting cognition in a specific fashion. Thus, this type of research can logically lead to the development of neuropharmacological models of different forms of syndrome-specific cognitive failure and could, in turn, provide new insights into our understanding of the unique mechanisms that determine different types of cognitive failure. However, these drug strategies will only be helpful if characterization of cognitive changes is systematic and precise. Third, many drugs that produce cognitive changes are also drugs with abuse potential. Understandably, the potential abuse of any class of drugs is dependent upon several different factors, but it certainly requires that the drug produces a qualitative shift in how individuals process information, perceive the world around them, and retrieve information from previous experience. A systematic evaluation of cognitive changes with and without drugs may provide some important new insights and strategies useful for examining the properties of these drugs of abuse.

REFERENCES

1. Tulving, E. (1985). How many memory systems? *Am. Psychol. 40*:385-398.
2. Squire, L.R., and Davis, H.P. (1981). The pharmacology of memory: A neurobiological perspective. *Annu. Rev. Pharmacol. Toxicol. 21*:323-356.
3. Weingartner, H., Grafman, J., Boutell, W., Kaye, W., and Martin, P.R. (1983). Forms of memory failure. *Science 221*:380-382.
4. Squire, L.R., and Zola-Morgan, S. (1983). The neurology of memory: The case for correspondence between the findings in man and the non-human primate. In *The Physiological Basis of Memory*, 2nd ed. Edited by J.A. Deutsch. New York, Academic Press, pp. 199-267.
5. Squire, L.R., and Butters, N. (1984). *Neuropsychology of Memory*. New York, Guilford Press.
6. Olton, D., and Gamzu, E. (1985). *New York Academy of Science 444*
7. Sunderland, T., Tariot, P.N., Cohen, R.M., Weingartner, H., Mueller, E.A., and Murphy, D.L. (1987). Anticholinergic sensitivity in patients with dementia of the Alzheimer type and age-matched controls: A dose-response study. *Arch. Gen. Psychiatr. 44*:418-426.
8. Tulving, W. (1982). *Elements of Episodic Memory*. New York, Oxford University Press.

9. Squire, L.R. (1982). Comparisons between forms of amnesia: Some deficits are unique to Korsakoff's syndrome. *J. Exp. Psychol. 8*:560-571.

10. Kahnemann, D. (1973). *Attention and Effort.* Englewood Cliffs, NJ, Prentice Hall.

11. Hasher, L., and Zacks, R.T. (1979). Automatic and effortful processes in memory. *J. Exp. Psycho. [Gen]. 108*:356-388.

12. Hasher, L., and Zacks, R.T. (1984). Automatic processing of fundamental information: The case of frequency of occurrence. *Am. Psychol. 39*:1372-1388.

13. Hirst, W., and Volpe, B.T. (1984). Automatic and effortful encoding in amnesia. In *Handbook of Cognitive Neuroscience.* Edited by M.S. Gazzaniga. New York, Plenum Press, pp. 369-386.

14. Weingartner, H., Burns, S., Diebel, R., and LeWitt, P.A. (1984). Cognitive impairments in Parkinson's disease: Distinguishing between effort-demanding and automatic cognitive processes. *Psychiatry Res. 11*:223-235.

15. Weingartner, H., Cohen, R.M., Sunderland, T., Tariot, P.N., and Thompson, K. (1987). Diagnosis and assessment of cognitive dysfunctions in the elderly. In *Psychopharmacology: The Third Generation of Progress.* Edited by H. Meltzer. New York, Raven Press, pp. 909-919.

16. Deutsch, J.A. (1971). The cholinergic synapse and the site of memory. *Science 174*:783-794.

17. Drachman, D.A., and Leavitt, J. (1974). Human memory and the cholinergic system. *Arch. Neurol. 30*:113-121.

18. Bartus, R.T., Dean, R.L., Beer, B., and Lippa, A.S. (1982). The cholinergic hypothesis of geriatric memory dysfunction. *Science 217*:408-417.

19. Ghoneim, M.M., and Mewaldt, S.P. (1975). Effects of diazepam and scopolamine on storage, retrieval, and organizational processes in memory. *Psychopharmacologia 44*:257-262.

20. Petersen, R.C. (1977). Scopolamine induced learning failures in man. *Psychopharmacology 52*:283-289.

21. Ghoneim, M.M., and Mewaldt, S.P. (1977). Studies on human memory: The interactions of diazepam, scopolamine, and physostigmine. *Psychopharmacology 52*:1-6.

22. Safer, D.J., and Allen, R.P. (1971). The central effects of scopolamine in man. *Biol. Psychiatry 3*:347-355.

23. Wolkowitz, O.M., Tinklenberg, J.R., and Weingartner, H. (1985). A psychopharmacological perspective of cognitive functions: II. Specific pharmacological agents. *Neuropsychobiology 14*:133-156.

24. Whitehouse, P.J., Price, D.L., Struble, R.G., Clark, A.W., Coyle, J.T., and DeLong, M.R. (1982). Alzheimer's disease and senile dementia: Loss of neurons in the basal forebrain. *Science 215*:1237-1239.

25. Davies, P., and Maloney, A.J. (1976). Selective loss of central cholinergic neurons in Alzheimer's disease. *Lancet 2*:1403-1405.

26. Perry, E.K., Tomlinson, B.E., Blessed, G., Bergmann, K., Gibson, P.H., and Perry, R.H. (1978). Correlation of cholinergic abnormalities with senile plaques and mental test scores in senile dementia. *Br. Med. J. 2*:1457-1459.

27. Mohs, R.C., Davis, B.N., Johns, C.A., Mathe, A.A., Greenwald, B.S., Horvath, T.B., and Davis, K.L. (1985). Oral physostigmine treatment of patients with Alzheimer's disease. *Am. J. Psychiatry 142*:28-33.

28. Summers, W.K., Majouski, L.V., March, Q.M., Tachiki, K., and Kling, A. (1986). Oral tetrahydroaminoacridine in long-term treatment of senile dementia of the Alzheimer type. *N. Engl. J. Med. 315*:1241-1245.

29. Block, R.I., DeVoe, M., Stanley, B., Stanley, M., and Pomara, N. (1985). Memory performance in individuals with primary degenerative dementia: Its similarity to diazepam-induced impairments. *Exp. Aging Res. 11*:151-155.

30. Flood, J.F., and Cherkin, A. (1985). Fluoxetine enhances memory processes in mice. *Psychopharmacology 93*:36-43.

31. Verloes, R., Scotto, A.M., Gobert, J., and Wulfert, E. (1988). Effects of nootropic drugs in a scopolamine-induced amnesia model in mice. *Psychopharmacology 95*:226-230.

32. Lister, R.B. (1985). The amnesic action of benzodiazepines in man. *Neurosci. Biobehav. Rev. 9*:87-94.

33. Wolkowitz, O.M., Weingartner, H., Thompson, K., Pickar, D., Paul, S.M., and Hommer, D.W. (1987). Diazepam induced amnesia: A neuropharmacological model of an "organic amnestic syndrome." *Am. J. Psychiatry 144*:25-29.

34. Petersen, R.C., and Ghoneim, M.M. (1980). Diazepam and human memory: Influence on acquisition, retrieval, and state-dependent learning. *Proc. Neuro-Psychopharmacol. 4*:81-89.

35. Braestro, P.C., and Mogens, N. (1982). Neurotransmitters and central nervous system anxiety disease. *Lancet 2*:1030-1034.

36. O'Boyle, C., Lambe, R., Darragh, A., Taffe, W., Brick, I., and Kenny, M. (1983). RO-15-1788 antagonizes the effects of diazepam in man without affecting its bioavailability. *Br. J. Anaesth. 55*:349-355.

37. Katz, R.J., and Lieber, L. (1978). GABA involvement in memory consolidation: Evidence from a post-trial amino-oxyacetic acid. *Psychopharmacology [Berlin] 56*:191-193.

38. Jobert, A., Thiebot, M.H., and Soubrie, P. (1979). A comparative study of the effects of muscimol and diazepam on the recall of noxious events. *Experientia 35*: 239-240.

39. Hinrichs, J.V., Ghoneim, M.M., and Mewaldt, S.P. (1984). Diazepam and memory: Retrograde facilitation produced by interference reduction. *Psychopharmacology 84*:158-162.

40. Hommer, D.W., Matsuo, V., Wolkowitz, O., Chrousos, G., Greenblatt, D.J., Weingartner, H., and Paul, S.M. (1986). Benzodiazepine receptor sensitivity in normal human subjects. *Arch Gen. Psychiatry 43*:542-551.

41. de Wied, D. (1971). Long-term effects of vasopressin on the maintenance of a conditioned avoidance response in rats. *Nature 232*:58-60.

42. Kovacs, G.L., Bohus, S., and Versteeg, D.H.G. (1979). The effects of vasopressin on memory processes: The role of noradrenergic neurotransmission. *Neuroscience 4*:1529-1537.

43. Beckwith, B.E., Petros, T., Kanaan-Beckwith, S., Couk, D.I., and Haug, R.J. (1982). Vasopressin analog (DDAVP) facilitates concept learning in human males. *Peptides 3*:627-630.

44. McGaugh, J.L. (1983a). Hormonal influences on memory. *Ann. Rev. Psychol. 34*:297-323.

45. McGaugh, J.L. (1983b). Preserving the presence of the past: Hormonal influences on memory storage. *Am. Psychol. 38*:161-174.
46. Tanaka, M., De Kloet, E.F., de Wied, D., and Versteeg, D.H.G. (1977). Arginine-8-vasopressin affects catecholamine metabolism in specific brain nuclei. *Life Sci. 20*:1799-1808.
47. Esposito, R.U., Parker, E.S., and Weingartner, H. (1984). Enkephalinergic-dopaminergic "reward" pathways: A critical substrate for the stimulatory, euphoric and memory enhancing actions of alcohol: A hypothesis. *Subst. Alcohol Actions 5*:111-119.
48. Oliveros, J.C., Jandali, M.K., Timsit-Berthier, M., Remy, R., Behghezal, A., Audibert, A., and Moeglan, J.H. (1978). Vasopressin amnesia. *Lancet 1*:41.
49. Tinklenberg, J.R., Pfefferbaum, A., and Berger, P.A. (1981). 1-Desamino-D-arginine vasopressin (DDAVP) in cognitively impaired patients. *Psychopharmacol. Bull. 17*:206-207.
50. Tinklenberg, J.R., Pigache, R., Pfefferbaum, A., Berger, P.A., and Kopell, B.S. (1982). 8-L-Arginine-9-desglycinamide-vasopressin (Organon 5667) and cognitively impaired patients. *Psychopharmacol. Bull. 18*:202-204.
51. Jenkins, J.S., Mather, H.M., Coughlin, A.K., and Jenkins, D.O. (1982). Desmopressin and desglycinamide vasopressin in post-traumatic amnesia. *Lancet 1*:39.
52. Weingartner, H., Gold, P., Ballenger, J.C., Smallberg, S.A., Summers, R., Rubinow, D.R., Post, R.M., and Goodwin, F.K. (1981). Effects of vasopressin on human memory function. *Science 211*:601-603.
53. Weingartner, H., Kaye, W., Gold, P., Smallberg, S., Petersen, R., Gillin, J.C., and Ebert, M. (1981). Vasopressin treatment of cognitive dysfunction in progressive dementia. *Life Sci. 29*:2721-2726.
54. Kovacs, G.L., Vecsei, L., Medve, L., and Telegdy, G. (1980). Effects of endogenous vasopressin content of the brain on memory processes: The role of catecholaminergic mechanisms. *Exp. Brain Res. 38*:357-361.
55. Parsons, O.A., Butters, N., and Nathan, P. (1987). *Neuropsychology of Alcoholism: Implications for Diagnosis and Treatment.* New York, Guildford Press.
56. Rosen, L.J., and Lee, C.L. (1976). Acute and chronic effects of alcohol use on organizational processes in memory. *J. Abnorm. Psychol. 85*:309-317.
57. Birnbaum, I.M., and Parker, E.S. (1977). *Alcohol and Human Memory.* Hillsdale, NJ, Lawrence Erlbaum Associates.
58. Hashtroudi, S., Parker, E.S., DeLisi, L.E., and Wyatt, R.J. (1983). On elaboration and alcohol. *J. Verb. Learn. Verb. Behav. 22*:164-173.
59. Williams, H.L., and Rundell, O.H. (1984). Effect of alcohol on recall and recognition as functions of processing levels. *J. Stud. Alcohol 45*:10-15.
60. Birnbaum, I.M., Parker, E.S., Hartley, J.T., and Noble, E.P. (1978). Alcohol and memory: Retrieval processes. *J. Verb. Learn. Verb. Behav. 17*:325-335.
61. McGaugh, J.L. (1973). Drug facilitation of learning and memory. *Annu. Rev. Psychol. 13*:229-241.
62. Alpern, H.P., and Jackson, S.J. (1978). Short-term memory: A neuropharmacologically distinct process. *Behav. Biol. 22*:133-146.
63. Weitzner, M. (1965). Manifest anxiety, amphetamine, and performance. *J. Psychol. 60*:71-79.

64. Hurst, P.M., Radlow, R., Chubb, N.C., and Bagley, S.K. (1969). Effects of d-amphetamine on acquisition, persistence, and recall. *Am. J. Psychol. 82*:307-319.
65. Weiss, B., and Laties, V.G. (1962). Enhancement of human performance by caffeine and the amphetamines. *Pharmacol. Rev. 14*:1-36.
66. Hamilton, M.J., Bush, M., Smith, P., and Peck, A.W. (1982). The effect of buspirone, a new antidepressant drug, and diazepam, and their interaction in man. *Br. J. Clin. Pharmacol. 14*:791-797.

6

Models of Memory and the Understanding of Memory Disorders

Daniel L. Schacter, Alfred W. Kaszniak, and John F. Kihlstrom

University of Arizona
Tucson, Arizona

In 1882, Theodule Ribot published one of the now classic treatises of 19th century psychology, *Diseases of Memory*. In addition to describing and integrating a large number of clinical studies of memory problems, Ribot also argued forcefully that these observations should not be viewed merely as "a collection of amusing anecdotes" (1, p. 10). Instead, he contended that the phenomena encountered in cases of memory disorders are "regulated by certain laws which constitute the very basis of memory, and from which its mechanism is easily laid bare" (1, p. 10). Ribot went on to suggest various ways in which the study of memory deficits could provide important insights into the nature of normal memory processes. Unfortunately, as pointed out by Schacter and Tulving (2), subsequent studies of memory pathology made little or no impact on experimental and theoretical analyses of normal memory function for most of the 100 years following the publication of Ribot's work; likewise, clinical observations of memory deficits were relatively uninfluenced by the techniques and ideas of experimental psychology for much of the same period. Schacter and Tulving have delineated some of the negative consequences attributable to the gulf that separated the study of normal and abnormal memory for nearly a century.

During the 1970s, however, there were signs that the gap between the two research areas had begun to narrow, and on that basis Schacter and Tulving (2, p. 2) predicted the coming of a "golden age" characterized by much more extensive and fruitful interactions between students of normal and abnormal memory than had existed previously. As Shimamura (3) points out, a number of developments during the past several years suggest that the "golden age" is upon us: empirical phenomena observed in memory-disordered patients have heavily influenced theorizing about normal memory; research concerning memory deficits has made extensive use of paradigms and theories from experimental psychology; and studies of memory-impaired populations have appeared with increasing regularity in the pages of mainstream experimental and cognitive journals.

In view of these encouraging recent developments, it seems appropriate and even necessary for a clinically oriented volume to include a chapter that focuses on the relation between models of normal memory and the understanding of memory disorders. The main purpose of our contribution is to summarize briefly some of the ways in which the analysis of memory disorders is currently being influenced by—as well as contributing to—contemporary thinking about normal memory. To accomplish this objective, we shall consider research concerning three different populations in which memory deficits are observed: amnesic patients, demented patients, and the normal elderly. Since it is not practically feasible to discuss all theoretical aspects of memory disorders in these populations, we limit ourselves to considering several distinctions between different *types* or *forms* of memory that have influenced thinking about memory disorders: the distinctions between primary and secondary memory (4,5), episodic and semantic memory (6,7), and implicit and explicit memory (8,9), respectively. The main reason for such a focus, as opposed to other sorts of models, is that they have been central to various debates and discussions about the nature of memory disorders in recent years. It should be noted, however, that a number of well-articulated and reasonably precise formal models of memory do exist (10-14). However, there has been little if any attempt to apply these models to clinical populations (for an exception, see Ref. 15). Although we think that formal modelling of memory disorders is a potentially valuable enterprise—and would even predict that this will constitute one of the next major theoretical trends—we restrict the present focus to ideas that have already played a role in shaping contemporary thinking about the nature of memory disorders.

THE AMNESIC SYNDROME

The amnesic syndrome is perhaps the most striking of all memory disorders, insofar as a profound inability to remember recent events occurs against a background of relatively intact cognitive, linguistic, and perceptual abilities (for review, see Refs. 16-18). Though observed as a consequence of various types of brain injury and disease, amnesia is usually attributable to damage in either the medial temporal and diencephalic brain regions (19,20). A good deal of research and theorizing during the past two decades has focused on distinguishing between preserved and impaired memory processes in amnesic patients.

PRIMARY AND SECONDARY MEMORY

One of the great debates in experimental psychology during the 1960s concerned the distinction between short-term and long-term memory. According to the modal model (cf., Refs. 5,21), it is necessary to draw a sharp distinction between two different memory stores or systems: a *short-term store* that is characterized by limited capacity, exclusive reliance on acoustic codes, and extremely rapid decay; and a *long-term store* that is characterized by unlimited capacity, reliance on semantic codes, and a slower rate of forgetting. Although the modal model was worked out in impressive quantitative detail and received experimental support, serious conceptual and empirical problems with this view were delineated during the 1970s—most notably by Craik and Lockhart (22), resulting in what Crowder (23) called the demise of the concept of short-term memory. Despite their rejection of the modal model, however, even Craik and Lockhart recognized the need to preserve some sort of distinction between immediate and delayed retention. *Primary memory* refers to the processes that support immediate retention, whereas *secondary memory* refers to processes that support retention across delays (4).

The distinction between primary and secondary memory fits nicely with, and receives empirical support from, studies of amnesic patients. One of the most consistently observed features of the amnesic syndrome is that even the most profoundly amnesic patients exhibit normal immediate retention of various kinds of information, as assessed by such tasks as digit span (e.g., 24, 25). If primary memory is equated with immediate retention, there can be little doubt that amnesic patients possess intact primary memory. Moreover, the primary/secondary distinction also receives support from studies of patients who exhibit normal long-term retention together with severely impaired immediate memory (e.g., 26). Controversy has arisen, however, concerning the ability of amnesic patients to retain information across relatively brief delays (i.e., 3-30 seconds) under conditions in which rehearsal is prevented, as in the classic Brown-Peterson short-term forgetting paradigm. Although normal forgetting by amnesic patients in this paradigm has been observed (24,27), impaired performance has also been reported (e.g., 28,29). The reasons for these discrepant findings are still not entirely clear (for discussion, see Refs. 16,27,30). Nevertheless, they indicate that any global statements about amnesic patients' ability to remember information across brief delays must be regarded cautiously. We can conclude unequivocally that primary memory is intact in amnesic patients only so long as "primary memory" is identified with immediate retention.

The most extensively investigated theoretical account of primary memory is found in the *working memory* model developed by Baddeley and his colleagues (see Ref. 31). According to Baddeley, working memory consists of three main components: a limited-capacity *central executive* that is involved in selection and control functions; the *articulatory loop*, a "slave subsystem" of the central executive that allows for temporary storage of up to three items of speech-based information; and the *visuospatial scratchpad*, which provides temporary storage of nonverbal information. Baddeley's group has reported a variety of elegant experiments using dual-task methodology that have supported the working memory model by teasing apart and delineating properties of the various subsystems. The model has been applied successfully to some memory-disordered populations (31), but as yet has not been systematically evaluated with respect to the amnesic syndrome. Research within the working memory framework might help to clarify further the nature of primary memory abilities of amnesic patients.

EPISODIC AND SEMANTIC MEMORY

According to Tulving (6), episodic memory entails recollection of specific autobiographical events that are unique to an individual and are defined by particular spatial and temporal contexts, whereas semantic memory involves general knowledge of the world; facts, vocabulary, rules, and the like that is common to many individuals. Although Tulving (6) initially put forward the episodic/semantic distinction as a heuristic device, he later took the stronger position that episodic and semantic memory represent distinct and dissociable memory systems (7). A good deal of controversy still exists concerning this latter, theoretically based version of the distinction (cf., Refs. 32,33).

With respect to the amnesic syndrome, the episodic/semantic distinction appears initially to provide a compelling account of patients' preserved and impaired abilities (29). After all, one of the most striking features of amnesia is the coexistence of a severe inability to remember recent events (episodic memory) with a normal ability to retrieve general knowledge and vocabulary (semantic memory). However, as pointed out by Huppert and Piercy (34) and Zola-Morgan et al. (35), this pattern of performance can be equally well described as an impairment in new learning together with intact access to old, premorbid knowledge acquired long before the onset of amnesia; that is, the distinction between episodic and semantic memory is confounded with the distinction between new and old learning. Thus, the critical questions for an episodic/semantic account of amnesia concern the status of new semantic learning (which should be intact) and old episodic memories (which should be impaired).

Consider first the question of whether amnesic patients can acquire new semantic knowledge, as would be expected if the semantic memory system is entirely preserved. On one hand, it is clear that *some* acquisition of new semantic knowledge occurs in densely amnesic patients. Thus, for example, Kinsborne and Wood (29) reported that Korsakoff amnesics learned and retained a new mathematical rule despite their impaired episodic memory. Schacter, Harbluk, and McLachlan (36) found that an etiologically mixed group of amnesic patients retained some fictitious facts about familiar and unfamiliar people, despite their inability to remember when and where they acquired the facts (see also Ref. 37). Glisky, Schacter, and Tulving (38-40) demonstrated that head-injured and other amnesic patients could learn, and retain across delays of up to nine months, new computer-related vocabulary as well as various complex computer commands and programming rules; even though some patients had no recollection that they had ever worked on a computer (see also Refs. 41,42). These results, as well as other similar reports (cf., 43,44), lend support to the episodic/semantic account. On the other hand, however, amnesic patients' semantic learning in the foregoing studies was consistently and sometimes severely impaired relative to the performance of control subjects; moreover, failure to observe any new semantic learning in amnesia has also been reported (e.g., Ref. 45). These studies thus do not provide strong support for the existence of a spared semantic memory system (for further discussion, see Refs. 2,19,44,46-48).

Studies concerning the status of old, premorbid episodic memories are also somewhat equivocal. Kinsbourne and Wood (29) claimed that amnesic patients could not retrieve any memories of autobiographical incidents in response to word cues (49), in contrast to their normal ability to retrieve old vocabulary and factual knowledge. However, Zola-Morgan et al. (35) reported that amnesic patients were no more impaired in gaining access to old episodic than old semantic memories. In a single-case study, Butters and Cermak (50) reported deficits in access to both premorbid episodic and semantic memories, although the episodic deficit appeared to be rather more severe than the semantic deficit. Tulving et al. (51) described a patient who showed excellent retention of factual knowledge that was acquired at a particular job he had performed prior to the onset of amnesia, yet could not recollect a single incident that occurred during the entire period that he performed the job. The data thus suggest the possibility of an episodic/semantic dissociation within the domain of premorbid knowledge, but the overall picture is still somewhat muddy and a good deal more pertinent evidence needs to be collected. Part of the problem here is that the criteria for distinguishing between episodic and semantic memories are not always stated explicit (for discussion see Refs. 46,51,52), nor is it entirely straightforward to determine what constitutes an "episodic" task and what constitutes a "semantic" task. These kinds of issues will have to be resolved in future attempts to evaluate the utility of the episodic/semantic distinction as an account of amnesia.

IMPLICIT AND EXPLICIT MEMORY

In traditional investigations of episodic memory, subjects initially study target materials and are then tested with recall and recognition tasks that require them to deliberately think back to the study episode and retrieve target information. During the past several years, however, experimental psychologists have assessed memory in a rather different way. Instead of instructing subjects to try to remember previously studied information, they are simply required to perform a task, such as completing a word fragment or identifying a word from a brief perceptual exposure; memory is inferred when task performance is facilitated by prior study of target materials. Graf and Schacter (8,9) used the term *explicit memory* to refer to conscious recollection of recent events on recall and recognition tests, and the term *implicit memory* to refer to facilitations of performance on completion, identification, and other such tests that do not require conscious or intentional recollection of a specific prior episode. Graf and Schacter emphasized that the implicit/explicit dichotomy is a descriptive distinction that does not imply the existence of two separate systems underlying implicit and explicit memory, respectively (for further discussion of definitional and conceptual issues surrounding the implicit/explicit distinction, see Refs. 9,53,54).

The major reason for advancing an implicit/explicit distinction stems from empirical observations of dissociations between performance of recall and recognition tests on the one hand, and completion, identification, and similar tasks on the other. Studies of normal subjects have revealed that a number of experimental variables, including level and type of study processing, retention interval, and study/test modality shifts, have different and even opposite effects on tasks that tap implicit and explicit memory (e.g., 9,55-62). Equally importantly, neuropsychological investigations have shown that amnesic patients show intact performance on various implicit memory tests that do not require conscious recollection of a previous episode. A number of studies have shown that amnesic patients can acquire various kinds of perceptual/motor skills in a normal or near normal manner, despite their inability to remember explicitly the episodes in which they acquired the skills (e.g., 63-66). It has also been established that amnesic patients show normal priming effects on such implicit memory tasks as word completion (67,68), free association (69,70), and category instance production (71,72), as well as various other implicit tests (for review, see 9,44,73).

A number of theoretical proposals have been put forward to account for dissociations between implicit and explicit memory in amnesia. It has been suggested, for example, that intact perceptual and motor skill learning can be attributed to a spared *procedural* memory system that entails on-line modification of processing operations, and that is distinct from a *declarative* system that represents the outcomes of particular processing operations (e.g., 19,74). With respect to priming effects, some investigators have argued that amnesics' intact performance can be attributed to an automatic and temporary activation of pre-existing semantic memory representations (e.g., 46,47, 67,75), whereas others have suggested that priming may reflect the influence of newly created episodic representations that are inaccessible to conscious remembering (e.g., 8,76-78). A related proposal has been put forward recently by Schacter (79), who suggested that many implicit memory phenomena in normal and amnesic subjects can be attributed to the activity of *perceptual representation systems*—processors that represent domain-specific information about the form and structure of words and objects (cf., 80,81), but do not store and retrieve the kinds of information that are necessary for explicit remembering of episodes. Perceptual representation systems are typically unimpaired in amnesic patients, and thus could underly at least some of the implicit memory phenomena that have been observed (see Schacter, 79, for further discussion).

Although the present chapter does not allow us to explore fully the complex issues surrounding implicit/explicit dissociations in amnesic patients, it should be emphasized that this is one area of investigation in which studies of normal and abnormal memory have been, and will likely continue to be, tightly linked to one another. Indeed, the implicit/explicit distinction (unlike the primary/ secondary and episodic/semantic distinctions) was directly motivated by empirical studies of amnesic patients.

MEMORY AND DEMENTIA

According to DSMIII-R, impairment of memory is an essential feature of dementia (82). During the past 15 years, there has been increasing research interest in the nature of memory deficit in various dementing illnesses (e.g., Alzheimer's disease, Huntington's disease). The largest body of this research has focused upon Alzheimer's disease (AD), the most prevalent cause of dementia among older adults (for comprehensive reviews, see Refs. 83-85). Longitudinal psychometric studies of AD patients (86,87) have supported clinical impressions that memory is impaired very early in the course of AD, and deteriorates progressively. We will limit our present discussion to those studies of AD patients relevant to the distinctions between primary/secondary, episodic/semantic, and implicit/explicit memory. It should be noted that conclusions drawn from these studies may not generalize to other dementing illnesses, such as Huntington's disease (e.g., 88).

PRIMARY AND SECONDARY MEMORY

In contrast to amnesic syndrome patients, AD patients show impairment of primary memory, as reflected in impairment on digit, word, and block span tasks, the Brown-Peterson short-term forgetting paradigm, and the recency component of the serial-position curve in list-learning tasks (for review see Refs. 89,90). Although digit span may be normal or only minimally reduced early in the course of AD, it becomes clearly compromised as the disease progresses (86,91). Measures thought to reflect secondary memory, in comparison with those of primary memory, show more severe impairment throughout the course of AD (see Ref. 89).

There have been several attempts to account theoretically for the primary memory deficit of AD patients. Wilson et al. (92) employed a verbal free recall paradigm, using the scoring method of Tulving and Colotla (93) to define primary and secondary memory components. In this scoring method, items recalled with less than seven items between presentation and recall are identified as representing primary memory, and the rest as secondary memory. AD patients, relative to matched healthy controls, showed primary memory impairment, with the size of this impairment increasing linearly with greater numbers of items between presentation and recall. The secondary memory score showed an even greater difference between the groups. Further, although the primary and secondary memory scores were independent in the healthy controls, they were significantly correlated in the AD patients. Finally, Wilson et al. observed a lack of proactive interference effects for the AD patient group, as indicated by no decline in free recall across four consecutive list presentations and by fewer prior list item intrusions than healthy controls (cf. Ref. 94). On the basis of these observations, Wilson et al. (92) proposed that both the primary and secondary memory deficits of AD patients are at least partially the result of initial processing and encoding failure, perhaps reflecting attentional deficit. Martin et al. (95) have suggested a similar explanation of primary and secondary memory deficits in AD.

More recently, Morris and Baddeley (90), using Baddeley's (31) working memory model as a theoretical framework, have argued for impairment in central executive control processes as a cause of the primary memory deficit in AD. In contrast to Wilson et al. (92), Morris and Baddeley propose that this central executive impairment has its major effect on the manipulation and maintenance of information, rather than on its initial encoding. This conclusion is based upon several lines of evidence. First, the documented reduction of digit span in AD does not appear due to impairment in the articulatory loop system. Two subsystems are hypothesized to comprise the articulatory loop system, a phonological store and an articulatory rehearsal mechanism (31). Integrity of the phonological store in AD is inferred from the observation that phonological similarity reduces memory span for letters to the same extent in AD patients as in normal subjects (96), despite the AD patients' moderate overall reduction in span. Integrity of the articulatory rehearsal mechanism in AD is inferred from demonstrations of a normal effect of word length (longer words are presumed to take longer to be recycled through the articulatory loop, leading to slower and less effective rehearsal), a normal rate of articulating a random list of visually presented digits (and hence presumably of subvocal rehearsal), and normal suppression of word and letter memory span by concurrent articulation of irrelevant material (96-99). Second, impairment in the central executive component of working memory is inferred from demonstrations of disproportionate AD patient impairment in performance of various dual tasks (97,100).

Wilson et al. (92), on the basis of their observation that primary and secondary memory scores were independent in healthy controls but were significantly correlated in the AD patients, suggested that the secondary memory impairment of AD may be at least partially attributable to their primary memory deficit. This raises the question of whether all of the memory impairment of AD might be due to a single factor (e.g., impairment of the central executive component of working memory). Recently, Becker (101) presented evidence in support of dissociable contributions of both working memory and secondary memory deficits in AD. The performance of AD patients on tests related to working memory/central executive dysfunction could be statistically dissociated from that on tests related to secondary memory. Further, Becker described individual AD cases for whom the difference between scores on tasks related to these two memory domains was large and in different directions.

In summary, recent research has provided evidence for dissociable contributions of both primary and secondary memory deficit to the progressive memory impairment of AD. Further, studies of AD patients that have employed the working memory model have provided support for the dissociability of hypothesized components of this model. Becker (101) suggests that the secondary memory deficit of AD may be due to the perihippocampal damage that serves to functionally disconnect much of hippocampus and cortex (102,103). Becker further suggests that impairment of the central executive component of working memory may be attributable to pathology of the frontal lobes or their afferent connections in AD (104). An important direction for future research will involve the testing of such hypotheses, particularly through the use of concurrent neuropsychological and regional brain metabolic measures within longitudinal research designs (e.g., 105).

EPISODIC AND SEMANTIC MEMORY

Much research has shown mildly demented AD patients to be comparable to amnesic syndrome (e.g., Korsakoff's) patients in their impairment on episodic memory tasks, such as recall of text passages (e.g., 106). However, unlike amnesic patients, AD patients also show impairment in the recall of previously acquired semantic knowledge. For example, on confrontation naming tasks, AD patients are impaired relative to healthy controls, with this impairment accounted for mostly by semantic errors (e.g., 107). Further, ability to retrieve items from within a given semantic category (e.g., animals) is progressively impaired in AD (87). AD patients produce fewer correct responses than do healthy controls, from fewer subcategories, and produce fewer responses per category (108,109). AD patients also are impaired in their memory for remote public events and public figures (110,111), information that is likely represented as semantic rather than episodic knowledge (46).

Several investigations have provided evidence consistent with the interpretation that semantic memory deficit contributes to the episodic memory impairment of AD. Inadequate semantic encoding of information has been suggested by such observations as the failure of AD patients to show the expected rare word advantage in verbal recognition memory (112), or to benefit from procedures designed to enhance elaborative semantic processing (113,114) and facilitate semantic organization (115) in episodic memory tasks. Significant intercorrelations have been found between episodic (e.g., free recall, selective reminding) and semantic (e.g., category generative naming) memory tasks for AD patients, but not for Korsakoff's amnesics, although both patient groups showed equally profound episodic memory impairment (116).

Although there is consensus that AD patients are impaired on tasks requiring retrieval from semantic memory, there is disagreement concerning the question of whether AD patients have an impairment in the representational structure of semantic memory (see Ref. 117 for a discussion of semantic memory models), or only in those processes necessary for its access (for review see Refs. 83,118). It has been argued (e.g., 119) that tasks such as category generative naming place heavy demands upon effortful processing, and that questions about the structural integrity of semantic memory in AD are more appropriately addressed by tasks involving automatic, implicit activation of lexical or semantic memory. Studies employing lexical and semantic priming paradigms will be discussed in the following section. Even among those studies relying upon explicit tasks, there remains disagreement. For example, some investigators (e.g., 108,120,121) have concluded that general categorical information (e.g., item membership in a superordinate semantic category) remains intact early in the course of AD, while ability to differentiate among items or attributes within a semantic category is impaired. These conclusions have been inferred on the basis of patterns of confrontation and generative naming errors, as well as AD patients' ability to select objects belonging to a specified functional category. Other investigators (122,123) have concluded that representation of the semantic attributes of concepts is intact in AD, based upon the performance of tasks requiring patients to determine whether various attributes (e.g., physical features, functions, actions) were related to a given concept.

In summary, there is general agreement that AD patients are impaired in their performance on tasks requiring episodic memory for recent experience, as well as on tasks requiring explicit retrieval of previously acquired semantic knowledge. Further, in AD patients, semantic memory deficit appears to contribute to the severity of their episodic memory impairment. Disagreement remains, however, concerning the question of whether the representational structure of semantic memory is disturbed in AD, or only those processes necessary for explicitly accessing semantic memory are impaired. An important task for future research is to resolve this controversy. It is possible that differences in dementia severity, or in AD patient sample heterogeneity, might contribute to apparently contradictory findings. Impairment of performance on semantic memory tasks is progressive over the course of AD, and various semantic memory tasks do not reveal equivalent impairment across levels of dementia severity (87,107). Further, the existence of AD patients with unusually severe linguistic/semantic deficits (and hemispherically asymmetric cerebral hypometabolism) early in their disease course have been documented (124,125). The presence of such "linguistic/semantic deficit" AD patients may contribute to variability in the results of prior studies, as they have been shown to demonstrate preserved semantic knowledge on a superordinate and category level but not at the level of object attributes (126).

Another possible contributor to the variability of conclusions within this literature may lie in the demands of the experimental tasks. As Nebes and Brady (123) point out, patients in the Martin and Fedio (108) study were asked explicit questions concerning properties of pictured objects (e.g., Is it used for cutting?), and thus had to search the semantic fields of concepts for particular attributes. In contrast, both Nebes and Brady, and Grober, et al. (122), AD patients were required to indicate whether given attributes were related to particular concepts, and thus had only to recognize that some association exists between the concept and attribute. It remains for future studies to contrast such differing experimental approaches within the same patient sample.

EXPLICIT AND IMPLICIT MEMORY

All of the research involving AD patients described above have used explicit memory tasks, and have documented marked impairment for most tasks. As already mentioned, another approach to the question of whether the structure of semantic memory is impaired in AD has been through the use of implicit memory tasks. Unfortunately, this approach has also failed to settle the controversy. Several investigators (119,127,128) have used semantic priming and semantic category decision tasks in studies of AD patients. They have concluded that the network of associations existing between semantic concepts and attributes remains intact in AD, provided that the patient's use and retrieval of this information is guided by the stimulus context. Other investigators (129-131) have used lexical decision, word-stem completion, and word-association priming tasks. These investigators have found AD patients impaired on these implicit memory tasks, and concluded that conceptual relationships within semantic memory are disrupted. At present, the reasons for these discrepancies between studies are unclear. As with the studies reviewed in the episodic and semantic memory section above, possibilities would appear to include both sample differences as well as differences in experimental methodology, and remain to be determined in future studies.

Studies investigating other implicit memory phenomena in AD patients have also recently begun to appear. Relatively intact motor-skill learning (132,133) has been demonstrated in AD patients. Implicit learning of a repeating sequence of digits (as indicated by a serial reaction time task) was also found for many, although not all, AD patients studied by Knopman and Nissen (134). Those patients who failed to show implicit learning of the sequence were similar to learners in age and overall dementia severity, but scored lower on some tasks of nonverbal reasoning.

In summary, it appears that at least some AD patients are able to demonstrate relatively intact performance on certain implicit memory tasks. Future research will need to clarify the characteristics of both AD patients and tasks that result in preserved implicit memory performance. Such research is of both theoretical and practical importance, since the potential exists for designing interventions and management strategies based upon preserved domains of implicit learning, as has already been done with amnesic patients (e.g., 41,42).

MEMORY AND NORMAL AGING

In addition to the memory loss associated with Alzheimer's disease and other dementias, even normally healthy elders claim to have difficulty learning new information and remembering recent events. Although some complaints about memory function may be related to depression, objective psychometric studies do indicate considerable but selective age-related impairments in memory function (for representative comprehensive reviews see Refs. 135-147). The selectivity of these impairments can be organized in terms of the three heuristic distinctions among forms of memory considered in the preceding sections.

PRIMARY AND SECONDARY MEMORY

There is almost universal agreement that normal aging has little or no deleterious effect on the operation of primary memory, or on the sensory information stores that hold information at a very early stage of processing (143, 148). For example, there are minimal differences in forward digit span, rate of forgetting in the Brown-Peterson paradigm, or the recency component of the serial-position curve. There are age effects on backwards digit span, however. This finding suggests an age-related deficit in working memory, in which the subject must actively manipulate and transform the material (140), presumably reflecting an underlying age-related difficulty with the controlled deployment of attention. By contrast, there is overwhelming evidence of age-related impairments in secondary memory (e.g., 136,137). Prima facie evidence for a specific age-related deficit in long-term memory comes from differences between young and old in single-trial free recall, and particularly in the primacy portion of the serial-position curve. The extent of the age deficit depends, of course, on the manner in which secondary memory is assessed. The modal finding in the literature is that the aged perform least well on tasks involving free recall, and best on tasks involving recognition (147). For example, Craik and McDowd (149) engaged subjects in a concurrent reaction-time task during tests of cued recall and recognition. They found no age-related differences in recognition (as measured by the signal-detection measure d'), but a substantial deficit in cued recall.

EPISODIC AND SEMANTIC MEMORY

Primary and secondary memory are both reflections of episodic memory, in that they tap the ability of the person to remember, after shorter or longer intervals of time, events that occurred in a specific spatiotemporal context. Thus, the aged clearly show an impairment in episodic memory, especially over long retention intervals and when retrieval cues are relatively impoverished; that is, free recall from secondary memory. By contrast, most evidence indicates that context-free semantic memory remains relatively intact in the healthy aged. For example, it has long been known that performance on "crystallized intelligence" tests involving vocabulary and general information—which might be called semantic memory in its purest form—shows relatively little decrement, and may actually *increase* with age—presumably because age provides more opportunities to acquire this sort of information (143,150,151). Similarly, young and old subjects show the same magnitude of priming effect in a category verification task (139). However, response latencies in such tasks, as well as word fluency in general, do decrease with age; again perhaps as a result of a general age-related slowing of cognitive functions.

As indicated earlier, however, a clear distinction must be made between the type of memory, episodic or semantic, and the age of the memory, distant or recent. Most tests of semantic memory involve information learned while the subject was young, while most tests of episodic memory involve events that occurred quite recently. There is surprisingly little research available on the comparative abilities of young and old subjects to acquire wholly new vocabulary or world knowledge. On the other hand, there is fairly good evidence that the elderly have difficulty retrieving both remote and recent personal recollections (152,153). Unfortunately, in these studies the age of the subject is confounded with retention interval. Thus, when asked to recognize high-school classmates, 70 year olds tend to do worse than 50 or 30 year olds. But it should be noted that the 70 year olds are being asked to retrieve memories from 55 years ago, while 50 year olds are being asked to retrieve memories that are only 35 years old. At present, we do not know whether the elderly are more forgetful of remote memories when the retention interval has been held constant.

EXPLICIT AND IMPLICIT MEMORY

Research comparing explicit and implicit memory in the elderly is at a very early stage, but there is already some evidence that implicit memory is relatively spared among the normal aged. For example, Light et al. (154) asked old and young subjects to study a list of target words, followed by an explicit test of yes/no recognition and an implicit test of word fragment completion. Elderly subjects showed poor recognition accuracy compared with younger subjects, especially after one week; however, there were no significant age-related effects on word fragment completion. Similar results have been obtained by Light and Singh (155), and by others using a variety of paradigms (e.g., 156,157).

Because explicit recollection is mediated by retrieval of the context in which the target event occurred, the dissociation between explicit and implicit memory observed in older adults suggests that contextual information may be relatively vulnerable to encoding and/or retrieval difficulties. In fact, the available evidence indicates that the elderly show impairments in processing at least three forms of contextual information: temporal context, spatial context, and external source of information (e.g., 136). For example, the elderly appear to be disadvantaged in remembering both the particular list in which an item was presented (e.g., 158), and the spatial location in which list items (both verbal and pictorial) are presented (e.g., 159,160), even when the items themselves are correctly recognized as belonging to a previously presented list, and even under intentional study conditions. With respect to source, the elderly have difficulty remembering the gender of the voice in which list items had been read (161), which of two experimenters provided them with new factual information (162), or whether a word had been presented visually or orally (163). Interestingly, however, the elderly appear to have little or no difficulty distinguishing between externally and internally generated list items (e.g., 163).

CONCLUDING COMMENTS

Although there was a time when theorizing about normal memory function and studying clinical memory disorders were independent enterprises, even our rather brief consideration of the literature confirms that this is clearly no longer the case. Ideas developed in the study of normal memory have become an almost ubiquitous component of clinical investigations concerning memory disorders observed in amnesia, dementia, and normal aging. The time when studies of memory disorders consisted solely of administering a theoretical test batteries or clincial protocols appears to be behind us. This development bodes well for both the clinical study of memory impairments, and the experimental study of normal memory. We have little doubt that if he were alive today, Theodule Ribot would have warmly applauded the emergence of the kind of studies that he had called for over a century ago.

ACKNOWLEDGMENTS

Preparation of this chapter was supported by National Institute of Aging Grant RO1 AG08441-01. We thank Mindy Tharan for valuable help in preparation of the manuscript.

REFERENCES

1. Ribot, T. (1882). *Diseases of Memory*. Appleton, New York.
2. Schacter, D.L., and Tulving, E. (1982). Amnesia and memory research. In *Human Memory and Amnesia*. Edited by L.S. Cermak. Lawrence Erlbaum Associates, Hillsdale, NJ, pp. 1-32.
3. Shimamura, A.P. (1989). Disorders of memory: The cognitive science perspective. In *Handbook of Clinical Neuropsychology*. Edited by F. Boller and J. Grafman. Elsevier Science Publishers, Amsterdam, pp. 35-74.

4. Craik, F.I.M., and Levy, B.A. (1976). The concept of primary memory. In *Handbook of Learning and Cognitive Processes*, Vol. IV. Edited by W.K. Estes. Academic Press, New York, pp. 133-175.

5. Waugh, N.C., and Norman, D.A. (1965). Primary memory. *Psychol. Rev. 72*: 89-104.

6. Tulving, E. (1972). Episodic and semantic memory. In *Organization of Memory*. Edited by E. Tulving and W. Donaldson. Academic Press, New York.

7. Tulving, E. (1983). *Elements of Episodic Memory*. The Clarendon Press, Oxford.

8. Graf, P., and Schacter, D.L. (1985). Implicit and explicit memory for new associations in normal subjects and amnesic patients. *J. Exp. Psychol. [Learn. Mem. cogn.] 11*:501-518.

9. Schacter, D.L. (1987). Implicit memory: History and current status. *J. Exp. Psychol. [Learn. Mem. Cogn.] 13*:501-518.

10. Anderson, J.R. (1983). *The Architecture of Cognition*. Harvard University Press, Cambridge.

11. Eich, J.M. (1982). A composite holographic associative recall model. *Psychol. Rev. 89*:627-661.

12. Gillund, G., and Shiffrin, R.M. (1984). A retrieval model for both recognition and recall. *Psychol. Rev. 19*:1-65.

13. Hinton, G., and Anderson, J.A. (1981). *Parallel Models of Associative Memory*. Erlbaum Associates, Hillsdale, NJ.

14. McClelland, J.L., and Rumelhart, D.E. (1985). Distributed memory and the representation of general and specific information. *J. Exp. Psychol. [Gen.] 114*: 159-188.

15. McClelland, J.L., and Rumelhart, D.E. (1986). *Parallel Distributed Processing*, Vol. 2. Bradford Books, Cambridge, MA

16. Cermak, L.S. (1982). *Human Memory and Amnesia*. Lawrence Erlbaum Associates, Hillsdale, NJ.

17. Hirst, W. (1982). The amnesic syndrome: Descriptions and explanations. *Psychol. Bull. 91*:435-460.

18. Parkin, A.J. (1987). *Memory and Amnesia: An Introduction*. Basil Blackwell Ltd., Oxford.

19. Squire, L.R. (1987). *Memory and Brain*. Oxford University Press, New York.

20. Weiskrantz, L. (1985). On issues and theories of the human amnesic syndrome. In *Memory Systems of the Brain: Animal and Human Cognitive Processes*. Edited by N. Weinberger, J. McGaugh, and G. Lynch. Guilford Press, New York.

21. Atkinson, R.C., and Shiffrin, R.M. (1968). Human memory: A proposed system and its control processes. In *The Psychology of Learning and Motivation*, Vol. II. Edited by K.W. Spence and J.T. Spence. Academic Press, New York, pp. 89-155.

22. Craik, F.I.M., and Lockhart, R.S. (1972). Levels of processing: A framework for memory research. *J. Verbal Learn. Verbal Behav. 11*:671-684.

23. Crowder, R.G. (1982). The demise of short-term memory. *Acta Psychologica 50*:291-323.

24. Baddeley, A.D., and Warrington, E.K. (1970). Amnesia and the distinction between long- and short-term memory. *J. Verbal Learn. Verbal Behav. 9*:176-189.

25. Milner, B. (1966). Amnesia following operation on the temporal lobes. In *Amnesia.* Edited by C.W.M. Whitty and O.L. Zangwill. Butterworths, London, pp. 109-133.

26. Shallice, T., and Warrington, E.K. (1970). Independent functioning of verbal memory stores: A neuropsychological study. *Q.J. Exp. Psychol. 22*:261-273.

27. Warrington, E.K. (1982). The double dissociation of short-term and long-term memory deficits. In *Human Memory and Amnesia.* Edited by L.S. Cermak. Erlbaum Associates, Hillsdale, NJ, pp. 61-76.

28. Cermak, L.S., Butters, N., and Goodglass, H. (1971). The extent of memory loss in Korsakoff patients. *Neuropsychologia 9*:307-315.

29. Kinsbourne, M., and Wood, F. (1975). Short term memory and the amnesic syndrome. In *Short-Term Memory.* Edited by D.D. Deutsch and J.A. Deutsch. Academic Press, New York, pp. 258-291.

30. Moscovitch, M. (1982). Multiple dissociations of function in amnesia. In *Human Memory and Amnesia.* Edited by L.S. Cermak. Lawrence Erlbaum Associates, Hillsdale, NJ, pp. 337-370.

31. Baddeley, A.D. (1986). *Working Memory.* Oxford University Press, Oxford.

32. McKoon, G., and Ratcliff, R. (1986). A critical evaluation of the semantic/episodic distinction. *J. Exp. Psychol.* [*Learn. Mem. Cogn.*] *12*:295-306.

33. Tulving, E. (1984). Multiple learning and memory systems. In *Psychology in the 1990's.* Edited by K.M.J. Lagerspetz and P. Niemi. Elsevier Science Publishers, Amsterdam, p. 163-184.

34. Huppert, F.A. and Piercy, M. (1982). In search of the functional locus of amnesic syndromes. In *Human Memory and Amnesia.* Edited by L.S. Cermak. Lawrence Erlbaum Associates, Hillsdale, NJ, pp. 123-137.

35. Zola-Morgan, S., Cohen, N.J., and Squire, L.R. (1983). Recall of remote episodic memory in amnesia. *Neuropsychologia 21*:487-500.

36. Schacter, D.L., Harbluk, J.L., and McLachlan, D.R. (1984). Retrieval without recollection: An experimental analysis of source amnesia. *J. Verbal Learn. Verbal Behav. 23*:593-611.

37. Shimamura, A.P., and Squire, L.R. (1987). A neuropsychological study of fact learning and source amnesia. *J. Exp. Psychol.* [*Learn Mem. Cogn.*] *13*:464-474.

38. Glisky, E.L., Schacter, D.L., and Tulving, E. (1986). Computer learning by memory-impaired patients: Acquisition and retention of complex knowledge. *Neuropsychologia 24*:313-328.

39. Glisky, E.L., Schacter, D.L. and Tulving, E. (1986). Learning and retention of computer-related vocabulary in memory-impaired patients: method of vanishing cues. *J. Clin. Exp. Neuropsychol. 8*:292-312.

40. Glisky, E.L., and Schacter, D.L. (1988). Long-term retention of computer learning by patients with memory disorders. *Neuropsychologia 26*:173-178.

41. Glisky, E.L., and Schacter, D.L. (1987). Acquisition of domain-specific knowledge in organic amnesia: Training for computer-related work. *Neuropsychologia 25*:893-906.

42. Glisky, E.L., and Schacter, D.L. (1989). Extending the limits of complex learning in organic amnesia: Computer training in a vocational domain. *Neuropsychologia 27*:107-120.

43. Parkin, A. (1982). Residual learning capability in organic amnesia. *Cortex 18*: 417-440.

44. Schacter, D.L. (1987). Implicit expressions of memory in organic amnesia: learning of new facts and associations. *Human Neurobiol. 6*:107-118.

45. Gabrielli, J.D.E., Cohen, N.J., & Corkin, S. (1983). The acquisition of lexical and semantic knowledge in amnesia. *Soc. Neurosci. Abstr. 9*:98-105.

46. Cermak, L.S. (1984). The episodic-semantic distinction in amnesia. In *Neuropsychology of Memory*. Edited by L.R. Squire and N. Butters. Guilford Press, New York, pp. 55-62.

47. Kinsbourne, M., and Wood, F. (1982). Theoretical considerations regarding the episodic-semantic memory distinction. In *Human Memory and Amnesia*. Edited by L.S. Cermak. Erlbaum Associates, Hillsdale, NJ, pp. 195-217.

48. Schacter, D.L., and Tulving, E. (1982). Memory, amnesia, and the episodic/semantic distinction. In *The Expression of Knowledge*. Edited by R.L. Isaacson. Plenum Press, New York, pp. 33-65.

49. Crovitz, H.F., and Shiffrin, H. (1974). Frequency of episodic memories as a function of their age. *Bull. Psychonomic Soc. 4*:517-518.

50. Butters, N., and Cermak, L.S. (1986). A case study of the forgetting of autobiographical knowledge: Implications for the study of retrograde amnesia. In *Autobiographical Memory*. Edited by D.C. Rubin. Cambridge University Press, Cambridge, pp. 33-65.

51. Tulving, E., Schacter, D.L., McLachlan, D.R., and Moscovitch, M. (1988). Priming of semantic autobiographical knowledge: A case study of retrograde amnesia. *Brain Cogn. 8*:3-20.

52. Schacter, D.L. (1987). Memory, amnesia, and frontal lobe dysfunction. *Psychobiology 15*:21-36.

53. Schacter, D.L., Bowers, J., and Booker, J. (1989). Intention, awareness, and implicit memory: The retrieval intentionality criterion. In *Implicit Memory: Theoretical Issues*. Edited by S. Lewandowsky, J. Dunn, and K. Kirsner. Erlbaum Associates, Hillsdale, N.J., pp. 47-65.

54. Graf, P., and Schacter, D.L. (1987). Selective effects of interference on implicit and explicit memory for new associations. *J. Exp. Psychol. [Learn. Mem. Cogn.] 13*:45-53.

55. Graf, P., and Mandler, G. (1984). Activation makes words more accessible, but not necessarily more retrievable. *J. Verbal Learn. Verbal Behav. 25*:553-568.

56. Jacoby, L.L., and Dallas, M. (1981). On the relationship between autobiographical memory and perceptual learning. *J. Exp. Psychol. [Gen.] 110*:306-340.

57. Jacoby, L.L. (1983). Perceptual enhancement: Persistent effects of an experience. *J. Exp. Psychol. [Learn. Mem. Cogn.] 9*:21-38.

58. Roediger, H.L., and Blaxton, T.A. (1987). Effects of varying modality, surface features, and retention interval on priming in word-fragment completion. *Mem. Cogn. 15*:379-388.

59. Schacter, D.L., and Graf, P. (1986). Effects of elaborative processing on implicit and explicit memory for new associations. *J. Exp. Psychol. [Learn. Mem. Cogn.] 12*:432-444.

60. Schacter, D.L., and Graf, P. (1989). Modality specificity of implicit memory for new associations. *J. Exp. Psychol.* [*Learn. Mem. Cogn.*] *15*:3-12.
61. Tulving, E., Schacter, D.L., and Stark, H.A. (1982). Priming effects in word-fragment completion are independent of recognition memory. *J. Exp. Psychol.* [*Learn. Mem. Cogn.*] *8*:336-342.
62. Richardson-Klavehn, A., and Bjork, R.A. (1988). Measures of memory. *Ann. Rev. Psychol. 36*:475-543.
63. Brooks, D.N., and Baddeley, A.D. (1976). What can amnesic patients learn? *Neuropsychologia 14*:111-122.
64. Cohen, N.J., and Squire, L.R. (1980). Preserved learning and retention of pattern analyzing skill in amnesia: Dissociation of "knowing how" and "knowing that." *Science 210*:207-209.
65. Milner, B., Corkin, S., and Teuber, H.L. (1968). Further analysis of the hippocampal amnesic syndrome: 14 year follow-up study of H.M. *Neuropsychologia 6*:215-234.
66. Nissen, M.J., and Bullemer, P. (1987). Attentional requirements of learning: Evidence from performance measures. *Cogn. Psychol. 19*:1-32.
67. Graf, P., Squire, L.R., and Mandler, G. (1984). The information that amnesic patients do not forget. *J. Exp. Psychol.* [*Learn. Mem. Cogn.*] *10*:164-178.
68. Warrington, E.K., and Weiskrantz, L. (1974). The effect of prior learning on subsequent retention in amnesic patients. *Neuropsychologia 12*:419-428.
69. Schacter, D.L. (1985). Multiple forms of memory in humans and animals. In *Memory Systems of the Brain.* Edited by N. Weinberger, J. McGaugh, and G. Lynch. Guilford Press, New York, pp. 351-379.
70. Shimamura, A.P., and Squire, L.R. (1984). Paired-associate learning and priming effects in amnesia: A neuropsychological study. *J. Exp. Psychol.* [*Gen.*] *113*:556-570.
71. Gardner, H., Boller, F., Moreines, J., and Butters, N. (1973). Retrieving information from Korsakoff patients: Effects of categorical cues and reference to the task. *Cortex 9*:165-175.
72. Graf, P., Shimamura, A.P., and Squire, L.R. (1985). Priming across modalities and priming across category levels: Extending the domain of preserved function in amnesia. *J. Exp. Psychol.* [*Learn. Mem. Cogn.*] *11*:385-395.
73. Shimamura, A.P. (1986). Priming effects in amnesia: Evidence for a dissociable memory function. *Q. J. Exp. Psychol.* 38A:619-644.
74. Cohen, N.J. (1984). Preserved learning capacity in amnesia: Evidence for multiple memory systems. In *Neuropsychology of Memory.* Edited by L.R. Squire and N. Butters. Guilford Press, New York, pp. 83-103.
75. Dimond, R., and Rozin, P. (1984). Activation of existing memories in the amnesic syndrome. *J. Abnorm. Psychol. 93*:98-105.
76. Jacoby, L.L. (1984). Incidental versus intentional retrieval: Remembering and awareness as separate issues. In *Neuropsychology of Memory.* Edited by L.R. Squire & N. Butters. Guilford Press, New York, pp. 145-156.
77. Moscovitch, M., Winocur, G., and McLachlan, D. (1986). Memory as assessed by recognition and reading time in normal and memory-impaired people with

Alzheimer's disease and other neurological disorders. *J. Exp. Psychol.* [*Gen.*] *115*:331-347.

78. Schacter, D.L. (1989). On the relation between memory and consciousness: Dissociable interactions and conscious experience. In *Varieties of Memory and Consciousness: Essays in Honor of Endel Tulving.* Edited by H.L. Roediger and F.I.M. Craik. Lawrence Erlbaum Associates, Hillsdale, NJ, pp. 355-389.

79. Schacter, D.L. (in press). Perceptual representation systems and implicit memory: Toward a resolution of the multiple memory systems debate. In *Development and Neural Bases of Higher Cognition.* Edited by A. Diamond. Annals of the New York Academy of Sciences, New York.

80. Riddoch, M.J., and Humphreys, G.W. (1987). Picture naming. In *Visual Object Processing: A Cognitive Neuropsychological Approach.* Edited by G.W. Humphreys and M.J. Riddoch. Lawrence Erlbaum, London, pp. 107-143.

81. Warrington, E.K., and Shallice, T. (1980). Word-form dyslexia. *Brain 103*:99-112.

82. American Psychiatric Association (1987). *Diagnostic and Statistical Manual of Mental Disorders*, 3rd ed. revised. American Psychiatric Association, Washington, DC.

83. Bayles, K.A., and Kaszniak, A.W. (1987). *Communication and Cognition in Normal Aging and Dementia.* College Hill/Little Brown, Boston.

84. Kaszniak, A.W. (1986). The neuropsychology of dementia. In *Neuropsychological Assessment of Neuropsychiatric Disorders.* Edited by I. Grant. Oxford University Press, New York, pp. 172-220.

85. Riege, W.H., and Metter, E.J. (1988). Cognitive and brain imaging measures of Alzheimer's disease. *Neurobiol. Aging 9*:69-86.

86. Botwinick, J., Storandt, M., and Berg, L. (1986). A longitudinal behavioral study of senile dementia of the Alzheimer type. *Arch. Neurol. 43*:1124-1127.

87. Kaszniak, A.W., Wilson, R.S., Fox, J.H., and Stebbins, G.T. (1986). Cognitive assessment in Alzheimer's disease: Cross-sectional and longitudinal perspectives. *Can. J. Neurol. Sci. 13*:420-423.

88. Moss, M.B., Albert, M.S., Butters, N., and Payne, M. (1986). Differential patterns of memory loss among patients with Alzheimer's disease, Huntington's disease, and alcoholic Korsakoff's syndrome. *Arch. Neurol. 43*:239-246.

89. Kaszniak, A.W., Poon, L.W., & Riege, W. (1986). Assessing memory deficits: An information processing approach. In *Handbook for Clinical Memory Assessment of Older Adults.* Edited by L.W. Poon. American Psychological Association, Washington, DC, pp. 168-188.

90. Morris, R.G., and Baddeley, A.D. (1988). Primary and working memory functioning in Alzheimer-type dementia. *J. Clin. Exp. Neuropsychol. 10*:279-296.

91. Wilson, R.S., Kaszniak, A.W., and Fox, J.H. (1981). Remote memory in senile dementia. *Cortex 17*:41-48.

92. Wilson, R.S., Bacon, L.D., Fox, J.H., and Kaszniak, A.W. (1983). Primary memory in dementia of the Alzheimer type. *J. Clin. Neuropsychol. 5*:337-344.

93. Tulving, E., and Colotla, V.A. (1970). Free recall of trilingual lists. *Cogn. Psychol. 1*:86-98.

94. Cushman, L.A., Como, P.G., Booth, H., and Caine, E. (1988). Cued recall and release from proactive interference in Alzheimer's disease. *J. Clin. Exp. Neuropsychol. 10*:685-692.

95. Martin, A., Brouwers, P., Cox, C., and Fedio, P. (1985). On the nature of the verbal memory deficit in Alzheimer's disease. *Brain Lang. 25*:323-341.
96. Morris, R.G. (1984). Dementia and functioning of the articulatory loop system. *Cogn. Neuropsychol. 1*:143-157.
97. Morris, R.G. (1986). Short-term forgetting in senile dementia of the Alzheimer's type. *Cogn. Neuropsychol. 3*:77-97.
98. Morris, R.G. (1987). Articulatory rehearsal in Alzheimer-type dementia. *Brain Lang. 30*:351-362.
99. Morris, R.G. (1987). The effect of concurrent articulation on memory span in Alzheimer-type dementia. *Br. J. Clin. Psychol. 26*:233-244.
100. Baddeley, A.D., Logie, R.H., Bressi, S., Della Sala, S., and Spinnler, H. (1986). Dementia and working memory. *Q. J. Exp. Psychol. 38A*:603-618.
101. Becker, J.T. (1988). Working memory and secondary memory deficits in Alzheimer's disease. *J. Clin. Exp. Neuropsychol. 10*:739-753.
102. Hyman, B.T., Van Hoesen, G.W., Damasio, A.R., and Barnes, C.L. (1984). Alzheimer's disease: Cell-specific pathology isolates the hippocampal formation. *Science 225*:2268-1170.
103. Hyman, B.T., Van Hoesen, G.W., Kromer, L.J., and Damasio, A.R. (1986). Perforant pathway changes and the memory impairment of Alzheimer's disease. *Ann. Neurol. 20*:472-481.
104. DeKosky, S.T., Scheff, S.W., and Markesbery, N.R. (1985). Laminar organization of cholinergic circuits in human frontal cortex in Alzheimer's disease and aging. *Neurology 35*:1525-1531.
105. Grady, C.L., Haxby, J.V., Horwitz, V., Sundaram, M., Berg, G., Schapiro, M., Friedland, R.P., and Rappoport, S.I. (1988). Longitudinal study of the early neuropsychological and cerebral metabolic changes in dementia of the Alzheimer type. *J. Clin. Exp. Neuropsychol. 10*:576-596.
106. Butters, N., Granholm, E., Salmon, D.P., Grant, I., and Wolfe, J. (1987), Episodic and semantic memory: A comparison of amnesic and demented patients. *J. Clin. Exp. Neuropsychol. 9*:479-497.
107. Bayles, K.A., and Tomoeda, C.K. (1983). Confrontation naming in dementia. *Brain Lang. 19*:98-114.
108. Martin, A., and Fedio, P. (1983). Word production and comprehension in Alzheimer's disease: The breakdown of semantic knowledge. *Brain Lang. 19*:124-141.
109. Ober, B.A., Dronkers, N.F., Koss, E., Delis, D.C., and Fredland, R.P. (1986). Retrieval from semantic memory in Alzheimer-type dementia. *J. Clin. Exp. Neuropsychol. 8*:75-92.
110. Beatty, W.W., Salmon, D.P., Butters, N., Heindel, W.C., and Granholm, E.P. (1988). Retrograde amnesia in patients with Alzheimer's or Huntington's disease. *J. Clin. Exp. Neuropsychol. 10*:78(Abstr.).
111. Wilson, R.S., Kaszniak, A.W., and Fox, J.H. (1981). Remote memory in senile dementia. *Cortex 17*:41-48.
112. Wilson, R.S., Bacon, L.D., Kramer, R.L., Fox, J.H., and Kaszniak, A.W. (1983). Word frequency effect and recognition memory in dementia of the Alzheimer type. *J. Clin. Neuropsychol. 6*:97-104.
113. Rissenberg, M., and Glanzer, M. (1986). Picture superiority in free recall: The effects of normal aging and primary degenerative dementia. *J. Gerontol. 41*:64-71.

114. Wilson, R.S., Kaszniak, A.W., Bacon, L.D., Fox, J.H., and Kelly, M.P. (1982). Facial recognition memory in dementia. *Cortex 18*:329-336.

115. Weingartner, H., Kaye, W., Smalling, S., Cohen, R., Ebert, M.H., Gillin, J.C. and Gold, P. (1982). Determinants of memory failure in dementia. In *Aging*, Vol. 19. *Alzheimer's Disease: A Report of Progress in Research*. Edited by S. Corkin, K.L. Davis, J.H. Growdon, and E. Usdin. Raven Press, New York, pp. 171-176.

116. Weingartner, H., Grafman, J., Boutelle, W., Kaye, W., and Martin, P.R. (1983). Forms of memory failure. *Science 221*:380-383.

117. Chang, T.M. (1986). Semantic memory: facts and models. *Psychol. Bull. 99*: 199-220.

118. Kaszniak, A.W. (1988). Cognition in Alzheimer's disease: Theoretic models and clinical applications. *Neurobiol. Aging 9*:92-94.

119. Nebes, R.D., Martin, D.C., and Horn, L.C. (1984). Sparing of semantic memory in Alzheimer's disease. *J. Abnorm. Psychol. 93*:321-330.

120. Flicker, C., Ferris, S.H., Crook, T., and Bartus, R.T. (1987). Implications of memory and language dysfunction in the naming deficit of senile dementia. *Brain Lang. 31*:187-200.

121. Huff, F.J., Corkin, S., and Growdon, J.H. (1986). Semantic impairment and anomia in Alzheimer's disease. *Brain Lang. 28*:235-249.

122. Grober, E., Buschke, H., Kawas, C., and Fuld, P. (1985). Impaired ranking of semantic attributes in dementia. *Brain Lang. 26*:276-286.

123. Nebes, R.D., and Brady, C.B. (1988). Integrity of semantic fields in Alzheimer's disease. *Cortex, 24*:291-300.

124. Grady, C.L., Haxby, J.V., Schlageter, N.L., Berg, G., and Rappoport, S.I. (1986). Stability of metabolic and neuropsychological asymmetries in dementia of the Alzheimer type. *Neurology, 36*:1390-1392.

125. Martin, A., Brouwers, P., Lalonde, F., Cox, C., Teleska, P., Fedio, P., Foster, N.L., and Chase, T.N. (1986). Towards a behavioral topology of Alzheimer's patients. *J. Clin. Exp. Neuropsychol. 8*:594-610.

126. Martin, A. (1987). Representation of semantic and spatial knowledge in Alzheimer's patients: Implications for models of preserved learning in amnesia. *J. Clin. Exp. Neuropsychol. 9*:191-224.

127. Brandt, J., Spencer, M., McSorley, M.F., and Folstein, M.F. (1986, February). *Memory Activation and Implicit Remembering in Alzheimer's Disease*. Paper presented at the meeting of the International Neuropsychological Society, Denver, CO.

128. Nebes, R.D., Boller, F., and Holland, A. (1986). Use of semantic context by patients with Alzheimer's disease. *Psychol. Aging 1*:261-269.

129. Ober, B.A., and Shenaut, G.K. (1988). Lexical decision and priming in Alzheimer's disease. *Neuropsychologia 26*:273-286.

130. Salmon, D.P., Shimamura, A.P., Butters, N., and Smith, S. (1988). Lexical and semantic priming deficits in patients with Alzheimer's disease. *J. Clin. Exp. Neuropsychol. 10*:477-494.

131. Shimamura, A.P., Salmon, D.P., Squire, L.R., and Butters, N. (1987). Memory dysfunction and word priming in dementia and amnesia. *Behav. Neurosci. 101*:347-351.

132. Butters, N. (1987, February). *Procedural Learning in Dementia: A Double Dissociation Between Alzheimer's and Huntington's Disease Patients on Verbal Priming and Motor Skill Learning.* Paper presented at the meeting of the International Neuropsychological Society, Washington, DC.

133. Eslinger, P.J., and Damasio, A.R. (1986). Preserved motor learning in Alzheimer's disease: Implications for anatomy and behavior. *J. Neurosci. 6*:3006-3009.

134. Knopman, D.S., and Nissen, M.J. (1987). Implicit learning in patients with probable Alzheimer's disease. *Neurology 37*:784-788.

135. Botwinick, J. (1984). *Aging and Behavior.* Springer, New York.

136. Burke, D.M., and Light, L.L. (1981). Memory and aging: The role of retrieval processes. *Psychol. Bull. 90*:513-546.

137. Craik, F.I.M. (1977). Age differences in human memory. In *Handbook of the Psychology of Aging.* Edited by J.E. Birren and K.W. Schaie. Van Nostrand Reinhold, New York, pp. 384-420.

138. Craik, F.I.M. (1984). Age differences in remembering. In *Neuropsychology of Memory.* Edited by L.R. Squire and N. Butters. Guilford Press, New York, pp. 3-12.

139. Craik, F.I.M., and Byrd, M. (1982). Aging and cognitive deficits: The role of attentional resources. In *Aging and Cognitive Processes.* Edited by F.I.M. Craik and S. Trehub. Plenum, New York, pp. 384-420.

140. Craik, F.I.M., and Rabionwitz, J. (1984). Age differences in the acquisition and use of verbal information. In *Attention and Performance X.* Edited by H. Bouma and D.G. Bouwhuis. Lawrence Erlbaum Associates, Hillsdale, NJ, pp. 191-212.

141. Craik, F.I.M., and Simon, E. (1980). Age differences in memory: The role of attention and depth of processing. In *New Directions in Memory and Aging: Proceedings of the George A. Talland Memorial Conference.* Edited by L.W. Poon, J.L. Fozard, L.S. Cermak, and D. Arenberg. Erlbaum Associates, Hillsdale, NJ, pp. 95-112.

142. Guttentag, R.E. (1985). Memory and aging: Implications for theories of memory development during childhood. *Dev. Rev. 5*:56-82.

143. Kausler, D.H. (1982). *Experimental Psychology and Human Aging.* Wiley, New York.

144. Poon, L.W. (1985). Differences in human memory with aging: Nature, causes, and clinical implications. In *Handbook of the Psychology of Aging.* Edited by K.W. Schaie and J.E. Birren. Van Nostrand Reinhold, New York, pp. 427-462.

145. Poon, L.W., Fozard, J.L., Cermak, L.S., Arenberg, D., and Thompson, L.W. (1980). *New Directions in Memory and Aging: Proceedings of the George Talland Memorial Conference.* Lawrence Erlbaum Associates, Hillsdale, NJ.

146. Rabinowitz, J.C., Craik, F.I.M., and Ackerman, B.P. (1982). A processing resource account of age differences in memory. *Can. J. Psychol. 36*:325-244.

147. Schonfield, D., and Stones, M.J. (1979). Remembering and aging. In *Functional Disorders of Memory.* Edited by J.F. Kihlstrom and F.J. Evans. Lawrence Erlbaum Associates, Hillsdale, NJ, pp. 103-139.

148. Craik, F.I.M. (1968). Short-term memory and the aging process. In *Human Aging and Behavior.* Edited by G.A. Talland. Academic Press, New York.

149. Craik, F.I.M., and McDowd, J.M. (1987). Age differences in recall and recognition. *J. Exp. Psychol. [Learn Mem. Cogn.]* *13*:474-479.
150. Denney, N.W. (1984). A model of cognitive development across the life span. *Dev. Rev. 4*:171-191.
151. Schaie, K.W. (1980). Cognitive development in aging. In *Language and Communication in the Elderly: Clinical, Therapeutic and Experimental Issues.* Edited by L.K. Ober and M.L. Albert. Lexington Books, Lexington, MA.
152. Bahrick, H.P., Bahrick, P.O., and Wittlinger, R.P. (1975). Fifty years of memory for names and faces: A cross-sectional approach. *J. Exp. Psychol. [Gen.]* *104*:54-75.
153. Warrington, E.K., and Sanders, H.I. (1971). The fate of old memories. *Q. J. Exp. Psychol. 23*:432-442.
154. Light, L.L., Singh, A., and Capps, J.L. (1986). Dissociation of memory and awareness in young and older adults. *J. Clin. Exp. Neuropsychol. 8*:62-74.
155. Light, L.L., and Singh, A. (1987). Implicit and explicit memory in young and older adults. *J. Exp. Psychol. [Learn Mem. Cogn.]* *13*:531-541.
156. Craik, F.I.M., Byrd, M., and Swanson, J.M. (1987). Patterns of memory loss in three elderly samples. *Psychol. Aging 2*:79-86.
157. Rabinowitz, J.C. (1986). Priming in episodic memory. *J. Gerontol. 41*:204-213.
158. Kausler, D.H., Lichty, W., and Davis, R.T. (1985). Temporal memory for performed activities: Intentionality and adult age differences. *Dev. Psychol. 21*:1132-1138.
159. Naveh-Benjamin, M. (1987). Coding of spatial location information: An automatic process. *J. Exp. Psychol. [Learn Mem. Cogn.]* *13*:595-605.
160. Zelinski, E.M., and Light, L.L. (1988). Younger and older adults' use of context in spatial memory. *Psychol. Aging 3*:99-101.
161. Kausler, D.H., and Puckett, J.M. (1981). Adult age differences in memory for modality attributes. *Exp. Aging Res. 7*:117-125.
162. McIntyre, J.S., and Craik, F.I.M. (1987). Age differences in memory for item and source information. *Can. J. Psychol. 41*:175-192.
163. Hashtroudi, S., Johnson, M.K., and Chrosniak, L.D. (1989). Aging and source monitoring. *Psychol. Aging 4*:106-112.

Part III

EVALUATION OF MEMORY FUNCTION

7

Memory Assessment at the Bedside

Ronald C. Petersen

Mayo Clinic and Mayo Foundation
Rochester, Minnesota

BASIC ISSUES IN MEMORY ASSESSMENT

The assessment of memory function at the bedside or in the office is a critical part of the mental status examination. Disorders of memory may be a major aspect of the patient's clinical condition, and occasionally, abnormal memory function is the only abnormality found on the entire medical or neurological examination. Consequently, an adequate assessment of memory function is a necessary part of the mental status/neurological examination.

In order for clinicians to perform an adequate memory assessment, certain familiarity with memory terminology is necessary. The terminology used in describing memory functions is discussed in Chapter 2, and hence will not be discussed in detail here. In brief, basic memory processes can be described in terms of input functions such as acquisition or storage and in terms of output functions such as recall or retrieval. Features of these fundamental processes need to be incorporated into the bedside testing procedure for an adequate assessment of memory function. Additionally, the clinician needs to be aware of the concepts of primary and secondary memory since the various memory tasks assess different aspects of each of these types of memory. These issues are discussed in more detail in Chapter 2.

Several questions should be addressed when performing a memory assessment:

1. Is memory function impaired?
2. Is memory function impaired in isolation or in relation to another specific cognitive deficit or as part of a more generalized defect in cognition?
3. If memory is impaired, what subprocesses are involved?

The answers to these questions can be helpful in diagnosing the patient's difficulties and in directing further evaluations.

IS MEMORY FUNCTION IMPAIRED?

This question is the primary focus of this chapter. In particular, what evaluations can we do at the bedside or in the office to determine if a problem with memory exists? Several factors neeed to be considered. If, based on the history (to be discussed later), you are not expecting a major memory problem, a screening test can be done involving a few verbal and nonverbal stimuli learned over multiple trials with recall testing at several delay intervals. based on the history, the next level of evaluation can be undertaken. This type of examination will involve more extensive verbal and nonverbal stimuli learned over multiple trials with recall testing at varying delay intervals. This level of analysis yields more specific information regarding the degree of impairment and the type of material involved (e.g., verbal or nonverbal).

IS MEMORY FUNCTION IMPAIRED IN ISOLATION OR IN RELATION TO ANOTHER COGNITIVE DEFICIT OR AS PART OF A MORE GENERALIZED COGNITIVE DYSFUNCTION?

This issue needs to be addressed early in the course of an evaluation for a memory deficit. Prior to concluding that a memory deficit exists, one must be certain that other cognitive impairments are not influencing the evaluation. For example, a patient with a significant attentional disorder, such as an acute confusional state, may not perform well on memory tests because of inattention rather than because of a fundamental memory disorder itself. Adequate attention is a prerequisite for most memory tasks, and disorders of attention can significantly influence performance. Erroneous conclusions regarding the presence or absence of memory disorders can be made in the setting of attentional disorders, and consequently, a total assessment of cognitive function is necessary as part of a memory evaluation.

Another cognitive function which can significantly alter the interpretation of memory tasks is language. An aphasic patient may have difficulty with memory tests, particularly verbal tests, because of a primary language deficit. An aphasic patient may not comprehend the instructions, may have difficulty providing verbal responses, may be unable to repeat well, or may have a variety of other problems which can interfere with memory testing. Hence, it is once again imperative that an overall assessment of cognitive function be conducted in addition to specific memory testing.

Finally, patients may not perform well on memory tests for other reasons including primary psychiatric disorders such as depression, psychosis, or personality disorders. These conditions may interfere with performance on the tests without necessarily implicating a major memory dysfunction. Several excellent reviews of general mental status testing are available (1-3).

IF MEMORY IS IMPAIRED, WHAT SUBPROCESSES ARE INVOLVED?

To address this issue, more extensive testing needs to be done. In particular, the memory task should involve both verbal and nonverbal materials, an acquisition phase over several learning trials, free recall, cued recall, and recognition testing preferably with varying delay intervals. Tasks containing these components will enable you to determine the degree of memory impairment and also provide some information regarding the anatomical localization of the disorder.

SELECTION OF MEMORY TESTS

Once the above questions have been addressed and it has been determined that a memory problem exists, the next decision involves the selection of appropriate memory tests. It is worth repeating that one must be careful in assessing memory to be certain to evaluate the several stages or subprocesses involved in memory function separately. Instruments that use a derived memory "index" or "quotient" such as the Wechsler Memory Scale (4) must be scrutinized carefully to be certain different memory functions are not being combined into a single measure. For example, an instrument that combines measures of primary memory with measures of secondary memory such as combining digit span with list learning over multiple trials may erroneously conclude a memory impairment is present when, in fact, there may just be a major defect in attention or primary memory. Consequently, by combining tasks which assess both primary and secondary memory into one measure, an overall memory index is derived which may lead the clinician to ascribe all of the deficits to "memory." On the other hand, primary memory or attention span measures are often preserved in many organic amnesias (e.g., Korsakoff's disease or temporal lobectomies), and a combined index of primary and secondary memory function will inflate the overall assessment of memory. If a pure measure of secondary memory were used in this instance, a much lower and more accurate assessment of the degree of impairment would be made. In general, whenever a single score is assigned to an aspect of mental status assessment, the clinician must understand the various subtests which contribute to the score.

In addressing the issue of selection of memory tests, one must consider the various subprocesses involved. This topic is discussed in more detail in Chapter 2. For example, primary memory should be assessed by a task such as forward digit span since inadequate performance on primary memory tests will also influence performance on other memory measures. However, in most memory disorders, primary memory is preserved since this aspect of memory function is largely based on attentional processes. That is, major deficits in primary memory function usually imply an attentional disorder (e.g., the acute confusional state). Therefore, by the general mental status examination suggested earlier, one can determine if a primary disorder of attention exists. Presuming this is not the case, then a more extensive evaluation of various memory functions themselves can be undertaken.

BACKGROUND INFORMATION
HISTORY

Prior to examining a patient for a possible memory deficit, several issues in the history should be explored. As indicated above, it is helpful to determine if the patient is actually describing a memory deficit or if the patient is referring to another cognitive dysfunction. Patients and observers typically ascribe all aberrations of mental function to memory, when in fact they may be describing another cognitive disorder. Consequently, these issues must be addressed in obtaining a history.

Occasionally when patients are asked about their memory, they state that it is "fine" indicating that they can remember events from 20 or 30 years ago without any problem. However, memory for more recent events may be patchy or incomplete. This piece of historical information can be important in indicating that a significant memory problem is present. Often the most labile aspect of memory function is the acquisition and retrieval of recently learned information. Consequently, this type of history can be quite informative regarding the presence of an actual memory defect. It is important to assess the impact of the memory disorder on daily activities, since this can be a meaningful index of the severity of the problem.

Some information regarding the patient's perceptions of his/her memory difficulties can be obtained from structured questions. It is usually helpful to initiate the interview with open-ended questions regarding the nature of the memory problems and then use more direct questioning for specific issues. For example, the patient can be asked if he/she has difficulties with names of acquaintances, recalling recent family events, recalling recent newspaper articles, remembering grocery lists, placement of objects, telephone messages, location of parked cars, etc. The clinician can ask the patient if he/she is having difficulties following conversations or television programs as well as having word-finding difficulties in mid-sentence. Of course, forgetting these types of information can be quite normal, but the frequency and severity of this type of forgetting are important to assess. Furthermore, since a failure to remember is a part of the disorder being investigated, it is necessary to take a corroborating history from a family member or friend since the patient may be unable to accurately assess his/her own difficulties. Several formal memory questionnaires are available for assessing one's opinion about his/her own memory function (5,6).

INFORMAL MEMORY ASSESSMENT

As an extension of the interview, the clinician can often gain important informal information regarding memory function. For example, the clinician can ask the patient if he/she reads the newspaper or watches television news programs. If they indicate "yes" then the clinician can quiz them about recent major events. Another type of questioning in a similar vein can be done concerning sporting events, if the patient is a sports fan. This assumes that the examiner has some knowledge of sports. This type of questioning can give the clinician an index of whether the patient has been acquiring recent major pieces of information. If the patient gives correct detailed information regarding recent news events, one can assume that the patient does not have a major defect in acquisition; however, if the patient is unsuccessful in reporting these events, he/she may have a acquisition problem. However, the examiner must be cautious in the interpretation of incorrect answers since one cannot be certain as to whether the patient was exposed to the material.

This type of questioning is one way of assessing episodic memory [see Chaps. 2 (Memory Nomenclature) and 6 (Models of Memory and the Understanding of Memory Disorders)] which can be important since this type of memory is often impaired in many organic memory impairments. Another way to assess this type of memory is to ask the patient to recount his activities of the past few days. This also assesses recent episodic memory, but one must have a family member or friend to corroborate the answers.

Finally, remote memory can also be assessed during the history. This can be difficult to examine in a formal fashion because of the uncertainty of the patient's exposure to historical information. Several formal tests of remote memory exist (7,8), but these instruments suffer from the problem of uncertain exposure and do not have norms against which to assess performance. Nevertheless, two types of remote memory can be assessed during the interview, one for personal information and one for nonpersonal information. To minimize the uncertainty of exposure to information, a personal history regarding schooling, occupational history, residences, etc., can be taken provided an informant is available. Most of this information should be resistant to disruption in many memory disorders except for more generalized cognitive disturbances such as dementia. A marked amnesia for personal information raises the suspicion of a functional disorder of memory (see Chapter 20, "Psychogenic Amnesias"). A more labile form of remote memory involves the recall of nonpersonal historical events. This may be clouded by a lack of exposure to material and is confounded by education. This type of questioning may involve the recall of major events in history such as World War I, World War II, the Vietnam conflict, John F. Kennedy's assassination, etc., and may be a sensitive index of an organic defect of remote memory. However, this type of memory may also be affected in a generalized dementing process.

The history can be important in directing one's further assessment of memory function. Certainly from the nature of the history described, the clinician can derive information regarding the nature of the memory deficit and its severity. This information will allow the clinician to determine what type of memory assessment tools should be used in the mental status examination.

SCREENING TESTS
SHORT WORD LISTS

As a summary test, often clinicians will use a short word list embedded in a more general mental status examination. For example, in the Mini-Mental State Exam (MMSE), three words are presented to the patient, and recall is tested a few minutes later after an intervening task involving counting backwards by 7's or spelling the word "world" backward (9). This is a crude, at best, index of memory function and is not sensitive. For example, it is uncertain what constitutes abnormal performance on this task. Is it abnormal if the patient recalls two of the three words or one of the three words?

Kokmen and colleagues improved this task when they introduced a four word learning procedure in their Short Test of Mental Status (10). In this instrument, four words are presented, and the number of learning trials up to a maximum of four is recorded. The remainder of the mental status test is completed, and delayed recall of the four words is then tested. Kokmen and colleagues have recently demonstrated that this technique involving four words increases the sensitivity of the memory testing and correlates better with other measures of memory function than does the three word subtest of the MMSE (11).

While these short memory tasks are useful as part of screening mental status exams, they do not suffice as an adequate assessment of memory. A screening test should involve, at least minimally, a sufficient amount of material to require the patient to take several trials to learn the information, thus obtaining an index of acquisition. The task should also have a delayed recall component to assess recall and retrieval functions. Finally, the task should involve both verbal and nonverbal material. Unfortunately, from a practical standpoint, the incorporation of these features into a test lengthens the overall examination procedure. However, if a memory dysfunction is a major part of the clinical disorder, this time is usually well spent.

THREE WORDS AND THREE SHAPES TEST

A task which can be used at the bedside or in the office which incorporates many of these features is the Three Words and Three Shapes Test described by Weintraub and Mesulam (1). This task involves the presentation of three words with low imagery value and three shapes (Fig. 1) to the patient with the instruction to copy the stimuli. The patient is not told to remember the stimuli at this point. After the patient has copied the three words and three shapes, the stimuli are removed, and the patient is asked to reproduce them. If the patient reproduces the words and shapes correctly, then delayed recall is tested approximately 15 minutes later. However, if the patient fails to reproduce all six stimuli correctly on the immediate recall trial, the stimulus materials are presented again for study, and the patient is instructed to study the stimuli without copying them again. After a 30 second study period, the stimuli are removed, and the patient must reproduce them. If the patient gets five or six items correct (of the total six items) then delayed recall is tested 15 minutes later. However, if recall after this first study period is unsuccessful, another study trial is given, and the process is repeated until the patient gets five or six items correct or five study trials have been given. At the delayed recall test, the patient is asked to reproduce the six items once again. If he or she fails to get all items correct, a recognition test is given.

This task incorporates several of the desirable features of memory tasks. An acquisition phase allows the patient to learn the stimuli over several trials which enables the patient to overcome mild attention deficits and provides an index of acquisition. This phase of learning/memory is frequently impaired in degenerative, vascular, or traumatic disorders involving the limbic system and, in particular, medial temporal lobe structures, the diencephalon and interconnecting pathways (see Chap. 3). Most patients under 65 years of age will learn the material in one study trial, while those over 65 may take more trials. This task also allows for the evaluation of free recall

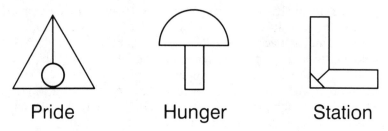

| Pride | Hunger | Station |

Figure 1 Three Word Three Shape Test. (From Ref. 1.)

which is sensitive to many of the disease processes mentioned above. Recognition testing in the setting of abnormal free recall allows for the assessment of retrieval deficits. Finally, the Three Word and Three Shapes Test involves both verbal and nonverbal stimuli which enables an approximate assessment of left hemisphere function (verbal material) and right hemisphere function (nonverbal material). Hence, this task takes more time to administer than simple word lists but yields significantly more information regarding memory function.

DRILLED WORD SPAN TEST

Weintraub and Mesulam have also described another task which involves several of the features described above for the adequate assessment of memory (1). The Drilled Word Span Test is meant to overcome difficulties with attention which may affect results on tests of recall. This task adjusts the list length for each patient as a function of the patient's own forward digit span. A list of common nouns whose list length is one fewer than the patient's forward digit span is presented to the patient in a free recall format until the patient recalls the entire list on three consecutive trials. Immediate recall is tested after each list presentation. Delayed recall is tested at three points in time:

after 60 seconds without distraction, after a second 60 second interval during which time the patient performs a distracting task such as subtracting serial 3s, and a final recall test following 3 minutes filled with other distracting activities. If the patient does not recall the entire list on either of the first two 60 second recall trials, further learning trials to the same initial criterion (three consecutive correct recall trials of the list) are given. Following the three minute recall, a recognition test is given if free recall is less than total.

The Drilled Word Span Test has several of the desirable features of learning and memory tasks described above. It has multiple learning trials, a delayed recall interval, and a recognition task. Weintraub and Mesulam contend that this task enables the clinician to differentiate between memory dysfunction characterized by defective acquisition, delayed recall and perhaps recognition, and a primary attentional dysfunction characterized by defective acquisition but relatively normal delayed recall and recognition. Presumably patients with disorders of attention will have difficulty acquiring the material initially, but once acquired, they will be able to recall it adequately; whereas a patient with a major memory disorder will not benefit from the Drilled Word Span Test procedure. This patient will perform poorly on acquisition, delayed recall, and recognition. This task can be useful but can be time consuming at the bedside. In addition, by using a subspan test which may minimize attentional difficulties, it does not stress the transfer of information from primary to secondary memory which is often the major difficulty encountered in many organic memory disorders. Nevertheless, the task has interesting theoretical properties and can be useful.

HIDDEN OBJECTS TEST

A task which is occasionally useful as a crude measure of nonverbal memory at the bedside or in the office is the Hidden Objects Test (2). This task simply involves hiding five or six objects around the hospital or examining room in view of the patient. The patient is initially asked to name the objects to be certain a significant anomia will not interfere with the task. After several objects, such as a comb, watch, spoon, dollar bill, or pencil, are hidden (e.g., in a drawer, under a pillow, etc.), the patient is asked to recall the names of the objects and their locations. If the patient is unsuccessful on the first trial, several learning trials are given. Then after a 15 minute delay filled with intervening activities, recall of the objects and their locations is tested. This is a reasonably simple test of nonverbal and verbal memory. Most patients should recall four or five objects and their locations without difficulty.

MORE EXTENSIVE MEMORY TESTS

Occasionally, if time permits, more detailed testing can be done at the bedside. In particular, if verbal materials are used, longer lists and different presentation techniques can be used. Tests such as the Rey Auditory Verbal Learning Test are described in Chapter 8, "Psychometric Memory Tests," and in general are too lengthy for an office procedure (12). However, certain modifications on these instruments can be used.

SELECTIVE REMINDING TEST

A procedure somewhat similar to the Rey Auditory Verbal Learning Test using a method of presentation involving selective reminding was originally described by Buschke and later by Buschke and Fuld (13,14). This task involves a multiple trial free recall procedure with several learning trials, and on each trial, the patient is presented only with the items he/she failed to recall on the immediately preceding trial. This is in contrast to other free recall procedures which involve the presentation of the entire list on each trial. This task allows for the assessment of several properties of memory and incorporates features of acquisition, delayed recall, and recognition. It, however, may be too lengthy to use as a bedside procedure.

FREE AND CUED SELECTIVE REMINDING TEST

Buschke described a variation on his selective reminding procedure in a task involving free and cued recall over several learning trials (15-17). This task is unique among learning procedures insofar as it involves a measure of free and cued recall on each learning trial, hence yielding an index of retrieval failure during the acquisition phase. Grober and Buschke have indicated that this task provides an index of a "genuine memory" deficit (16,17). They state that a genuine memory deficit exists if a patient fails both free recall and cued recall. That is, patients may perform poorly on free recall for a variety of reasons, but when cues are given to enhance their memory performance, most people with normal memory function will be able to use the cues to enhance their performance. If, however, recall is incomplete even with cuing on this task, Grober and Buschke argue that a significant memory impairment may be present and one should suspect an organic memory disorder.

The procedure for this task involves presenting the stimuli to the patients in the form of line drawings of the objects. The patient is then instructed to point to each item as it is described by the examiner and to label it verbally. Examples of items are as follows: "Which one is an article of clothing?" (sweater) or "Which one a part of the body?" (hand). Sixteen items are presented in this fashion. After each of these items has been pointed to and named by the patient, the pictures are removed. The examiner next asks the patient to list as many items as he/she can recall. The examiner then moves to the cued recall test after the free recall trial has been completed. In this condition, the descriptors of the items not retrieved on free recall are presented to the patient, and the patient is asked if he/she can remember the specific item. For example, the patient is cued with the following statement: "What was the article of clothing?" The patient is then required to answer "sweater" if this item had not been produced spontaneously on free recall. On the second and all subsequent trials, the patient is reminded only of the items not retrieved on free recall on the previous trial, that is, all of the items that required cued recall. However, the patient is instructed that each time he/she will have to try to remember all of the items. For trial 2 and all subsequent trials, the pictures are placed in front of the patient again, and the patient is asked to point to and name the items described by the examiner. Following this reminder trial, free recall and cued recall are repeated as described above. This procedure is repeated for six trials. Following the sixth trial, no more presentations of stimulus items are given, and free and cued recall are tested 10 minutes after trial 6.

This procedure generates two learning curves: one for free recall over trials and one for free plus cued recall over trials. A sample of these data for control subjects and for patients with dementia of the Alzheimer type is shown in Figure 2. From these data, it is apparent that in using a 16 item list most normal elderly individuals will obtain nearly maximal performance on the free plus cued recall tasks, but patients with dementia of the Alzheimer type are unable to recall the entire list in spite of the use of the cues. Presumably this implies that the neuroanatomical substrait required in free recall and cued recall is not functioning well enough to support normal learning and remembering in the patients with dementia. Grober and Buschke claim that this represents a genuine memory deficit. In general, this task has interesting theoretical properties for the assessment of memory function and may be a useful task. One problem with the test, however, is the length of time involved in its administration. The time invested approachs that of other instruments used in the neuropsychological laboratory such as the Rey Auditory Verbal Learning Test, and consequently, the task may be more useful in that setting than at the bedside. Nevertheless, it may have use in more extensive office evaluations.

DELAYED WORD RECALL TEST

Knopman and Ryberg have developed a test which has several of the features of the instrument described by Grober and Buschke, yet it is brief and more

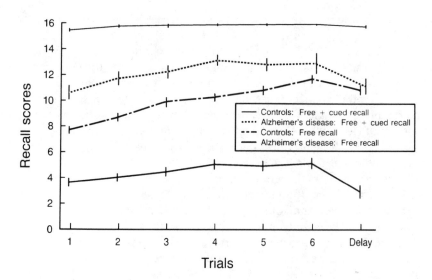

Figure 2   Typical performance on free and cued selective reminding test in a group of patients with dementia of the Alzheimer's type and an age-matched control group.

efficient for bedside use (18). The Delayed Word Recall Test involves the presentation of a set of ten common nouns, one word at a time. In response to reading each word on a 3 × 5 index card, the patient is then required to generate a sentence using the word. A second exposure of the list using this same format follows immediately. The patients are again asked to generate a sentence using the word even if it is the same sentence as the one they generated on the previous trial. This aspect of the task is meant to induce the patient to process the words semantically. After a 5-minute interval filled with other mental status examination activities, free recall of the ten word list is tested. No cues or prompts are given to the patient.

Using this procedure, Knopman and Ryberg reported preliminary results in 55 normal elderly subjects and 28 patients with possible or probable Alzheimer's disease (18). They found that scores on the test were not correlated with education or age and that the test had a high predictive accuracy with regard to dementia. This test incorporates two learning trials, semantic elaboration of the material, a delayed recall component, and is brief and efficient. Consequently, it should be useful as a bedside tool to help in identifying patients with memory deficits. It is, however, restricted to verbal materials.

REY-OSTERRIETH COMPLEX FIGURE

A commonly used nonverbal memory task which has a fair degree of complexity is the Rey-Osterrieth Complex Figure or a similar task involving the Taylor Figure (19). The Rey-Osterrieth Figure is shown in Figure 3. This task requires the patient to copy the complex design comprised of 18 elements (19,20). The initial copy of the figure provides an index of constructional abilities against which subsequent memory performance can be compared. Poor performance on the copy task could be due to constructional difficulties or inattention. Some variations in the procedure of administration exist, but generally, most examiners recommend an immediate recall test and a delayed recall test 20 to 40 minutes later. Variations in scoring procedures have recently been discussed by Loring and colleagues (20). This task is sufficiently difficult to permit an adequate assessment of nonverbal memory and can be useful at the bedside.

PARAGRAPH RECALL

A verbal memory task which is used by some examiners at the bedside is Paragraph Recall. This type of testing is modelled after the Wechsler Memory Scale (4,21). In this task, a paragraph is read to the patient, and the patient

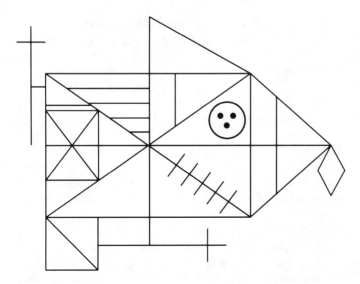

Figure 3 Rey-Osterrieth complex figure.

is instructed to remember the information. The paragraph contains a certain number of scorable items, and recall is typically tested immediately and after a 30-minute delay. It is probably best to avoid using the actual paragraphs from the Wechsler Memory Scale or Wechsler Memory Scale-Revised since this may contaminate later neuropsychological testing. Alternative paragraphs such as the "Babcock Story" or the "Cowboy Story" are available (19).

FIGURE MEMORY

A similar nonverbal task is also commonly used at the bedside. This task is also adapted from the Wechsler Memory Scale and Wechsler Memory Scale-Revised (18,19) and involves copying four line drawings of increasing complexity. The patient is asked to reproduce each of four designs on a piece of paper after a 5-second exposure and a 10-second delay. The patients are instructed to copy the designs and remember them. Typically, a 4-point scoring scale is used to evaluate performance (2). Most patients should recall all four designs with a reasonable degree of accuracy. Again, figures from published neuropsychological tests should be avoided. This task is also useful at the bedside and can give an estimate of nonverbal memory function.

SUMMARY

This chapter has provided a brief rationale for bedside memory testing. The essential components of memory function were described, and several illustrative instruments or tests were outlined for the use at the bedside or in the office. This list is incomplete, and several other testing procedures may be suitable as well. A reasonable recommendation for the clinician is for him/her to become familiar with a few memory tasks which incorporate several of the features felt to be desirable at varying levels of complexity and use these tests on appropriate patients. Once the clinician has become accustomed to using these instruments, he/she can choose those which best suit his/her need for a particular patient. That is, a particular patient may require assessment of both verbal and nonverbal memory skills, and depending on the degree of impairment, a task with an appropriate level of complexity can be selected.

The tests described here vary in their complexity and time of administration. The selection of tests should be governed by the nature of the problem and the clinical context. If the clinician has extensive neuropsychological expertise available to him/her, then the clinician can defer more detailed testing to the neuropsychologist. It is still beneficial, however, for the clinician to assess the problem adequately to enable him/her to characterize the problem for the neuropsychologist. However, if neuropsychological testing is not readily available to the clinician, several of the more detailed procedures described here may be worthwhile. The tasks described in this chapter will allow the clinician to answer the three questions posed at the beginning of this chapter and subsequently aid in the diagnosis of the patient and the selection of further evaluation procedures.

REFERENCES

1. Weintraub, S., and Mesulam, M.M. (1985). Mental state assessment of young and elderly adults in behavioral neurology. In *Principles of Behavioral Neurology*. Edited by M.M. Mesulam. F.A. Davis, Philadelphia.
2. Strub, R.L., and Black, F.W. (1985). *The Mental Status Examination in Neurology* (Second Edition). Edited by F.L. Strub, F.W. Black. F.A. Davis, Philadelphia.
3. Evaluation of mental status. (1990). In *Clinical Examinations in Neurology*. Mosby Yearbook, Chicago.
4. Wechsler, D. (1945). A standardized memory scale for clinical use. *J. Psychol. 19*:87-95.
5. Crook, T.H., and Larrabee, G.J. (1990). A self-rating scale for evaluating memory in everyday life. *Psychol. Aging 5*:48-57.
6. Herrmann, D.J. (1982). Know thy memory: The use of questionnaires to assess and study memory. *Psychol. Bull. 92*:434-452.
7. Albert, M.S., Butters, N., and Levin, J. (1979). Temporal gradients in the retrograde amnesia of patients with alcoholic Korsakoff's disease. *Arch. Neurol. 36*:211-216.
8. Squire, L.R., and Fox, M.M. (1980). Assessment of remote memory: Validation of the television test by repeated testing during a 7-day period. *Behav. Res. Meth. Instrum. 12*:583-586.
9. Folstein, M.F., Folstein, S.E., and McHugh, P.R. (1975). Mini-mental state: A practical method for grading the cognitive state of patients for the clinician. *J. Psychiatr. Res. 12*:189-198.
10. Kokmen, E., Naessens, J.M., and Offord, K.P. (1987). A short test of mental status: Description and preliminary results. *Mayo Clin. Proc. 62*:281-188.
11. Kokmen, E., Smith, G.E., Petersen, R.C., Tangalos, E.G., and Ivnik, R.J. (1990). The short test of mental status: Correlation with standardized psychometric testing. (submitted for publication).
12. Rey, A. (1964). *L'examen clinique en psychologie*. Presses Universitaries De France, Paris.
13. Buschke, H. (1973). Selective reminding for analysis of memory and learning. *J. Verbal Learn. Verbal Behav. 12*:543-550.
14. Buschke, H., and Fuld, P.A. (1974). Evaluating storage, retention, and retrieval in disordered memory and learning. *Neurology 24*:1019-1025.
15. Buschke, H. (1984). Cued recall in amnesia. *J. Clin. Exp. Neuropsych. 6*:433-440.

16. Grober, E., and Buschke, H. (1987). Genuine memory deficits in dementia. *Dev. Neuropsychol. 3*:13-36.
17. Grober, E., Buschke, H., Crystal, H., Bang, S., and Dresner, R. (1988). Screening for dementia by memory testing. *Neurology 38*:900-903.
18. Knopman, D.S., and Ryberg, S. (1989). A verbal memory test with high predictive accuracy for dementia of the Alzheimer type. *Arch. Neurol. 46*:141-145.
19. Lezak, M.D. (1983). *Neuropsychol. Assessment.* Oxford University Press, New York.
20. Loring, D.W., Martin, R.C., and Meador, K.J. (1990). Psychometric construction of the Rey-Osterrieth complex figure: Methodological considerations and interrater reliability. *Arch. Clin. Neuropsychol. 5*:1-14.
21. Wechsler, D. (1987). *Wechsler Memory Scaled-Revised. Manual.* Psychological Corporation, New York.

8

Memory Testing

Robert J. Ivnik
Mayo Clinic and Mayo Foundation
Rochester, Minnesota

INTRODUCTION

The complaint, "My memory isn't as good as it used to be," confronts medical practitioners of all specialties, but especially those who care for older adults. Whether this complaint represents memory change due to age, or whether it is a symptom of pathology, can present a difficult diagnostic dilemma.

Evaluating reported memory impairment involves many sources of information, and psychological testing is frequently necessary. Testing is important in the work-up of memory complaints because testing can establish the integrity of learning and memory skills within the context of the patient's overall cognitive status. Psychological testing documents the patient's memory skills and measures the degree to which an individual patient's learning and memory deviate from "normal for age."

As presented, the complaint of memory difficulty appears straightforward. However, "memory problems" expressed by patients often represent cognitive decline in any of several areas: speech, language, general intelligence, learning, recall, etc. Psychological testing can distinguish one cognitive deficit from another, but different tests are required to make these determinations. Consequently, thorough psychological testing incorporates measures of learning and memory within the broader examination of multiple cognitive functions.

Learning and memory are components of a process, not isolated abilities. That process involves alertness, orientation, concentration, information acquisition (i.e., learning), and information retrieval (i.e., recall). Several of these component processes can be further subdivided. For example, data retrieval can reflect recall at various points in time (immediate, short-term or delayed memory), under differing conditions (free vs. cued recall), for different types of data (verbal, nonverbal, or procedural) with differing formal characteristics (logical information vs. unstructured data). Consequently, psychological testing directed to assess complaints of memory impairment can become quite complex. Several different approaches have been developed by psychologists to address this complexity.

MEMORY TESTS: THE BATTERY APPROACH

Tests selected to examine a patient's memory complaints will vary from one setting to another. Test selection reflects the training and experience of the psychologist more than anything else. However, most tests contain similar elements. This chapter highlights those elements by reviewing the most commonly used memory measures. Often a memory "test battery" is used to assess the component processes of learning and recall. The general "test battery" approach may be augmented with other tests of specific learning or memory features. The additional tests are frequently taken from the experimental psychology literature and better delineate the features of a given person's memory problem.

Several available memory tests take the "battery" approach. The best known, best developed, and most up-to-date is *The Wechsler Memory Scale— Revised* (WMS-R) (1). Other common "batteries" are the *Denman Neuropsychology Memory Scale* (2), the *Memory Test* (3), and the *Rivermead Behavioral Memory Test* (4). These procedures are termed "batteries" because they are a collection of several different short tests, each of which is designed to examine different aspects of the learning and recall process. The hallmark features of the "battery" approach to memory testing will be discussed here by considering only the WMS-R; however, the general features of this test are similar to others in this genre.

WECHSLER MEMORY SCALE-REVISED

The WMS-R includes 12 separate subtests which are grouped to produce five summary indices of "memory" function: Alertness & Concentration, Verbal Memory, Visual Memory, General Memory, and Delayed Recall. These WMS-R summary indices are constructed to be similar to the I.Q. scores of the Wechsler Intelligence Scales (5,6). Their means are 100 and their standard deviations are 15. The intent was to make the WMS-R comparable to the *Wechsler Adult Intelligence Scale* (WAIS) (5) and the *Wechsler Adult Intelligence*

Scale-Revised (WAIS-R) (6), which are the most frequently administered tests of overall intellectual ability used by psychologists.

TESTABILITY

The first portion of the WMS-R does not contribute to any of the general indices. A series of orientation and information questions are asked to establish the patient's capability for testing. Significantly impaired individuals may experience difficulty answering these questions, suggesting that valid completion of the remaining WMS-R items is doubtful.

This brings us to the first important consideration for any psychological testing referral. Psychological testing is a standardized and structured interpersonal exchange. Standardization and structure allow measurement of importnat cognitive features. Nevertheless, psychological testing always requires *interaction* with the patient. Psychotic, confused, marginally alert, disoriented, or uncooperative patients may not be capable of valid testing. Unlike tests of physical health, psychological testing is done *with*—not to— the patient.

ATTENTION AND CONCENTRATION

Having established that the patient is testable, three WMS-R subtests assess alertness and concentration by testing (a) the speed with which the patient executes sequential tasks that place minimal demands on cognitive processing of data (i.e., counting backward, reciting the alphabet, adding serial threes), (b) the ability to recite digits forward and in reverse, and (c) the ability to mimic in either the same or reverse order the sequence in which the examiner points to randomly placed squares on a paper. At first glance these tasks may appear to require "memory"; however, due to their brevity and lack of encoding demand such tasks actually test concentration. Concentration is required for both learning and recall. Along with adequate orientation, concentration is a prerequisite to valid "memory" testing. The patient's overall level of alertness, attention, and concentration are summarized in the Attention/Concentration Index on the WMS-R.

The remaining WMS-R subtests are divided along two dimensions: type of data and presentation-recall interval. The WMS-R presents both verbal and nonverbal data to the patient. Data recall is requested immediately after presentation and again after a 30-minute delay. By using both verbal and nonverbal materials the WMS-R incorporates research relating these two types of information to preferential processing by the left and right cerebral hemispheres, respectively. By varying the presentation-recall interval (immediate vs. delayed), the WMS-R reflects research showing that delayed recall tasks are more sensitive to early or subtle neurologic memory deficits than immediate memory tests. Also, the presentation-recall interval consideration carries implications for the patient's daily functioning.

VERBAL MEMORY

Two WMS-R subtests assess verbal data acquisition and recall, and serve as the basis for computing the Verbal Memory Index. The first, Logical Memory, requires verbatim recitation of two stories immediately following a single reading of each. The second, Verbal Paired Associates, presents eight word pairs (e.g., baby-cries) during a learning phase after which the subject must provide the second word of each pair when the examiner says the first word. The words are grouped into two categories based upon the obviousness of their association: easy (e.g., fruit-apple) and hard (e.g., obey-inch). This procedure is repeated 3-6 times until mastery is attained, allowing an estimate of the capacity to improve performance with repetition. These tasks present verbal information that can be distinguished either based on the amount of inherent logic (paragraphs vs. word pairs) or the presence of learning trials. However, neither of these design characteristics is considered when computing the Verbal Memory Index. These features provide data that can only be considered as qualitative information from testing.

VISUAL MEMORY

Three WMS-R subtests assess visual memory and provide the basis for the Visual Memory Index. Figural Memory asks the patient to study a geometric drawing and then select the identical design from a series of highly similar designs; this is a nonverbal *recognition* task. Visual Reproduction requires drawing geometric figures immediately after studying them for ten seconds; a nonverbal *recall* task. Lastly, Visual Paired Associates presents six abstract line drawings, each paired with a different color, for learning and requires identification of the color when later shown the abstract drawings alone; this procedure is repeated 3-6 times until mastery is attained. Since each of these tasks deals with line drawings and/or color they are considered "nonverbal"; however, the design characteristics of many items are amenable to verbal description.

The Verbal and Visual Memory Indices provide age-specific, nationally normed estimations of content-specific memory. The WMS-R is a significant improvement in psychological test construction. Prior to its 1987 release no single, well-standardized, and adequately normed test allowed comparison of verbal versus nonverbal capabilities on tasks that had been developed on the same well-defined population.

The WMS-R was further organized such that the separate Verbal and Visual Memory Indices could then be combined into a General Memory Index. The General Memory Index summarizes the Verbal and Visual Memory Indices only, excluding the subtests that relate to alertness, concentration or delayed memory. Accordingly the General Memory Index only reflects *immediate* memory without distraction.

DELAYED RECALL

A Delayed Recall Index is also computed from four subtests (two verbal and two nonverbal: Logical Memory, Visual Reproduction, and both Verbal and Visual Paired Associates) which request data recall after a 30 minute delay. The Delayed Recall Index does not differentiate verbal from visual recall, which is unfortunate since research in both neurology and psychology suggests that delayed recall skills are differentially influenced by the hemispheric lesion lateralization, just as for immediate memory tasks.

MEMORY TESTS-LIST LEARNING APPROACHES

The WMS-R, and tests of similar design, provides a solid basis for the clinical examination of memory complaints. However, a feature that is not well captured by the "battery" approach is the person's ability to learn over trials. Therefore, many psychologists turn to the psychology research literature regarding list learning to construct testing procedures that better address processes that underlie learning across trials. There are a number of tests in this category. Again, they share many common features. This discussion focuses upon most recently published test, the *California Verbal Learning Test* (CVLT) (7), as representative of this category. Other popular measures include the *Auditory-Verbal Learning Test* (AVLT) (8), and the procedure of *Selective Reminding* (SR) (9).

CALIFORNIA VERBAL LEARNING TEST (CVLT)

The CVLT presents to the patient a list of 16 words for learning and memory. Five consecutive learning trials occur with the list being read in its entirety before each. Recall of the complete list is requested on each of the five trials. The 16 words on the list can be grouped into four semantic categories of four words each (i.e., spices & herbs, tools, articles of clothing, fruits), although this is not immediately pointed out to the patient.

When the five learning trials have been completed a second list of 16 words is read and recall is requested; this second list serves as "interference" to the consolidation of the first list. Two of the four semantic grouping categories for the second list are the same as those on the first list, which allows comparison of the patient's resistance to interference based upon shared versus unshared categorizations. When recall of the second list is complete, the patient is asked to recall all of the words from the first list without that list being read again; an index of short-term free recall after interference is thus obtained.

Next the examiner asks for recall of words from the first list *by category*. The patient is told, "Tell me all of the items from the first list that are tools (or spices & herbs, etc.).'' This provides a measure of free versus cued recall; however, the cuing procedure also identifies the fact that the words can be categorized. This has the potential of suggesting an organizational strategy to those patients who may not have recognized the feature of categorical organization on their own. This latter consideration becomes important because the free and cued recall testing procedures are repeated again after a delay interval of 20 minutes during which other testing occurs. The ability to organize new information is known to improve later recall of that data. Therefore, the first cued recall trial may suggest the use of categorical grouping to the patient, and in so doing may protect the patient's delayed free recall skills from deterioration that could have occurred without such prompting. Finally, the CVLT's delayed free and cued recall scores can be compared to the similar scores obtained immediately after the reading an recall of the interference task.

Much information is obtained from the CVLT. Most person's immediate memory span (i.e., the number of words likely to be recalled after the first learning trial) does not extend beyond 6 to 9 words; therefore, the 16 words presented by the CVLT exceed just about everyone's single trial learning. The five learning trials provide adequate repetition of the task for most persons to learn a majority of the items. Thus, learning efficiency is reflected in the learning curve that a given patient produces.

The second list briefly distracts the patient from the content of the first list, and presents similar data for learning which may interfere with consolidation of the first list. This interference can be measured by comparing free recall of the first list after interference with free recall of that same list immediately before interference (i.e., at trial 5). Likewise, repeating each recall task after a 20 minute delay measures the decay that occurs for the memory traces (i.e., forgetting) while the subject is engaged in completely unrelated activities.

Additional data (e.g., serial learning and recall strategies, vulnerability to proactive interference, false positive recognition) can also be determined on the CVLT. Consideration of these features go beyond the intended scope of this discussion, however. Suffice it to say that the CVLT has been designed to incorporate many of the most desirable features of verbal list-learning tasks into a single test.

AUDITORY-VERBAL LEARNING TEST (AVLT)

The CVLT provides much data, but it may be unnecessarily complicated for some clinical situations. The *Auditory-Verbal Learning Test* (AVLT) (8) is a 15-item, 5-trial learning task with recall after each presentation, recall after interference, delayed recall, and recognition memory features. The AVLT is a similar, but less complex, task than the CVLT and serves many of the same assessment purposes. The CVLT is thoughtfully designed, but due to its recent release the clinical utility of many of its intended features remains to be demonstrated. Also, the CVLT norms are modest; statistical manipulations were conducted on data obtained from 273 "neurologically intact individuals" generating "smoothed" age- and sex-specific norms. In contrast, normative data are more solid for the AVLT. Wiens et al. (10) provide AVLT norms derived from 222 "healthy young adults," and Ivnik et al. (11) have extended the AVLT to older ages with norms of 394 randomly solicited elderly normals age 55 to 97.

SELECTIVE REMINDING

Another common list learning task is the *Selective Reminding* procedure (9). Selective Reminding is a variation on testing "procedure," rather than a specific alternative test. The selective reminding procedure has been applied to word lists of varying lengths and compositions. No single "test" has been developed, validated, normed, and applied to both patient and healthy control populations.

Selective reminding deviates from the more common administration formats of the CVLT and AVLT. In selective reminding the patient is read the entire list-to-be-learned only once—during the first reading. On all subsequent trials the words reread to the patient are only those words that he or she failed to remember during the immediately preceding recall trial. The selective reminding procedure assumes that once a word has been recalled it has been learned. Only unlearned (i.e., unrecalled) words need to be presented again. Hence, the "selective" reminding. If a word is recalled after the first reading of the list it is not read to the patient again *unless* the patient fails to recall it on a later trial.

The selective reminding procedure structures the list-learning task in a manner intended to differentiate word storage (i.e., learning) from word retrieval (i.e., recall). Selective reminding produces four summary scores: "long-term storage," (words recalled on each learning trial), "total long-term storage," (sum of words recalled across all learning trials), "consistent long-term retrieval" (number of words recalled at any specific trial that were recalled on all preceding trials), and "total consistent long-term retrieval" (sum of the "consistent long-term retrieval" scores across trials).

Experimentation with selective reminding has shown it to differentiate among neurologic patients and normal controls. Some psychologists apply selective reminding tasks to the clinical examination of individual patients. However, until the psychometric properties (e.g., normative information) are better established, caution is advised when using any specific selective reminding task in the clinical examination of individual patients.

VISUAL SPATIAL LEARNING TEST (VSLT)

Verbal data lend themselves well to incorporation into learning over trials testing procedures. However, finding a truly nonverbal task with similar characteristics is more difficult. The chief difficulty is that although information may be presented visually—in the forms of pictures, designs, or objects—almost any visual stimulus can be verbally *described*. Tasks which are intended to be "nonverbal" may actually be verbally processed. Therefore, the intended nonverbal learning test may have a significant verbal component.

Several factor analytic studies of theoretically "verbal" and "nonverbal" memory tests with normal subjects have failed to identify specific verbal and nonverbal factors. Rather, these studies suggest that most memory tests correlate best with each other without regard to the type of information being used. The failure to identify specific verbal and nonverbal memory capacities *may* relate to the verbal encoding capabilities already mentioned.

In addition to the significant problem of possible verbal encoding of intended nonverbal stimuli, nonverbal tests must rely on a nonspoken response. Drawing responses have most commonly been required. However, drawing demands motor coordination and the absence of either constructional or motor apraxia, all of which are common correlates to neurologic conditions. Also, if a nonverbal test is to incorporate the "learning over trials" feature that has proven useful in verbal tasks, the material to be assimilated must be sufficiently complex. Many purportedly nonverbal learning and recall tests fail one or more of these considerations.

A new nonverbal test of learning and recall is the *Visual Spatial Learning Test* (VSLT) (12). The VSLT was designed with all of the above considerations in mind, and is intended to be a nonverbal CVLT or AVLT analog. The VSLT requires that the subject (a) learn to recognize 7 of 15 designs which are difficult to encode verbally, and (b) recall the correct placement of these designs on a 6 by 4 matrix. Patients are given five learning and recall trials; recall is also examined after a 30-minute delay. Three sets of scores are generated for each trial: the number of designs correctly recognized, the number of positions correctly recalled, and the number of designs recalled in their correct position. Research using the VSLT shows that it works better as a nonverbal memory test than many of its predecessors, given the design characteristics specified above. Factor analyses indicate that it functions as a learning and memory task distinct from verbal procedures. Furthermore, when given to temporal lobectomy patients before and after surgery the VSLT successfully detects deterioration of nonverbal learning and memory due to right temporal resections; other "nonverbal" memory tests have failed in this regard. The VSLT therefore appears to be an improved nonverbal learning and memory test for use in a variety of clinical situations.

Hopefully, this discussion of the CVLT, AVLT, VSLT and selective reminding has highlighted the manner in which procedures taken from the learning research literature augment the "battery" approach to memory testing.

ADVANTAGES AND LIMITATIONS OF MEMORY TESTS

The preceding discussion has presented the major aspects of clinical memory tests. The intent of the discussion has been to provide a better understanding of the procedures and rationale behind psychometric measurements of learning and memory. As such, this presentation has been largely descriptive at a very pragmatic, "how-to" level. Both the strengths and limitations of the psychometric approach to memory testing should be apparent. The strengths related primarily to the well-structured, highly standardized, well-normed, and proven sensitivity of psychometric memory testing to pathologic memory disorders. Standardization of testing procedures allows comparability of scores obtained at one institution or at one point in time to the scores earned by the same person at another place or time. Well-normed tests, such as the WMS-R and AVLT, control for the effects of age on learning and memory in their normative bases.

Psychometric tests assist the clinician by (1) assessing the validity of memory complaints, (2) delineating the cognitive processes underlying learning and recall disorders, (3) examining learning and memory within the context of other cognitive capabilities, and (4) measuring the severity of learning and memory problems.

Along with these advantages, psychometric testing possesses several inherent limitations, which must also be kept in mind. In order to differentiate one cognitive process from another, psychometric testing introduces structure and standardization into the testing process which thereby causes that process to become somewhat artificial. Psychometric testing cannot fully replicate the situations in which cognitive difficulties are experienced by persons in their daily lives. Also, the adequacy of norms vary across tests. Tests are usually normed by age, measured IQ, and/or sex. However, even the best normed measures contain limitations. It is impossible to account for all of the personal, social, and cultural factors that influence cognitive functioning in real life (e.g., education, occupation, cultural emphasis placed upon analytical thinking, English as a second language, etc.). Also, as already noted, testing is an interactive process. Any individual who either cannot or will not cooperate fully with testing introduces uncontrolled variability (i.e., error) into the testing situation.

COMPUTERIZED MEMORY ASSESSMENT

The standard psychometric approach to memory assessment, described above, has been recently challenged by the creative application of electronic technology to memory testing (13). Crook and associates have developed a memory assessment system that utilizes an AT&T microcomputer, a Panasonic videodisc player, a SONY touch-sensitive television, and a specially adapted telephone. Using the customized hardware and software, these researchers present an entirely new approach to memory testing. This approach translates aspects of traditional memory testing (e.g., learning and recalling narrative information or word lists) to new data presentation modes (e.g., a television newscast) which have the stimulus properties of real-life learning situations (e.g., watching the evening news). Many of their memory tasks have tremendously enhanced face validity when compared to the previously described traditional testing procedures.

The application of microcomputer technology to memory testing also opens a door of opportunity that has been heretofore closed to standard clinical tests: the reliable assessment of alertness with reaction time tests. Traditional memory tests, such as the *Wechsler Memory Scale-Revised*, include timed cognitive processing tasks (e.g., set repetition, serial additions or subtractions) to evaluate attention and concentration. Although useful, the fact that the testing process is dependent upon an examiner's hand-held stopwatch introduces error unrelated to the subject's status. For many traditional attention and concentration tests, the task being timed is dependent in part upon the response accuracy of the examiner, which may itself be affected by the examiner's own alertness, fatigue, boredom, distraction, health, etc. With computer-based technology reaction time tests are completed with no examiner confound. Stimuli presentation, timing, and response scoring are all performed by computer; error introduced by examiner variables are effectively removed. Furthermore, the response-required (i.e., moving a finger from one box on the touch sensitive television screen to another box) allows division of the patient's response into two components: reaction time (i.e., the interval between stimulus presentation and response initiation) and motor speed (i.e., the interval between response initiation and response completion). These reaction time and motor speed components of the patient's response are measured in milliseconds; an impossible task for a human examiner.

The use of a touch-sensitive television screen for task presentation and subject response expands the range of potential memory tasks as well. The experimental psychology literature on "working memory" has been adapted to the television presentation and response modality in a test that requires the patient to develop his or her own personal strategy for placing common items (i.e., keys, gloves, pens, medications) in a stylized house. The computer "remembers" which items were placed in which room of the stylized house. At a later point the subject is asked to recall where they placed each item, and the computer scores the subject's recall for accuracy. The unique aspect of this task is that it requires the subject to develop and apply their own personalized strategy to performing a task (i.e., placing the items in different "rooms" based upon whatever criteria they choose) and then later tests the subject's recall of their own prior placements. The recall that is required is recall of their own uniquely designed strategy, not an arbitrary or artificial set of materials determined by someone else.

Patient's reports of other problems in everyday living created by memory disorders can also be better assessed with this technology. For example, problem with learning peoples' names is examined by actors introducing themselves to the patient via the television, and the subject being asked at a later time to recall the actor's name when he or she reappears on the television screen speaking to the patient. The use of a video format simulates real life by providing relevant visual (the actor's image) and audio (the sound of the actor's voice) information that might influence name recall. In another test, difficulties remembering telephone numbers of varying length and with or without interruptions (i.e., getting a busy signal) are tested by use of a real telephone.

Crook and colleagues have shown impressive creativity in their adaptation of microcomputer technology to clinical evaluation of memory complaints. Nevertheless, much work needs to be done before these procedures can be recommended for general use. The normative basis for the computer tests is presently limited to data accumulated on highly motivated, well-educated, healthy, and usually occupationally accomplished elderly volunteers living in the Washington, D.C. region. Efforts to norm the computer tests in other geographic regions and with more representative community samples are underway. Also, despite the enhanced face validity of these tests, their true value as measures of meaningful cognitive constructs needs to be established. It also has not yet been demonstrated that the computer tests are any more sensitive to pathologic cognitive conditions (e.g., dementia) than traditional testing procedures. Finally, although the tests are exceptionally well conceived and designed, their reliance upon a microcomputer, videodisc player, touch-sensitive television, and custom designed hardware and software introduces cost considerations that will affect their acceptance by psychologists wishing to use them in either clinical or research undertakings.

CONCLUSION

Psychological tests can assist health care specialists working with patients who complain of memory difficulties. Psychological testing is designed to examine the cognitive processes that constitute learning and remembering new information. Testing usually examines these abilities within the broader context of the patient's overall cognitive status. By reviewing the design features of the most common memory tests we have discussed the rationale underlying memory testing. The strengths and the weaknesses associated with this type of examination have been presented. Psychological testing is shown to be a complex, sometimes time consuming, but valuable undertaking that contributes information for both diagnostic and treatment planning purposes. This presentation introduces the nonpsychologist, health care specialist to the memory testing basics. Persons interested in additional information are referred to Lezak's *Neuropsychological Assessment* (14), where a more comprehensive presentation of all types of cognitive tests can be found.

REFERENCES

1. Wechsler, D. (1987). *Wechsler Memory Scale-Revised. Manual.* Psychological Corporation, New York.
2. Denman, S.B. (1984). *Denman Neuropsychology Memory Scale.* S.B. Denman, Charleston, SC.
3. Randt, C.T., Brown, E.R., Osborne, D.P., et al. *Memory Test.* Department of Neurology, NYU Medical Center, New York.
4. Wilson, B.A., Cockburn, J., and Baddeley, A. (1985). *The Rivermead Behavioral Memory Test.* Thames Valley Test Co., Reading, England.
5. Wechsler, D. (1955). *Wechsler Adult Intelligence Scale. Manual.* Psychological Corporation, New York.
6. Wechsler, D. (1981). *Wechsler Adult Intelligence Scale-Revised. Manual.* Psychological Corporation, New York.
7. Delis, D.C., Kramer, J.H., Kaplan, E., and Ober, B.A. (1987). *The California Verbal Learning Test.* Psychological Corporation, San Antonio, TX.
8. Rey, A. (1964). *L'examen clinique en psychologie.* Presses Universitaires de France, Paris.
9. Buschke, H., and Fuld, P.A. (1974). Evaluating storage, retention, and retrieval in disordered memory and learning. *Neurology 24*:1019-1025.
10. Wiens, A.N., McMinn, M.R., and Crossen, J.R. (1988). Rey Auditory-Verbal Learning Test: development of norms for healthy young adults. *Clin. Neuropsychol. 2*:1, 67-87.
11. Ivnik, R.J., Malec, J.F., Tangalos, E.R., Peterson, R.C., Kokmen, E., and Kurland, L.T. (In press). The Auditory-Verbal Learning Test (AVLT): Norms for Age 55 and Above. *Psychol. Assess.*
12. Malec, J.F., Ivnik, R.J., and Hinkeldey, N.S. (In press). The Visual Spatial Learning Test (VSLT). *Psychol. Assess.*
13. Crook, T.H., and Larrabee, G.J. (1988). Interrelationships among everyday memory tests: stability of factor structure with age. *Neuropsychology 2*:1-12.
14. Lezak, M.D. (1983). *Neuropsychological Assessment,* 2nd ed. Oxford University Press, New York.

9

Neuropsychological Testing of Memory Disorders

Marilyn S. Albert
and
Ginette Lafleche

Massachusetts General Hospital
Harvard Medical School
Boston, Massachusetts

As reflected by the content of the current volume, numerous neurologic and psychiatric disorders can produce a memory impairment. The methods by which these memory-impaired patients can be differentiated from one another have been of increasing interest in recent years. This is probably the case for several reasons. First, the theoretical foundation of cognitive research, as it pertains to memory, has achieved a high degree of sophistication. This provides an extensive range of techniques and concepts that can be applied to testing memory-impaired populations (see Models of Memory and the Understanding of Memory Disorders, Chap. 6, for a discussion of this issue). Second, sophistication in the neurosciences has been expanding at a geometric rate, permitting both more accurate diagnostic procedures and a more detailed delineation of brain-behavior relationships. Lastly, the mean age of the population has increased dramatically in recent years, and with that has come an increased prevalence of the disorders that produce a memory impairment and therefore an increased interest in trying to understand them. Due to the interactions of these factors, it is now possible to use neuropsychological testing to improve the differential diagnosis of patients with memory deficits. A judicious use of testing results can also be used to guide patient management.

The main purpose of the present chapter is to summarize the neuropsychological differences in the presentation of the most common amnesic and dementing disorders. Issues related to differentiating among patient groups that are of theoretical, rather than practical, relevance are largely omitted, since they are described in detail elsewhere in this volume. Instead, the emphasis is on how one can use the wealth of knowledge that has recently emerged from neuropsychological examinations of amnesic and dementing patients to improve the clinical diagnosis of individuals with these disorders. Actual clinical examples are also provided to emphasize the practical application of this information. Wherever possible, the neuropathological and neurochemical underpinnings of the cognitive deficits will be briefly described in order to emphasize the fact that clinicopathologic correlations exist and may provide important insights into the nature of the patient's cognitive impairments.

THE AMNESIC SYNDROME

Although rare, amnesic syndromes represent the most striking pattern of memory disorder. That is because amnesic patients have an intact general fund of knowledge but a severe disability in learning new information. Thus, as pointed out in the chapter on alcoholic Korsakoff's syndrome (Chap. 12), the traditional psychometric hallmark of the amnesic syndrome is a normal IQ, as typically measured by the Wechsler Adult Intelligence Scale (WAIS or WAIS-R) (1,2), coupled with a memory quotient (MQ) at least 20 points lower (3), typically measured by the Wechsler Memory Scale (WMS or WMS-R) (4-5). It seems almost counterintuitive for such a pattern of deficits to exist, since it would seem that one could not remember things learned in the past if one did not have a good "memory." However, it is now clear that circumscribed damage to medial temporal regions (6-8) can produce a profound and lasting deficit in anterograde memory (the ability to learn and retain new verbal and nonverbal information) while leaving retrograde memory (the retrieval of previously learned information) largely or partially intact (9).

Although a variety of disorders can produce an amnesic syndrome (e.g., alcoholic Korsakoff syndrome, herpes encephalitis, surgical excision, etc.), the broad nature of the anterograde memory deficit is common across conditions. That is, primary memory is preserved, while secondary memory is impaired. Primary memory refers to the ability to retain information immediately after exposure to it. Information stored in primary memory (also referred to as immediate or short-term memory), begins to fade after several seconds unless it is rehearsed. Due to this limitation, the average capacity of primary memory is 7 (± 2) units (10). The most commonly used measure of primary memory is digit span forward (11) since it assesses the number of unrelated units, in this case numbers, one can retain. Thus, digit span forward has been shown to be normal in patients with alcoholic Korsakoff's syndrome (12), postencephalitis (13), and surgical excisions of the temporal lobes (14).

Secondary memory (sometimes referred to as long-term memory) refers to the ability to retain information across delays. Although there is controversy over whether amnesic patients demonstrate impairments over very brief delays when rehearsal is prevented (i.e., 3-30 seconds) (see Chap. 6), there is complete agreement that retention across longer intervals is severely deficient. Thus, Wechsler Memory Scale scores are 2-3 standard deviations below the norm in patients with alcoholic Korsakoff's syndrome (5), postencephalitis (15), and surgical excisions (14). Such patients are also impaired in other standard memory tasks such as the California Verbal Learning Test (16), the Delayed Recognition Span Test (17), and the Rey Auditory Verbal Learning Test (18).

The severity of this secondary memory deficit is reflected by the fact that on clinical memory tests, amnesic patients demonstrate a more rapid rate of forgetting compared with controls. While a continuous recognition paradigm administered over several days does not demonstrate this experimentally (19,20), standard clinical tests, such as the Wechsler Memory Scale-Revised, highlight this aspect of behavior. For example, on the WMS-R, the Delayed Memory Index for an alcoholic Korsakoff patient is generally 8-10 points lower than the General Memory Index (see Chap. 12). The former score primarily reflects delayed recall while the latter is more reflective of immediate recall.

Amnesic patients also typically demonstrate a considerable amount of proactive interference, that is, information which the patient is exposed to first will interfere with the patient's ability to retain later information. Thus, for example, prior item intrusion errors are commonly observed in patients with alcoholic Korsakoff's syndrome (21,22), postencephalitis (13), and surgical excisions (14).

Although, as described above, amnesic patients show severe secondary memory deficits when they are asked to consciously recall information, there are certain types of secondary memory tests on which amnesic patients perform normally. These are tests that evaluate the implicit, rather than the explicit, retention of information. As described in greater detail in Chapter 6, implicit memory is assessed by asking the subject to perform a task and then evaluating their performance on a different, but related, task on which savings from the former task can be inferred. For example, patients may be asked to rate the degree to which they like certain words (e.g., MOTEL), then later asked to complete word stems of words they previously rated (e.g., MOT--) and words to which they were not previously exposed (e.g., COM--). If they complete the word stems with the words they were exposed to earlier at a rate significantly greater than chance, then their retention of this earlier information can be inferred. A variety of tasks, from word priming (such as that described above), to perceptual motor skill learning (e.g., a pursuit rotor task), have demonstrated that many amnesic patients perform normally on implicit memory tasks.

Despite these commonalities among amnesic patients, there are clear differences among them, reflected in their neuropsychological profiles. These differences are attributable to the etiology of their disorder and the consequent neuropathological and neurochemical deficits produced.

ALCOHOLIC KORSAKOFF'S SYNDROME

Alcoholic Korsakoff's syndrome develops in a small percentage (5%) of persons who have been chronic alcoholics for many years (i.e. 10-20 years). It is most likely the result of both the direct effects of alcohol on the brain and a thiamine deficiency (22). In the vast majority of patients there is an acute onset, typified by a confusional state which is accompanied by a gait disorder and abnormal eye movements. If these symptoms are treated by large doses of thiamine, most of the symptoms improve but the patient is left with a profound and stable amnesia (23). The amnesia is secondary to hemorrhagic lesions of the diencephalon, primarily the dorsomedial nucleus of the thalamus and the mammillary bodies of the hypothalamus (24). It is also likely that the noradrenergic (25) and cholinergic deficiencies in these patients (26) contribute to their amnesic syndrome.

Although alcoholic Korsakoff patients have a normal IQ, reflecting a preservation of their general fund of knowledge, they do have subtle cognitive deficits when compared with normal controls. They have difficulty on tasks associated with the initiation and maintenance of sets, such as the Wisconsin Card Sorting Task (27,28), and the Controlled Word Association Task (29). Korsakoff patients are also impaired on complex visuoperceptual tasks, such as embedded figures (28,30). These later difficulties are, however, also seen in chronic alcoholics and have been attributed to damage to the anterior association cortex from alcohol abuse (31). A clinical example of an alcoholic Korsakoff patient is provided below.

PATIENT 1

The patient was an 80-year-old male with a 2-year history of cognitive disturbance. He worked at a responsible managerial position until the age of 70 when company policy required him to retire. Always a moderately heavy social drinker, he then began drinking a minimum of 6-7 2 oz. alcohol-containing drinks a day. This pattern continued for about 10 years. During the last two years he had not been eating properly because his wife had become ill and he relied on her to prepare his meals. He therefore was continuing to drink very heavily while getting poor nutrition. When he became suddenly confused and agitated he was admitted to the hospital. His gait was markedly abnormal and he developed cogwheeling, which later abated. When he recovered it became clear that he had a memory deficit. He repeated himself in conversation, could not keep track of day to day events and could not find his way around unfamiliar environments.

At the time of his evaluation his general physical examination was normal. His blood pressure was 140/90. His psychiatric evaluation was normal. His neurologic examination revealed a fine action tremor in both hands, a slightly stooped posture, reduced vibration sense bilaterally, and an inability to walk in tandem. His CT scan showed cerebral and cerebellar atrophy and his EEG was normal.

Neuropsychologic testing indicated that his IQ was in the normal range (ie., 110) but his memory was very impaired. He could not remember a simple sentence ten minutes after hearing it. He could not recall a three-word list after 5 minutes. Testing on the Delayed Recognition Span Test (17) confirmed a striking difficulty with memory. The patient's delayed verbal recognition span was 8, which is within normal limits. However, his immediate recall (after 15 seconds) was 1, and his delayed recall (after 2 minutes) was 1. He had no difficulty with simple calculations, and could perform serial 7s easily and quickly. His figure copying was adequate, though somewhat asymmetric, and his proverb interpretations were excellent. For example, for "Rome wasn't built in a day" he said, "Great enterprises are hard to come by and take a long time to mature." His verbal fluency was good but probably reduced from premorbid levels. His naming was normal (81st percentile).

During 3 years of follow-up this pattern of cognitive performance remained stable. He continued to have striking difficulty retaining information but showed no other major cognitive deficits. Due to the patient's memory problem he was unable to care for himself independently and required daily supervision. He rarely drank alcohol. This picture of sudden onset of confusion in a chronic alcoholic, which clears, leaving a profound memory deficit with other cognitive abilities relatively intact, is the typical picture of alcoholic Korsakoff's syndrome.

Patients with alcoholic dementia have a substantially different clinical picture. While they have a memory deficit, they show substantial declines in other cognitive areas as well. Their general fund of knowledge is deficient, as reflected in depressed IQ scores. They frequently have difficulty with confrontation naming and figure copying. The cause of alcoholic dementia is thought to be the multiple central nervous system (CNS) insults that are concomitants of alcoholism (e.g., head injury, liver function abnormalities, vitamin deficiency, etc.). Thus, if a patient who has developed alcoholic dementia stops drinking, his/her cognitive deficits do not progress (32). However, if a patient is actively drinking, the cognitive impairment is likely to become more severe. Under these circumstances, it is almost impossible to differentiate an alcoholic who has developed Alzheimer's disease from an alcoholic who has become demented from alcohol abuse and its attendant CNS injuries.

POSTENCEPHALITIS

The herpes simplex virus can, on rare occasions, produce an encephalitis. The factors that permit this common virus to attack the brain are unknown. The encephalitis comes on acutely and, if not treated successfully, can result in death. Some patients recover completely, others have multiple cognitive deficits. The unusual patient is left with a profound amnesic syndrome which, like alcoholic Korsakoff's disease, remains stable over time. Because such patients are rare, there are few existing systematic studies describing their characteristics. Those that are available suggest that secondary memory tasks with very brief delays are less disrupted by distraction in postencephalitics than in patients with alcoholic Korsakoff's disease (33). The pattern of remote memory loss also differs between these two groups. Postencephalitic patients have a severe loss of remote memories that has much less of a temporal gradient than that of alcoholic Korsakoff patients; in other words, remote events are almost as hard to recall as recent events (34). The overall severity of the loss can also be greater in postencephalitic patients than in alcoholic Korsakoff's.

The differences between these two patient groups are most likely related to their differing etiologies. The herpes simplex virus appears to have a predilection for the medial temporal lobe, a region that remains relatively undamaged in alcoholic Korsakoff patients. Furthermore, the temporal gradient of the alcoholic Korsakoff patient is most likely the result of an anterograde memory deficit, namely difficulty establishing new memories during the many years of alcohol abuse and a remote memory deficit that develops acutely with the onset of the disorder, while the postencephalitic develops a remote memory loss acutely at the time of medial temporal damage from the virus (34). The patient described below has the typical presentation of an amnesic postencephalitic patient.

PATIENT 2

The patient was a 44-year-old male who presented with a 6-month history of cognitive impairment. Six months earlier he had developed weakness, fever, and headache and then became comatose. The coma lasted for approximately one month with very high fever. On recovering consciousness, he had a right hemiparesis, incoherent speech, and a memory disturbance. Within two weeks the right hemiparesis and speech disturbance had cleared entirely but the memory impairment remained. He could not remember daily events and had difficulty remembering events from both his recent and remote past.

At the time of his evaluation his general physical and psychiatric examination were normal. His neurologic examination was unremarkable, with the exception that his left eye was less reactive to light than his right and he had no sense of smell.

His CT scan showed enlarged ventricles and marked atrophy of the temporal lobes, greater on the left than the right. His EEG showed increased slowing, primarily on the left.

Neuropsychologic testing revealed an IQ of 133 (he had 18 years of education). His memory quotient, based on the Wechsler Memory Scale, was 84, representing an almost 40 point discrepancy with his IQ. Since a person's MQ and IQ should be approximately equal, this discrepancy, in the presence of a normal IQ and no other major cognitive deficits confirmed his amnesic disorder. Furthermore, more detailed testing revealed a discrepancy between his verbal and nonverbal memory abilities. When given very brief amounts of information and asked to recall it after a very brief delay (2-20 s), he performed within the normal range when the material was verbal but had considerably more difficulty with nonverbal material. He performed normally, however, on all tests of spatial ability, on confrontation naming and on concept formation tasks.

During the 10 years of follow-up the cognitive deficits of the patient remained entirely stable. He continued to have great difficulty learning anything new and remembering events from the remote past but performed well in other cognitive domains.

SURGICAL EXCISIONS

The most famous amnesic patients are those who became amnesic after surgical removal of portions of the hippocampus and amygdala to relieve intractable seizures (35). These procedures were carried out before the essential role of the amygdala and hippocampus in memory performance was understood. The patient HM had tissue removed bilaterally and therefore, has remained densely amnesic for both verbal and nonverbal material (36). The patients who received left unilateral excisions have difficulty with verbal information only, and right unilateral lesions produce nonverbal memory deficits (35). Case reports of patients with circumscribed traumatic brain injury (36,37) have repeatedly confirmed this pattern of impairment. Lesions confined to the right or left hippocampal/amygdala complex produce little other than a dense anterograde amnesia and a remote memory loss of varying lengths of time (6,7,35-36). Additional cognitive impairments are evident, of course, if the lesions extend beyond this brain region, and are unique to that individual patient.

ANTERIOR COMMUNICATING ARTERY ANEURYSMS

Strokes can produce an amnesic syndrome. The rupture of an anterior communicating artery (ACoA) aneurysm is a stroke syndrome that has been most commonly associated with amnesia (39). The most likely cause of this amnesia is an ischemic lesion of the medial septum, a structure that has large numbers of acetylcholine-containing neurons and projects to the hippocampus (40).

The amnesia demonstrated by ACoA aneurysm rupture can be relatively "pure," i.e., digit-span forward is normal, WAIS subtests reflective of general knowledge are preserved, verbal and nonverbal memory tasks are severely impaired (39,40). Some patients, however, demonstrate difficulty on tasks related to frontal lobe functions. These patients also typically have long periods of confusion and confabulation following disease onset, and these additional difficulties have been attributed to the medial frontal damage that can occur following rupture of an ACoA aneurysm. Below is a description of a patient who became amnesic after rupture of an ACoA aneurysm.

PATIENT 3

The patient was a 31-year-old male who presented with a 5-month history of cognitive dysfunction. Five months earlier he developed a very severe headache that came and went over several days. An ACoA aneurysm was diagnosed and surgery was performed to clip it. The patient was confused and disoriented for several days, but this cleared within a week. It then became evident that although he was oriented to time and place, he had great difficulty retaining information over delays. He could not remember who he had seen from one day to the next and could not learn how to find his way around new surroundings.

His general physical examination, psychiatric evaluation, and neurologic examination were normal. His CT scan was normal, as was his EEG.

Neuropsychologic testing showed that his IQ was normal (i.e., 109). On tests of immediate memory he performed relatively well but on delayed recall he was very impaired. For example, his immediate recall of two stories was normal but after a 40 minute delay he remembered nothing. Similarly, he performed slightly below normal on a task that required him to draw figures from memory (16/26), but after a delay could recall almost nothing (1/26). Figure copying and the construction of block designs was, however, normal. Confrontation naming and abstraction tasks were also performed well.

During the two years of follow-up the cognitive impairments of this patient remained stable. Because of his memory problems he was unable to resume his former job but regularly helped out with household duties and found his way around his immediate neighborhood with ease.

It should also be noted that infarction of the medial thalamus as a result of basilar artery occlusion can produce isolated memory deficits, though rarely. Infarcts in the region of the angular gyrus are more likely to mimic a dementia. These patients typically develop a marked memory deficit and difficulty with confrontation naming. If the abrupt onset of the symptoms is unclear, this clinical picture can be mistaken for a dementia.

THE DEMENTIA SYNDROME

Dementia is a general term used to describe a chronic and substantial decline in two or more areas of cognitive function. This is unlike the amnesic patient who has a severe and striking deficit in only one area of cognitive function (i.e., memory). Some dementias are nonprogressive (e.g., alcoholic dementia), but most are progressive. While all dementias are accompanied by a memory impairment, the nature of the impairment differs substantially among patients of differing etiologies. For example, patients with Alzheimer's disease demonstrate a very rapid rate of forgetting over brief delays (17,41) while Pick's patients do not (42); patients with Huntington's disease show a preservation of verbal recognition memory, in comparison to nonverbal recognition memory (43). The other cognitive deficits that accompany these memory impairments also vary widely among patient groups.

The nature of the onset and progression of the cognitive deficits also differs greatly among the major dementing disorders. A carefully collected cognitive history is therefore an essential adjunct to a dementia work-up and often makes the difference between an accurate and inaccurate diagnosis. Most of the dementias have an insidious onset and develop slowly and gradually. These include Alzheimer's disease, Pick's disease, Parkinson's dementia, and progressive supranuclear palsy. The most virulent dementing disorder, Creutzfeldt-Jakob disease, develops insidiously but is known for its rapid rate of progression from onset to death (often 1 year's duration). The initial symptoms of a multi-infarct dementia develop acutely, but since multiple large or small cerebral infarcts are the cause of the cognitive decline, the ultimate clinical picture can take many years to develop, albeit in a stepwise and stuttering fashion.

Thus each dementing disorder has a unique cognitive history and a unique pattern of spared and impaired function which can help the clinician to identify it.

ALZHEIMER'S DISEASE

The first and most noticeable symptom generally observed in patients with Alzheimer's disease (AD) is a severe anterograde memory deficit. Early in the course of disease, this is primarily confined to an impairment of secondary memory, but as the disease progresses, primary memory deficits develop. The striking aspect of this difficulty in acquiring new information is the rapid rate at which information is forgotten in secondary memory. Comparisons of dementias of differing etiologies suggest that patients with AD lose more information over a brief delay than patients with Huntington's disease (17), Pick's disease (42), or progressive supranuclear palsy (44). It has recently been demonstrated by the use of a continuous recognition paradigm that this rapid rate of forgetting is primarily evident during the initial 10 minutes following exposure to new material (41). Therefore, retention intervals that fall within this time interval are most useful diagnostically. Recall paradigms with relatively brief intervals between exposure to information and its immediate and delayed recall (e.g., 15 seconds vs. 2 minutes, respectively) are thus best in accentuating differences among patients. There are many standard memory tests that can be readily adapted to these constraints.

It is likely that the rapid rate of forgetting seen in AD is the result of the striking damage to the hippocampal complex seen in this disorder. There is a high density of neurofibrillary tangle and neuritic plaque formation in the medial temporal lobe, particularly the afferent neurons of the entorhinal cortex and the efferent neurons of the subiculum (45). This appears to functionally disconnect the hippocampal formation from the rest of the cerebral cortex. The large declines in choline acetyltransferase (ACh) seen in AD (46) probably contribute to this memory impairment of AD patients. However, since the alteration in ACh levels is thought to result from neuronal loss in the basal forebrain (47) and basal forebrain damage is seen in other dementing disorders with a less severe memory impairment early in the course of disease (48), it is unlikely that the cholinergic deficit alone is responsible for the AD patient's particularly severe pattern of memory impairment.

Recent data suggest that, in addition to a memory impairment, the other cognitive deficit most commonly seen in the early stages of AD is difficulty with sequencing, monitoring, and shifting behavior (49,50). These abilities have typically been associated with frontal lobe function (51-53) but it has been suggested that problems with complex attentional mechanisms (secondary to parietal lobe abnormalities) may be responsible for these impairments (49).

In the most typical presentation of AD language deficits (e.g., difficulty with confrontation naming) and spatial deficits (e.g., difficulty with figure copying) develop after the onset of memory dysfunction (54,55). These have been attributed to neurofibrillary tangle and neuritic plaque formation in multimodal association cortices (56,57). The patient below is an example of this typical type of presentation.

PATIENT 4

The patient was a 78-year-old female who presented with a 4-year history of declining memory. The initial symptoms were very subtle; the patient began repeating herself, forgot names and appointments, and began having trouble handling her finances. She had been a very active and lively person, but had begun to lose interest in many of her previous activities. In the words of her son, "her horizons have shrunk." She was aware of these difficulties but tended to minimize them. She was widowed and lived in an apartment on her own. She was able to prepare her meals, though they were on a much simpler scale than before, she could shop but frequently duplicated items; she drove, but only in restricted local areas because she had gotten lost several times driving in places with which she was not thoroughly familiar. There was no history or psychiatric illness, alcohol abuse, or major head trauma. Her sister had died in her early 80s with memory problems.

The patient's general medical examination was normal. CT scan showed mild cerebral atrophy. Blood pressure was 106/60. The neurological examination showed a slight limitation of upward gaze.

Neuropsychological testing revealed a variety of deficits. Though the patient's estimated IQ, using the reduced WAIS-R (42), was still in the normal range (i.e., 110), she had substantial difficulty with memory, set-shifting, and conceptualization, and slight difficulty with naming. Her memory quotient, based on the Wechsler Memory Scale, was 90 out of a possible 143 points. Since a person's MQ should be approximately equal to their IQ, this represented a 20 point discrepancy from her expected level. It also represented an extremely low score for a person with 16 years of education. Her delayed recall performance on the Delayed Recognition Span Test was also impaired. While here verbal recognition span was 8, which is in the low normal range, after 15 seconds she could only recall 2 words and after 2 minutes she could recall only 1 word. Impairments in set-shifting and abstraction were revealed by her performance on the Trail Making Test. This task requires an individual to first connect a series of numbers in order (Trails A) and then alternate between connecting a number and a letter (e.g., 1-A, 2-B, etc.) (Trails B). She performed extremely slowly on both Trails A and Trails B (taking almost 2 minutes and 3 minutes, respectively, to complete the tasks), and she made 1 error on Trails B. She was also impaired on the Similarities subtest of the WAIS-R. All of her responses were concrete (e.g., she said that an apple and an orange were alike because they both had peels). Her performance on the Mattis Dementia Rating Scale (DRS) reflected these difficulties. She received a score of 121 out of a possible 144 on the DRS, which is in the mild range of impairment. Most of her credit was lost on the memory and conceptualization subtests of the DRS. She also had difficulty on 10 items from the Boston Naming Test (this task consists of a series of line drawings that patients are asked to name). The patient failed to spontaneously name 3 of the 10 drawings, giving either category descriptions or semantic associates of the target word (e.g., "ladle" for "funnel," "musical instrument" for "accordion," and "not plier" for "tongs"). Despite these obvious difficulties, her Mini-Mental State Exam score was relatively good (28 out of 30). The Mini Mental State Exam (MMSE) is the most commonly used screening tool among the elderly. Predictably, her two errors were on the recall portion, where she failed to recall 2 of the 3 words.

A slight and gradual decline in mental status was observed over the two years of follow-up. The patient's memory declined, as did her naming, and she began to have difficulty copying moderately difficult two-dimensional drawings.

In addition to this typical presentation of Alzheimer's disease (i.e., where the patient's earliest symptom consists of a gradual and progresssive memory deficit), there have been increasing reports of autopsy-proven AD patients who developed severe impairments in either spatial ability (58,59) or language function (60) prior to the onset of their memory deficit. The cause of these differential patterns of presentation is unclear but may be of important etiologic significance. Two such patients are described below.

PATIENT 5

This patient was a 53-year-old man who presented with a 2-year history of cognitive dysfunction. He was a chemical engineer who had an administrative job in a large company. His initial symptoms related to spatial difficulty. He began to have great difficulty driving and had several minor accidents and many near misses in the previous two years. Apropos of this his wife had said, "we saw the whites of many people's eyes." Difficulty in the spatial domain was also evident in leisure activities. Once an avid golfer, he could no longer play with any reasonable skill. When he noticed that his spatial skills were declining, he had his glasses checked but the ophthalmologist said his vision was adequately corrected. He also became more forgetful, having difficulty keeping track of appointments and forgetting to complete parts of his monthly reports. There was no history of major medical illness, psychiatric illness, alcohol abuse, or major head trauma.

The patient's physical examination and laboratory tests were within the normal range. His CT scan showed slightly enlarged ventricles and his EEG was normal. Both his psychiatric examination and neurologic examination were unremarkable.

Neuropsychological testing confirmed the presence of both spatial difficulties and memory problems, with the former being of much greater severity. On the Mattis DRS for example, he could only copy 3 of 6 simple two-dimensional figures but got a score of 24 out of 25 on the memory subtest. His spatial difficulties were evident on even the simplest tasks. When asked to cross out all the letter "As" that were scattered among other letters irregularly arranged on a page, he only identified 37 of the 50 letters correctly. His score on the Wechsler Memory Scale was 80, clearly indicating that his memory was abnormal. His naming ability was also impaired. He received a score of 41 out of 60 on the Boston Naming Test. Although he occasionally misperceived the line drawings, most of his errors consisted of giving an associate of the target word ("hippopotamus" for "rhinoceros") or describing the function of an object correctly without being able to name it ("you blow on it" for "harmonica").

During the five years of follow-up the patient's cognitive abilities gradually declined. At first the declines were most evident in relation to spatial function. He began to develop problems with depth perception and would reach for things incorrectly. He broke objects with some frequency either because he was not holding them correctly or did not see them. He began to have trouble dressing himself because he could not manipulate his clothing in space and had trouble buttoning and zipping. These difficulties were reflected in his drawings, which became almost unrecognizable. Ultimately, he became almost functionally blind. He often did not see objects directly in front of him and could not see his food on his plate. His memory also declined, but less precipitously. His delayed verbal recognition span went from 12 to 7 over the course of three years. Following these declines, his language abilities began to deteriorate. His word finding became severely impaired (i.e., his Boston Naming Test score was 6/60, 4 years after his initial visit), and he began to have difficulty understanding what was said to him. His Mini Mental score, which had been 25 initially, plummeted to 9. While this patient has not yet come to autopsy, there is no report to date of patients with this pattern of disease who do not turn out to have AD on autopsy. Patients with a prominent language disturbance can have other disorders, however, the one described below has autopsy-proven AD.

PATIENT 6

The patient was a 58-year-old woman who presented with a 3-year history of cognitive decline. Her earliest symptoms related to a decreased ability to express herself in conversation. Over time this word finding deficit became gradually worse. She also developed memory impairments. She would forget appointments and had trouble with orientation. She continued to drive without difficulty and was reported to have an excellent sense of direction. There was no history of psychiatric illness, or alcohol abuse. She had a major head trauma in a car accident 10 years earlier. There were no reports of family members with memory problems.

Her general medical examination was normal. Her CT scan showed substantial cortical atrophy but her EEG was normal. Blood pressure was 130/80. Both her neurologic and psychiatric examinations were normal.

Neuropsychological testing revealed a prominent language deficit and memory problems. Her naming was quite impaired as reflected by a score of 5 out of 10 on selected items from the Boston Naming Test. She described some of the things she could not name ("they're in the water" for "sea horse"), but also made paraphasic errors ("comical" for "unicorn"). Much of her conversational speech was empty and she frequently used filler words or phrases, such as "some situation" or "something." Comprehension of simple conversation was adequate but sentences that were lengthy or complex were difficult for her to understand. Reading was intact but writing was abnormal (e.g., her sentence on the Mini Mental State Exam was "I would like to a boy"). Difficulties with memory were more evident on verbal memory tasks than nonverbal tasks. Her verbal delayed recognition span was 5 whereas her spatial span was 7. This discrepancy between verbal and nonverbal tasks was also evident on the WAIS, where she had a verbal IQ of 79 and a performance IQ of 106. Figure copying was good but abstractions were severely impaired, verbal much more so than nonverbal.

Within two years of her initial evaluation the patient had become completely aphasic. Although other cognitive functions had gradually declined as well, the patient was still reported to recognize immediate family members. The patient then developed cancer and died. Autopsy confirmed AD.

DEMENTIA OF THE FRONTAL LOBE TYPE

Several pathologic entities have been associated with a progressive dementing process that involves the frontal lobes. Recently these disorders have been called dementia of the frontal lobe type (DFT) (61) to differentiate them from dementia of the Alzheimer type. To date, three different pathologic entities have been described. These include Pick's disease (62), progressive subcortical gliosis (PSG) (63), and frontal lobe degeneration (FLD) (64,65). PSG has also been called Type II Pick's disease (66).

All of these disorders begin with changes in personality (61). Lack of impulse control, stereotyped behavior, and inappropriate affect have been described in most cases. Speech that is either hypophonic or excessively loud has also been noted. Alterations in pain sensitivity may occur.

Although memory function is abnormal early in the course of disease, it is less severely affected than in AD. DFT patients remember less than normals immediately after being exposed to it, but do not forget it at as rapid a rate thereafter (42). It is therefore of considerable interest that the hippocampus has been reported as spared in some DFT patients (66), though not invariably (67). Spatial ability is typically reported as relatively intact, even in advanced disease (61), which has been attributed to the relative absence of pathological changes in the parietal cortex. It is also noteworthy that the EEG remains normal until late in the course of disease (61).

The accurate identification of this group of syndromes is particularly important for good patient management. Early in the course of disease, DFT patients give the appearance of having much preserved ability due to their relatively mild memory deficit. However, their inappropriate behavior makes them severe management problems and families who are not prepared for this can become distraught (64). In many cases, DFT patients must be treated like psychiatric patients, with whom they are sometimes confused (61). Enabling families to understand that the cause of the disorder is a brain disease generally helps them to adapt to the extremes of behavior DFT patients display. One such patient is described below.

PATIENT 7

A 55-year-old female presented with a 6-year history of cognitive and personality change. The initial episodes that raised concern related to a series of car accidents in which the patient was involved. In each case she hit another car and drove away, apparently unconcerned about the accident and its consequences for the other driver. At the same time she was becoming more emotionally labile and irritable. She developed increasing difficulty in switching from one task to another. For example, if she was involved in doing something around the house and the phone rang, she would pick up the phone but then have trouble speaking. She began to be socially inappropriate; she would shout across a room at formal functions or have loud arguments in a public place. She also showed evidence of increasing difficulty with memory. She repeatedly lost things around the house and appeared to have trouble concentrating. Nevertheless, she remained independent in activities of daily living and continued to take care of routine household chores. There was no history of psychiatric illness, alcohol abuse, or major head trauma.

CT scan, MRI, and EEG were normal. Her blood pressure was 120/70. Her neurologic examination was normal. Despite her personality change, there was no evidence of major psychiatric illness on examination.

Neuropsychological testing revealed an estimated verbal IQ of 104, a memory quotient of 118, and a Mini-Mental score of 29. Despite the apparent normality of these scores, the patient had clear cognitive deficits. She had great difficulty with proverb interpretation. For example, when asked to explain the proverb "Barking dogs seldom bite," she said "They try to act fiercer to cover up the fact that they're really gentle." Her set-shifting abilities were also compromised. She was slow on the Trail Making Test but, more importantly, made three errors. Her naming was impaired; she received a score of 49 out of 60 on the Boston Naming Test. Her errors consisted primarily of semantic associates of the target word (e.g., "fancy fish" for "seahorse" or "harmonica" for "accordion"). Although her Wechsler Memory Scale score was well within the normal range, her memory performance was quite variable. On the Delayed Recognition Span Test, her verbal recognition span was 11 (which is normal), but after both the 15-second and 2-minute delay, she recalled only 4 words (considerably less than one would have pre-dicted given her good recognition span). The one item she missed on the Mini-Mental State Exam was the recall of 1 of the 3 items, and on an earlier ad-ministration of the Wechsler Memory Scale (given prior to her evaluation) she had obtained an MQ of 97. This variability, both within and across test sessions, suggested that the patient's memory deficit was at least partially the result of declines in concentration.

During the 4-year follow-up period, the patient continued to demonstrate a gradual decline in function, with personality changes continuing to be prom-inent. Her behavior was increasingly unpredictable and inappropriate. Her behavior became more childlike and temper tantrums were increasingly com-mon. Her word finding deficits increased and her language became very de-liberate and slow. Despite these impairments, she continuted to carry out many leisure activities and household duties for several years; she read and did crossword puzzles for 3 years after her diagnosis and continued to cook, though not as well as previously.

To complicate the foregoing emphasis on personality change in frontal lobe dementia, patients with a gradually progressive language deficit have also been found to have autopsy-confirmed Pick's disease (68,69) or pro-gressive subcortical gliosis (70). As mentioned earlier, patients with a grad-ually progressive language deficit have also been reported to have a pathologic diagnosis of AD. In addition to the cognitive uniqueness of this patient group, it should be noted that they also require special care. Since the early symptoms of disease mimic a gradually progressive aphasia, these patients benefit from nonverbal communication strategies rather than the mnemonic aids often recommended for AD patients. An example of a patient with a gradually pro-gressive language deficit who had progressive subcortical gliosis on autopsy is presented below.

PATIENT 8

This 68-year-old male presented with a 4-year history of cognitive dysfunc-tion. The earliest symptom of change was a slight apathy and withdrawal. Shortly after that he began having difficulty with language. He first had word finding problems (e.g., he could not provide the names of the labels under which his factory canned goods). His speech became halting and he had trouble understanding what people said to him. He became more forgetful and frequently forgot things that were said to him. He was forced to retire and soon lost even the ability to help with household tasks. He was, how-ever, able to find his way around the neighborhood and 3 months prior to his evaluation had gone to the store and returned without difficulty. His only medication was hydrodiuril to control his hypertension. There was no history of psychiatric illness, alcohol abuse, or major head trauma. His parents had died in their 70s, both of cancer. He had five siblings, none with evidence of cognitive dysfunction.

The patient's general medical examination was normal. His CT scan showed substantial cerebral atrophy, greater on the left than the right. His EEG was normal. His blood pressure was 150/80. His psychiatric evaluation was unremarkable. His neurologic examination showed a positive sucking and snout reflex and en bloc turning.

Neuropsychological testing revealed a profound language deficit. His communication consisted primarily of single word utterances such as "yeah, yeah" or "very good." He could name simple common objects to confrontation (e.g., pen, tie, belt) but could not name any body parts or more uncommon objects (e.g., plug). He received a score of 13 out of 85 on the Boston Naming Test. His comprehension appeared to be better than his spontaneous speech (e.g., he could follow single step commands such as "raise your right hand"). He could read simple sentences and could repeat single words and three word sentences but failed on more difficult reading and repetition tasks. He could write his name but could not communicate information in writing. His memory was impaired but less severely than his language ability. His spatial delayed recognition span was 7 (i.e., he could point to the new position of a disc added one-at-a-time to a series of discs until 7 discs were on the board). He could correctly identify 3 out of 3 coins hidden around a room. His visuospatial abilities were also moderately impaired. He could draw a diamond, square, and cross but had problems drawing more complex figures (e.g., a diamond in a square, a clock, etc.). He was also very perseverative. He was completely unable to draw alternating figures (e.g., the alternation of a triangle and a square), and on several occasions drew directly on top of a figure when asked to copy it.

During the two years of follow-up the patient's linguistic difficulties continued to progress. Within one year he was totally nonverbal and shortly after that developed difficulty chewing and swallowing. He became bedridden and died. Autopsy was consistent with the diagnosis of progressive subcortical gliosis (63).

PARKINSON'S DEMENTIA

A significant number of patients with Parkinson's disease (PD) develop a dementia syndrome. Prevalence rates vary from 25% to 40% (71), but appear to be higher than would be explained by the co-occurrence of AD and PD. Indeed, some demented PD patients have neuritic plaques and neurofibrillary tangles on autopsy (the pathological hallmark of AD) while others do not (72).

Given this complex pathological picture, it is not surprising that the neuropsychological deficits associated with demented PD patients is varied and heterogeneous. Most have the cognitive deficits associated with PD itself, specifically, visuospatial dysfunction and difficulty with concept formation and set shifting (73-75). These have been most commonly ascribed to cell loss in the basal ganglia, which projects to the prefrontal cortex, and to the declines in dopamine, which accompany the neuronal loss in the basal ganglia (76).

When dementia develops in PD patients, it generally includes substantial difficulty with memory (77) and occasionally with linguistic skills such as confrontation naming. Recently, implicit memory problems, both in motor skill learning (i.e., pursuit rotor), and in verbal priming have been reported in demented PD patients (78). Since AD patients have preserved motor skill learning, but impaired verbal priming (78), it may be that a subgroup of demented PD patients with preserved motor skill learning and impaired verbal priming identifies the subgroup of demented PD patients with coexistent Alzheimer's disease.

PROGRESSIVE SUPRANUCLEAR PALSY

Though progressive supranuclear palsy (PSP) is an extremely rare disorder, it is being studied with increasing frequency. This is largely due to the fact that it represents a dementia in which damage is restricted almost entirely to subcortical areas (79). Patients with Huntington's disease ultimately develop neocortical damage (80) as do demented patients with Parkinson's disease (76), thus, PSP is considered the classic subcortical dementia. Pathologic damage in PSP appears to be limited to the basal ganglia, brain stem, and cerebellar nuclei. It is therefore striking that memory function in the early stages of PSP is near normal levels, even when tasks requiring initiation and sequencing, such as verbal fluency, are devastated (44). PSP patients also have difficulties with so-called "frontal" tasks, such as card sorting, which is thought to result from a disconnection of the frontal lobes from subcortical structures (81). This hypothesis has received some recent support from single photon emission computed tomography data (SPECT) showing frontal metabolic declines in PSP patients (82). Though it has not been examined, it may be that memory remains relatively intact in PSP patients until late in the course of disease if it is assessed in a manner that minimizes the profound initiation and conceptualization deficit of PSP patients.

The neurologic deficits of PSP (i.e., ophthalmoplegia, gait disturbance, etc.) are generally diagnostic of the disorder. Thus, memory testing may not be needed to establish the diagnosis with certainty. However, a demonstration of relatively preserved memory in the face of profound initiation and conceptualization deficits will greatly assist caregivers in patient management. A patient with PSP is described below.

PATIENT 9

The patient was a 71-year-old male with a 1-year history of cognitive problems. The primary complaint related to language. The patient had developed very slow speech and word finding difficulties which had gotten gradually worse over time. There was also a recent history of falls which the patient described as "my leg just buckles and gives out." This was not associated with dizziness or vertigo. At the time of his evaluation he was still handling his finances, driving, and helping with chores around the house. There was no history of psychiatric illness, alcohol abuse or major head trauma. He had an older brother who was in good health; a younger brother had died of cancer at 44.

The patient's general medical examination was normal. CT scan showed mild cerebral atrophy, MRI revealed both cerebral, brain stem, and cerebellar atrophy. The brain stem atrophy, particularly evident in the pons and cerebral peduncles, was greater on the left than on the right. His EEG showed slowing, left greater than right. Blood pressure was 150/70. The psychiatric examination showed no evidence of psychiatric illness. The neurologic examination was, however, strikingly abnormal. There was a masked face, reduced spontaneous blinking, a positive snout and glabellar reflex, hypokinesia and bradykinesia, as well as an abnormal gait and markedly abnormal eye movements. There were no vertical eye movements and horizontal eye movements were limited.

Neuropsychological testing showed striking impairments in abstraction, response initiation, and motoric set shifting tasks. Naming and memory were also deficient but less so. His estimated verbal IQ was 80, primarily because of difficulty with the Similarities and Vocabulary subtests of the WAIS. For example, he could not say how North and West were alike but knew that the distance from New York to Paris is about 3,000 miles. Proverb interpretation was, likewise, dramatically concrete. Difficulty with response initiation was most dramatic on verbal tasks. Spontaneous speech showed immense latencies. During critical points in a narrative, usually over substantive words or action verbs, he would stop for as long as two minutes before continuing. This greatly reduced initiation was reflected in a markedly impaired performance on word list generation. For example, when asked to name all the words he could think of in 1 minute beginning with the letter "S," he could produce only 3, which is in the 0 percentile of performance. On verbal tasks, where the stimulus for the response was provided, such as on confrontation naming, he was less impaired than on tasks where he had to spontaneously generate his response. He received a score of 67 out of 85 on the Boston Naming Test, which was below the norm for his age. His memory was also abnormal but irregularly so. For example, he failed to recall all 3 of the words on the Mini-Mental State Exam but recalled both sentences on the Mattis Dementia Rating Scale. His score on the Wechsler Memory Scale was clearly impaired (i.e., 81) but his delayed recall of the stories and figures on the WMS was not substantially worse than his immediate recall, suggesting that he did not have a particularly rapid rate of forgetting.

During the three years of follow-up there was a striking decline in neurologic status. His eye movements became even more reduced and he began falling almost daily. Amantadine was tried but with little effect and eventually he lost almost all mobility. Relative to this severe disability, his cognitive function declined more slowly. But eventually all aspects of his cognitive function was severely compromised.

HUNTINGTON'S DISEASE

Huntington's disease (HD) is another dementing disorder that is generally diagnosed by the presence of a characteristic neurologic abnormality (i.e., chorea) (83). A history of HD in other family members is, of course, also sought since HD is a genetic disorder (84). However, occasionally there is no family history of HD (perhaps because of illegitimacy) and the choreic movements are atypical. In these instances neuropsychologic testing can be very helpful.

Huntington's disease patients have poor verbal and nonverbal recall and poor nonverbal recognition. However, as mentioned earlier, verbal recognition is relatively well preserved early in the course of disease (17,43). Furthermore, HD patients also have impaired motor skill learning but preserved verbal priming, as mentioned earlier (78), so that tasks that assess implicit memory may also be useful in difficult diagnostic situations. Early HD patients also have good confrontation naming ability and relative preservation of many of the verbal tasks on the WAIS, e.g., Information, Vocabulary, Similarities (85). Several studies have demonstrated many of the WAIS subtests that deal with spatial and arithmetic ability are impaired early in the disease process, i.e., Arithmetic, Digit Span, Picture Arrangement, Digit-Symbol (85,86). A combination of this pattern of preserved and impaired function should be diagnostic. A patient with a strong family history and a typical course of HD is presented below.

PATIENT 10

The patient was a 38-year-old female who presented with a 1-year history of motor and cognitive dysfunction. She developed "hand spasms" and began tripping, even on smooth surfaces. She had very mild difficulty with memory that was less evident to others than it was to the patient herself. She had no history of major medical illness, psychiatric illness, alcohol abuse, or major head trauma. Her mother and her maternal grandmother had had Huntington's disease. Her brother had no history of motor or cognitive disturbance.

Her general medical examination and her psychiatric evaluation were normal. The neurologic examination, however, showed the characteristic choreic movements of HD in both her arms and legs. She often was able to incorporate them into what appeared to be purposeful actions.

Neuropsychological testing revealed an estimated verbal IQ of 99 (100 being the average for the population). This may have represented a slight decline from her premorbid level since she had completed 14 years of education. Her memory quotient, based on the Wechsler Memory Scale, was 90. Thus, there was a 9 point differential between her MQ and IQ which was suggestive of memory difficulties. Additional testing revealed that her verbal recognition span, which was 12, was selectively preserved in comparison to her recognition span for faces or spatial positions, which were 7 and 6, respectively. She also had difficulty with a variety of tasks that required speed, sequential planning, and set formation. She was impaired on the Digit Symbol Substitution test, a task that requires one to match a series of symbols that go with a set of numbers. On the Trail Making Test she performed poorly, i.e., in the 10th percentile on Trails A and in the 25th percentile on Trails B. When asked to generate as many words as possible within 1 minute beginning with a specified letter (i.e., verbal fluency), she performed in the 27th percentile. Spatial tasks, such as figure copying, were accurate but demonstrated slight difficulty with planning. Naming was within normal limits.

During 5 years of follow-up the patient showed significant, but slowly progressive, declines in cognitive function. Her memory declined substantially (e.g., MQ = 50) as did tasks assessing speed and sequencing (e.g., verbal fluency dropped to the 1st percentile). She developed difficulty with spatial tasks and with confrontation naming. Despite these declines she remained at home and functional. She did minor housekeeping, took long walks, and drove her car to carry out errands. Her choreic movements increased, they affected her trunk and her facial expressions, but they were not disabling.

MULTI-INFARCT DEMENTIA

Cerebrovascular disease most commonly presents clinically as the "stroke syndrome" (87). Although not all forms of vascular disease in the central nervous system involve stroke (e.g., cardiac arrest, prolonged hypotension), the disorders that produce dementia are generally the result of multiple strokes over time. These have recently been labeled multi-infarct dementia (88) to emphasize the fact that the deficits result from actual infarcts and not from diffuse narrowing of blood vessels.

These dementias are characterized by at least two clinical pictures. When large vessel disease produces multiple cerebral emboli, large discrete cerebral infarcts typically occur. The focal cognitive deficits that result include aphasia, apraxia, agnosia and amnesia, depending on the anatomic distribution of the lesion. Repeated strokes lead to a stepwise development of multiple cognitive deficits.

Medium or small vessel disease, secondary to arteriosclerosis of the small vessels that penetrate subcortical white matter, produces more incomplete, diffuse infarction of brain tissue. Defined in this manner, the latter encompasses the syndromes known as 'etat lacunaire', or lacunar state (89) and Binswanger's disease (90). These disorders produce a more insidious decline and are harder to differentiate from progressive primary dementias, such as Alzheimer's disease, than those produced by large vessel disease. Since the cognitive deficits that occur depend upon the location and size of the damaged tissue, it has been difficult to identify a consistent cognitive profile associated with it (91,92). Neuroimaging procedures, such as magnetic resonance imaging, can also be inconclusive due to the fact that multiple regions of high signal intensity do not always reflect infarction (93) and are often seen in cognitively high functioning individuals as well as in those with dementia (94). At the present time, a very careful cognitive history and neurologic examination, in combination with neuroimaging procedures, tend to provide the most useful information in the diagnosis of lacunar disease and other associated disorders. An example of a patient with lacunar disease is provided below.

PATIENT 11

The patient was a 61-year-old male who presented with a 2-year history of gradual cognitive decline. He had had a left hemisphere stroke 15 years earlier that produced a transient right sided weakness and difficulty with speech. Two years before his evaluation he fell off a ladder and broke his hip. From that time on he appeared slower and less sharp and attentive. About one year before his evaluation he had an episode of headache and dizziness which lasted for a few hours. Following this, his memory was impaired, and it continued to deteriorate over time. He got lost while driving and forgot conversations and appointments. His language also became impaired; his speech was slurred and he had word finding problems. Subsequently, he developed pseudobulbar affect; he both cried and giggled with little provocation. His only previously noted medical illness was the stroke 15 years earlier. Since that time he had been taking aspirin and dipyridamole. He had no history of psychiatric illness, alcohol abuse or head trauma. His parents died in their late 70s, one had a stroke and one a heart attack. Three of his five siblings had had strokes.

His physical examination was generally normal, but he had elevated triglycerides (45 mg/dl). CT scan showed generalized atrophy and multiple lacunar infarcts. His MRI showed multiple lacunar infarcts and diffuse white matter abnormalities. There was also decreased signal intensity in the substantia nigra and basal ganglia. The corpus callosum was markedly thin. The EEG showed increased theta activity with paroxysmal components, maximal over frontal regions. The neurological examination showed increased reflexes, more on the right than the left. He had a positive jaw jerk and a glabellar response. His gait was broadbased and shuffling. He could not stand on heels or toes or perform a tandem walk. His face was somewhat expressionless and his posture was stooped. His psychiatric evaluation was, however, unremarkable.

Neuropsychological testing demonstrated prominent difficulties with language, initiation and set shifting. He could not write single words (e.g., he wrote "squar" for "square" and "scoss" for "cross"). His sentence on the Mini-Mental State Exam was "I came your by automobile." He had difficulty reading simple sentences and misnamed letters of the alphabet. Repetition was impaired. His naming was below normal but less impaired than reading, writing, or repetition. He was severely impaired on word list generation. When asked to name in one minute all the things one can buy in a supermarket, he only produced three items. Even simple alternating movements were impossible (e.g., He could not perform even alternate taps with the index finger of each hand). Drawings that involved alternation were also impaired. However, other drawings were surprisingly good; he could draw a key to command and could copy moderately complex two-dimensional drawings with ease. Only the simplest verbal and visual abstractions were performed correctly. His memory impairment was variable. Orientation was mildly impaired; he knew the month, the year, the president, the governor, the name of the hospital, and the city. He recalled a simple sentence after 10 minutes, but could not recall any of the three words on the Mini-Mental State Exam. Despite the range and severity of his impairments his MMSE score was 19.

During the two years of follow-up he remained relatively stable, with the exception that his language difficulty became slightly worse.

CONCLUSION

In summary, it is apparent that memory disorders can be a major feature of many neurologic and psychiatric disorders. This chapter compared and contrasted a variety of neuropsychological memory test patterns in several of these disorders. The profile of neuropsychological tests can be quite distinctive in various disorders and can aid in the diagnosis of these disorders. Furthermore, the neuropsychological profile can have implications for anatomical structures involved in each disorder, as presented in this chapter.

REFERENCES

1. Wechsler, D. (1955). *Wechsler Adult Intelligence Scale Manual*. Psychological Corporation, New York.
2. Wechsler, D. (1981). *Wechsler Adult Intelligence Scale-Revised Manual*. Psychological Corporation, New York.
3. Butters, N., and Cermak, L.S. (1980). *Alcoholic Korsakoff's Syndrome: An Information Processing Approach to Amnesia*. Academic Press, New York.
4. Wechsler, D. (1945). A standardized memory scale for clinical use. *J. Psychol. 19*:87-95.
5. Wechsler, D. (1987). *Wechsler Memory Scale-Revised*. Psychological Corporation, New York.
6. Scoville, W.B., and Milner, B. (1957). Loss of recent memory after bilateral hippocampal lesions. *Neuropsychologia 20*:11-21.
7. Corkin, S. (1984). Lasting consequences of bilateral medial temporal lobectomy: Clinical course and experimental findings in H.M. *Semin. Neurol. 6*:249-259.
8. Mishkin, M., and Appenzeller, T. (1987). The anatomy of memory. *Sci. Am.* June:80-89.
9. Albert, M.S. (1984). Implications of different patterns of remote memory loss for the concept of consolidation. In *Memory Consolidation: Psychobiology of Cognition*. Edited by H. Weingartner and E.S. Parker. Lawrence Erlbaum Associates, Hillsdale, NJ, pp. 211-230.
10. Miller, G.A. (1956). The magical number seven, plus or minus two: Some limits on our capacity for processing information. *Psychol. Rev. 63*:81-97.
11. Lezak, M. (1983). *Neuropsychological Assessment*. Oxford, New York.
12. Baddeley, A.D., and Warrington, E.K. (1970). Amnesia and the distinction between long- and short-term memory. *J. Verb. Learn. Verb. Behav. 9*:176-189.
13. Cermak, L.S. (1976). The encoding capacity of a patient with amnesia due to encephalitis. *Neuropsychologia 14*:311-326.
14. Milner, B. (1966). Amnesia following operation on the temporal lobes. In *Amnesia*. Edited by C.W.M. Whitty and O.L. Zangwill. Butterworths, London, pp. 109-133.
15. Cermak, L.S., and O'Connor, M. (1983). The anterograde and retrograde retrieval ability of a patient with amnesia due to encephalitis. *Neuropsychologia 21*:213-234.
16. Delis, D.C., Kramer, J.H., Kaplan, E., and Ober, B.A. (1987). *California Verbal Learning Test*. Psychological Corporation, New York.
17. Moss, M., Albert, M.S., Butters, N., and Payne, M. (1986). Differential patterns of memory loss among patients with Alzheimer's disease, Huntington's disease and alcoholic Korsakoff's syndrome. *Arch. Neurol. 43*:239-246.
18. Rey, A. (1964). *L'examen clinique en psychologie*. Presses Universitaires de France, Paris.
19. Huppert, F.A., and Piercy, M. (1979). Normal and abnormal forgetting in organic amnesia: Effects of locus of lesion. *Cortex 15*:385-390.
20. Squire, L.R. (1981). Two forms of human amnesia: An analysis of forgetting. *J. Neurosci. 1*:635-640.

21. Meudell, P.R., Butters, N., and Montgomery, K. (1978). Role of rehearsal in the short-term memory performance of patients with Korsakoff's and Huntington's disease. *Neuropsychologia 16*:507-510.
22. Salmon, D.P., and Butters, N. (1987). The etiology and neuropathology of alcoholic Korsakoff's syndrome: Some evidence for the role of the basal forebrain. In *Recent Developments in Alcoholism*. Edited by M. Galanter. Plenum Press, New York, pp. 27-58.
23. Victor, M., Adams, R.D., and Collins, G.H. (1971). *The Wernicke-Korsakoff Syndrome*. F.A. Davis Co., Philadelphia.
24. Adams, R.D., Collins, G.H., and Victor, M. (1962). Troubles de la memoire et de l'apprentissage chez l'homme: Leurs relations avec les lesions des lobes temporaux et du diencephale. In *Physiologie de l'Hippocampe*. Centre National de la Recherche Scientifique, Paris, pp. 273-297.
25. McEntee, W.J., and Mair, R.G. (1978). Memory impairments in Korsakoff's psychosis: a correlation with brain noradrenergic activity. *Science 202*:905-907.
26. Arendt, T., Bigl, V., Arendt, A., and Tennstedt, A. (1983). Loss of neurons in the nucleus basalis of Meynert in Alzheimer's disease, Paralysis agitans and Korsakoff's disease. *Acta Neuropathol. 61*:101-108.
27. Moscovitch, M. (1982). Multiple dissociations of function in amnesia. In *Human Memory and Amnesia*. Edited by L.S. Cermak. Lawrence Erlbaum Associates, Hillsdale, NJ, pp. 337-370.
28. Talland, G.A. (1965). *Deranged Memory*. Academic Press, New York.
29. Butters, N. (1985). Alcoholic Korsakoff's syndrome: Some unresolved issues concerning etiology, neuropathology, and cognitive deficits. *J. Clin. Exp. Neuropsychol. 7*:181-210.
30. Kapur, N., and Butters, N. (1977). An analysis of the visuoperceptual deficits in alcoholic Korsakoff's and long-term alcoholics. *J. Stud. Alcohol. 38*:2025-2035.
31. Ryback, R. (1971). The continuum and specificity of the effects of alcohol on memory: A review. *Q. J. Stud. Alcohol 32*:995-1016.
32. Seltzer, B., and Sherwin, I. (1978). "Organic brain syndromes": An empirical study and critical review. *Am. J. Psychiatry, 135*:13-21.
33. Cermak, L.S. (1976). The encoding capacity of a patient with amnesia due to encephalitis. *Neuropsychologia 14*:311-326.
34. Butters, N., Miliotis, P., Albert, M.S., and Sax, D. (1984). Memory assessment: Evidence of the heterogeneity of amnesic symptoms. In *Advances in Clinical Neuropsychology*, Vol. 1. Edited by G. Goldstein. Plenum Press, New York, pp. 127-159.
35. Milner, B. (1971). Interhemispheric difference in the localization of psychological processes in man. *Br. Med. Bull. 27*:272-277.
36. Milner, B. (1968). Visual recognition and recall after right temporal-lobe excision in man. *Neuropsychologia 6*:191-209.
37. Teuber, H.L., Milner, B., and Vaughn, H. (1968). Persistent anterograde amnesia after stab wound of the basal brain. *Neuropsychologia 6*:267-282.
38. Squire, L.R., and Slater, P.C. (1978). Anterograde and retrograde memory impairment in chronic amnesia. *Neuropsychologia 16*:312-322.

39. Vilkki, J. (1985). Amnesic syndromes after surgery of anterior communicating artery aneurysms. *Cortex 21*:431-444.

40. Corkin, S. (1982). Some relationships between global amnesias and the memory impairments in Alzheimer's disease. In *Alzheimer's disease: Report of Progress*, Vol. 19, *Aging*. Edited by S. Corkin, R.L. Davis, J.H. Growdon, E. Usdin, and R.J. Wurtman. Raven Press, New York, pp. 149-164.

41. Hart, R.P., Kwentus, J.A., Harkins, S.W., and Taylor, J.R. (1988). Rate of forgetting in mild Alzheimer's type dementia. *Brain Cognition 7*:31-38.

42. Moss, M.B., and Albert, M.S. (1988). Alzheimer's disease and other dementing disorders. In *Geriatric Neuropsychology*. Edited by M.S. Albert and M.B. Moss. Guilford Press, New York, pp. 145-178.

43. Butters, N., Albert, M.S., Sax, D.S., Miliotis, P., Nagode, J., and Sterste, A. (1983). The effect of verbal mediators on the pictorial memory of brain-damaged patients. *Neuropsychologia 21*:307-323.

44. Milberg, W., and Albert, M. (1989). Cognitive differences between patients with Progressive Supranuclear Palsy and Alzheimer's disease. *J. Clin. Exp. Neuropsychol. 11*:605-614.

45. Hyman, B.T., Van Hoesen, G.W., Damasio, A.R., and Barnes, C.L. (1984). Alzheimer's disease: Cell specific pathology isolates the hippocampal formation. *Science 225*:1168-1170.

46. Davies, P., and Maloney, A.J.R. (1976). Selective loss of central cholinergic neurons in Alzheimer's disease. *Lancet 2*:1403.

47. Whitehouse, P.J., Price, D.L., Clark, A.W., Coyle, J.P., and DeLong, M.R. (1981). Alzheimer's disease: Evidence for selective loss of cholinergic neurons in the nucleus basalis. *Ann. Neurol. 10*:122-126.

48. Tagliavini, F., and Pilleri, I. (1983). Basal nucleus of Meynert: A neuropathological study in Alzheimer's disease, simple senile dementia, Pick's disease, Huntington's chorea. *J. Neurol. Sci. 62*:243-260.

49. Grady, G.L., Haxby, J.V., Horwitz, B., Sundaram, M., Berg, G., Schapirom, M., Friedland, R.P., and Rapoport, S.I. (1989). Longitudinal study of the early neuropsychological changes in dementia of the Alzheimer type. *J. Clin. Exp. Neuropsychol. 10*:576-596.

50. Morris, J.C., and Fulling, K. (1983). Early Alzheimer's disease: Diagnostic considerations. *Arch. Neurol. 45*:345-356.

51. Damasio, A. (1985). The frontal lobes. In *Clinical Neuropsychology*. Edited by K. Heilman and E. Valenstein. University Press, New York, pp 339-375.

52. Milner, B. (1964). Some effects of frontal lobectomy in man. In *The Frontal Granular Cortex and Behavior*. Edited by J.M. Warren and K. Akert. McGraw-Hill, New York, pp. 313-334.

53. Stuss, D.T., and Benson, D.F. (1986). *The Frontal Lobes*. Raven Press, New York.

54. Rosen, W.G. (1983). Neuropsychological investigation of memory, visuoconstruction, visuoperceptual, and language abilities in senile dementia of the Alzheimer type. In *The Dementias*. Edited by R. Mayeux and W.G. Rosen. Raven Press, New York, pp. 65-73.

55. Bayles, K.A., and Kaszniak, A.W. (1987). *Communication and Cognition in Normal Aging and Dementia*. Little, Brown, Boston.

56. Kemper, T. (1984). Neuroanatomical and neuropathological changes in normal aging and dementia. In *Clinical Neurology of Aging*. Edited by M.L. Albert. Oxford University Press, New York, pp. 9-52.

57. Pearson, R.C.A., Esiri, M.M., Hiorns, R.W., Wilcock, G.K., and Powell, T. P.S. (1985). Anatomical correlate of the distribution of the pathologic changes in the neocortex in Alzheimer's disease. *Proc. Natl. Acad. Sci. (USA) 82*:4531-4534.

58. Faden, A.I., and Townsend, J.J. (1976). Myoclonus in Alzheimer's disease. *Arch. Neurol. 33*:278-280.

59. Crystal, H.A., Horoupian, D.S., Katzman, R., and Seymour, J. (1982). Biopsy-proved Alzheimer disease presenting as a right parietal lobe syndrome. *Ann. Neurol. 12*:186-188.

60. Kirshner, H.S., Webb, W.G., Kelly, M.P., and Wells, C.E. (1984). Language disturbance: An initial symptom of cortical degeneration and dementia. *Arch. Neurol. 41*:491-496.

61. Neary, D., Snowden, J.S., Northen, B., and Goulding, P. (1988). Dementia of frontal lobe type. *J. Neurol. Neurosurg. Psychiat. 51*:353-361.

62. Picks, A. (1977). On the relation between aphasia and senile atrophy of the brain. In *Neurological Classics in Modern Translation*. Edited by D.A. Rottenberg and F.H. Hochberg. Hasper Press, New York, pp. 35-40.

63. Neumann, M., and Cohn, R. (1967). Progressive subcortical dementia. *Brain 90*:405-418.

64. Gustafson, L. (1987). Frontal lobe degeneration of non-Alzheimer type. II. Clinical picture and differential diagnosis. *Arch. Gerontol. Geriatr. 6*:209-223.

65. Brun, A. (1987). Frontal lobe degeneration of non-Alzheimer type: 1. Neuropathology. *Arch. Gerontol. Geriatr. 6*:193-208.

66. Constantinidis, J., Richard, J., and Tissot, R. (1974). Pick's disease: Histological and clinical correlation. *Eur. J. Neurol. 11*:208-217.

67. Seitelberger, F., Gross, H., and Pilz, P. (1983). Pick's disease. A neurological study. In *Neuropsychiatric Disorders in the Elderly*. Edited by A. Hirano and K. Miyashi. Igaku-Shoin Medical Publishers Inc., New York, pp. 87-117.

68. Wechsler, A.F., Verity, M.A., Rosenschein, S., Fried, I., and Scheibel, A.B. (1982). Pick's disease: A clinical, computed tomographic and histologic study with golgi impregnation observations. *Arch. Neurol. 39*:287-290.

69. Cole, M., Wright, D., and Banker, B.Q. (1979). Familial aphasia due to Pick's disease. *Ann. Neurol. 6*:158.

70. Moss, M.B., Albert, M.S., and Kemper, T. The dementia of progressive subcortical gliosis: A case study. Submitted.

71. Brown, R.G., and Marsden, C.D. (1984). How common is dementia in Parkinson's disease? *Lancet 2*:1262-1265.

72. Jellinger, K. (1987). Neuropathological substrates of Alzheimer's disease and Parkinson's disease. *J. Neural. Transm. 24*(suppl):109-129.

73. Taylor, A.E., Saint-Cyr, J.A., and Lang, A.E. (1986). Frontal lobe dysfunction in Parkinson's disease. *Brain 109*:845-883.

74. Boller, F., Passafiume, D., Keefe, N., Rogers, K., Morrow, L., and Kim, Y., (1984). Visual impairment in Parkinson's disease. *Arch. Neurol. 41*:485-490.

75. Hovestadt, A., deJong, G.J., and Meerwaldt, J.D. (1987). Spatial disorientation as an early symptom of Parkinson's disease. *Neurology 37*:485-487.
76. Divac, I. (1972). Neostriatum and functions of the prefrontal cortex. *Acta Neurobiol. Exp. 32*:461-477.
77. El-Awar, M., Becker, J.T., Hammond, K.M., Nebes, R.D., and Boller, F. (1987). Learning deficit in Parkinson's disease: Comparison with Alzheimer's disease and normal aging. *Arch. Neurol. 44*:180-184.
78. Heindel, W.C., Salmon, D.P., Shults, C.W., Walicke, P.A., and Butters, N. (1989). Neuropsychological evidence for multiple implicit memory systems: A comparison of Alzheimer's, Huntington's and Parkinson's disease patients. *J. Neurosci. 9*:582-587.
79. Steele, J.C., Richardson, J.C., and Olszewiski, J. (1964). Progressive Supranuclear Palsy. *Arch. Neurol. 10*:333-359.
80. Bruyn, G.W., Bots, G., and Dom, R. (1979). Huntington's chorea: Current neuropathological status. In *Advances in Neurology, Vol. 23: Huntington's Disease.* Edited by T. Chase, N. Wexter, and A. Barbeau. Raven Press, New York, pp. 83-94.
81. Pillon, B., Dubois, B., Lhermitte, F., and Agid, Y. (1986). Heterogeneity of cognitive impairment in progressive supranuclear palsy, Parkinson's disease, and Alzheimer's disease. *Neurology 36*:1179-1185.
82. Goffinet, A.M., DeVolder, A.G., Gillain, C., Rectem, D., Bol, A., Michel, C., Cogneau, M., Labar, D., and Laterre, C. (1988). Positron tomography demonstrates frontal lobe hypometabolism in progressive supranuclear palsy. *Ann. Neurol. 25*:131-139.
83. Huntington, G. (1872). On chorea. *Med. Surg. Reporter 26*:317.
84. Pratt, R.T.C. (1967). *The Genetics of Neurological Disorders: Oxford Monographs on Medical Genetics.* Oxford University Press, New York.
85. Josiassen, R.C., Curry, L., Roemer, R.A., DeBease, C., and Mancall, E.L. (1982). Patterns of intellectual deficit in Huntington's disease. *J. Clin. Neuropsychol. 4*:173-183.
86. Butters, N., Sax, D., and Tarlow, S. (1978). Comparison of the neuropsychological deficits associated with early and advanced Huntington's disease. *Arch. Neurol. 35*:585-589.
87. Mohr, J.P., Fisher, C.M., and Adams, R.D. (1980). Cerebrovascular diseases. In *Harrison's Principles of Internal Medicine.* Edited by K. Isselbacher, et al. McGraw-Hill, New York, pp. 1911-1941.
88. Hachinski, V.C., Lassen, N.A., and Marshall, J. (1974). Multi-infarct dementia: A cause of mental deterioration in the elderly. *Lancet 2*:207-209.
89. Marie, P. (1901). Des foyers lacunaires de desintegration et de differents autres etats cavetaures du cerveau. *Rev. Med. 21*:281-298.
90. Fisher, C.M. (1982). Lacunar strokes and infarcts: A review. *Neurology 32*: 871-876.
91. Perez, F.I., Rivera, V.M., and Meyer, J.S. (1975). Analysis of intellectual and cognitive performance in patients with multi-infarct dementia, vertebrobasillar insufficiency with dementia and Alzheimer's disease. *J. Neurol. Neurosurg. Psychiat. 38*:533-540.

92. Cummings, J.L., Miller, B., Hill, M.A., and Neskes, R. (1987). Neuropsychiatric aspects of multi-infarct dementia and dementia of the Alzheimer type. *Arch. Neurol. 44*:389-393.

93. Johnson, K.A., Davis, K.R., Buonanno, F.S., Brady, T.J., Rosen, J., and Growden, J.H. (1987). Comparison of magnetic resonance and roentgen ray computed tomography in dementia. *Arch. Neurol. 44*:1075-1080.

94. Brand-Zawadski, M., Fein, G., Van Dyke, C., Kiernan, R., Davenport, L., and deGroot, J. (1985). Magnetic resonance imaging of the aging brain: patchy white matter lesions and dementia. *AJNR 6*:675-682.

Part IV

MEMORY DYSFUNCTION IN NEUROPSYCHIATRIC DISORDERS

10

Memory Disorders in Cerebral Vascular Diseases

Takehiko Yanagihara

Mayo Clinic and Mayo Foundation
Rochester, Minnesota

A memory disorder associated with cerebrovascular disease was described as early as 1900 by von Bechterew (1), who observed softening of the mesial temporal lobes including the hippocampal formations in a 60-year-old patient with memory impairment and apathy of many years duration. Since then, numerous publications have appeared dealing with memory dysfunction in cerebrovascular diseases. While pure amnesia may occur, memory disorders in cerebrovascular diseases are often associated with other behavioral or neurologic abnormalities. Three anatomical locations have been implicated for memory dysfunction: the hippocampus, dorsomedial nucleus of the thalamus, and basal frontal cortex. While these anatomic structures are often damaged in patients with memory disorders in association with cerebrovascular diseases, damage in other anatomic structures also occurs. This chapter examines the characteristics of memory disorders seen in patients with cerebrovascular diseases by reviewing memory disorders associated with cerebral thromboembolism, intracerebral hemorrhage, and subarachnoid hemorrhage as well as those associated with hypoxic-ischemic encephalopathy and amnesias encountered in migraine. Transient global amnesia will be presented in another chapter; therefore only its relationship to cerebrovascular disease will be discussed briefly.

MEMORY DISORDERS
ASSOCIATED WITH THROMBOEMBOLISM

Whether amnesia is caused by thrombosis of a major intracranial artery or embolization from the heart or an extracranial artery, identification of the involved arterial territory is important for understanding of the pathophysiologic mechanism of the memory impairment. The majority of amnestic episodes occur with cerebral ischemic events in the posterior part of the cerebral hemisphere and the thalamus supplied by the basilar circulation. However, amnesia occasionally results from thromboembolism in the carotid circulation. In patients with multi-infarct dementia and Binswanger's disease, the memory disorder occurs as a part of dementia.

THROMBOEMBOLISM IN THE TERRITORY OF THE
POSTERIOR CEREBRAL ARTERY

The posterior cerebral artery (PCA) supplies a major part of the hippocampus through the hippocampal artery, which arises from the trunk of the PCA distal to the posterior communicating artery (Fig. 1). It is grouped as a part of the inferior temporal arteries by Zeal and Rhoton (2) together with the arterial branches supplying the inferior surface of the temporal lobe (Fig. 1). However, it may also arise from the lateral posterior choroidal artery (3), another branch of the PCA. The anterior part of the hippocampus is often supplied by the anterior choroidal artery (4).

Memory impairment was observed in ischemic infarction of both temporal lobes, including the hippocampus, by von Bechterew (1) as well as by Glees and Griffith (5) and in ischemic infarction of bilateral lingual gyri by Dide and Botcazo (6). However, the importance of the hippocampus and the temporal lobe for memory function did not draw further attention until Scoville and Milner (7) observed a profound loss of recent memory following bilateral resection of the medial temporal lobes. Further observations in autopsy studies have confirmed the association of bilateral hippocampal infarction with amnesia (8,9). However, the infarcted areas in those cases were not confined to the hippocampal formation, but involved the parahippocampal gyrus, lingual gyrus, fusiform gyrus, and fornix (Fig. 1) as the earlier authors had observed (1,5). Victor et al. (8) and Delay et al. (10) observed the presence of old thrombosis in the dominant or both PCAs, indicating that occlusion of the PCA was responsible for infarction. The patient reported by DeJong et al. (9) might have had embolic stroke to both PCA distributions. In another patient with amnesia, infarction of both parahippocampal gyri and hippocampi as well as the left lingual gyrus were observed (11). Woods et al. (12) also observed bilateral hippocampal infarcts in one patient at autopsy, where the infarct on the dominant side extended to the parahippocampal gyrus and

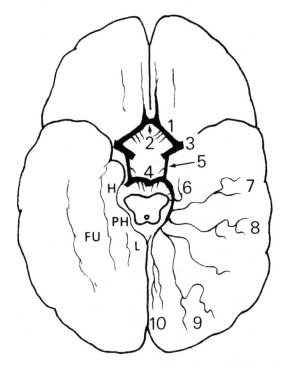

Figure 1   The inferior surface of the cerebral hemisphere showing the cerebral gyri affected in patients with memory dysfunction and the arterial distribution patterns. *Cerebral gyri*: PH, parahippocampal gyrus; FU, fusiform gyrus; L, lingual gyrus; H, hippocampus (buried inside the PH). *Arterial branches*: (1) anterior cerebral artery; (2) anterior communicating artery (pointed by an arrow); (3) middle cerebral artery; (4) posterior cerebral (basilar communicating) artery; (5) posterior communicating artery (pointed by an arrow); (6) hippocampal artery; (7-9) anterior, middle and posterior temporal arteries of the inferior temporal artery (Zeal and Rhoton, ref. 2); (10) calcarine artery.

the fusiform gyrus. Thus, there has been no patient whose amnesia was caused by thromboembolism resulting in unilateral or bilateral infarction limited to the hippocampus alone without damage to the adjacent anatomical structures supplied by the PCA, although this has been observed following global hypoxic-ischemic events (see Memory Disorders Associated with Global Ischemia and Hypoxia).

Ischemic infarction in the dominant PCA distribution may result in amnesia and alexia without agraphia (13-15). In those cases an infarct was found in the hippocampus and the inferior temporal lobe extending to the calcarine cortex. Amnesia was transient in the case reported by Geschwind and Fusillo

(13) and improved to a certain extent in the case reported by Caplan and Hedley-Whyte (15), while it persisted for three months in the case reported by Mohr et al. (14). Neuropsychologically, recent memory was more affected but some impairment of remote memory was also present (14) and visual recall was better preserved than verbal recall (15).

Occlusive disease of the PCA has been investigated in many patients with cerebral angiography and imaging procedures such as cranial computerized tomography (CT scan) and magnetic resonance imaging (MRI scan). Mones et al. described a memory disorder in 3 of 10 patients with angiographic evidence of unilateral or bilateral stenosis or occlusion of PCA (16). Benson et al. reported 10 patients with amnesia associated with unilateral or bilateral visual field defects (17). Four patients had unilateral involvement, all on the dominant side, and they also had alexia without or with minimal agraphia. Fisher also observed the involvement of the dominant side in 14 of 25 patients with memory impairment and PCA occlusion, while the dominant side was affected only in 13 of 45 patients without memory impairment (18). An acute confusional state may occur when the dominant side is affected (18,19). De Renzi et al. (20) observed that impairment of verbal memory was most frequently associated with infarcts in the left PCA territory regardless of the presence or absence of alexia. With analysis of CT lesions, Von Cramon et al. observed the association between severe memory deficit and the location of the infarct along the left collateral sulcus affecting the posterior parahippocampal gyrus and the collateral isthmus, where the bidirectional pathways connecting the posterior parahippocampal gyrus and various association areas traverse (21). However, they did not observe constant involvement of the hippocampus. A CT scan and a brief history of a patient who experienced transient memory impairment and confusion after sustaining an embolic infarct to the dominant PCA territory are shown in Figure 2.

Memory impairment has been observed following infarction in other locations in the PCA territory. Ischemic destruction of the splenum and the posterior part of the corpus callosum (22) has resulted in transient memory impairment. Transient amnesia also has occurred following dissection of the vertebral artery (23); the mechanism may have been distal embolization.

Thus memory disorders have been observed after ischemic infarctions in the PCA territory. While earlier autopsy studies demonstrated damage to the hippocampus on each side, the surrounding areas including the parahippocampal, fusiform, and lingual gyri were also affected. More recent investigations have shown that unilateral infarction in the dominant PCA territory can cause memory impairment, often accompanied by homonymous hemianopsia and alexia without agraphia. Once it occurs, memory impairment is often persistent. It is not clear why a unilateral lesion on the dominant side is sufficient in some patients to have impairment of recent memory, while other patients are affected only by bilateral lesions. Investigations with CT

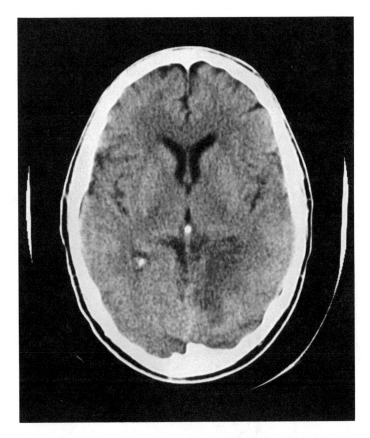

Figure 2 A CT scan showing an acute infarct in the left inferior temporal and occipital region. This 60-year-old man experienced an episode of confusion, memory impairment (for new information), blurring of vision on the right side, and left occipital headache. An examination 3 days later revealed moderate impairment of recall after 5 minutes. He was found to have a small apical aneurysm in the left ventricle of the heart. He has been asymptomatic for 2 years while on oral anticoagulant therapy.

scans suggest that memory impairment can occur without damage to the hippocampus if a part of the posterior inferior temporal lobe is affected, although this should be confirmed by future pathologic examination.

THALAMIC INFARCTS
CAUSED BY THROMBOEMBOLISM

Arterial supply to the thalamus is quite variable depending on the sources and three different sets of terminology have been used to describe arterial supplies to the thalamic nuclei. The artery which stems from the basilar communicating artery and supplies the midline thalamic structure (Fig. 3) has been called the paramedian thalamic artery by Percheron (3,24) and Castaigne et al. (25,26), the interpeduncular profundus artery by Schlesinger (27) and the thalamoperforating artery by Stephens and Stilwell (4) as well as by Saeki and Rhoton (28). This artery originates from the left and right side separately but sometimes the artery on one side supplies both sides (3,26). Another artery, which originates from the posterior communicating artery and supplies the anterior part of the thalamus (Fig. 3), has been called the polar artery by Percheron (3), the tuberothalamic artery by Schlesinger (27) and the premamillary artery by Stephens and Stilwell (4). Sometimes this artery originates from the basilar communicating artery (29). When this artery is absent or hypoplastic, the paramedian thalamic artery may supply the ventroanterior, ventrolateral, and ventroposterior nuclei of the thalamus

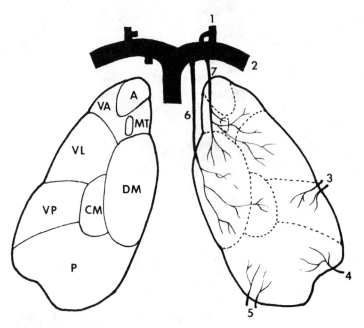

Figure 3   A schematic presentation of the transaxial view of the thalamic nuclei and their arterial supplies. *Thalamic nuclei and tract*: A, anterior nucleus; VA, ventroanterior nucleus; VL, ventrolateral nucleus; VP, ventroposterior nucleus; DM, dorsomedial nucleus; CM, centrum medianum; P, pulvinar; MT, mammillothalamic tract. *Arterial branches*: (1) posterior communicating artery; (2) posterior cerebral artery; (3) thalamogeniculate artery; (4) lateral posterior choroidal artery; (5) medial posterior choroidal artery; (6) paramedian thalamic artery; (7) tuberothalamic artery.

(30). In this chapter, the terms "paramedian thalamic artery" and "tubero-thalamic artery" will be used. The general symptom complex of thalamic infarcts has been reviewed by Graff-Radford et al. (31) and Bogousslavsky et al. (32). Behavioral disorders, particularly amnesia, are mainly caused by thromboembolism and lacunar infarcts in the territories supplied by the para-median thalamic and tuberothalamic arteries. Participation of the anterior choroidal artery to diencephalic amnesia is controversial (31,32).

ISCHEMIC INFARCTS IN THE TERRITORY OF THE TUBEROTHALAMIC ARTERY

When the tuberothalamic artery is occluded, an ischemic infarct may occur in the ventroanterior, ventrolateral, and/or dorsomedial nucleus of the thal-amus. Many patients have a transient or relatively mild hemiparesis, some-times restricted to the lower face and only associated with emotional expres-sion (31-33). However, the main clinical feature is the neuropsychological abnormalities. If the left (dominant) side is affected, patients often have aphasia with slow spontaneous speech and commit paraphasic errors (31, 32,34,35). Along with intellectual deficits, both verbal and visual memory impairments may occur but the verbal one is predominant (31,32,36,37). When the right (nondominant) side is affected, visual memory impairment become apparent and visuospatial performance is also impaired. Anterograde memory is affected regardless of the involved side but retrograde memory is affected less severely (31). Memory impairment is believed to be caused by the lesion in the dorsomedial nucleus but disruption of the mamillothalamic tract (32) and involvement of a part of the anterior nucleus (30) may also contribute. It is sometimes difficult to differentiate this group of patients from those having ischemic infarcts in the territory of the paramedian thalamic artery if the infarct involves a small area. Such patients will be described in the next section.

ISCHEMIC INFARCTS IN THE TERRITORY OF THE PARAMEDIAN THALAMIC ARTERY

This artery mainly supplies the dorsomedial nucleus, centrum medianum, and other medial thalamic nuclei (31,32). This artery may also supply the ventrolateral, ventroanterior, and ventroposterior nuclei (30). Depending on whether the paramedian thalamic artery exists on each side or has a com-mon origin for both sides, unilateral, or bilateral infarcts occur (24,26). Be-cause of the close proximity to the counterpart at the mesencephalic level, the clinical signs indicative of the mesencephalic lesions often accompany the thalamic manifestations. The clinicopathologic correlation of thrombo-embolic infarction in the territory of the paramedian thalamic artery was in-vestigated in detail by Castaigne et al. (26). Both thrombosis and embolism were observed. Depending on the involved arterial territories, they divided 28 patients into unilateral paramedian thalamic infarct, bilateral paramedian thalamic infarct, and paramedian thalamopeduncular infarct.

After unilateral paramedian infarct, agitation and confusion may occur during the acute stage, while hypersomnia, apathy, and psychomotor retardation may manifest at a later stage (26). No clear description of memory impairment was provided for this group by Castaigne et al. Without anatomic confirmation, a unilateral paramedian infarct may be difficult to distinguish from ischemic damage in the territory of the tuberothalamic artery, unless the clinical signs indicative of involvement of the superior paramedian mesencephalic artery are present. This is particularly true if amnesia is a sole manifestation of a small infarct in the left dorsomedial nucleus (38). Two other patients with an ischemic lesion in the left medial thalamus may have had thromboembolism in the left paramedian thalamic and/or the tuberothalamic artery (39,40). Both verbal and nonverbal memory were affected in those patients with a unilateral left medial thalamic lesion, although verbal functions were more severely affected. When the dorsomedial nucleus on the right (nondominant) side sustains ischemic damage, impairment of visual memory occurs without affecting verbal memory (41).

Among patients with bilateral paramedian thalamic infarcts, Castaigne et al. observed a disturbance of consciousness ranging from hypersomnia to coma during the acute stage and apathy and prostration later (26). A severe memory impairment was commonly observed (26). Bilateral paramedian thalamic infarcts without mesencephalic signs have also been observed as verified by CT scan (42,43). Confusion and coma were present at the onset and severe memory impairment became apparent after improvement of alertness and attention. Severe anterograde amnesia often persisted, but sometimes retrograde amnesia was also present. Both verbal and nonverbal memory functions were affected. While focal neurologic signs such as hemiparesis and Babinski sign are usually present, pure amnesia also may occur (44). Ischemic lesions in the medial thalamic regions including the dorsomedial nucleus and the mamillothalamic tract have been demonstrated on CT scan and the anatomic regions supplied by the tuberothalamic artery were also affected in some patients (45).

Paramedian thalamopeduncular infarcts are caused by occlusion of the paramedian thalamic and paramedian mesencephalic arteries. The latter originates separately or together with the paramedian thalamic artery sharing a common trunk and supplies the interpeduncular nucleus, the medial part of the red nucleus, the oculomotor nucleus, and the anterior part of the periaqueductal gray (26). The clinical characteristics of these lesions include coma, akinetic mutism, and hypersomnia initially and confusion and amnesia after improvement of alertness. Ocular palsies including supranuclear palsy, oculomotor palsy, and total ophthalmoplegia were present in 13 of 17 patients described by Castaigne et al., while abnormal clonic or athetotic movement of the arms or face was observed in 6 of 17 patients at a later stage (26). In addition to another autopsy case (46), a fair number of patients with memory loss and vertical gaze palsy have been observed to have thalamic lesions with CT (31,32,47-55) and MRI scans (49,55). These imaging procedures invariably revealed unilateral or bilateral infarcts in the dorsomedial nucleus or in the medial thalamus with extension to the mesencephalon in some instances. A MRI scan and a brief history of such a patient is shown in Figure 4. Vertical gaze palsy and oculomotor paresis were common, but some patients were free of oculomotor signs (26,56). As observed after ischemic infarcts in the

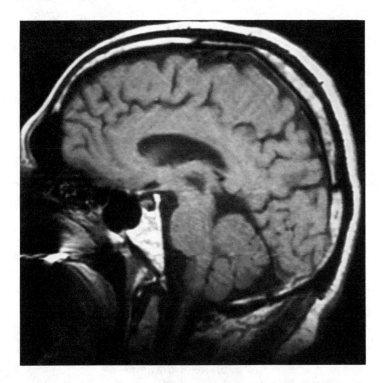

Figure 4 A parasagittal view of a T_1-weighted MRI scan showing a chronic infarct in the midline structure of the left thalamus extending to the pulvinar. This 57-year-old man was hospitalized comatose 5 years earlier. Upon regaining alertness, he was found to have profound memory impairment with inability to retain new information. He also had vertical gaze palsy. CT scan 10 days after the onset showed an enhanced area in the midline structure of each thalamus. His memory performance and vertical gaze palsy have not improved in 5 years.

territory of the tuberothalamic artery, both verbal and nonverbal memory impairment were apparent when the left (dominant) side was affected (51,55), but impairment of nonverbal memory was more prominent with the lesion on the right (nondominant) side (31,32). Severe impairment of recent memory commonly occurred, while remote memory was also affected in some patients. Stuss et al. observed one patient with severe retrograde amnesia who retained intact generic facts but lost personal remote memory (57), implicating more selective impairment of episodic memory as compared to semantic memory. In another patient with bilateral thalamic infarcts, however, Nichelli et al. (58) observed a lack of dissociation between impairment of episodic and semantic memory or declarative and procedural memory, and concluded that diencephalic amnesia was a disconnection syndrome between the frontal and temporal lobe as proposed earlier by Warrington and Weiskrantz (59).

It appears that paramedian thalamic infarcts tend to result in persistent impairment of recent memory and variable impairment of remote memory. The extent of memory impairment and recovery appear to depend on the extent and location of damage. Involvement of the dorsomedial nucleus and the mamillothalamic tract together may cause severe memory impairment with poor recovery.

THROMBOEMBOLISM IN THE CAROTID CIRCULATION

It is uncommon to encounter memory disorders in patients with thromboembolism of the carotid circulation. Occasionally memory impairment occurs after ischemic damage to the territory of the anterior cerebral artery or the anterior choroidal artery. Memory and mental dysfunction is also occasionally encountered in patients with occlusion of the internal carotid artery. While the acute confusional state and agitated delirium may occur after infarction in the territory of the nondominant middle cerebral artery (60,61), amnesia has not been observed following ischemic damage in the territory of the middle cerebral artery.

THROMBOEMBOLISM IN THE TERRITORY OF THE ANTERIOR CEREBRAL ARTERY

In 1913, Mabille and Pitres (62) observed bilateral prefrontal white matter infarcts at autopsy of a patient who suffered from amnesia following stroke 23 years earlier. In 1930, Critchley stated that profound loss of memory could occur in patients with occlusion of the main trunk of the (dominant) anterior cerebral artery (63). Subsequently Brion et al. reported a patient with Korsakoff syndrome who, at autopsy, was found to have ischemic infarcts in the left basal ganglia and both fornices as the result of the left anterior cerebral artery occlusion (64). Laplane et al. also observed a patient with inattention, amnesia, and confabulation who was found at autopsy to have ischemic infarcts bilaterally in the cingulate gyri and the underlying white matter as well as the fornices (65). While destruction of both fornices could be the cause of amnesia in the cases reported by Brion et al. (64) and Laplane et al. (65), the case reported by Mabille and Pitres (62) and another case reported by Laplane et al. (65) also suggested destruction of both cingulate gyri or disconnection of the limbic circuit between the thalamus and the cingulate gyrus and back to the hippocampus to be the cause of memory impairment.

THROMBOEMBOLISM IN THE TERRITORY OF THE ANTERIOR CHOROIDAL ARTERY

The anterior choroidal artery originates from the intracranial portion of the internal carotid artery, passes posterolaterally, and traverses the choroid fissure to anastomose with the lateral posterior choroidal artery. It supplies blood to the choroid plexus in the temporal horn but also supplies blood to the uncus, anterior hippocampus, striatum, and lateral thalamus. While the neuropsychological evidence of verbal and nonverbal memory impairment has been documented in patients with ischemic infarct of the lateral thalamus and the posterior limb of the internal capsule (31), clinically obvious amnesia is rare. A patient with an ischemic lesion in the posterior limb of the left internal capsule suffered from amnesia, but he also had an additional lesion in the left temporal lobe on CT scan, suggesting that the lesion in the medial temporal lobe could be the cause of amnesia (66). Another patient with verbal amnesia and right hemiparesis had an ischemic lesion in the posterior limb of the left internal capsule and nearby white matter on CT scan (67). The authors stated that the infarct was in the territory of the anterior choroidal artery and raised the possibility of disconnection of the dorsomedial nucleus of the thalamus from the amygdaloid and prefrontal regions. Additional information is necessary to identify the cause of amnesia in those cases, but the available information suggests that damage to the medial temporal lobe or its connecting pathway to the thalamus can cause memory dysfunction instead of direct damage to the thalamic nuclei.

OCCLUSION OF THE INTERNAL CAROTID ARTERY

Memory impairment and dementia are encountered occasionally in patients with occlusion or severe stenosis of the internal carotid artery, usually involving both sides. As we observed in one patient (68), and others have observed in another (69), memory impairment may be accompanied by other cognitive dysfunction and behavioral disorder. Our study with electroencephalogram (68) and a recent study with positron emission tomography (70) indicated the presence of hemodynamic ischemia in the dominant cerebral hemisphere. Carotid endarterectomy (69) and superficial temporal to middle cerebral artery anastomosis (68,70) resulted in excellent recovery of memory function.

MULTI-INFARCT DEMENTIA

Memory impairment may occur as a part of dementia in patients with multi-infarct dementia (MID) and it can be the main complaint in some patients. The memory function may be more selectively affected if a battery of neuropsychological examinations are performed (71). Neuropathologically, patients with MID have scattered cerebral infarcts without typical findings for Alzheimer's disease such as neurofibrillary tangles and senile plaques. While Tomlinson et al. (72) observed a correlation between dementia and the volume of multiple infarcts measuring over 50 milliliter, dementia can occur with lesser amount of cerebral infarction (71,73). It is difficult to separate Alzheimer's disease and MID based on neuropsychological examination alone. However, patients with MID may be identified by the presence in the history of abrupt onset, stepwise deterioration, previous stroke, focal neurologic signs, and emotional incontinence (73-75). Clinical and neuropsychological evaluations cannot separate patients with MID and those with mixed dementia (a combination of multi-infarcts and Alzheimer disease). Functional imaging procedures may be helpful in distinguishing those patients.

LACUNAR DEMENTIA

Dementia associated with multiple lacunar infarcts (the lacunar state) as a separate entity is debatable, since some lacunea are caused by thromboembolism and it may be difficult to separate the lacunar state and multiple embolic infarcts on CT or MRI scan alone. Román observed dementia in 36 of 100 patients with autopsy-proven lacunea (76). Loss of memory may be the main feature in some patients with relative preservation of personality. In the study of 30 patients with dementia and the lacunar state, Ishii et al. (77) found lacunar infarcts most commonly in the periventricular white matter around the anterior horn of the lateral ventricles, the head of the caudate nucleus and the putamen. Histopathologic examination revealed fibrohyaline degeneration of the deep penetrating arteries and arterioles as well as diffuse incomplete softening of the white matter, suggesting transition to subcortical arteriosclerotic encephalopathy (Binswanger disease).

BINSWANGER DISEASE
(SUBCORTICAL ARTERIOSCLEROTIC ENCEPHALOPATHY)

In Binswanger disease, decreased attenuation occurs widely in the centrum semiovale on CT scan. It often occurs in the periventricular areas early. Microscopic examination of the affected areas shows fibrohyaline thickening of the small arterial and arteriolar walls and loss of myelin staining, and lacunar infarcts are often present. Caplan and Schoene (78) observed mental abnormalities in all five autopsy-proven patients but in variable degrees. Memory loss was also variable. A more recent review by Babikian and Ropper (79) showed an insidious progression of memory deficit being most common and an amnestic syndrome being a dominant feature of the early illness in 55% of patients. Other mental symptoms ranged from loss of judgment to abulia (78,79). Gait disturbance was often present and many patients were hypertensive. However, patients with the same pathologic findings may not have dementia or memory impairment (80). The pathogenesis is not well established but chronic ischemia due to hypoperfusion in the periphery of the perforating arteries arising from the surface of the cerebral hemisphere has received support as a plausible cause.

Leukoencephalopathy in the centrum semiovale has been recognized in increasing numbers of elderly hypertensive or normotensive people who are asymptomatic or have clinical symptoms indistinguishable from those with autopsy-proven Binswanger disease (81,82). The term "leukoaraiosis" has been proposed to describe patchy or diffuse lucencies seen in the white matter of those people with CT scan (83). The extent of cognitive dysfunction including memory impairment appears to be quite variable when the subjects are selected on the basis of CT and MRI findings (84,85), possibly reflecting the stage of the pathologic process.

MEMORY DISORDERS ASSOCIATED WITH INTRACEREBRAL HEMORRHAGE

The majority of patients with memory disorders in this group have had thalamic hemorrhage. This probably reflects the higher incidence of parenchymal hemorrhage in this area than other anatomical locations important for memory function such as the temporal lobe and basal frontal region.

THALAMIC HEMORRHAGE

After thalamic hemorrhage on the left (dominant) side, amnesia has been accompanied by confusion, disorientation, language impairment, including paraphasic errors and perseveration, hemiparesis, acalculia, and astereognosis (86-88). Both verbal and nonverbal memory may be affected. While anterograde amnesia is predominant, retrograde amnesia may be present (86). Hemorrhage has been found in the medial thalamus with CT scan (86,88) and in the anterior nucleus disrupting the mammillothalamic tract at autopsy (87). Amnesia after thalamic hemorrhage on the right (nondominant) side has been accompanied by hemineglect, hemiparesis, and hemianopia (89-91), but hypersomnia, apathy and psychotic behavior may be the prominent manifestation (90,91). While impairment of verbal memory has been noted in these patients, the assessment of nonverbal memory is often difficult because of the presence of hemineglect. Hemorrhage is variable in size with CT scan but often involves the medial thalamus.

HEMORRHAGE IN OTHER INTRACEREBRAL LOCATIONS

Amnesia has been observed in patients with intracerebral hemorrhage in locations outside the thalamus (92-95). A patient developed amnesia after hemorrhage from an arteriovenous malformation which damaged the splenium of the corpus callosum, the retrosplenial cortex and the cingulate cortex on the left side (92). Anterograde amnesia was profound and persistent and milder retrograde amnesia was also present. Verbal memory was severely affected and nonverbal memory more mildly. It was postulated that amnesia was caused by disruption of the pathway from the subiculum of the hippocampus to the anterior nucleus of the thalamus in the retrosplenial cortex and/or by damage of the cingulate bundle disrupting the pathway from the anterior nucleus of the thalamus to the medial temporal lobe. Another patient sustained hemorrhage in the left (dominant) parieto-occipital region. After surgical evacuation, she was found to have profound and persistent impairment of recent memory affecting both verbal and nonverbal memory in addition to visual agnosia, alexia, impaired color naming, and right hemianopia (93). Transient amnesia with impairment of learning has occurred in one patient after having hemorrhage in the left posterior inferior temporal region (94) and in another patient after having hemorrhage in the left lentiform nucleus (95).

Reduplicative paramnesia (a false belief that more than one place with identical appearance exist) has been observed in a patient after suffering right frontal hemorrhage (96). He had visual inattention and his memory impairment was more severe with nonverbal memory. Another patient also developed reduplicative paramnesia after damage to the right cerebral hemisphere which could have been hemorrhagic in nature (97). It was postulated that partial impairment of visual perception, nonverbal memory and integration of information are necessary for development of reduplicative paramnesia.

Thus, intracerebral hemorrhage in the thalamus and temporo-occipital region elicits clinical profiles similar to those seen in patients with ischemic damage to the corresponding areas. However, memory impairment also occurs after intracerebral hemorrhage in other locations. Compression of the surrounding structures by hematoma may be responsible for memory impairment in some patients.

MEMORY DISORDERS ASSOCIATED WITH
SUBARACHNOID HEMORRHAGE

Subarachnoid hemorrhage (SAH) has been known for years to cause amnesia and dementia. Vasospasm, intracerebral hemorrhage, hydrocephalus, and surgical repairs of intracranial aneurysms are responsible for memory and behavioral disorders. Korsakoff syndrome associated with SAH was reviewed by Tarachow in 1939 (98) and by Walton in 1953 (99). Psychiatric disorders associated with SAH secondary to ruptured intracranial aneurysms have been studied in detail (100). Confusion and disorientation are common among those recovering from coma or stupor and impairment of recent memory and, sometimes, of remote memory are obvious in some patients. While confabulation is frequent, it is relatively shortlived and amnesia often improves within months. Transient amnesia lasting only for hours without major neurologic deficits has been reported (101). Among various causes, ruptured aneurysms of the anterior communicating artery (ACoA) and surgical repair are by far the most frequent etiology of amnesia and Korsakoff syndrome following SAH.

RUPTURED ANEURYSMS OF THE ANTERIOR COMMUNICATING ARTERY

The anatomy of the anterior cerebral artery (ACA) and ACoA is important for understanding of the pathogenesis of neuropsychiatric manifestations (102,103). The perforating arteries from the most proximal portion of the ACA supply blood to the genu and the contiguous posterior limb of the internal capsule, rostral thalamus and much of the hypothalamus (102). Heubner's recurrent artery originates just proximal to the ACoA, directly from the ACoA, or just distal to the ACoA and supplies blood to the anterior part of the striatum and the anterior limb of the internal capsule. It is now recognized that perforating arteries also arise from the ACoA itself and supply blood to the corpus callosum, anterior cingulate gyrus, lamina terminalis, fornix, septal region, and hypothalamus (102). While most patients develop the amnestic syndrome after surgical repair of the aneurysms, amnesia and Korsakoff syndrome have been observed even without surgery or prior to surgery (100,102-107). Okawa et al. (107) observed psychiatric symptoms in 61% of patients with ruptured ACoA aneurysms. Amnesia was noted in 16% of patients. Psychiatric symptoms were more severe among patients with multiple episodes of SAH, prolonged periods of unconsciousness and neurologic deficits. Impairment of learning new information was common and both anterograde and retrograde amnesia occurred. The structural damage and functional impairment are probably caused by vasospasm and parenchymal hemorrhage in the same anatomical sites as encountered following surgical repair.

SURGICAL REPAIR OF THE ANTERIOR COMMUNICATING ANEURYSMS

Memory and behavioral disorders are known to occur in some patients following surgical repair of the ACoA aneurysms. The perforating arteries from the ACoA, Heubner's recurrent artery and even the trunk of the ACA can be damaged during surgery or occluded at the time of aneurysm clipping. Since Norlén and Olivecrona observed memory impairment following surgical repair of the ACoA aneurysms in 1953 (108), a fair number of patients with this disorder have been reported (100,104-107,109-115). Characteristically, impairment of recent memory and learning becomes apparent after patients regain alertness after surgery, but impairment of remote memory and confabulation may also occur. Other personality changes include lethargy, agitation, and confusion soon after surgery and apathy, inattention, aggression, and euphoria later. Amnesia and Korsakoff syndrome have been observed postoperatively in 37 to 56% of patients by some (100,107,109) and general neuropsychiatric symptoms in 14% of patients by others at the time of discharge from hospital (110). Memory impairment has occurred more often following trapping of the aneurysm instead of clipping (111). Confabulation is mostly transient, clearing in 1 to 3 months (107) and amnesia also improves, although 15-17% may have persistent memory impairment (107,109).

The presence of perforating arteries originating from the ACoA (102) and the visualization of hematomas and infarcts in the basal forebrain areas by CT scans (112,113,115) have suggested that the anatomical sites responsible for amnestic syndrome and other behavioral disorders are in the medial septal nuclei, nucleus basalis of Meyert, nucleus accumbens, anterior cingulum, and anterior hypothalamus (113,115). Indeed, an autopsy examination of such a patient revealed damage to the precommissural gray matter, septal area, nucleus of the diagonal band of Broca, and nucleus accumbens (116). Since the septohippocampal and septoamygdaloid pathways traverse this area, disruption of the limbic circuit in the basal forebrain area may be the cause of memory impairment. A positron emission tomographic examination of such patients demonstrated reduced oxygen utilization in the medial temporal lobes (117). The cerebral disconnection syndrome with memory impairment and defects in the interhemispheric transfer of information has been observed in a patient who underwent surgical clipping of the ACoA aneurysm (118). Another patient with a ruptured aneurysm of the right pericallosal artery also developed the hemispheric disconnection syndrome with transient memory impairment (119). Damage to the anterior corpus callosum and the surrounding frontal lobe was believed to be the cause. Memory impairment and Korsakoff syndrome have also occurred after removal of an arteriovenous malformation from the medial and basal frontal region (119).

Thus, the ACoA aneurysms have accompanied the amnesic and Korsakoff syndrome as well as other behavioral disorders in a considerable number of patients both before and after surgical repairs. Vasospasm, parenchymal hemorrhage, and surgical obliteration of the branch arteries originating from the ACoA appear to be responsible and amnesia may be caused by disruption of the limbic circuit in the basal forebrain area. After introduction of the microsurgical technique, those behavioral disorders have occurred less frequently (107).

RUPTURED ANEURYSMS OF THE BASILAR ARTERY

Neuropsychiatric disorders also may occur after rupture or surgical repair of aneurysms in the vertebrobasilar circulation. Takaku et al. observed neuropsychiatric disorders in 32% of such patients postoperatively (110). While amnesia may be prominent following surgical repair of the basilar aneurysms, it may be due to inattention. Since the number of patients who have undergone surgical repair of the basilar aneurysms is still limited, the information is scanty. The pathophysiological mechanism for memory impairment and other behavioral disorders may be very similar to those seen in patients with paramedian thalamic syndrome.

MEMORY DISORDERS ASSOCIATED WITH GLOBAL ISCHEMIA AND HYPOXIA

Cardiopulmonary arrest or failure from acute myocardial ischemia or cardiac arrhythmia is the most common cause of global cerebral ischemia/hypoxia. However, global ischemia/hypoxia has also been encountered following sustained systemic hypotension, apnea, severe chest injury, attempted suicide by hanging, drowning, and carbon monoxide poisoning. If the ischemic/hypoxic condition is severe, patients may remain comatose even if they survive. On the other hand, some patients exhibit no neuropsychiatric abnormalities after recovery. A variable degree of intellectual dysfunction is common and amnesia may be a prominent feature. Following earlier reviews by Fletcher (120) and Allison (121), Brierley and Cooper reported a clinicopathological correlation in a patient who developed Korsakoff's syndrome following a hypotensive episode during general anesthesia (122). Since then a considerable amount of information has been accumulated from the neuropsychological and clinicopathological point of view, particularly for memory and intellectual dysfunction following cardiopulmonary arrest (123-131).

 After profound global ischemia/hypoxia, patients typically present with marked impairment of new learning and recent memory and a variable degree of impairment of remote memory. Confabulation, mild dementia, and apathy are sometimes present. Volpe et al. observed preservation of recognition memory even in the presence of severe impairment of recall (127,130). Amnesia could be transient resolving within 1 to 2 weeks, but could persist (125). Chronic hypoperfusion and hypoxia seen in patients with congestive heart failure and chronic pulmonary diseases without a catastrophic cardiopulmonary arrest can also lead to dementia with memory and intellectual impairment (132,133).

While Brierley and Cooper found widespread neuronal damage in the cerebral cortex and anterior thalamus with minimal damage to the hippocampus at autopsy (122), Cummings et al. observed anoxic neuronal damage almost exclusively in the CA1 region of the hippocampus (128). For patients with amnesia and dementia, Volpe and Petito observed neuronal damage not only in the CA1 region of the hippocampus but also in the subiculum, inferior temporal cortex, parahippocampal gyrus and amygdala (132). Of importance is that Zola-Morgan et al. found anoxic neuronal damage confined to the CA1 region of the hippocampus in a postmortem examination of a patient who had experienced multiple hypotensive/hypoxic episodes and suffered persistent amnesia (131). Thus, damage to the hippocampus appears to be the cause of memory impairment following hypoxic/ischemic events, but damage to the anterior thalamus may contribute in some patients.

MEMORY DISORDER ASSOCIATED WITH MIGRAINE

Patients with classic migraine (migraine with aura) may develop neurologic symptoms particularly during the prodromal stage. Neurologic abnormalities often include hemianopia, hemiparesis, paresthesia, ophthalmoplegia, and aphasia. By one account, 3.5% of patients with migraine headaches experience mental confusion as a manifestation of migraine (134). An acute confusional state is known to occur in association with migraine in children (135-137) and occasionally in adults with familial hemiplegic migraine (138,139).

Association of amnestic episodes with migrainous attacks has been known for many years. Moersch described a patient with amnesia associated with migraine in 1924 (140) and the patient described by von Bechterew in 1900 (141) may have had migraine. The memory impairment during migraine attack consists of inability to form new memories with a variable degree of remote memory impairment. If the sensorium is clear and there are no focal neurologic deficits, the profile is consistent with the diagnosis of transient global amnesia (TGA) (142-145). While the presence of headache alone during the TGA episodes does not necessarily link TGA to migraine (146), TGA episodes during typical attacks of classic migraine (134,145) indicate that some TGA episodes are actually caused by a migrainous mechanism. Lauritzen et al. (147) observed reduced blood flow in the posterior head region during classic migraine attacks and postulated "spreading depression of Leao" (148) as the cause of focal symptoms and hypoperfusion during classic migraine attacks. The same mechanism has also been proposed as the cause of TGA (149). The amnestic episodes associated with classic or complicated migraine therefore may represent TGA episodes, but the majority of TGA episodes are not associated with migraine (146).

TRANSIENT GLOBAL AMNESIA. AND CEREBROVASCULAR DISEASE

Patients with TGA experience a transient inability to form new memory without impairment of consciousness, higher cognitive dysfunction or focal neurologic deficits. Many theories have been proposed as the pathophysiologic mechanism of TGA such as transient ischemic attack (TIA) or stroke (95, 150-156). This theory stems from the presence of the past history of cerebral ischemic episodes prior to TGA, the presence of the risk factors for cerebrovascular disease in many patients with TGA and transient or persistent neurologic events subsequent to TGA. While amnestic episodes have been observed in association with ischemic and hemorrhagic events and called TGA (88, 94,95,101,150-153,156), those without any other focal neurologic deficits or sustained headaches are very rare. The presence of hypodense CT lesions in the medial thalamus or medial temporal lobe alone should be interpreted with caution unless they occurred in association with the amnestic episodes. Stroke and TIA subsequent to a TGA episode appear to occur in the series where TGA episodes were accompanied by focal neurologic signs and symptoms (152,153).

Measurement of cerebral blood flow and metabolism during TGA episodes has not been helpful in distinguishing TGA from thromboembolic events. A unilateral temporal lobe abnormality has been observed by Raichle with positron emission tomography during a TGA episode (cited in ref. 146). Unilateral temporal hypoperfusion has also been observed in two patients during TGA episodes by Trillet et al. (157), but they also appeared to have marked bilateral global hypoperfusion. Because of the benign nature of TGA, postmortem examination is rarely available. One patient had diffuse atherosclerosis throughout cerebral arteries but no infarction existed in the temporal lobe or medial thalamus (146). Kadota et al. reported a patient who experienced transient amnestic episode and later was found to have widespread nerve cell atrophy, neuronophagia, and severe atherosclerosis of cerebral arteries (158). While those abnormalities were more notable in the temporal lobe, Sommer's sector of the hippocampus was relatively well preserved. This patient probably had an amnestic stroke since he had dysarthria during the episode and focal neurologic deficits afterward.

The available information therefore does not support the contention that most TGA episodes without other neurologic signs and symptoms are the thromboembolic events in the vertebrobasilar circulation. On the contrary, a low incidence of stroke subsequent to TGA suggests that the vast majority of TGA episodes are not thromboembolic TIA (146). Thus, most TGA episodes should not be considered as a manifestation of cerebrovascular disease and patients with amnestic episodes with obvious neurologic deficits or evidence of an ischemic or hemorrhagic event by history and laboratory procedures should be separated from TGA.

CONCLUSION

Memory impairment can be seen in patients with cerebral thromboembolism, intracerebral hemorrhage, subarachnoid hemorrhage, or global ischemic/ hypoxic events as a sole manifestation or as a part of dementia and other behavioral disorders. While the mechanism may be different, amnestic episodes also occur during migrainous attacks. The autopsy examination as well as CT and MRI examination have demonstrated three discrete anatomical areas to be involved in memory disorders: the medial temporal lobe, the medial thalamus, and the basal forebrain. Within the medial temporal lobe, the hippocampus is often affected in patients with severe memory impairment and the CA1 region is particularly vulnerable. However, it is also common to observe cerebral infarction in the posterior inferior temporal lobe in these patients, including the parahippocampal, fusiform and lingual gyri. In the thalamus, a memory impairment is often found in patients with ischemic or hemorrhagic lesions in the dorsomedial nucleus but damage to the mammillothalamic tract or the anterior nucleus may also produce a memory impairment. In the frontal lobe, damage to the anterior cingulate cortex and the medial septal nucleus as well as the connecting pathways such as the fornix and those from the anterior nucleus of the thalamus to the cingulate cortex and back to the amygdala and the hippocampus have been implicated in memory impairments. The findings suggest that injury to any of those structures and connecting pathways constituting the limbic circuit may be sufficient to cause a memory impairment. The findings also suggest that extensive damage to the limbic circuit may result in severe memory impairment, particularly when the damage is bilateral.

The resulting memory impairment is predominantly anterograde amnesia with a variable degree of retrograde amnesia, implying that the structures in the limbic circuit are more pertinent for new memory formation or learning than for retrieval of the consolidated information. While the neocortical association areas have been implicated for storage of information, no definite anatomical location has been identified for this function from patients with cerebrovascular diseases. The lateralization of verbal and nonverbal memory impairment exists both in the medial temporal lobe and thalamus, where damage to the dominant side primarily produces an impairment of verbal memory and to a lesser extent nonverbal memory, while damage to the nondominant side results in impairment of nonverbal memory. The nature of the memory impairment caused by damage to the medial temporal lobe, medial thalamus or basal forebrain is indistinguishable based on the information reviewed in this chapter.

It appears that damage to hippocampal neurons, particularly when bilateral, can cause memory impairment. Damage to any interconnecting pathways within the network of the limbic circuit including the basal forebrain region may also be sufficient to cause memory impairment. It is not certain, however, from analysis of patients with cerebrovascular diseases, whether the thalamic nuclei possess unique memory functions or act as interconnecting nuclei within the limbic circuit.

REFERENCES

1. Bechterew, W.v. (1990). Demonstration eines Gehirns mit Zerstörung der vorderen und inneren Theile der Hirnrinde beider Schläfenlappen. *Neurol. Zentbl. 19*:990-991.
2. Zeal, A.A., and Rhoton, A.L., Jr. (1978). Microsurgical anatomy of the posterior cerebral artery. *J. Neurosurg. 48*:534-559.
3. Percheron, G. (1973). The anatomy of the arterial supply of the human thalamus and its use for the interpretation of the thalamic vascular pathology. *Z. Neurol. 205*:1-13.
4. Stephens, R.B., and Stilwell, D.L. (1969). *Arteries and Veins of the Human Brain.* Charles C Thomas, Springfield, pp. 96-99.
5. Glees, P., and Griffith, H.B. (1952). Bilateral destruction of the hippocampus (cornu ammonis) in a case of dementia. *Psychiat. Neurol. 123*:193-204.
6. Dide, M., and Botcazo (1902). Amnesie continue, cécité verbale pure, perte du sens topographique, ramollissement double du lobe lingual. *Rev. Neurol. 10*:676-680.
7. Scoville, W.B., and Milner, B. (1957). Loss of recent memory after bilateral hippocampal lesions. *J. Neurol. Neurosurg. Psychiat. 20*:11-21.
8. Victor, M., Angevine, J.B. Jr., Mancall, E.L., and Fisher, C.M. (1961). Memory loss with lesions of hippocampal formation. *Arch. Neurol. 5*:244-263.
9. DeJong, R.N., Itabashi, H.H., and Olson, J.R. (1969). Memory loss due to hippocampal lesions. *Arch. Neurol. 20*:339-348.
10. Delay, J., Brion, S., Escourolle, R., and Marques, J.M. (1961). Démences artériopathiques. Lésions du système hippocampo-mamillo-thalamique dans le déterminisme des troubles mnésiques. *Rev. Neurol. 105*:22-32.
11. Van Buren, J.M., and Borke, R.C. (1972). The mesial temporal substratum of memory. Anatomical studies in three individuals. *Brain 95*:599-632.
12. Woods, B.T., Schoene, W., and Kneisley, L. (1982). Are hippocampal lesions sufficient to cause lasting amnesia? *J. Neurol. Neurosurg. Psychiat. 45*:243-247.
13. Geschwind, N., and Fusillo, M. (1966). Color-naming defects in association with alexia. *Arch. Neurol. 15*:137-146.
14. Mohr, J.P., Leicester, J., Stoddard, L.T., and Sidman, M. (1971). Right hemianopia with memory and color deficits in circumscribed left posterior cerebral artery territory infarction. *Neurology 21*:1104-1113.
15. Caplan, L.R., and Hedley-Whyte, T. (1974). Cuing and memory dysfunction in alexia without agraphia. A case report. *Brain 97*:251-262.
16. Mones, R.J., Christoff, N., and Bender, M.B. (1961). Posterior cerebral artery occlusion. A clinical and angiographic study. *Arch. Neurol. 5*:68-76.

17. Benson, D.F., Marsden, C.D., and Meadows, J.C. (1974). The amnestic syndrome of posterior cerebral artery occlusion. *Acta Neurol. Scand. 50*:133-145.
18. Fisher, C.M. (1986). The posterior cerebral artery syndrome. *Can. J. Neurol. Sci. 13*:232-239.
19. Devinsky, O., Bear, D., and Volpe, B.T. (1988). Confusional states following posterior cerebral artery infarction. *Arch. Neurol. 45*:160-163.
20. De Renzi, E., Zambolin, A., and Crisi, G. (1987). The pattern of neuropsychological impairment associated with left posterior cerebral artery infarcts. *Brain 110*:1099-1116.
21. Von Cramon, D.Y., Hebel, N., and Schuri, U. (1988). Verbal memory and learning in unilateral posterior cerebral infarction. A report on 30 cases. *Brain 111*: 1061-1077.
22. Degos, J.D., Gray, F., Louarn, F., Ansquer, J.C., Poirier, J., and Barbizet, J. (1987). Posterior callosal infarction. Clinicopathological correlations. *Brain 110*:1155-1171.
23. Laterra, J., Gebarski, S., and Sackellares, J.C. (1988). Transient amnesia resulting from vertebral artery dissection. *Stroke 19*:98-101.
24. Percheron, G. (1976). Les artères du thalamus humain. II. Artéres et territoires thalamiques paramédians de l'artère basilaire communicante. *Rev. Neurol. 132*:309-324.
25. Castaigne, P., Buge, A., Cambier, J., Escourolle, R., Brunet, P., and Degos, J.D. (1966). Démence thalamique d'origine vasculaire par ramollissement bilatéral, limité au territoire du pédicule rétromamillaire. *Rev. Neurol. 114*: 89-107.
26. Castaigne, P., Lhermitte, F., Buge, A., Escourolle, R., Hauw, J.J., and Lyon-Caen, O. (1981). Paramedian thalamic and midbrain infarcts: clinical and neuropathological study. *Ann. Neurol. 10*:127-148.
27. Schlesinger, B. (1976). *The Upper Brainstem in the Human. Its Nuclear Configuration and Vascular Supply.* Springer-Verlag, Berlin, Heidelberg, New York, pp. 92-93.
28. Saeki, N., and Rhoton, A.L., Jr. (1977). Microsurgical anatomy of the upper basilar artery and the posterior circle of Willis. *J. Neurosurg. 46*:563-578.
29. Percheron, G. (1976). Les artères du thalamus human. I. Artère et territoire thalamiques polaires de l'artère communicante posterieure. *Rev. Neurol. 132*: 297-307.
30. Graff-Radford, N.R., Eslinger, P.J., Damasio, A.R., and Yamada, T. (1984). Nonhemorrhagic infarction of the thalamus: behavioral, anatomic, and physiologic correlates. *Neurology 34*:14-23.
31. Graff-Radford, N.R., Damasio, H., Yamada, T., Eslinger, P.J., and Damasio, A.R. (1985). Nonhaemorrhagic thalamic infarction. Clinical, neuropsychological and electrophysiological findings in four anatomical groups defined by computerized tomography. *Brain 108*:485-516.
32. Bogousslavsky, J., Regli, F., and Uske, A. (1988). Thalamic infarcts: Clinical syndromes, etiology, and prognosis. *Neurology 38*:837-848.
33. Bogousslavsky, J., Regli, F., and Assal, G. (1986). The syndrome of unilateral tuberothalamic artery infarction. *Stroke 17*:434-441.

34. Cohen, J.A., Gelfer, C.E., and Sweet, R.D. (1980). Thalamic infarction producing aphasia. *Mt. Sinai J. Med. 47*:398-404.

35. Archer, C.R., Ilinsky, I.A., Goldfader, P.R., and Smith, K.R. Jr. (1981). Aphasia in thalamic stroke: CT sterotactic localization. *J. Comp. Assist. Tomograph. 5*:427-432.

36. Biller, J., Merchut, M., and Emanuele, M. (1984). Nonhemorrhagic infarctions of the thalamus. *Neurology 34*:1269-1270.

37. Goldenberg, G., Wimmer, A., and Maly, J. (1983). Amnestic syndrome with a unilateral thalamic lesion. A case report. *J. Neurol. 229*:79-86.

38. Speedie, L.J., and Heilman, K.M. (1982). Amnestic disturbance following infarction of the left dorsomedial nucleus of the thalamus. *Neuropsychol. 20*:597-604.

39. Gorelick, P.B., Amico, L.L., Ganellen, R., and Benevento, L.A. (1988). Transient global amnesia and thalamic infarction. *Neurology 38*:496-499.

40. Michel, D., Laurent, B., Foyatier, N., Blanc, A., and Portafaix, M. (1982). Infarctus thalamique paramédian gauche. Étude de la mémoire et du language. *Rev. Neurol. 138*:533-550.

41. Speedie, L.J., and Heilman, K.M. (1983). Antegrade memory deficits for visuospatial material after infarction of the right thalamus. *Arch. Neurol. 40*:183-186.

42. Schott, B., Mauguière, F., Laurent, B., Serclerat, O., and Fischer, C. (1980). L'amnésie thalamique. *Rev. Neurol. 136*:117-130.

43. Barbizet, J., Degos, J.D., Louarn, F., Nguyen, J.P., and Mas, J.L. (1981). Amnésie par lésion ischémique bi-thalamique. *Rev. Neurol. 137*:415-424.

44. Winocur, G., Oxbury, S., Roberts, R., Agnetti, V., and Davis, C. (1984). Amnesia in a patient with bilateral lesions to the thalamus. *Neuropsychol. 22*:123-143.

45. von Cramon, D.Y., Hebel, N., and Schuri, U. (1985). A contribution to the anatomical basis of thalamic amnesia. *Brain 108*:993-1008.

46. Bogousslavsky, J., Miklossy, J., Deruaz, J.P., Regli, F., and Assal, G. (1986). Unilateral left paramedian infarction of thalamus and midbrain: a clinicopathological study. *J. Neurol. Neurosurg. Psychiat. 49*:686-694.

47. Mills, R.P., and Swanson, P.D. (1978). Vertical oculomotor apraxia and memory loss. *Ann. Neurol. 4*:149-153.

48. Guberman, A., and Stuss, D. (1983). The syndrome of bilateral paramedian thalamic infarction. *Neurology 33*:540-546.

49. Swanson, R.A., and Schmidley, J.W. (1985). Amnestic syndrome and vertical gaze palsy: Early detection of bilateral thalamic infarction by CT and NMR. *Stroke 16*:823-827.

50. Vighetto, A., Confavreux, Ch., Boisson, D., Aimard, G., and Devic, M. (1986). Paralysie de l'abaissement du regard et amnésie globale durables par lésion thalamo-sous-thalamique bilatérale. *Rev. Neurol. 142*:449-455.

51. Mori, E., Yamadori, A., and Mitani, Y. (1986). Left thalamic infarction and disturbance of verbal memory: a clinicoanatomical study with a new method of computed tomographic stereotaxic lesion localization. *Ann. Neurol. 20*:671-676.

52. Meissner, I., Sapir, S., Kokmen, E., and Stein, S.D. (1987). The paramedain diencephalic syndrome: a dynamic phenomenon. *Stroke 18*:380-385.

53. Katz, D.I., Alexander, M.P., and Mandell, A.M. (1987). Dementia following strokes in the mesencephalon and diencephalon. *Arch. Neurol.* 44:1127-1133.
54. Gentilini, M., De Renzi, E., and Crisi, G. (1987). Bilateral paramedian thalamic artery infarcts—report of 8 cases. *J. Neurol. Neurosurg. Psychiat.* 50:900-909.
55. Fensore, C., Lazzarino, L.G., Nappo, A., and Nicolai, A. (1988). Language and memory disturbances from mesencephalothalamic infarcts. *Eur. Neurol.* 28:51-56.
56. Poirier, J., Barbizet, J., Gaston, A., and Meyrignac, C. (1983). Démence thalamique. Lacunes expansives du territoire thalamo-mésencéphalique paramedian. Hydrocéphalie par sténose de l'aqueduc du sylvius. *Rev. Neurol.* 139:349-358.
57. Stuss, D.T., Guberman, A., Nelson, R., and Larochelle, S. (1988). The neuropsychology of paramedian thalamic infarction. *Brain Cogn.* 8:348-378.
58. Nichelli, P., Bahmanian-Behbahani, G., Gentilini, M., and Vecchi, A. (1988). Preserved memory abilities in thalamic amnesia. *Brain* 111:1337-1353.
59. Warrington, E.K., and Weiskrantz, L. (1982). Amnesia: a disconnection syndrome? *Neuropsychologia* 20:233-248.
60. Mesulam, M.-M., Waxman, S.G., Geschwind, N., and Sabin, T.D. (1976). Acute confusional states with right middle cerebral artery infarctions. *J. Neurol. Neurosurg. Psychiat.* 39:84-89.
61. Mori, E., and Yamadori, A. (1987). Acute confusional state and acute agitated delirium. Occurrence after infarction in the right middle cerebral artery territory. *Arch. Neurol.* 44:1139-1143.
62. Mabille, H., and Pitres, A. (1913). Sur un cas d'amnésie de fixation post-apoplectique ayant persisté pendant vingt-trois ans. *Rev. Med.* 33:257-279.
63. Critchley, M. (1930). The anterior cerebral artery, and its syndromes. *Brain* 53: 120-165.
64. Brion, S., Pragier, G., Guérin, R., nad Teitgen, M. (1969). Syndrome de Korsakoff par ramollissement bilatéral du fornix. Le problème des syndromes amnésiques par lésion vasculaire unilatérale. *Rev. Neurol.* 120:255-262.
65. Laplane, D., Degos, J.D., Baulac, M., and Gray, F. (1981). Bilateral infarction of the anterior cingulate gyri and of the fornices. *J. Neurol. Sci.* 51:289-300.
66. Amarenco, P., Cohen, P., Roullet, E., Dupuch, K., Kurtz, A. and Marteau, R. (1988). Syndrome amnésique lors d'un infarctus du territoire de l'artère choroidienne antérieure gauche. *Rev. Neurol.* 144:36-39.
67. Kooistra, C.A., and Heilman, K.M. (1988). Memory loss from a subcortical white matter infarct. *J. Neurol. Neurosurg. Psychiat.* 51:866-869.
68. Yanagihara, T., Houser, O.W., and Klass, D.W. (1981). Computer tomography and EEG in cerebrovascular disease. *Arch. Neurol.* 38:597-600.
69. Paulsen, G.W., Kapp, J., and Cook, W. (1966). Dementia associated with bilateral carotid artery disease. *Geriatrics* 21:159-166.
70. Leblanc, R., Tyler, J.L., Mohr, G., Meyer, E., Diksic, M., Yamamoto, L., Taylor, L., Gauthier, S., and Hakim, A. (1987). Hemodynamic and metabolic effects of cerebral revascularization. *J. Neurosurg.* 66:529-535.
71. Loeb, C., Gandolfo, C., and Bino, G. (1988). Intellectual impairment and cerebral lesions in multiple cerebral infarcts. A clinical-computed tomography study. *Stroke* 19:560-565.

72. Tomlinson, B.E., Blessed, G., and Roth, M. (1970). Observations on the brains of demented old people. *J. Neurol. Sci. 11*:205-242.

73. Erkinjuntti, T., Haltia, M., Palo, J., Sulkava, R., and Paetau, A. (1988). Accuracy of the clinical diagnosis of vascular dementia: a prospective clinical and postmortem neuropathological study. *J. Neurol. Neurosurg. Psychiat. 51*:1037-1044.

74. Hachinski, V.C., Iliff, L.D., Zilhka, E., Du Boulay, G.H., McAllister, V.L., Marshall, J., Ross Russel, R.W., and Symon, L. (1975). Cerebral blood flow in dementia. *Arch. Neurol. 32*:632-637.

75. Rosen, W.G., Terry, R.D., Fuld, P.A., Katzman, R., and Peck, A. (1979). Pathological verification of ischemic score in differentiation of dementia. *Ann. Neurol. 7*:486-488.

76. Román, G.C. (1985). Lacunar dementia. In *Senile Dementia of the Alzheimer Type*. Edited by J.T. Hutton and A.D. Kenny. Alan R. Liss, Inc., New York, pp. 131-151.

77. Ishii, N., Nishihara, Y., and Imamura, T. (1986). Why do frontal lobe symptoms predominate in vascular dementia with lacunes? *Neurology 36*:340-345.

78. Caplan, L.R., and Schoene, W.C. (1978). Clinical features of subcortical arteriosclerotic encephalopathy (Binswanger disease). *Neurology 28*:1206-1215.

79. Babikian, V., and Ropper, A.H. (1987). Binswanger's disease: a review. *Stroke 18*:2-12.

80. De Reuck, J., Crevits, L., De Coster, W., Sieben, G., and vander Eecken, H. (1980). Pathogenesis of Binswanger chronic progressive subcortical encephalopathy. *Neurology 30*:920-928.

81. Loizou, L.A., Kendall, B.E., and Marshall, J. (1981). Subcortical arteriosclerotic encephalopathy: a clinical and radiological investigation. *J. Neurol. Neurosurg. Psychiat. 44*:294-304.

82. Kinkel, W.R., Jacobs, L., Polachini, I., Bates, V., and Heffner, R.R. Jr. (1985). Subcortical arteriosclerotic encephalopathy (Binswanger's disease). Computed tomographic, nuclear magnetic resonance, and clinical correlations. *Arch. Neurol. 42*:951-959.

83. Hachinski, V.C., Potter, P., and Merskey, H. (1987). Leuko-araiosis. *Arch. Neurol. 44*:21-23.

84. Steingart, A., Hachinski, V.C., Lau, C., Fox, A.J., Diaz, F., Cape, R., Lee, D., Inzitari, D., and Merskey, H. (1987). Cognitive and neurologic findings in subjects with diffuse white matter lucencies on computed tomographic scan (leuco-araiosis). *Arch. Neurol. 44*:32-35.

85. Rao, S.M., Mittenberg, W., Bernardin, L., Haughton, V., and Leo, G.J. (1989). Neuropsychological test findings in subjects with leukoaraiosis. *Arch. Neurol. 46*:40-44.

86. Choi, D., Sudarsky, L., Schachter, S., Biber, M., and Burke, P. (1983). Medial thalamic hemorrhage with amnesia. *Arch. Neurol. 40*:611-613.

87. Hankey, G.J., and Stewart-Wynne, E.G. (1988). Amnesia following thalamic hemorrhage. Another stroke syndrome. *Stroke 19*:776-778.

88. Moonis, M., Jain, S., Prasad, K., Mishra, N.K., Goulatia, R.K., and Maheshwari, M.C. (1988). Left thalamic hypertensive hemorrhage presenting as transient global amnesia. *Acta Neurol. Scand. 77*:331-334.

89. Watson, R.T., and Heilman, K.M. (1979). Thalamic neglect. *Neurology 29*: 690-694.

90. Waxman, S.G., Ricaurte, G.A., and Tucker, S.B. (1986). Thalamic hemorrhage with neglect and memory disorder. *J. Neurol. Sci. 75*:105-112.

91. Guard, O., Bellis, F., Mabille, J.P., Dumas, R., Boisson, D., and Devic, M. (1986). Démence thalamique aprés lésion hémorragique unilatérale du pulvinar droit. *Rev. Neurol. 142*:759-765.

92. Valenstein, D., Bowers, D., Verfaellie, M., Heilman, K.M., Day, A., and Watson, R.T. (1987). Retrosplenial amnesia. *Brain 110*:1631-1646.

93. Benke, Th. (1988). Visual agnosia and amnesia from a left unilateral lesion. *Eur. Neurol. 28*:236-239.

94. Landi, G., Giusti, M.C., and Guidotti, M. (1982). Transient global amnesia due to left temporal hemorrhage. *J. Neurol. Neurosurg. Psychiat. 45*:1062-1063.

95. Bogousslavsky, J., and Regli, F. (1988). Transient global amnesia and stroke. *Eur. Neurol. 28*:106-110.

96. Kapur, N., Turner, A., and King, C. (1988). Reduplicative paramnesia: possible anatomical and neuropsychological mechanisms. *J. Neurol. Neurosurg. Psychiat. 51*:579-581.

97. Patterson, M.B., and Mack, J.L. (1985). Neuropsychological analysis of a case of reduplicative paramnesia. *J. Clin. Exp. Neuropsychol. 7*:111-121.

98. Tarachow, S. (1939). The Korsakoff psychosis in spontaneous subarachnoid hemorrhage. *Am. J. Psychiat. 95*:887-889.

99. Walton, J.N. (1953). The Korsakoff syndrome in spontaneous subarachnoid haemorrhage. *J. Ment. Sci. 99*:521-530.

100. Maeda, S., Okawa, M., and Aiba, T. (1974). Psychiatric symptoms in intracranial arterial aneurysms—before and after surgery and their prognosis at follow-up. *Clin. Neurol. (Tokyo) 14*:1-9.

101. Sandyk, R. (1984). Transient global amnesia: a presentation of subarachnoid hemorrhage. *J. Neurol. 231*:283-284.

102. Dunker, R.O., and Harris, A.B. (1976). Surgical anatomy of the proximal anterior cerebral artery. *J. Neurosurg. 44*:359-367.

103. Perlmutter, D., and Rhoton, A.L., Jr. (1976). Microsurgical anatomy of the anterior cerebral-anterior communicating-recurrent artery complex. *J. Neurosurg. 45*:259-272.

104. Norlén, G., and Lindqvist, G. (1964). The anatomy of memory. *Lancet 1*:335.

105. Talland, G.A., Sweet, W.H., and Ballantine, H.T. Jr. (1967). Amnestic syndrome with anterior communicating artery aneurysm. *J. Nerv. Ment. Dis. 145*: 179-192.

106. Logue, V., Durward, M., Pratt, R.T.C., Piercy, M., and Nixon, W.L.B. (1968). The quality of survival after rupture of an anterior cerebral aneurysm. *Br. J. Psychiat. 114*:137-160.

107. Okawa, M., Maeda, S., Nukui, H., and Kawafuchi, J. (1980). Psychiatric symptoms in ruptured anterior communicating aneurysms: social prognosis. *Acta Psychiat. Scand. 61*:306-312.

108. Norlén, G., and Olivecrona, H. (1953). The treatment of aneurysms of the circle of Willis. *J. Neurosurg. 10*:404-415.

109. Lindqvist, G., and Norlén, G. (1966). Korsakoff's syndrome after operation on ruptured aneurysm of the anterior communicating artery. *Acta Pyschiat. Scand. 42*:24-26,1966.

110. Takaku, A., Tanaka, S., Mori, T., and Suzuki, J. (1979). Postoperative complications in 1000 cases of intracranial aneurysms. *Surg. Neurol. 12*:137-144.

111. Gade, A. (1982). Amnesia after operations on aneurysms of the anterior communicating artery. *Surg. Neurol. 18*:46-49.

112. Volpe, B.T., and Hirst, W. (1983). Amnesia following the rupture and repair of an anterior communicating artery aneurysm. *J. Neurol. Neurosurg. Psychiat. 46*:704-709.

113. Alexander, M.P., and Freedman, M. (1984). Amnesia after anterior communicating artery aneurysm rupture. *Neurology 34*:752-757.

114. Vilkki, J. (1985). Amnestic syndromes after surgery of anterior communicating artery aneurysms. *Cortex 21*:431-444.

115. Damasio, A.R., Graff-Radford, N.R., Eslinger, P.J., Damasio, H., and Kassell, N. (1985). Amnesia following basal forebrain lesions. *Arch. Neurol. 42*: 263-271.

116. Phillips, S., Sangalang, V., and Sterns, G. (1987). Basal forebrain infarction. A clinicopathologic correlation. *Arch. Neurol. 44*:1134-1138.

117. Volpe, B.T., Herscovitch, P., and Raichle, M.E. (1984). Positron emission tomography defines metabolic abnormality in mesial temporal lobes of two patients with amnesia after rupture and repair of anterior communicating artery aneurysm. *Neurology 34 (Suppl.1)*:188.

118. Beukelman, D.R., Flowers, C.R., and Swanson, P.D. (1980). Cerebral disconnection associated with anterior communicating artery aneurysm: Implications for evaluation of symptoms. *Arch. Phys. Med. Rehab. 61*:18-23.

119. Levin, H.S., Goldstein, F.C., Ghostine, S.Y., Weiner, R.L., Crofford, M.J., and Eisenberg, H.M. (1987). Hemispheric disconnection syndrome persisting after anterior cerebral artery aneurysm rupture. *Neurosurgery 21*:831-838.

120. Fletcher, D.E. (1945). Personality disintegration incident to anoxia: Observations with nitrous oxide anesthesia. *J. Nerv. Ment. Dis. 102*:392-403.

121. Allison, R.S. (1961). Chronic amnestic syndromes in the elderly. *Proc. Roy. Soc. Med. 54*:961-965.

122. Brierley, J.B., and Cooper, J.E. (1962). Cerebral complications of hypotensive anaesthesia in a healthy adult. *J. Neurol. Neurosurg. Psychiat. 25*:24-30.

123. McNeill, D.L., Tidmarsh, D., and Rastall, M.D. (1965). A case of dysmnesic syndrome following cardiac arrest. *Br. J. Psychiat. 111*:697-699.

124. Berlyne, N., and Strachan, M. (1968). Neuropsychiatric sequelae of attempted hanging. *Br. J. Psychiat. 114*:411-422.

125. Finklestein, S., and Caronna, J.J. (1978). Amnestic syndrome following cardiac arrest. *Neurology 28*:389.

126. Muramoto, O., Kuru, Y., Sugishita, M., and Toyokura, Y. (1979). Pure memory loss with hippocampal lesions. A pneumoencephalographic study. *Arch. Neurol. 36*:54-56.

127. Volpe, B.T., and Hirst, W. (1983). The characterization of an amnestic syndrome following hypoxic ischemic injury. *Arch. Neurol.* 40:436-440.

128. Cummings, J.L., Tomiyasu, U., Read, S., and Benson, D.F. (1984). Amnesia with hippocampal lesions after cardiopulmonary arrest. *Neurology* 34:679-681.

129. Della Sala, S., and Spinnler, H. (1986). 'Indifférence amnésique' in a case of global amnesia following acute brain hypoxia. *Eur. Neurol.* 25:98-109.

130. Volpe, B.T., Holtzman, J.D., and Hirst, W. (1986). Further characterization of patients with amnesia after cardiac arrest: Preserved recognition memory. *Neurology* 36:408-411.

131. Zola-Morgan, S., Squire, L., and Amaral, D.G. (1986). Human amnesia and the medial temporal region: Enduring memory impairment following a bilateral lesion limited to field CA1 of the hippocampus. *J. Neurosci.* 6:2950-2967.

132. Volpe, B.T., and Petito, C.K. (1985). Dementia with bilateral medial temporal lobe ischemia. *Neurology* 35:1793-1797.

133. Grant, I., Prigatano, G., Heaton, R.K., McSweeny, A.J., Wright, E.C., and Adams, K.M. (1987). Progressive neuropsychologic impairment and hypoxemia. Relationship in chronic obstructive pulmonary disease. *Arch. Gen. Psychiat.* 44:999-1006.

134. Selby, G., and Lance, J.W. (1960). Observations on 500 cases of migraine and allied vascular headache. *J. Neurol. Neurosurg. Psychiat.* 23:23-32.

135. Gascon, G., and Barlow, C. (1970). Juvenile migraine, presenting as an acute confusional state. *Pediatrics* 45:628-635.

136. Emery, E.S. III (1977). Acute confusional state in children with migraine. *Pediatrics* 60:110-114.

137. Ehyai, A., and Fenichel, G.M. (1978). The natural history of acute confusional migraine. *Arch. Neurol.* 35:368-369.

138. Symonds, C. (1951). Migrainous variants. *Trans. Med. Soc. Lond.* 67:237-250.

139. Feely, M.P., O'Hare, J., Veale, D., and Callaghan, N. (1982). Episodes of acute confusion of psychosis in familial hemiplegic migraine. *Acta Neurol. Scand.* 65:369-375.

140. Moersch, F. (1924). Psychic manifestations in migraine. *Am. J. Psychiat.* 80:697-716.

141. Bechterew, W.v. (1900). Ueber periodische Anfälle retroactiver Amnesie. *Monatschrift Psychiat. Neurol.* 8:353-358.

142. Gilbert, J.J., and Benson, D.F. (1972). Transient global amnesia: report of two cases with definite etiologies. *J. Nerv. Ment. Dis.* 154:461-464.

143. Olivarius, B. deF., and Jensen, T.S. (1979). Transient global amnesia in migraine. *Headache* 19:335-338.

144. Caplan, L., Chedru, F., Lhermitte, F., and Mayman, C. (1981). Transient global amnesia and migraine. *Neurology* 31:1167-1170.

145. Crowell, G.F., Stump, D.A., Biller, J., McHenry, L.C. Jr., and Toole, J.F. (1984). The transient global amnesia-migraine connection. *Arch. Neurol.* 41:75-79.

146. Miller, J.W., Petersen, R.C., Metter, E.J., Millikan, C.H., and Yanagihara, T. (1987). Transient global amnesia: Clinical characteristics and prognosis. *Neurology 37*:733-737.

147. Lauritzen, M., Olsen, T.S., Lassen, N.A., and Paulson, O.B. (1983). Changes in regional cerebral blood flow during the course of classic migraine attacks. *Ann. Neurol. 13*:633-641.

148. Leao, A.A.P., and Morrison, R.S. (1945). Propagation of spreading cortical depression. *J. Neurophysiol. 8*:33-46.

149. Olesen, J., and Jørgensen, M.B. (1986). Leao's spreading depression in the hippocampus explains transient global amnesia. A hypothesis. *Acta Neurol. Scand. 73*:219-220.

150. Steinmetz, E.F., and Vroom, F.Q. (1972). Transient global amnesia. *Neurology 22*:1193-1200.

151. Shuttleworth, E.C., and Wise, G.R. (1973). Transient global amnesia due to arterial embolism. *Arch. Neurol. 29*:340-342.

152. Mathew, N.T., and Meyer, J.S. (1974). Pathogenesis and natural history of transient global amnesia. *Stroke 5*:303-311.

153. Jensen, T.S., and Olivarius, B. deF. (1980). Transient global amnesia as a manifestation of transient cerebral ischemia. *Acta Neurol. Scand. 61*:115-124.

154. Shuping, J.R., Rollinson, R.D., and Toole, J.F. (1980). Transient global amnesia. *Ann. Neurol. 7*:281-285.

155. Cattaino, G., Querin, F., Pomes, A., and Piazza, P. (1984). Transient global amnesia. *Acta Neurol. Scand. 70*:385-390.

156. Kushner, M.J., and Hauser, W.A. (1985). Transient global amnesia: A case-control study. *Ann. Neurol. 18*:684-691.

157. Trillet, M., Croisile, B., Philippon, B., Vial, C., Laurent, B., and Guillot, M. (1987). Ictus amnésique et débits sanguins cérébrauz. *Rev. Neurol. 143*: 536-539.

158. Kadota, E., Irino, T., Nishide, M., Kaneda, H., and Hashimoto, S. (1981). Pathological findings in an autopsied case of transient global amnesia. *Brain and Nerve (Tokyo) 33*:399-406.

11

Alcoholic Korsakoff's Syndrome

William C. Heindel
David P. Salmon
and
Nelson Butters

San Diego Veterans Administration Medical Center
La Jolla
and
University of California School of Medicine at San Diego
San Diego, California

GENERAL CLINICAL FEATURES

Approximately 5% of all chronic alcoholics eventually develop alcoholic Korsakoff's syndrome. This neurologic disorder is characterized by a severe inability to learn and retain new information and to remember events that occurred prior to the acute onset of the syndrome. Despite this severe amnesia, the alcoholic Korsakoff patients' general intellectual capacities, as measured by standardized intelligence tests, are relatively preserved. However, detailed neuropsychological assessments indicate that these patients also have significant impairments in problem solving and visuoperceptual processes.

The first detailed descriptions of alcoholic Korsakoff's syndrome emanate from the writings of Carl Wernicke and of S.S. Korsakoff in the 1880s. Wernicke described three patients with a neurological syndrome that included a gait disorder (i.e., ataxia), abnormal eye movements, and a state of psychological confusion. He attributed this disorder to an inflammatory disease of subcortical brain structures and noted that the symptoms were progressive and led to death within approximately five weeks. Six years following the publication of Wernicke's paper, Korsakoff published the first of a series of reports in which he described the amnesic symptoms that often accompany the neurological symptoms described previously by Wernicke. In addition to long-term alcoholism, Korsakoff noted that these mental changes were associated with a number of other conditions, such as persistent vomiting and intestinal obstruction. Although neither Wernicke nor Korsakoff was specific with regard to etiology, and both seemed unaware that their two syndromes often occurred sequentially in the same patients, their clinical descriptions of the symptomatology of the patients were accurate and represented important initial steps in the identification of the Wernicke-Korsakoff syndrome.

Clinical studies conducted during the twentieth century have demonstrated that if a patient in the Wernicke state (i.e., confusional stage) of the syndrome is not treated with large doses of thiamine he is in danger of having fatal midbrain hemorrhages. If, however, the patient does receive proper vitamin therapy, his confusional state will clear and his ophthalmoplegia, peripheral neuropathies, and gait disorder will show marked improvement within 2-4 weeks. The patient can now maintain a coherent conversation with his physician and cooperate with the administration of mental status and other neuropsychological examinations. At this point, the patient has passed through the acute Wernicke phase and entered the chronic Korsakoff stage which is marked by a severe, permanent amnesic condition. Very few patients (fewer than 25%) with Wernicke's encephalopathy, especially when their medical histories include long-term alcoholism, show a complete return to their premorbid intellectual state.

The traditional psychometric hallmark of the amnesic syndrome of alcoholic Korsakoff patients has been the the scatter between their normal IQ as measured by the Wechsler Adult Intelligence Scale (WAIS or WAIS-R) (1,2) and their severely impaired memory quotient (MQ) as measured by the Wechsler Memory Scale (WMS) (3). Butters and Cermak (4) have reported 20 to 30 points scatter between IQ and MQ (e.g., IQ = 100; MQ = 75) in Korsakoff patients. However, given the severity of the patients' amnesia, this amount of scatter seems to grossly underestimate the difference between intelligence and memory. The discrepancy between the dramatic clinical presentation of amnesia and the moderately impaired MQ is likely due to the WMS' inclusion of attention and concentration tasks (i.e., Digit Span, Mental Control) that are usually unimpaired in amnesia, and to the exclusion of highly sensitive measures of delayed recall for the Logical Memory and Visual Reproduction tests. Butters et al. (5) have recently demonstrated that the revised version of the Wechsler Memory Scale (WMS-R) (6), which provides five separate memory indices (i.e., Attention/Concentration, Verbal Memory, Visual Memory, General Memory and Delayed Memory), more accurately estimates the severe retention problems of Korsakoff patients (Table 1). Instead of MQs in the 70-80 range, Korsakoff patients earned General and Delayed Memory Indices of 65 and 57, respectively.

Besides general memory and cognitive changes, alcoholic Korsakoff patients demonstrate dramatic changes in personality. They often have premorbid histories of antisocial behavior characterized by impulsive aggressive

Table 1 WMS-R Memory Index Scores for Normal Control (NC) and Alcoholic Korsakoff (AK) Groups: Mean ± SD

	NC (n = 28)	AK (n = 11)
Attention/concentration	106.18 ± 11.91	96.91 ± 19.20
Verbal	114.29 ± 16.01	68.00 ± 9.65
Visual	116.54 ± 13.88	76.64 ± 18.48
General	117.79 ± 15.50	65.36 ± 12.14
Delayed	122.64 ± 14.51	56.64 ± 5.71

acts and petty crimes designed to support their chronic alcoholism. Many were "barroom brawlers" who also violently attacked members of their immediate families. With the onset of Korsakoff's syndrome, a dramatic change occurs in these motivational-affective characteristics. Impulsivity, aggression, and severe alcohol abuse are replaced by apathy, passivity, a lack of initiative, and a virtual disinterest in alcohol. The patient is also unable to formulate, organize, and initiate a series of plans. Left to his own devices, the Korsakoff patient is likely to remain seated before a television set or even in bed for long periods of time. He makes few demands or inquiries of hospital staff and will obey all instructions in a passive indifferent manner. Since these personality changes are apparent as soon as the patient enters the chronic Korsakoff stage, they cannot be attributed to the consequence of institutionalization.

Another common clinical feature of alcoholics with Korsakoff's syndrome is their tendency to confabulate when faced with questions they cannot answer (7-9). When asked to recall his activities of the previous day, an alcoholic Korsakoff patient may "fill in" a gap in his memory with a story concerning a trip to his home or to a sporting event that may (or may not) actually have occurred many years ago. This tendency is not a constant or necessarily permanent feature of amnesic patients, and there are marked individual differences among amnesic populations. In general, confabulation is most apparent during the acute stages of the illness and becomes progressively less noticeable as the patient adjusts to his disorder. It is relatively easy to elicit confabulation from a patient in a Wernicke-Korsakoff confusional state, but such responses are less frequent in chronic Korsakoff patients who have had this disorder for five or more years.

Kopelman (7) has categorized the confabulation of alcoholic Korsakoff patients into two types: spontaneous and provoked. The spontaneous form is typically emitted without any probing or queries by the examiner, and may be due to some "frontal lobe" disinhibition superimposed on the patient's organic amnesia. In contrast, provoked confabulations, which occur during examination of the patient's memory capacities, may represent an attempt to conceal or compensate for a severely deficient memory. As noted by both Kopelman (7) and by Butters and his associates (10,11), the Korsakoff patient's attempted recall of prose passages is often characterized by the intrusion of episodes, objects, and individuals not included in the original story. Such extra-story intrusion errors may be confabulations provoked by the recall demands of the task and the patient's faulty memory.

ANTEROGRADE AMNESIA

The most striking feature of the alcoholic Korsakoff patient's severe memory impairment is *anterograde amnesia*, which refers to an inability to acquire new verbal and nonverbal information. Learning the names of his physicians and nurses, the name and location of the hospital, and the location of his bed may require weeks or months of constant repetition and rehearsal. Events that transpired minutes or even seconds before are forgotten by the Korsakoff patient. Not only does the patient fail to learn the names of important people and places, but often he will not remember previous encounters with these individuals. If the patient spends three hours completing a battery of intelligence and memory tests, he will usually fail to recall the entire test session two hours after it has ended.

These anecdotal examples of Korsakoff patients' memory failures can all be characterized as impairments in *episodic memory* (12). Tulving (13) has defined episodic memories as memories for specific events which are dependent upon temporal and/or spatial cues for their retrieval. Experimentally, this severe episodic memory deficit is exemplified by the severe difficulty the Korsakoff patient has in learning even short lists of five or six verbal paired-associates (14,15). When the Korsakoff patient is shown a list of word pairs (e.g., man-hammer) in which he must learn to associate the second word with the first, the acquisition of these associations may require 30 or 40 trials instead of the three or four presentations needed by normal subjects (Fig. 1).

Although a few studies have found Korsakoff patients to have intact short-term memories (16-18), most investigations have reported these patients to be impaired in retention if a few seconds of distractor activity intervene between presentation and recall (for review, see Refs. 4,19,20). For example, if presented (visually or orally) with three words (e.g., apple, pen, roof), and then required to count backward from 100 by three's to prevent rehearsal (a distractor task), Korsakoff patients will be impaired in the recall of the three words after only 9 or 18 seconds of such counting activity. Similarly, these patients are unable to retain nonverbal materials (such as geometric patterns) for 18 seconds if a demanding distractor activity intervenes between presentation and recognition testing (21).

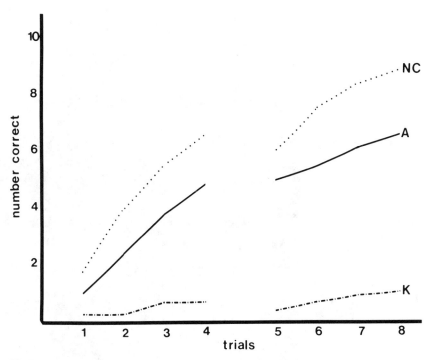

Figure 1 Mean number of words recalled on eight trials of a verbal paired-associate task for normal controls (NC), alcoholics (A) and alcoholic Korsakoff patients (K). (From Ref. 14).

In contrast to their impaired performance on episodic memory tasks, Korsakoff patients have been found to perform relatively well on tests of *semantic memory* (12). Semantic memories have been defined as memories for general principles, associations, rules, etc. which are totally independent of contextual cues for their retrieval. The observations that Korsakoff patients perform normally on verbal fluency tests (22), and do not forget the meaning of words, the rules of syntax, or basic arithmetical skills (23) support the notion of an intact semantic memory in Korsakoff patients.

Although Korsakoff patients do encounter more difficulty with episodic than with semantic memory tasks, their performances on both are marked by an increased sensitivity to proactive interference (i.e., the interference from previously learned material in learning new information). Korsakoff patients have been shown to perform normally (e.g., correctly recalling up to 90% of the items) on the first trials of a short-term memory distractor task, but then deteriorate very rapidly (e.g., recalling fewer than 50% of the items on the fifth trial) on subsequent trials (24). Since Korsakoff patients

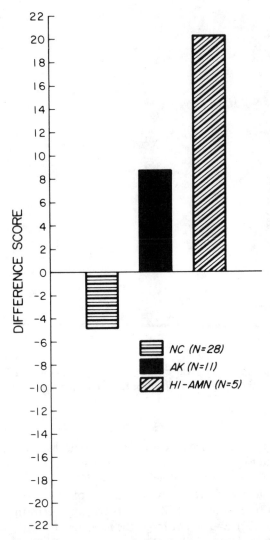

Figure 2 Mean differences between General and Delayed Memory Indices of the Wechsler Memory Scale-Revised for normal controls (NC), alcoholic Korsakoff patients (AK), and amnesic patients with presumed hippocampal damage (HI-AMN). (From Ref. 5.)

on Trial 5 often continue to recall information presented on Trials 1 and 2, it would appear that the successful learning of material on the first two trials severely hinders the patients' attempted recall on succeeding trials. Numerous investigations have noted that alcoholic Korsakoff patients are also highly prone to prior-item intrusion errors on verbal paired-associate learning (15), recall of short passages (10), and verbal fluency tests (10).

In addition to being severely impaired in their ability to acquire new information, Korsakoff patients may also show rapid forgetting of what little they do learn. Butters et al. (5) found that alcoholic Korsakoff patients showed a large difference between General and Delayed Memory indices and very little savings over a 30 minute delay on the Logical Memory and Visual Reproduction tests of the WMS-R (Figs. 2 and 3). Although apparent on most clinical tests of memory, rapid forgetting rates in Korsakoff patients generally have not been observed on experimental tests (25-27). One reason for this discrepancy may be that, on some experimental tests, initial levels of performance were equalized in the amnesic and control subjects by manipulating the duration of stimulus exposure (i.e., longer and/or more frequent exposure for the amnesic subjects). This increased exposure for the Korsakoff patients

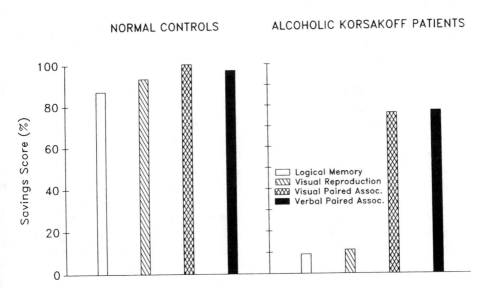

Figure 3   Mean savings scores for normal controls (NC) and alcoholic Korsakoff patients (AK) on the Logical Memory, Visual Recognition, Visual Paired Associate and Verbal Paired Associate tests of the Wechsler Memory Scale-Revised. (Adapted from Ref. 5.)

may have resulted in an overlearning of materials and subsequently to a masking of differences in forgetting rates between patients and control subjects. Butters et al.'s (5) finding of normal forgetting rates for Korsakoff patients on the Verbal and Visual Paired-Associate tests of the WMS-R supports this conclusion. On both of these paired-associate tasks the Korsakoff patients were administered up to three more learning trials than were their intact control subjects.

RETROGRADE AMNESIA

The second main feature of the alcoholic Korsakoff patients' severe memory impairment is their inability to recall events that occurred prior to the onset of their illness (i.e., *retrograde amnesia*). When asked who was President of the United States before Mr. Reagan, an alcoholic Korsakoff patient might answer "Nixon" or "Kennedy." He will admit that Lyndon Johnson was once President, but be unable to specify whether Johnson's presidency preceded or followed Kennedy's. In general, this difficulty in retrieving old memories is usually more pronounced for events just prior to the onset of the illness, while very remote events from the patients' childhood are relatively (but not perfectly) preserved. Most 55-65-year-old alcoholic Korsakoff patients who served in World War II or Korea can describe their tours of duty in great detail but are unable to recall any of the major public events (e.g., the assassination of the Kennedys, Watergate, the Iranian hostage crisis, the bombing of Libya) of the past three decades.

This temporal "gradient" has also been observed in numerous experimental studies of retrograde amnesia (28-31). Albert, Butters, and Levin (28), for example, developed a retrograde amnesia test battery that included a famous persons (i.e., faces) test, a recall questionnaire, and a multiple-choice recognition questionnaire. Each test consisted of items from the 1930s to the 1970s that had been assessed on a population of normal controls before the inclusion in the final test battery. Half of the items were "easy" as judged by the performance of the standardization group; the other half were difficult or "hard" judged by the same criterion. For both the faces test and the recall test of public events, the alcoholic Korsakoff patients identified more items from the 1930s and 1940s than from the 1960s (Fig. 4). This same pattern emerged regardless of whether the items were easy or hard. Similar temporal gradients were reported for the recognition test of public events (28).

In addition to providing a detailed description of the alcoholic Korsakoff patients' loss of remote memories, many investigations have demonstrated that the retrograde amnesia of alcoholic Korsakoff patients differs significantly from that of amnesics with other etiologies (e.g., viral, vascular, trauma) and constellation of brain lesions (e.g., the mesial regions of the temporal

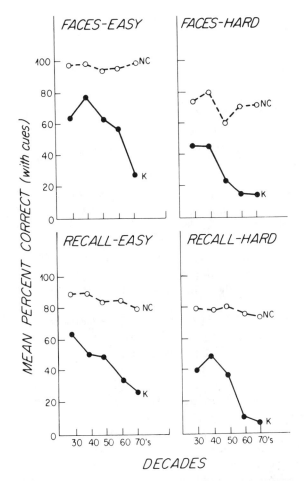

Figure 4 Performance of alcoholic Korsakoff patients (K) and nonalcoholic control subjects (NC) on the Famous Faces Test and Public Events Recall Questionnaire. Results for easy and hard items are shown separately. (From Ref. 28.)

lobes). For example, the temporary retrograde amnesia of depressed patients receiving bilateral ECT (electroconvulsive shock treatment) has been found to be limited to the four-year period immediately preceding shock treatment (29). Scoville and Milner's (32) patient HM, who had bilateral mesial temporal lobe ablations to relieve life-threatening epileptic seizures, was originally reported to have a retrograde amnesia limited to the 3-5 year period prior to his surgery (33).

Given that the retrograde amnesia of many amnesic patients is relatively brief, how can the alcoholic Korsakoff patient's extended, graded loss of old memories be explained? One factor may be a primary defect in establishing new memories (i.e., anterograde amnesia) during the 15-30 years of severe alcoholism that precede the acute onset of the Wernicke-Korsakoff syndrome. Recent studies with detoxified, long-term (non-Korsakoff) alcoholics have shown that these seemingly intact patients have mild but significant deficits on a variety of learning tasks (for review, see Ref. 34). Consequently, if chronic alcoholics are learning and retaining less information about public and private events each year due to a progressive anterograde memory problem, then at the time an alcoholic develops Korsakoff's syndrome, a mild retrograde amnesia with a temporal gradient would be expected. A second factor which may account for the severity of the alcoholic Korsakoff patient's retrograde amnesia involves an acute loss of access to old memories with the onset of the Wernicke stage of the illness. Presumably, this storage or retrieval problem would affect all periods of the patient's life equally. Since this acute loss would be superimposed upon a depleted amount of information about the most recent decades of the patient's life (i.e., factor one), the resulting severe retrograde amnesia would be characterized by what appears to be a relative sparing of events from childhood and early adulthood (i.e., the period before the patient began to drink heavily).

There is some evidence for this two-factor model of the Korsakoff patients' retrograde amnesia. When non-Korsakoff detoxified alcoholics were administered questionnaires about public events and tests of famous faces (i.e., persons), they exhibited a deficit in their knowledge of important events that occurred during the past 10-15 years (29,35). Although this impairment in remote memory was much milder than that observed in alcoholic Korsakoff patients, it demonstrated that long-term alcoholics do have an inadequate store of information about the very recent past. The detrimental effects of alcohol on the patients' ability to learn new materials did, as predicted, become more apparent as the length of alcoholism increased.

Evidence of a very severe acute loss of old memories with the onset of Wernicke's encephalopathy emanates from a single-case study of patient PZ, an eminent scientist and university professor who developed alcoholic Korsakoff's syndrome at the age of 65 (36,37). PZ had authored several hundred research papers and numerous books and book chapters, including an extensive autobiography three years prior to the acute onset of his Wernicke-Korsakoff syndrome in the fall of 1981. To determine whether PZ had also lost access to his autobiographical material that was well-known to him just before his illness, a retrograde amnesia test based upon his autobiography was developed. PZ was found to have a very severe retrograde amnesia for autobiographical events, with considerable sparing of information from the remote past (Fig. 5). Since all the questions were taken from his own autobiography, PZ's retrograde amnesia cannot be secondary to a deficiency in

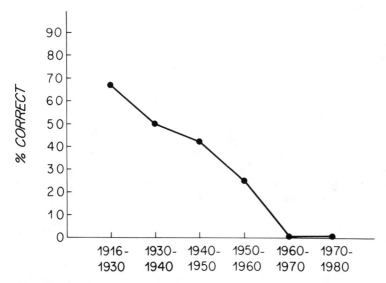

Figure 5   Patient P.Z.'s retrograde amnesia for information from his published autobiography (From Ref. 37.)

original learning. Furthermore, the relatively more severe impairment for the most recent decades suggests that autobiographical information acquired during these time periods was not as stable as that acquired earlier in PZ's lifetime.

Cermak (12) has proposed that this relative sparing of PZ's and other Korsakoff patients' very remote memories may be due to a transfer of information from an episodic to a semantic memory store. That is, newly acquired information may be episodic in nature, but with time and continued rehearsal the memories become independent of specific temporal and spatial contexts (i.e., semantic memory). From this viewpoint, the gradients evidenced by alcoholic Korsakoff patients are due to the greater vulnerability of episodic than of semantic memory to extensive damage to diencephalic or mesial temporal lobe structures. This hypothesis, stressing the loss of episodic memory, is unique among theories of amnesia because it attempts to account for both the patients' anterograde and retrograde amnesias.

It is also possible that the extended retrograde amnesia of alcoholic Korsakoff patients may be due to impaired problem solving, initiation, and planning abilities associated with damage to the anterior association cortices. Alcoholic Korsakoff patients have previously been found to be impaired on the Wisconsin Card Sorting Test (WCST), tests of verbal fluency, embedded figures tests, and tasks requiring temporal order judgments (4,38-40). Although some retrograde amnesias may be a consequence of cortically mediated cognitive deficits beyond the domain of the amnesic syndrome, there now have been several reports of non-Korsakoff amnesic patients without prominent cognitive impairments who still exhibit extended retrograde amnesias (41-45).

PRESERVED MEMORY

Despite their severe anterograde and retrograde memory deficits, alcoholic Korsakoff patients demonstrate an intact capacity to acquire and retain rule-based motor and cognitive skills. Korsakoff patients, like all amnesic patients, show normal learning on visuomotor tasks such as mirror tracing and pursuit rotor (46,47). This preserved learning ability is also observed on skills which require some utilization of cognitive processes. Cohen and Squire (48) found that the ability of amnesic patients to read mirror-reversed words improved at a normal rate over three test sessions, and this ability was retained over a 3-month period, even though the patients could remember neither the test sessions nor the specific words read. Based on these results, Squire and his colleagues (48,49) have proposed that alcoholic Korsakoff patients are severely impaired in learning specific data-based *declarative knowledge* (e.g., recognizing the words employed in the mirror-reading task) but are capable of normal acquisition and retention of rule-based *procedural knowledge* (e.g., learning to read mirror-reflected words).

A recent study (50) comparing the mirror-reading and recognition memory capacities of alcoholic Korsakoff patients and patients with progressive dementia due to atrophy of the basal ganglia (i.e., patients with Huntington's disease) provides further confirmation of the dissociation between procedural and declarative memory. While Korsakoff patients again demonstrated an intact rate of acquisition of mirror-reading and impaired recognition of verbal stimuli, the demented patients were retarded in their acquisition of the mirror-reading skill despite normal recognition of the words employed in the task. Based upon this dissociation, it appears that limbic (i.e., hippocampal-diencephalic) structures may mediate the learning of declarative knowledge while the basal ganglia may be critical for the acquisition of procedural knowledge.

In addition to normal skill learning ability, alcoholic Korsakoff patients have also demonstrated intact performance on a wide variety of priming tasks. Priming is defined as the temporary (and unconscious) facilitation of performance via prior exposure to specific stimuli (51). For example, both amnesic patients and intact control subjects have a strong tendency (relative to chance) to complete three-letter words stems (e.g., MOT) with previously presented words (e.g., MOTEL) despite the failure of the amnesic patients to recall or recognize these words on standard memory tests (52-54). Similar normal priming effects have been observed in alcoholic Korsakoff patients on tasks in which subjects are asked to generate exemplars of particular categories (55,56), identify words flashed for short durations (e.g., 35 ms) on a computer screen (57,58), and identify incomplete (i.e., "fragmented") line drawings of animate and inanimate objects (53,54). In all instances, subjects showed an increased tendency to complete the task with items presented earlier.

In an attempt to integrate the skill learning and priming literature, Graf and Schacter (59) proposed that the types of memory that are preserved in amnesia can all be characterized as *implicit* in nature. Implicit memory represents an unconscious facilitation or change in task performance that is attributable to information acquired during a previous study episode (60). Implicit memory would therefore encompass both procedural learning and priming. *Explicit* memory, in contrast, requires the conscious, deliberate recollection of prior study episodes and is impaired in amnesia.

Although all explicit memory abilities are cleary dependent upon the integrity of the mesial temporal and diencephalic structures damaged in amnesia (20), it is likely that different forms of implicit memory are mediated by distinct neuroanatomical systems. A recent study comparing the implicit memory abilities of patients with different dementing illnesses (i.e., Alzheimer's, Huntington's, and Parkinson's diseases) suggests that, while skill learning may be mediated by a corticostriatal system, verbal priming may depend upon the integrity of the neocortical association areas involved in the storage of semantic knowledge (61). To the extent that the brain damage in alcoholic Korsakoff patients is restricted to the diencephalic regions, one would expect their memory deficit to be limited to the explicit domain. If, as in the case of demented patients, the damage extends beyond the explicit memory system, one would anticipate additional deficits in one or more forms of implicit memory.

OTHER COGNITIVE DEFICITS

Although the amnesic syndrome is the alcoholic Korsakoff patients' most obvious deficit, impairments on other cognitive tasks have also been observed. As mentioned previously, Korsakoff patients have been found to be impaired on problem-solving tasks such as the Wisconsin Card Sorting Test (39,40). Oscar-Berman (62) found that Korsakoff patients also utilized inefficient and insufficient strategies on other tests of hypothesis formation.

Becker et al. (63) examined the problem-solving abilities of both alcoholic Korsakoff patients and long-term (non-Korsakoff) alcoholics using a modification of the old parlor game "20 Questions" (64). The subjects were shown a presentation card with 42 stimuli (e.g., outlined drawings of objects) arranged in a 6 × 7 matrix (Fig. 6), and were asked to "figure out" which object

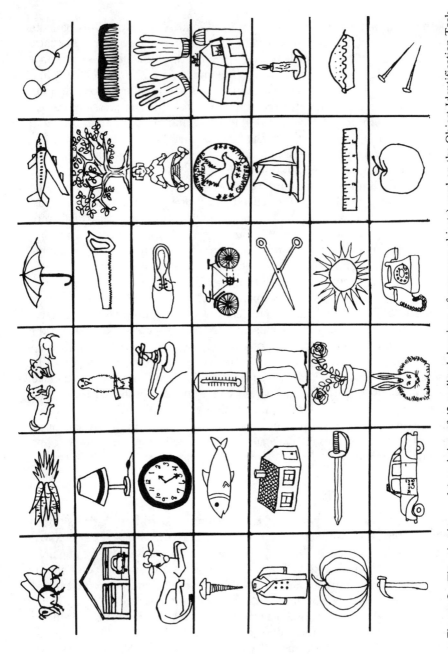

Figure 6 The stimulus card (consisting of 42 outlined drawings of common objects) used on the Object Identification Task (i.e., "20 Questions") (From Ref. 64.)

the examiner was thinking of at that time. The subjects could ask any question as long as the examiner could answer it with a "yes" or "no" response. The subjects' goal was to identify the preselected object in as few questions as possible.

Figure 7 shows the results for three trials with this identification task. Nonalcoholic control subjects adopted the efficient strategy of first asking "constraint-seeking" questions, which reduced by as much as 50% the number of possible alternatives (objects), regardless of a "yes" or "no" answer (e.g., "Is it a tool?"). Only when two or three alternative objects remained did a nonalcoholic subject ask a "hypothesis-scanning" question, which referred to a single object (e.g., "Is it the saw?"). In contrast, both the Korsakoff patients and detoxified long-term alcoholics quickly abandoned the efficient use of constraint-seeking questions and shifted to hypothesis scanning and even "pseudoconstraint" questions, which superficially seemed to be general questions but actually referred to only one object on the card (e.g., The question "Is it something to tell time with?" was only relevant to the drawing of a clock and not to any other alternative).

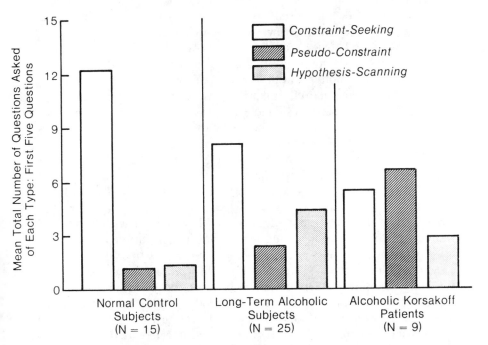

Figure 7   The performance of normal controls, long-term alcoholics, and alcoholic Korsakoff patients on the Object Identification Task. The mean number of constraint-seeking, hypothesis-scanning, and pseudo-constraint questions asked during the first five questions are plotted. (From Ref. 64.)

These findings, like those of Oscar-Berman (62), indicate that both Korsakoff patients and chronic alcoholics are unable to initiate and maintain an optimal strategy for identifying the preselected objects. Such deficiencies in planning and problem solving have often been associated with damage to the frontal association cortex (65,67).

In addition to their problem-solving abilities, alcoholic Korsakoff patients are usually impaired on tasks requiring complex visuoperceptual and visuospatial processing (40). These deficits are most evident on digit-symbol and symbol-digit substitution tests (68,69) and on embedded figures tests (40,69). Similar perceptual deficits have been observed in chronic (non-Korsakoff) alcoholics (for review, see Ref. 34).

NEUROPSYCHOLOGICAL EXAMINATION

Given the particular pattern of memory, problemsolving, and perceptual symptoms associated with alcoholic Korsakoff's syndrome, a minimal neuropsychological examination should include the WAIS-R, the National Adult Reading Test (NART) (70), the WMS-R, the California Verbal Learning Test (CVLT) (71), the Boston Naming Test (BNT) (72), the Wisconsin Card Sorting Test (WCST) (73), Benton's test of verbal fluency (74), and either an embedded figures test (e.g., Ref. 75), or the Visual Search Test (76).

The WAIS-R and NART provide indicators of present (WAIS-R) and premorbid (NART) estimates of overall intelligence. If the WAIS-R is one or more standard deviations below the NART, general alcoholic dementia (8,77) instead of (or in addition to) Korsakoff's syndrome must be considered. Also, alcoholic Korsakoff patients should evidence no impairments on the BNT. If naming deficiencies are noted, the role of other etiologies such as Alzheimer's disease and head injuries should be explored.

Performance on the General and Delayed Memory Indices of the WMS-R should be severely impaired, with scores ranging between 50 and 70. Due to the Korsakoff patients' rapid rate of forgetting, the Delayed Memory Index is usually 8-10 points lower than the General Memory Index. Also, savings scores computed for the Logical Memory and Visual Reproduction tests should be less than 20% after a 30 minute delay. Prior-item intrusion errors are frequently noted on these two tests.

As anticipated, alcoholic Korsakoff patients' performance on the CVLT is usually 3 or more standard deviations below the norms for *both* recall and recognition measures. Due to deficits in encoding (4,78), the patients show little clustering of semantically related words. Because the CVLT utilizes a second list as a distractor, measures of proactive interference (i.e., the intrusion of words from List 1 when attempting recall of List 2) are available. Compared with normal controls, alcoholics (non-Korsakoff), and many forms of dementia, alcoholic Korsakoff patients usually evidence considerable proactive interference on this task.

Since the WCST and the fluency tests are sensitive to "frontal lobe" dysfunction, alcoholic Korsakoff patients are mild to moderately impaired on these tasks. On the WCST, Korsakoff patients have difficulty initiating and then maintaining an appropriate sorting strategy. When the examiner shifts reinforcement contingencies, thereby requiring the adoption of a new sorting strategy, alcoholic Korsakoff patients continue to use their most current strategy and compile a large number of perseverations. On letter fluency tasks, Korsakoff patients frequently show a 25% reduction from established norms (79).

In comparison to intact individuals, the Korsakoff patients' visuoperceptual deficits should be evident from the long temporal intervals needed to locate embedded figures and a particular black-white configuration on the Visual Search Test. The patients' age-correct scaled scores on the Digit-Symbol subtest (WAIS or WAIS-R) are usually between 4 and 7, and are far below scaled scores on the Vocabulary and Information subtests.

Although standardized remote memory batteries for assessing retrograde amnesia are not readily available, the clinician should attempt to assess informally the patients' recall of major historical events that have occurred during their lifetime. If spouses or close relatives are available to provide details about the personal life of patients, assessment of autobiographical memories should also be attempted. As described previously, patients with alcoholic Korsakoff's syndrome have an extended, temporally graded loss of remote memories for both public and personal (i.e., autobiographical) events.

This suggested neuropsychological test battery not only will prove useful in confirming Korsakoff's syndrome in alcoholic patients with a clear history of Wernicke's encephalopathy, but also can help the clinician differentiate Korsakoff's syndrome from other forms of dementia. For instance, patients with alcoholic dementia show a general decline in all cognitive functions (including IQ), with memory being only moderately impaired (8,77). Although patients in the early stages of Alzheimer's disease show many of the same severe memory and problem-solving deficits as do Korsakoff patients (for review, see Ref. 79), they usually exhibit some anomia on the BNT and/or the Vocabulary subtest of the WAIS-R.

NEUROLOGIC BASES

The majority of neuropathological studies of the Wernicke-Korsakoff syndrome support the notion that the neurologic symptoms of Wernicke's encephalopathy are related to lesions of the brainstem and cerebellum, whereas the amnesic symptoms of the chronic Korsakoff state involve damage to several thalamic and hypothalamic structures surrounding the third ventricle of the brain. The dorsomedial nucleus of the thalamus and the mammillary bodies of the hypothalamus are the specific structures most often associated with the alcoholic Korsakoff patients' amnesic symptoms (for review, see Refs. 9,80,81).

Several studies suggest that the mammillary bodies are the crucial structure for the amnesic syndrome. Gamper (82) studies the brains of 16 alcoholic Korsakoff patients and found that, although there was wide variation with lesions extending from the thalamus to lower brainstem, all 16 patients had extensive atrophy of the mammillary bodies. Riggs and Boles (83) examined 29 brains of patients who had "Wernicke's disease" due to various causes, and noted that the mammillary bodies were affected in 21 of 23 cases, the dorsomedial nucleus of the thalamus in 23 of 27, and the pulvinar of the thalamus in 10 of 14. Of 8 Korsakoff patients with both anterograde and retrograde memory deficits examined neuropathologically by Delay and co-workers (84,85), atrophy of the mammillary bodies was common to all cases whereas significant thalamic involvement was noted in only one brain.

Adams et al. (86) found that the severe memory disorder of 54 Korsakoff patients was correlated with the presence of lesions not only in the mammillary bodies but also in several thalamic nuclei (dorsomedial, anteroventral, and pulvinar) as well. Victor et al. (9) noted extensive atrophy of the dorsomedial nucleus in 38 out of 43 brains of alcoholic Korsakoff patients, but in the five brains with no atrophy there had been no lasting memory disorder during life. Since all five of these "negative" cases showed severe atrophy of the mammillary bodies, Victor et al. concluded that the dorsomedial nucleus, and not the mammillary bodies, is the critical structure. It is possible, however, that since all 38 cases with amnesia also had lesions in both the mammillary bodies and the dorsomedial nucleus, a combined thalamic-hypothalamic lesion is the one that is both necessary and sufficient for Korsakoff's syndrome.

Two recent neuropathological studies (87,88) suggest that the atrophic and vascular diencephalic changes associated with the Wernicke-Korsakoff syndrome may also be common among nonamnesic, long-term alcoholics. In one investigation of 51 cases of Wernicke's encephalopathy diagnosed at necropsy, only seven had been diagnosed clinically during life (87). In a second, more extensive study, Harper (88) found that 83% of 131 brains of alcoholics evidenced significant medial diencephalic changes (including atrophy of the mammillary bodies, hemorrhagic lesions of the thalamus, dilatation of the third ventricle) even though only 20% of the cases had been reported to have signs of Wernicke's encephalopathy prior to death.

One explanation of Harper's findings rests upon quantitative differences in neurologic damage between alcoholics with and without the clinical signs of the Wernicke-Korsakoff syndrome. That is, non-Korsakoff alcoholics may simply have less atrophy and fewer hemorrhagic lesions than do alcoholics with Korsakoff's syndrome. For an alcoholic to progress to the Wernicke's state the amount of diencephalic damage may have to exceed a critical threshold necessary for the maintenance of neurological and neuropsychological functioning. A second explanation of Harper's findings concerns the presence of other neuropathology in the Wernicke-Korsakoff syndrome. Arendt et al. (89) found that the number of neurons in the basal forebrain (the major source of cholinergic input to the cerebral cortex and hippocampus) was reduced by 47% in the brains of 3 Korsakoff patients, whereas there was no significant loss of neurons for 5 chronic alcoholics. In addition, McEntee and Mair (90-92) have suggested that alcoholic Korsakoff patients' anterograde memory deficits may be associated with a deficiency in norepinephrine.

A recent study employing computer-generated measures derived from CT scans of living alcoholics (with and without Korsakoff's syndrome) suggests that cortical abnormalities may also be involved in the Wernicke-Korsakoff's syndrome. Shimamura's group (93) examined seven alcoholic Korsakoff patients, seven detoxified alcoholics, and seven intact (nonalcoholic) control subjects. The Korsakoff patients were found to have lower density values in the region of the thalamus and greater fluid volumes in the third ventricle than did the alcoholic and intact subjects. Signs of anterior cortical atrophy (e.g., increased sulcal size) were noted in both groups of alcoholics. For the Korsakoff patients several cognitive measures, including indices of memory functioning, correlated significantly with density measures of the thalamus and fluid volumes in the region of the frontal lobes. The authors conclude that dysfunction of both midline thalamic and anterior cortical structures contribute to the Korsakoff patients memory and other cognitive problems.

ETIOLOGY

Despite the numerous neuropathological studies, the etiology of the brain damage in alcoholic Korsakoff patients remains obscure. Victor et al. (9) and Dreyfus (94) have reviewed considerable data pointing to thiamine deficiency as the primary factor in this disease. Since chronic alcoholics often fail to eat nutritionally balanced diets, malnutrition and avitaminosis are common correlates of chronic alcohol abuse. According to this nutritional theory, the diencephalon, the brainstem, and the cerebellum of Korsakoff patients either atrophy or become prone to hemorrhagic lesions due to their high sensitivity to thiamine deficiency.

Three principal forms of evidence lend support to this theory of avitaminosis. First, the symptoms of Wernicke's stage occur commonly in disorders (e.g., chronic gastritis, intestinal obstruction, protracted vomiting during pregnancy) that interfere with food metabolism and absorption. Second, treatment of Wernicke-Korsakoff patients with large amounts of thiamine often alleviates the symptoms associated with the Wernicke stage (confusional state, ophthalmoplegia, nystagmus, ataxia), but usually does not alleviate the memory and personality disorders of the Korsakoff stage. Third, experimental studies with animals (95-97) have shown that prolonged thiamine deprivation will result in the major neurological symptoms of Wernicke's encephalopathy and that these symptoms are subsequently alleviated by the administration of thiamine.

Although most textbooks of neurology accept avitaminosis as the primary cause of the Wernicke-Korsakoff disorder, there is now impressive evidence that prolonged alcohol ingestion, unaccompanied by malnutrition, does result in some permanent learning deficits and in significant brain lesions. This evidence suggests the need for some reevaluation of the etiology of the Wernicke-Korsakoff syndrome. In a review of the literature, Freund (98) has concluded that there is virtually no documented evidence of a permanent memory disorder in patients with thiamine deficiencies unaccompanied by alcohol abuse. Most likely, the amnesic syndrome of Korsakoff patients results from an interaction of thiamine deficiency and the direct neurotoxic effects of alcohol.

Given that ethanol has a direct toxic effect on cortical and subcortical brain structures regardless of the nutritional status of the organism, one must consider the possibility that the memory and cognitive disorders of Korsakoff patients may not appear acutely, but rather, may develop slowly over decades of severe alcoholism. This "continuity hypothesis" (99) suggests that there is a continuum of cognitive impairment between the Korsakoff patient on the one hand and the heavy social drinker on the other, and would predict that a given individual's degree of cognitive deficit is determined by his drinking history (i.e., quantity, frequency, and duration).

The most impressive evidence favoring this continuity hypothesis emanates from comparisons of the visuoperceptive and problem-solving deficits (i.e., cortical dysfunctions) of Korsakoff patients and long-term alcoholics. As noted previously, long-term alcoholics demonstrate impairments on digit-symbol and symbol-digit substitution tasks (68,69) and on hypothesis formation tasks (62,63) that are qualitatively similar to that of Korsakoff patients. It therefore seems likely that the cortical dysfunctions of Korsakoff patients may develop slowly during many years of alcohol abuse and do not appear suddenly with the onset of Wernicke's encephalopathy.

In contrast to the cortical dysfunctions of Korsakoff patients, their memory deficits do not appear to develop slowly over a period of time. Although non-Korsakoff alcoholics do demonstrate some anterograde memory dysfunction, these deficits are relatively mild (100,101), often material-specific (102,103), and do not seem to involve the same processes characteristic of Korsakoff patients (100,104). Similarly, as mentioned previously, while some of their remote memory impairments may be attributable to a mild deficit in original learning during the 20 years of alcohol abuse that preceded the diagnosis of the amnesic syndrome, the major factor in the development of the Korsakoff patients' retrograde amnesia appears to involve an acute loss of memories for episodes that occurred before the onset of their illness (37).

In summary, it appears that the continuity hypothesis has quite different merits when applied to cortical and subcortical dysfunctions. The Korsakoff patients' visuoperceptual and problem-solving deficits, which presumably reflect the cortical abnormalities (e.g., widening of cortical sulci) frequently seen on CT scans of the brains of Korsakoff and alcoholic patients (e.g., Refs. 8,77,105-108) develop slowly during the patients' 20-30 year history of alcohol abuse. Since alcohol may have a direct neurotoxic effect on association cortex, a normal nutritional status may not protect the alcoholic patient from eventual visuoperceptual and analytical deficiencies. However, the Korsakoff patients' memory deficits, which have been associated with medial diencephalic (and perhaps basal forebrain) lesions, become very apparent following acute, severe malnutrition combined with the chronic neurotoxic effects of ethanol.

ACKNOWLEDGMENTS

Some of the research cited in this chapter was supported by funds from the Medical Research Service of the Veterans Administration and by NIAAA grant AA-00187 to Boston University.

Some of the material covered in this chapter has been reviewed previously in two articles: (1) N. Butters, "Alcoholic Korsakoff's syndrome: An update," *Seminars in Neurology*, 1984, pp. 226-244; and (2) D. Salmon and N. Butters, "The etiology and neuropathology of alcoholic Korsakoff's syndrome: Some evidence for the role of the basal forebrain," In M. Galanter (Ed.), *Recent Developments in Alcoholism*, Vol. 5, 1987, Plenum Press, New York, pp. 27-58.

REFERENCES

1. Wechsler, D. (1955). *Wechsler Adult Intelligence Scale Manual*. Psychological Corporation, New York.

2. Wechsler, D. (1981). *Wechsler Adult Intelligence Scale—Revised Manual*. Psychological Corporation, New York.
3. Wechsler, D. (1945). A standardized memory scale for clinical use. *J. Psychol.* 19:87-95.
4. Butters, N., and Cermak, L.S. (1980). *Alcoholic Korsakoff's Syndrome: An Information Processing Approach to Amnesia*. Academic Press, New York.
5. Butters, N., Salmon, D., Cullum, C.M., Cairns, P., Troster, A., Jacobs, D., Moss, M., and Cermak, L. (1988). Differentiation of amnesic and demented patients with the Wechsler Memory Scale-Revised. *Clin. Neuropsychol.* 2:133-148.
6. Wechsler, D. (1987). *Wechsler Memory Scale—Revised*. Psychological Corporation, New York.
7. Kopelman, M. (1987). Two types of confabulation. *J. Neurol. Neurosurg. Psychiatry* 50:1482-1487.
8. Lishman, W.A. (1987). *Organic Psychiatry*, 2nd Ed. Blackwell Scientific Publications, London.
9. Victor, M., Adams, R.D., and Collins, G.H. (1971). *The Wernicke-Korsakoff Syndrome*. F.A. Davis, Philadelphia.
10. Butters, N., Wolfe, J., Granholm, E., and Martone, M. (1986). An assessment of verbal recall, recognition and fluency abilities in patients with Huntington's disease. *Cortex* 22:11-32.
11. Butters, N., Granholm, E., Salmon, D., Grant, I., and Wolfe, J. (1987). Episodic and semantic memory: a comparison of amnesic and demented patients. *J. Clin. Exp. Neuropsychol.* 9:479-497.
12. Cermak, L.S. (1984). The episodic-semantic distinction in amnesia. In *Neuropsychology of Memory*. Edited by L. Squire and N. Butters. Guilford Press, New York, pp. 55-62.
13. Tulving, E. (1983). *Elements of Episodic Memory*. Oxford University Press, New York.
14. Ryan, C., and Butters, N. (1980). Further evidence for a continuum-of-impairment encompassing male alcoholic Korsakoff patients and chronic alcoholic men. *Alcoholism (NY)* 4:190-198.
15. Winocur, G., and Weiskrantz, L. (1976). An investigation of paired-associate learning in amnesic patients. *Neuropsychologia* 14:97-110.
16. Baddeley, A.D., and Warrington, E.K. (1970). Amnesia and the distinction between long- and short-term memory. *J. Verb. Learn. Verb. Behav.* 9:176-189.
17. Kopelman, M. (1985). Rates of forgetting in Alzheimer-type dementia and Korsakoff's syndrome. *Neuropsychologia* 23:623-638.
18. Mair, W.G., Warrington, E.K., and Weiskrantz, L. (1979). Memory disorder in Korsakoff's psychosis: a neuropathological and neuropsychological investigation of two cases. *Brain* 102:749-783.
19. Goodglass, H., and Butters, N. (1988). Psychology of cognitive processes. In *Stevens' Handbook of Experimental Psychology*. 2nd Ed. Vol. 2, *Learning and Cognition*. Edited by R.C. Atkinson, R.J. Herrnstein, G. Lindzey, and R.D. Luce. John Wiley & Sons, New York, pp. 863-952.
20. Squire, L.R. (1987). *Memory and Brain*. Oxford University Press, New York.

21. DeLuca, D., Cermak, L.S., and Butters, N. (1975). An analysis of Korsakoff patients' recall following varying types of distractor activity. *Neuropsychologia* 13:271-279.
22. Weingartner, H., Grafman, J., Boutelle, W., Kaye, W., and Martin, P.R. (1983). Forms of memory failure. *Science* 221:380-382.
23. Kinsbourne, M., and Wood, F. (1975). Short-term memory processes and the amnesic syndrome. In *Short-Term Memory*. Edited by D. Deutsch and J.A. Deutsch. Academic Press, New York.
24. Cermak, L.S., Butters, N., and Moreines, J. (1974). Some analyses of the verbal encoding deficit of alcoholic Korsakoff patients. *Brain Lang.* 1:141-150.
25. Huppert, F.A., and Piercy, M. (1979). Normal and abnormal forgetting in organic amnesia: effects of locus of lesion. *Cortex* 15:385-390.
26. Moss, M., Albert, M.S., Butters, N., and Payne, M. (1986). Differential patterns of memory loss among patients with Alzheimer's disease, Huntington's disease and alcoholic Korsakoff's syndrome. *Arch. Neurol.* 43:239-246.
27. Squire, L.R. (1981). Two forms of human amnesia: an analysis of forgetting. *J. Neurosci.* 1:635-640.
28. Albert, M.S., Butters, N., and Levin, J. (1979). Temporal gradients in the retrograde amnesia of patients with alcoholic Korsakoff's disease. *Arch. Neurol. 36*: 211-216.
29. Cohen, N., and Squire, L.R. (1981). Retrograde amnesia and remote memory impairment. *Neuropsychologia* 19:337-356.
30. Marslen-Wilson, W.D., and Teuber, H.L. (1975). Memory for remote events in anterograde amnesia: recognition of public figures from news photographs. *Neuropsychologia* 13:347-352.
31. Seltzer, B., and Benson, D.F. (1974). The temporal pattern of retrograde amnesia in Korsakoff's disease. *Neurology* 24:527-530.
32. Scoville, W.B., and Milner, B. (1957). Loss of recent memory after bilateral hippocampal lesions. *Neuropsychologia* 20:11-21.
33. Corkin, S. (1984). Lasting consequences of bilateral medial temporal lobectomy: clinical course and experimental findings in H.M. *Semin. Neurol.* 6:249-259.
34. Ryan, C., and Butters, N. (1986). The neuropsychology of alcoholism. In *The Neuropsychology Handbook*. Edited by D. Wedding, A. Horton, and J. Webster. Springer Publishing Co., New York, pp. 376-409.
35. Albert, M.S., Butters, N., and Brandt, J. (1980). Memory for remote events in alcoholics. *J. Stud. Alcohol 41*:1071-1081.
36. Butters, N. (1984). Alcoholic Korsakoff's syndrome: an update. *Sem. Neurol.* 4:226-244.
37. Butters, N., and Cermak, L.S. (1986). A case study of the forgetting of autobiographical knowledge: implications for the study of retrograde amnesia. In *Autobiographical Memory*. Edited by D. Rubin, Cambridge University Press, New York, pp. 253-272.
38. Squire, L.R. (1982). Comparisons between forms of amnesia: some deficits are unique to Korsakoff's syndrome. *J. Exp. Psychol. [Learn. Mem. Cogn.]* 8:560-571.

39. Moscovitch, M. (1982). Multiple dissociations of function in amnesia. In *Human Memory and Amnesia*. Edited by L.S. Cermak. Lawrence Erlbaum Assoc., Hillsdale, NJ, pp. 337-370.
40. Talland, G.A. (1965). *Deranged Memory*. Academic Press, New York.
41. Cermak, L.S. (1976). The encoding capacity of a patient with amnesia due to encephalitis. *Neuropsychologia 14*:311-326.
42. Cermak, L.S., and O'Connor, M. (1983). The anterograde and retrograde retrieval ability of a patient with amnesia due to encephalitis. *Neuropsychologia 21*:213-234.
43. Beatty, W., Salmon, D., Bernstein, N., and Butters, N. (1987). Remote memory in a patient with amnesia due to hypoxia. *Psychol. Med. 17*:657-665.
44. Salmon, D.P., Lasker, B., Butters, N., and Beatty, W. (1988). Remote memory in a patient with circumscribed amnesia. *Brain Cogn. 7*:201-211.
45. Stuss, D.T., Guberman, A., Nelson, R., and Larochelle, S. (1988). The neuropsychology of paramedian thalamic infarction. *Brain Cogn. 8*:348-378.
46. Brooks, D.N., and Baddeley, A.D. (1976). What can amnesic patients learn? *Neuropsychologia 14*:111-112.
47. Cermak, L.S., Lewis, R., Butters, N., and Goodglass, H. (1973). Role of verbal mediation in performance of motor tasks by Korsakoff patients. *Percept. Motor Skills 37*:259-262.
48. Cohen, N., and Squire, L.S. (1980). Preserved learning and retention of pattern analyzing skills in amnesia: dissociation of knowing how and knowing that. *Science 210*:207-210.
49. Squire, L.R. (1982). The neuropsychology of human memory. *Annu. Rev. Neurosci. 5*:241-273.
50. Martone, M., Butters, N., Payne, M., Becker, J., and Sax, D.S. (1984). Dissociations between skill learning and verbal recognition in amnesia and dementia. *Arch. Neurol. 41*:965-970.
51. Shimamura, A. (1986). Priming effects in amnesia: evidence for a dissociable memory function. *Q. J. Exp. Psychol. [A] 38*:619-644.
52. Graf, P., Squire, L.R., and Mandler, G. (1984). The information that amnesic patients do not forget. *J. Exp. Psychol. [Learn. Mem. Cogn.] 10*:164-178.
53. Warrington, E.K., and Weiskrantz, L. (1968). New method of testing long-term retention with special reference to amnesic patients. *Nature 217*:972-974.
54. Warrington, E.K., and Weiskrantz, L. (1970). Amnesic syndrome: consolidation or retrieval? *Nature 228*:628-630.
55. Gardner, H., Boller, F., Moreines, J., and Butters, N. (1973). Retrieving information from Korsakoff patients: effects of categorical cues and reference to the task. *Cortex 9*:165-175.
56. Shimamura, A., and Squire, L.R. (1984). Paired-associate learning and priming effects in amnesia: a neuropsychological study. *J. Exp. Psychol. [Gen.] 113*: 556-570.
57. Cermak, L.S., Talbot, N., Chandler, K., and Wolbarst, L.R. (1985). The perceptual priming phenomenon in amnesia. *Neuropsychologia 23*:615-622.
58. Jacoby, L.L., and Dallas, M. (1981). On the relationship between autobiographical memory and perceptual learning. *J. Exp. Psychol. [Gen.] 3*:306-340.

59. Graf, P., and Schacter, D. (1985). Implicit and explicit memory for new associations in normal and amnesic subjects. *J. Exp. Psychol. [Learn. Mem. Cogn.]* *11*:501-518.

60. Schacter, D.L. (1987). Implicit memory: history and current status. *J. Exp. Psychol. [Learn. Mem. Cogn.]* *13*:501-518.

61. Heindel, W.C., Salmon, D.P., Shults, C.W., Walicke, P.A., and Butters, N. (1989). Neuropsychological evidence for multiple implicit memory systems: a comparison of Alzheimer's, Huntington's and Parkinson's disease patients. *J. Neurosci.* *9*:582-587.

62. Oscar-Berman, M. (1973). Hypothesis testing and focusing behavior during concept formation by amnesic Korsakoff patients. *Neuropsychologia* *11*:191-198.

63. Becker, J., Butters, N., Rivoira, P., and Miliotis, P. (1986). Asking the right questions: problem solving in male alcoholics and male alcoholics with Korsakoff's syndrome. *Alcoholism: Clin. Exp. Res.* *10*:641-646.

64. Laine, M., and Butters, N. (1982). A preliminary study of the problem solving strategies of detoxified long-term alcoholics. *Drug Alcohol Depend.* *10*:235-242.

65. Damasio, A. (1985). The frontal lobes. In *Clinical Neuropsychology*, 2nd Ed. Edited by K.M. Heilman and E. Valenstein. Oxford University Press, New York, pp. 339-402.

66. Luria, A.R. (1973). *The Working Brain*. Basic, New York.

67. Milner, B. (1964). Some effects of frontal lobectomy in man. In *The Frontal Granular Cortex and Behavior*. Edited by J.M. Warren and K. Akert. McGraw-Hill, New York, pp. 313-334.

68. Glosser, G., Butters, N., and Kaplan, E. (1977). Visuoperceptual processes in brain-damaged patients on the digit-symbol substitution test. *Int. J. Neurosci.* *7*:59-66.

69. Kapur, N., and Butters, N. (1977). Visuoperceptive deficits in long-term alcoholics with Korsakoff's psychosis. *J. Stud. Alcohol* *38*:2025-2035.

70. Nelson, H.E. (1982). *National Adult Reading Test (NART) Test Manual*. NEFR-NELSON Publishing Co., Windsor.

71. Delis, D.C., Kramer, J.H., Kaplan, E., and Ober, B.A. (1987). *California Verbal Learning Test*. Psychological Corporation, New York.

72. Kaplan, E., Goodglass, H., and Weintraub, S. (1983). *Boston Naming Test*. Lea & Febiger, Philadelphia.

73. Heaton, R.K. (1981). *Wisconsin Card Sorting Test Manual*. Psychological Assessment Resources, Inc., Odessa, FL.

74. Benton, A.L. (1973). The measurement of aphasic disorders. In *Aspectos Patologicos del Lengage*. Edited by A. Caceres Velasquez. Centro Neuropsicologico, Lima.

75. Witkin, H., Oltman, P.K., Raskin, E., and Karp, S. (1971). *A Manual for the Embedded Figures Tests*. Consulting Psychologists Press, Palo Alto.

76. Rennick, P.M. (1979). *The Color Naming and Visual Search Tests*. Axon Publishing Co., Grosse Pointe Park, MI.

77. Lishman, W.A. (1981). Cerebral disorder in alcoholism: syndromes of impairment. *Brain* *104*:1-20.

78. Cermak, L.S., and Butters, N. (1973). Information processing deficits of alcoholic Korsakoff patients. *Q. J. Stud. Alcoholism 34*:1110-1132.

79. Butters, N. (1985). Alcoholic Korsakoff's syndrome: some unresolved issues concerning etiology, neuropathology, and cognitive deficits. *J. Clin. Exp. Neuropsychol. 7*:181-210.

80. Markowitsch, H.J. (1982). Thalamic mediodorsal nucleus and memory. A critical evaluation of studies in animals and man. *Neurosci. Biobehav. Rev. 6*:351-380.

81. Markowitsch, H.J., and Pritzel, M. (1985). The neuropathology of amnesia. *Prog. Neurobiol. 25*:189-287.

82. Gamper, E. (1928). Zur frage der polioencephalitis haemorrhagic der chronischen alcoholiker. Anatomische befunde beim alkoholischen Korsakov undihre Beziehungen zum klinischen bild. *Dtsch. Z. Nervenheilk. 102*:122-129.

83. Riggs, H., and Boles, H.S. (1944). Wernicke's disease: a clinical and pathological study of 42 cases. *Q. J. Stud. Alcohol 5*:361-370.

84. Delay, J., Brion, S., and Elissalde, B. (1958). Corps mamillaires et syndrome Korsakoff. Etude anatomique de huit cas de syndrome de Korsakoff d'origine alcoolique sans alterations significative du cortex cerebral. I. Etude anatomo-clinique. *Presse. Med. 66*:1849-1852.

85. Delay, J., Brion, S., and Elissalde, B. (1958). Corps mamillaires et syndrome Korsakoff. Etude anatomique de huit cas de syndrome de Korsakoff d'origine alcoolique sans alterations significative du cortex cerebral. II. Tubercules mammillaires et mecanisme de le memoire. *Presse. Med. 66*:1965-1968.

86. Adams, R.D., Collins, G.H., and Victor (1962). Troubles de la memoire et de l'apprentissage chez l'homme; leurs relations avec des lesions des lobes temporaux et du diencephale. In *Physiologie de l'Hippocampe*. Centre National de la Recherche Scientifique, Paris.

87. Harper, C. (1979). Wernicke's encephalopathy: a more common disease than realized. *J. Neurol. Neurosurg. Psychiatry. 42*:226-231.

88. Harper, C. (1983). The incidence of Wernicke's encephalopathy in Australia—a neuropathological study of 131 cases. *J. Neurol. Neurosurg. Psychiatry 46*:593-598.

89. Arendt, T., Bigl, V., Arendt, A., and Tennstedt, A. (1983). Loss of neurons in the nucleus basalis of Meynert in Alzheimer's disease, paralysis agitans and Korsakoff's disease. *Acta Neuropathol. 61*:101-108.

90. McEntee, W.J., and Mair, R.G. (1978). Memory impairments in Korsakoff's psychosis: a correlation with brain noradrenergic activity. *Science 202*:905-907.

91. McEntee, W.J., and Mair, R.G. (1980). Memory enhancement in Korsakoff's psychosis by clonidine: further evidence for a noradrenergic deficit. *Ann. Neurol. 7*:466-470.

92. Mair, R.G., and McEntee, W.J. (1986). Cognitive enhancement in Korsakoff's psychosis by clonidine: a comparison with L-dopa and ephedrine. *Psychopharmacology 88*:374-380.

93. Shimamura, A., Jernigan, T., and Squire, L.R. (1988). Korsakoff's syndrome: radiological (CT) findings and neuropsychological correlates. *J. Neurosci. 8*: 4400-4410.

94. Dreyfus, P.M. (1974). Diseases of the nervous system in chronic alcoholics. In *The Biology of Alcoholism: Clinical Pathology.* Vol. 3. Edited by B. Kissin and H. Begleiter. Plenum Press, New York.

95. Mesulam, M.-M., Van Hoesen, G., and Butters, N. (1977). Clinical manifestations of chronic thiamine deficiency in the rhesus monkey. *Neurology (Minneap.)* 27:239-245.

96. Witt, E.D., and Goldman-Rakic, P.S. (1983). Intermittent thiamine deficiency in the rhesus monkey I. Progression of neurological signs and neuroanatomical lesions. *Ann. Neurol. 13*:376-395.

97. Witt, E.D., and Goldman-Rakic, P.S. (1983). Intermittent thiamine deficiency in the Rhesus monkey II. Evidence for memory loss. *Ann. Neurol. 13*:396-401.

98. Freund, G. (1973). Chronic central nervous system toxicity of alcohol. *Annu. Rev. Pharmacol. 13*:217-227.

99. Ryback, R. (1971). The continuum and specificity of the effects of alcohol on memory: a review. *Q. J. Stud. Alcohol 32*:995-1016.

100. Becker, J., Butters, N., Hermann, A., and D'Angelo, N. (1983). Learning to associate names and faces: Impaired acquisition on an ecologically relevant memory task by male alcoholics. *J. Nerv. Ment. Dis. 171*:617-623.

101. Brandt, J., Butters, N., Ryan, C., and Bayog, R. (1983). Cognitive loss and recovery in long-term alcohol abusers. *Arch. Gen. Psychiatry 40*:435-442.

102. Parsons, O.A., and Prigatano, G.P. (1977). Memory functioning in alcoholics. In *Alcohol and Human Memory.* Edited by M. Birnham and E.S. Parker. Lawrence Erlbaum, Hillsdale, NJ, pp. 185-194.

103. Ryan, C., and Butters, N. (1983). Cognitive deficits in alcoholics. In *The Biology of Alcoholism*, Vol. 7, *The Pathogenesis of Alcoholism: Biological Factors.* Edited by B. Kissin and H. Begleiter. Plenum Press, New York, pp. 485-538.

104. Salmon, D., and Butters, N. (1987). The etiology and neuropathology of alcoholic Korsakoff's syndrome: some evidence for the role of the basal forebrain. In *Recent Developments in Alcoholism 5.* Edited by M. Galanter. Plenum Press, New York, pp. 27-58.

105. Bergman, H. (1987). Brain dysfunction related to alcoholism: some results from the KARTAD project. In *Neuropsychology of Alcoholism: Implications for Diagnosis and Treatment.* Edited by O. Parsons, N. Butters, and P. Nathan. Guilford Press, New York, pp. 21-44.

106. Jacobson, R., and Lishman, W.A. (1987). Selective memory loss and global intellectual deficits in alcoholic Korsakoff's syndrome. *Psychol. Med. 17*:649-655.

107. Ron, M. (1987). The brain of alcoholics: an overview. In *Neuropsychology of Alcoholism: Implications for Diagnosis and Treatment.* Edited by O. Parsons, N. Butters, and P. Nathan. Guilford Press, New York, pp. 11-20.

108. Wilkinson, D.A. (1987). CT scan and neuropsychological assessments of alcoholism. In *Neuropsychology of Alcoholism: Implications for Diagnosis and Treatment.* Edited by O. Parsons, N. Butters, and P. Nathan. Guilford Press, New York, pp. 76-102.

12

Memory Disorders After Closed Head Injury

Felicia C. Goldstein
Emory University
Atlanta, Georgia

Harvey S. Levin
The University of Texas Medical Branch
Galveston, Texas

Memory disturbance is one of the most frequent and disabling consequences of closed head injury (CHI), persisting for varying durations depending on the severity of acute cerebral insult. More than half the survivors of severe CHI (i.e., injury producing coma persisting at least until hospital admission) manifest a chronic deficit in learning and retrieving new information as reflected by neuropsychological tests and reports by the patients and their families (1-5). Posttraumatic memory deficit, along with information processing speed, is the best predictor of return to gainful employment (6) following severe CHI. Moreover, Stuss and co-workers (7) observed that CHI patients who had an apparently good recovery without obvious neurologic or cognitive deficits demonstrated problems in delayed recall of material when tested at least five months postinjury. Mild head injury (i.e., momentary or no loss of consciousness, absence of focal neurologic deficits, and no intracranial lesions) is also notable for producing memory difficulties particularly during the first month (8,9).

In this chapter, we characterize the aspects of memory typically affected in survivors of CHI. The relationship of neurologic indices to outcome and the types of impairments seen in the acute and long-term stages of recovery will be addressed. Finally, evidence for preserved memory and the potential of utilizing intact abilities to restore adaptive functioning will be examined. Our review covers memory disorders in adults. For a survey of such problems in children and adolescents, the reader is referred to articles by Gaidolfi and Vignolo (10) and Levin et al. (11,12).

SEVERITY INDICES RELATED TO
OUTCOME OF MEMORY PERFORMANCE

Investigators have utilized a variety of indices of severity of head injury to examine the effects on memory functioning. The presence and localization of hemispheric lesion, degree and duration of impaired consciousness, the integrity of ocular responses, and length of posttraumatic amnesia (PTA) have been analyzed in different studies. As Dikmen and co-workers (13) note, while it is clear from the research literature that more severe injuries are associated with more devastating and persistent deficits, less is known about the relationships among acute neurologic variables and how their contributions to memory disorder change over time.

Mild CHI is characterized by brief or no loss of consciousness, an initial Glasgow Coma Scale (14) score in the 13-15 range (implying the ability to obey commands), no focal neurologic deficits, and the absence of mass lesions or complications requiring neurosurgery. The postconcussional syndrome (PCS) encompasses a variety of somatic, affective, and cognitive symptoms such as headaches, depression, and concentration/memory disturbances. PCS can occur in the absence of direct insult to the head as in a whiplash injury (15). Studies have also noted that mild CHI is more frequently associated with traumatic spinal cord damage than previously realized (16,17). In a three-center study of outcome, Levin and colleagues (8) found that 85% of mild head injured patients performed below the mean control value on a test of verbal memory requiring learning and retention of words over 12 trials (18). Consistent with the impression of Figure 1, the performance of patients at one week postinjury across all three centers was impaired relative to controls. By one and three months, however, patients performed within control values, suggesting that verbal memory had recovered. The investigators concluded that a single mild head injury in the absence of premorbid complications (e.g., neuropsychiatric disturbance, substance abuse) is unlikely to produce deficits that persist over three months. Patients with previous injuries, however, may not recover at the same rate given the evidence for cumulative effects of repeated mild head injuries on outcome (19).

The prominence of memory deficit after CHI, occurring across the spectrum of severity, undoubtedly reflects the vulnerability of the temporal lobes to focal hematomas and contusions. Consistent with neuropathologic studies of fatal CHI (20), the preponderance of brain lesions revealed by magnetic resonance imaging (MRI) are situated in the frontotemporal region (21-24). In a study of 20 patients with mild and moderate head injuries (24), MRI detected lesions in 17 cases that were undisclosed by computed tomography (CT),

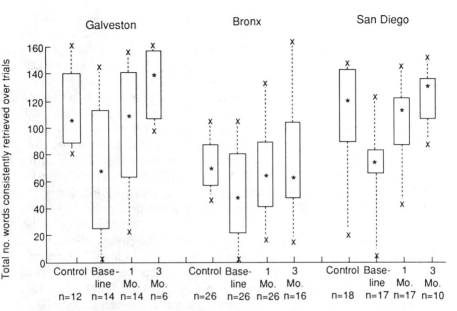

Figure 1 Box plots showing the distribution of verbal memory retrieval for control and CHI patients studied in Galveston, the Bronx, and San Diego. Each asterisk denotes the median, whereas the upper and lower horizontal lines of each bar indicate the 75th and 25th percentile scores, respectively. Maximum and minimum scores are depicted by an "x." Scores for CHI patients are presented at baseline (1 week postinjury) and at 1 and 3 months after injury. N = number of controls and patients. Adapted from Ref. 8, reprinted with permission of publisher.

and the majority of these lesions were located in the frontal and temporal lobes. Improvement in performance on tests measuring divergent thinking, problem solving, and memory was correlated with decreased lesion size on follow-up testing. Apart from focal lesions, cerebral ventricular enlargement is also related to impairments in memory functioning (25,26). Langfitt and co-workers (27) reported that areas of cerebral dysfunction not seen by CT or MRI could be characterized by positron emission tomography (PET). The investigators observed decreased metabolism in the bilateral anterior temporal lobes in three patients. The use of such technology may allow for a better understanding of links between neuroanatomic-neuropsychological features in CHI patients.

Other clinical indices, including the degree and duration of impaired consciousness, have been found to predict the presence of memory deficit (13, 28-32). The Glasgow Coma Scale (GCS) (14) score is an index of the depth of impaired consciousness as reflected by eye opening (none to spontaneous), motor response (none to obeying commands), and verbal response (none to oriented). As a general rule, acute GCS scores of less than 8 (indicating coma) are prognostic of residual memory deficits. In a series of consecutive admissions for CHI to the neurosurgery service in Verona, Alexandre and co-workers (28) reported that only 4% of patients with initial GCS scores within the 3-4 range (i.e., the lowest ratings possible) had relatively normal cognitive and memory functioning two years postinjury in contrast to 84% of patients with GCS scores of 8 or greater. The investigators found that the best GCS scores obtained within 24 hours of injury were also predictive of outcome. Only three percent of patients in the 3-4 range were relatively spared of cognitive problems versus 80% of patients with GCS scores of 8-15. Consistent with the results of the Italian study, Dikmen et al. (13) noted an ordering of the degree of memory impairment at one month as a function of the GCS scores documented within 24 hours of injury. Patients with GCS scores of 8 or less were most impaired on a test of verbal learning and memory followed next by improved functioning of patients with scores of 9-11 and 12 or greater. In addition to the initial and 24 hour GCS score, duration of the inability to follow commands is related to memory outcome (13,31). Vilkki et al. (31) recently reported that patients with coma persisting for greater than six hours were more impaired on delayed recall measures of verbal and visual memory than patients with coma durations less than six hours. Differences between the groups were not attributable to generalized cognitive disturbances (e.g., performance on a test of intellectual functioning). Dikmen and colleagues (13) found that coma durations of greater than one day were related to persisting memory deficits one year postinjury.

The presence of nonreactive pupils and oculomotor abnormalities, which are indicative of brainstem dysfunction, are similarly predictive of residual memory and intellectual deficits (28-30). Table 1 shows the relationship between measures of ocular functioning and memmory performance in patients with: (1) impaired memory but preserved intellectual outcome; (2) normal memory and intellectual outcome; or (3) deficient memory and intellectual outcome (i.e., globally impaired). At 5 to 15 months after injury, the presence of nonreactive pupils and abnormal oculocephalic/oculovestibular responses characterized patients with generalized memory/intellectual disturbances as compared to recovered patients. At 15 to 42 months, nonreactive pupils on admission were again associated with a persisting memory disturbance (regardless of whether intellectual functioning was preserved). Levin and colleagues (30) also found that severely injured CHI patients with acute oculovestibular deficits obtained lower memory and IQ scores than those without such impairments. Alexandre et al. (28) noted that of 58 patients with impaired oculomotor responses, only five were spared from a significant degree of cognitive disturbance. Similar to the GCS score obtained with 24 h, oculomotor function served as the strongest predictor of eventual outcome.

Table 1   Neurologic Indices of Injury in Memory Impaired Versus
Unimpaired Head Injured Patients[a]

	Pupillary reactivity		Oculocephalic/oculovestibular Response	
	Normal	Abnormal	Normal	Abnormal
5-15 Months Postinjury				
Memory impaired (n = 9)	5	4	6	3
Memory unimpaired (n = 34)	30	4[a]	29	5[b]
Globally impaired (n = 22)	11	11[a]	11	11[b]
> 15-42 Months Postinjury				
Memory impaired (n = 8)	3	5[c]	5	3
Memory unimpaired (n = 21)	18	3[c,d]	17	4
Globally impaired (n = 13)	5	8[d]	6	7

[a]A common superscript letter denotes a significant difference between groups of 0.05 or less.
Source: Adapted From Ref. 29, reprinted with permission of the publisher.

The length of PTA (i.e., the period of confusion and lack of consolidation of ongoing events immediately after injury) has been examined in relation to memory performance (6,13,32). In general, PTA durations of two or more weeks are predictive of residual cognitive deficits (6,13). Gronwall and Wrightson (32) isolated a specific memory impairment involving difficulty in storing information which was related to the duration of PTA. The inconsistent findings regarding lower ranges of PTA duration as prognostic indicators may reflect difficulties in measuring this amnesic period (e.g., retrospective patient reports) or variability in the types of memory functions that are examined (storage versus retrieval).

To summarize, research has identified severity variables predictive of memory outcome. The GCS score (particularly within 24 hours) and integrity of ocular responses are strongly related to residual memory performance, with patients sustaining the most severe acute injuries exhibiting long-lasting deficits. Longitudinal research examining the interactions among numerous early indices will enhance the ability to predict outcome and to plan early rehabilitation interventions.

ASPECTS OF MEMORY FUNCTIONING FOLLOWING CLOSED HEAD INJURY

Amnesia is a salient aspect of both the acute and chronic stages of recovery from CHI (Fig. 2). The amnesic disorder in the early period is characterized by difficulty in remembering events prior (retrograde amnesia) and immediately subsequent (posttraumatic amnesia) to the injury, whereas an enduring

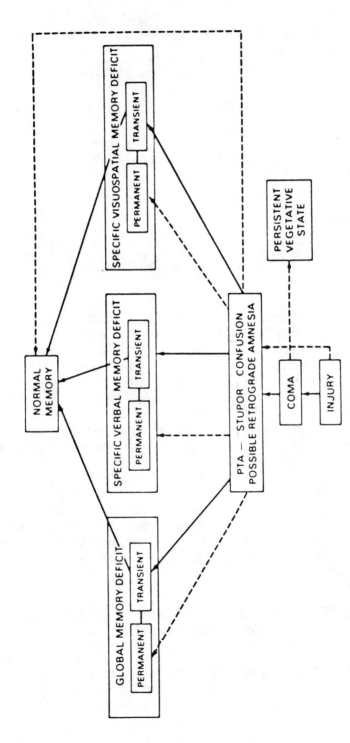

Figure 2   Residual memory functioning following closed head injury. From Ref. 2, reprinted with permission of publisher.

anterograde amnesia frequently persists after the clearing of gross confusion and disorientation. As seen in Figure 2, the memory disorder may be global (encompassing both verbal and visual information) or specific for one type of material. Furthermore, a subset of patients (e.g., cases of mild to moderate trauma) may exhibit a transient as opposed to a more permanent deficit.

Memory disturbances after CHI are distinct from etiologies such as Alzheimer's disease in their abrupt versus insidious onset, the stable or gradual improvement (although not necessarily to premorbid levels) versus progressive deterioration, and severity dependent upon the impairment of consciousness (mild, moderate, severe) versus the stage of illness (early, middle, late). The term "amnesia" should also be distinguished from the amnesic disorder resulting from such conditions as Korsakoff's syndrome in which memory is disproportionately impaired relative to preserved intellectual functioning (33). While approximately one-fourth of the survivors of head injury demonstrate a relatively isolated memory impairment, there are patients with neuropsychological disturbances (e.g., intellectual deficit) that coexist with their memory problems (29).

ACUTE MANIFESTATIONS OF MEMORY IMPAIRMENT

POSTTRAUMATIC AMNESIA

Posttraumatic amnesia, a common manifestation during the acute stages of recovery, refers to difficulty in the acquisition and retrieval of new information, that is, a failure to commit to memory an ongoing, continuous record of daily activities (2,34-36). This memory deficit is frequently accompanied by disorientation, agitated and disinhibited behavior, confabulation, and lack of sustained and focused attention. Early concepts emphasized the total duration of disturbed consciousness and included the period during which the patient was in coma (37). More recent definitions of PTA have stressed defective storage of information about ongoing events (36) distinct from coma. Although the duration of PTA is generally related to the interval of unconsciousness, it is prolonged in approximately 10-15% of patients sustaining mild or moderate CHI (i.e., brief or no loss of consciousness) (38). Cases of severe CHI may also show a disparity between the length of coma and duration of PTA (39).

Assessment of PTA has included both retrospective and prospective measures. Interviewing recovered patients to estimate when they first experienced continuous memory for events (e.g., 35) may be inaccurate because of the inherent difficulty in recalling material from a period when memory was impaired. Gronwall and Wrightson (40) found that approximately 25% of survivors of mild head injury changed their initial estimates made in the first hours when interviewed up to three months later. The investigators proposed that patients may have difficulty separating their own recollections from reports of others regarding their amnesic period.

Prospective techniques entail following the recovery of continuous memory during the acute stages. The Galveston Orientation and Amnesia Test (GOAT) (41) involves serial measurement of orientation to person, place, and time as well as memory for events before and after injury. Davidoff and colleagues (42) demonstrated the sensitivity of the GOAT in detecting PTA in patients with spinal cord injuries. Whereas PTA was noted in the medical records for seven out of 34 patients, administration of the GOAT increased the estimate to 15, thus detecting cases of occult CHI missed by clinical impression alone. Alternative measures to the GOAT have assessed new learning (43,44). The Westmead PTA scale (44), in addition to asking questions concerning orientation, requires that the patient remember three objects and the examiner's face and name over three days.

Recovery of orientation during PTA was recently examined by High and colleagues (45). Eighty-four CHI survivors of mild, moderate, and severe CHI were administered serial GOATs during their acute hospitalization. As shown in Figure 3, orientation recovered in the order of person, place, and time in the majority (70%) of patients. Moreover, estimates of the date were

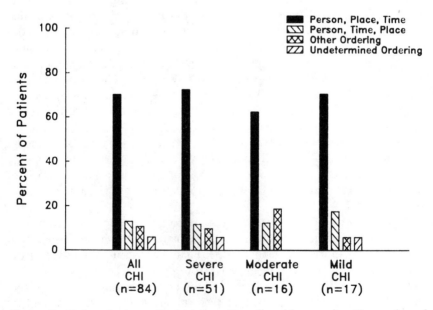

Figure 3 Order of return of orientation: Overall and by severity. N = number of patients. From Ref. 45.

displaced backward in time (up to five years for severe injuries), and the discrepancy between the estimates and the actual date became smaller as orientation improved. "Shrinkage" was observed for moderate and severe but not mild head injuries. High and colleagues proposed that orientation to person is least disrupted because it represents older and more rehearsed material. Additionally, orientation to place may recover earlier than time because the former information remains constant. Finally, backward displacement of time may shrink in parallel with the resolution of loss of information for events preceding the injury. These features are similar to recovery of orientation in patients undergoing electroconvulsive (ECT) therapy. Daniel et al. (46) observed that orientation following ECT returned predominantly in the order of person, place, and time and that shrinkage occurred in the temporal estimates.

Accelerated forgetting has also been found to characterize memory disturbance during PTA. Levin and colleagues (47) administered a recognition memory test to patients in or out of PTA and subjects without head injuries. The groups were equated for initial learning ability by varying the exposure duration (longest for PTA patients) of to-be-remembered stimuli. Retention was measured at 10 minutes, 2 hours, and 32-hour intervals. Patients in PTA evidenced more rapid forgetting over the 32-hour period than the other groups. This accelerated forgetting appeared to be unrelated to the types and areas of mass lesions detected on CT.

Finally, there is evidence that patients in PTA exhibit new learning and retention of skills that carry over when PTA resolves. Neuropsychologists have distinguished two types of memory. Procedural memory refers to retention of skills and procedures and is not dependent on remembering specific conditions or facts. In contrast, declarative memory must be stated or explicitly rehearsed following learning such as recalling words or recognizing pictures and is highly dependent on strategies including elaboration and organization (48-50). Investigations of amnesics performing maze learning (51) and mirror reading (52) indicate improvement in performance (e.g., decreased reaction times) over sessions despite an inability to remember being tested or the stimulus materials. Ewert et al. (53) examined procedural memory for skills (i.e., reading words presented as mirror images, maze learning, and keeping a stylus on a moving target) while CHI patients were in PTA and on a follow-up session after PTA ended. Despite their inability to remember the examiner, previous testing, or the words on the mirror-reading task, the patients showed improved learning over sessions and retention of skills when PTA resolved. Extrapolating from these findings would support the feasibility of teaching physical or occupational therapy skills during PTA.

RETROGRADE AMNESIA

In addition to problems in registering new information, patients often exhibit a memory disturbance for events preceding the injury. This retrograde amnesia (RA) shares features similar to what is observed during PTA. First, patients may demonstrate "islands of memory," that is, memory for isolated events during an otherwise amnesic period (54). Second, RA may shrink from a loss of memory that extends far back in time to a shorter period up to a few seconds or minutes before the injury (54,55), a phenomenon analogous to shrinkage of temporal disorientation. Difficulty in remembering events concerning the injury may reflect a lack of consolidation of this material at the time of impact.

Attempts have been made to establish a relationship between the relative durations of PTA and RA. In one study of CHI patients in whom RA and PTA were assessed retrospectively, Russel and Nathan (54) found that longer PTA durations coincided with longer periods of RA. Patients without reported PTA denied a period of RA, whereas patients with PTA greater than seven days reported RA for events preceding the injury. Recently, Crovitz and colleagues (56,57) developed regression equations to predict the length of RA. College students were administered questionnaires to identify individuals who had previously sustained a head injury resulting in loss of consciousness. The investigators found that RA was more common with PTA of longer duration, and was more likely to be reported the closer in time patients were to their injuries, suggesting a forgetting factor as time elapsed.

Research assessing the nature and extent of retrograde memory loss has examined a temporal gradient to the amnesia and the vulnerability of recent versus more remote memories. According to Ribot's "law of regression," older memories are less susceptible to disruption due to their repetition and organization than more recently acquired memories (58). Consequently, memories acquired long before onset of amnesia should be better preserved than those closer in time to the disease process. Numerous studies in populations including Korsakoff patients and those undergoing ECT have utilized questionnaires to test memory from various time periods of the patient's life such as names of television shows or public events (59-62). Levin et al. (63) applied this procedure with CHI patients to examine the extent of RA and whether older memories are better preserved. A questionnaire sampling names of television programs from five time periods was given to patients during and after PTA and neurologically intact controls. As shown in Figure 4, although the RA of patients was more extensive than that of controls, there was no compelling evidence for relative preservation of older versus recent memories. Levin et al. proposed that the failure to find support for Ribot's hypothesis in head-injured patients might reflect the abrupt onset of the memory disorder. In contrast, insidious conditions such as Korsakoff's syndrome might produce a more pronounced deficit for recent material since this information would have been acquired during a period when overall memory functioning was generally degraded.

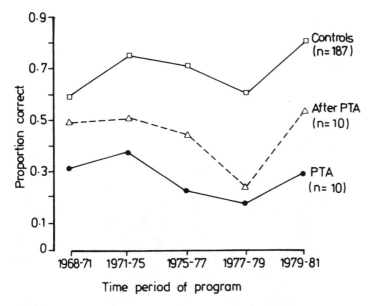

Figure 4 Mean proportion of correctly recognized television program titles across time periods of broadcast for oriented (after PTA) and amnesic (PTA) CHI patients and controls. From Ref. 63, reprinted with permission of publisher.

After the relative clearing of PTA and RA, many survivors are left with a persistent inability to register and/or retrieve material, a finding characteristic of conditions including dementia, epilepsy, and alcoholic Korsakoff's syndrome. Studies have indicated that memory is often affected along a number of dimensions involving the ability to retain information over time, to remember material as a function of whether it emphasizes visual or verbal relations, and to take advantage of features present at both encoding and retrieval (e.g., semantic relations). In the following sections, we review the aspects of memory that are frequently affected.

CHRONIC MANIFESTATIONS OF MEMORY IMPAIRMENT

IMMEDIATE VERSUS DELAYED RECALL

A consistent finding in survivors of CHI is a dissociation between relatively preserved immediate recall versus deficient recall of the same material following a delay period (7,13,64-67). This trend is similar to the performance of amnesic populations (e.g., Korsakoff patients) who exhibit intact retrieval over a short period of time with deficits present after an elapsed interval (68). Tests of digit span (e.g., WAIS-R; 69) are sensitive to the presence of a dissociation. Brooks (64) found that CHI patients were comparable to controls in their recall of digits in a forward order (e.g., immediately repeating the sequence 3-7-9 after presentation) but not when patients had to reverse the sequence before recall (e.g., examiner presents 3-7-9 and patient recalls 9-7-3). We recently examined a 31-year-old patient 10 years after injury who sustained a severe CHI in a motor vehicle accident and was unable to obey motor commands until seven weeks. Although the patient performed within normal limits (7 ± 2) on forward span, he was unable to consistently recall more than three digits backward (expected = four to five). Apart from digit recall, investigators (13,66,70) have also reported clear differences between patients and controls in delayed but not immediate conditions of prose recall, paired associate learning, and memory for individual words or pictures.

One explanation for disparities between immediate and delayed recall entails the distinction between short-term (STM) versus long-term (LTM) memory stores. STM is assumed to be capacity-limited and to hold information for a brief interval (i.e., 30 seconds) whereas LTM is able to hold large amounts of information for extended periods. According to this distinction, patients can retain information for less than a minute but have difficulty in delayed recall either because information has not transferred into LTM or it is difficult to retrieve. However, psychologists have recently embraced a more dynamic view that stresses interactions among numerous subsystems (e.g., working memory; 71) and the importance of how information is processed rather than the quantitative single store models of memory.

The finding of deficient delayed recall may also reflect the heightened susceptibility of memory to interference. Stuss and co-workers (7) reported that the Brown-Peterson task (72,73) had the most discriminating power between CHI patients with "good" recoveries (e.g., back to work, no obvious neurologic deficits) and normal controls. In this procedure, patients recall three consonants after varying delays filled with interference such as counting backward. Stuss and colleagues (7) attributed the poor performance by their patients to difficulty in maintaining consistent directed attention when confronted with interference, and they proposed that performance might reflect underlying damage to the frontal-limbic reticular-activating system.

Finally, it is possible that CHI patients forget disproportionately more material than neurologically intact individuals during the delay period between learning and recall (64,67). Levin et al. (47) reported that rapid forgetting of pictures tended to occur in patients out of PTA who had temporal lobe lesions (although inconsistencies were noted). Rapid forgetting may be attributable to temporal lobe pathology, a premise that could be substantiated by investigating forgetting over extended intervals and neuroimaging techniques such as MRI.

MATERIAL-SPECIFIC VERSUS
GLOBAL MEMORY IMPAIRMENTS

In addition to impairments in remembering information over time, patients may exhibit material specific deficits (i.e., isolated problems in remembering verbal or visual information) or more generalized disturbances extending across numerous modalities. Studies of patients undergoing temporal lobectomies for the treatment of epilepsy have implicated the role of the language dominant temporal lobe for processing verbal material and the right nondominant temporal lobe for visuospatial information (74-76). While dissociations in memory performance have been noted in head-injured patients as a function of type of material, a clear link between side/site of lesion and functioning is less compelling, perhaps reflecting limitations in neuroimaging techniques or the diffuseness of injuries.

In a study examining the prevalence of generalized impairments in both verbal and visual memory versus a material-specific deficit, we characterized recovery at less than five months postinjury and again at 6 to 15 months in survivors or moderate to severe CHI (77). Patients were administered the Selective Reminding Memory Test (18), a 12 word, 12 trial list learning procedure in which the patient is reminded only of words not recalled on a previous trial. Visual memory was evaluated using Continuous Recognition Memory (78) requiring identification of drawings as old (previously seen) or new (never encountered). Based upon normal control group data, performance was defined as intact, globally impaired (both verbal and visual deficits), or specifically impaired for one type of material. Of 51 patients examined initially, 12 were not impaired, whereas 39 patients exhibited some form of memory deficit (19 with a global deficit, 20 with a specific impairment). As seen in Table 2, patients with global memory impairments had significantly longer durations of impaired consciousness and lower acute GCS scores than those who demonstrated performance within preserved limits. Patients with a specific memory deficit were intermediate between these two groups. Furthermore, the presence of nonreactive pupils or abnormal oculocephalic/oculovestibular responses on hospital admission was related to a residual, generalized memory impairment.

Follow-up data on 29 patients between 6 to 15 months were obtained for patients who exhibited some form of memory disturbance at the earlier occasion. Eight of these patients were now performing within normal limits, whereas over two-thirds continued to exhibit deficits (11 with a global deficit, 10 with a specific impairment). Acute nonreactive pupils and oculocephalic/oculovestibular disturbances were again associated with the continued presence of memory impairment. No patient in the recovered memory group had an acute deficit. Although bilateral mass lesions were more commonly associated with a global memory deficit, diffuse injuries (e.g., absence of mass lesions) were also noted in all the groups.

Table 2 Type of Memory Deficit as a Function of Neurologic Indices[a]

	Duration of impaired consciousness	Lowest GCS score	Pupillary reactivity Normal	Abnormal	Oculovestibular responses Normal	Abnormal
<5 Months Postinjury						
Not impaired (n=12)	Median = .125 days[a] Range = 0-16	Median = 11.0[c] Range = 7-15	11	1[d]	11	1[f]
Specific deficit (n=20)	Median = 1.0 days[b] Range = 0-24	Median = 7.5 Range = 3-15	19	1[e]	17	3[g]
Global deficit (n=19)	Median = 5.0 days[a,b] Range = 0-56	Median = 7.0[c] Range = 4-15	10	9[d,e]	10	9[f,g]
6-15 Months Postinjury						
Not impaired (n=8)	Median = 2.0 days[h] Range = 0-15	Median = 7.0[j] Range = 3-14	8	0[l,m]	8	0[n,o]
Specific deficit (n=10)	Median = 5.0 days[i] Range = 0-26	Median = 7.0[k] Range = 5-15	6	4[l]	5	5[n]
Global deficit (n=11)	Median = 10.0 days[h,i] Range 0-24	Median = 5.0[j,k] Range = 4-15	7	4[m]	7	4[o]

[a]A common superscript letter denotes a significant difference or a trend approaching significance of 0.08 or less.
Source: From Ref. 77.

Tabbador and colleagues (79) examined differential recovery of various components of cognitive functioning following CHI. The researchers found that nonverbal recall (reproductive memory for pictures after an exposure of 10 seconds) improved from baseline to six months, but there was no additional recovery at one year in patients with moderate and severe CHI. In contrast, verbal recall and recognition showed improvement. The long-term prediction of early versus later recovery of memory for specific types of material could be useful for directing remediation efforts (80).

CHARACTERISTICS OF ENCODING AND RETRIEVAL

One difference that has been hypothesized to distinguish normal memory from amnesia concerns the relative intactness of processes requiring automatic and effortful encoding. According to Hasher and Zacks (81,82), certain features of to-be-learned material are processed without active strategies, intention, or draining of attentional resources. These "automatic" processes include encoding of frequency information (the number of times events occur), temporal location (the order in which events occur), and spatial location (the relative position of events). On the other hand, "effortful" processes (e.g., remembering specific words or pictures) require deliberate strategies involving organization and rehearsal. Hasher and Zacks argue that the act of remembering depends not only on registering the target material (an effortful process), but also encoding automatically acquired information concerning frequency, temporal, and spatial qualities. For example, while being introduced to someone, we not only encode the name but also register features such as the frequency of the name in the English language. The results of automatic encoding may then be used to aid future recall as in trying to remember the name by cuing oneself to whether it was common or uncommon (81,82).

Studies have examined if certain memory impaired groups show a deficit in automatic processing. Automatic processing of frequency information appears to be preserved in patients with depression or Parkinson's disease despite impairments in recall of material (effortful processing) relative to controls (81,83-85). This finding suggests that deficits become apparent when tasks require the use of strategies and directed attention. On the other hand, patients with Alzheimer's disease and Korsakoff syndrome have difficulty on both automatic and effortful tasks, implicating a more functional disturbance extending beyond the use of active mnemonic skills and poor attentional capacity (86,87).

Recently, we examined the relative preservation of automatic versus effortful encoding following severe closed head injury (88). Survivors of CHI at least one year postinjury who were enrolled in rehabilitation and neurologically intact controls were administered tasks emphasizing effortful (word recall) and automatic (frequency judgment) processes. There were significant differences between the groups on the recall task. Out of 50 possible words (10 unique words for each of five trials), controls recalled an average of 32 words (range = 19-39) versus 23 words (range = 17-30) for patients. We also observed impairments on the automatic processing task. Subjects were asked to estimate the number of times they heard words presented at frequencies zero (never heard), two, four, and six times. Figure 5 depicts the estimates as a function of actual frequency presentation. The slope was greater for controls, indicating that they were more sensitive than patients to frequency changes. Impaired automatic processing in survivors of severe CHI may underlie their memory disturbance. Hirst (89) has suggested that amnesics have a deficit in automatic encoding such that ordinarily effortless activities now require increased effort. As a result, there is less capacity available for registering the to-be-learned material. The head-injured patient may be required to divide attention between two types of information in an already impaired attentional system, thus resulting in overall poorer memory performance.

Along with deficits in automatic encoding, intrusion of extraneous material may characterize retrieval processes following CHI. Levin and Goldstein (90) reported a tendency of survivors of severe CHI to make more extralist intrusions in verbal free recall than controls. It has also been found that patients make an excessive number of false alarms (i.e., reporting a stimulus shown

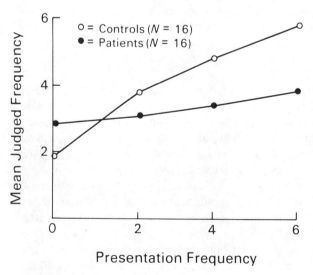

Figure 5   Mean judged frequency as a function of presentation frequency for CHI patients and controls. From Ref. 88, reprinted with permission of publisher.

for the first time as previously encountered) on a visual recognition memory procedure (78,91). This tendency of a subset of CHI patients to report irrelevant material may reflect deficient separation of various memory systems and difficulty in screening information. The phenomenon may also signify a tendency of patients to be less cautious in responding than individuals with intact memory.

Finally, we have found that survivors of severe CHI utilize inactive retrieval strategies (90). Twelve severely injured patients enrolled in rehabilitation and 10 controls were asked to learn unrelated words, words that belonged to categories (e.g., fruits, animals) but were unclustered at input, and words that belonged to categories but were presented in a grouped fashion (all animals, all fruits, etc.). Although patients, similar to controls, showed a benefit in remembering semantically related words, they failed to take advantage of the conceptual relations in structuring their recall. Control subjects sequentially recalled items belonging to the same semantic category whereas this feature was unimpressive in patients. Moreover, all the controls consistently accessed words from the three categories in contrast to only nine patients who were employing all the categories on the final recall trial. Analysis of qualitative features of recall may be useful to further characterize memory performance following head injury.

EVIDENCE FOR PRESERVED LEARNING AND MEMORY

Although much of this chapter has described features of memory that are disrupted in survivors, there is evidence suggesting that amnesic patients are capable of learning and retaining skills that could potentially be adapted for job-related tasks. The work of Schacter and Glisky (92-94) on teaching domain-specific knowledge (i.e., knowledge relevant to a particular task) has demonstrated that memory-disordered patients, including those with head injuries, can acquire the vocabulary and techniques necessary to operate a computer. These investigators have employed the "method of vanishing cues" to help patients learn technical jargon. In this technique, a specific computer term (e.g., SAVE) is initially paired with a definition, and the number of target letters are gradually increased (e.g., S---; SA--; SAV-) until patients can identify the correct vocabulary term. On subsequent trials, fewer letters are provided until ultimately the definition itself elicits the correct term. Schacter and Glisky (92) compared this training technique with a simple rote rehearsal procedure that simply presented the terms and the definitions in a repeated fashion. Relative to a group that received rote rehearsal, patients in the vanishing cue condition demonstrated greater retention of the target terms after a six-week interval.

In a second phase of training, Schacter and Glisky examined the ability of patients to utilize their knowledge to interact with a computer, that is, to learn basic operating terms and to write simple programs. Training consisted of graded steps involving the acquisition of relevant vocabulary and implementation of these terms on the computer. Again, patients with severe memory deficits were able to effectively interact with the computer.

As Schacter and Glisky note (92), the teaching of domain-specific knowledge could be employed in a number of relevant areas including management of household duties and specific job-related tasks. Although much of their research has been conducted in the laboratory, a recent report by these investigators (94) indicates that an amnesic patient has been trained to learn the skills of a data-entry job and is now actively employed. These preliminary results are encouraging in terms of the potential for restoring adaptive functions in CHI patients.

Coupled with the acquisition of new vocabulary terms and skills, there is also evidence that head-injured patients show a relative preservation of the ability to access and recognize semantic relations and to use these relationships to guide their learning and recall (95,96). We have conducted research indicating that survivors of severe CHI who are enrolled in rehabiliation spontaneously encode the semantic features of words (e.g., category membership), remember more words that belong to categories than unrelated words, and exhibit improved retention when they are required to encode the conceptual as opposed to the physical or acoustic qualities of to-be-remembered stimuli (90,97-98). These preserved abilities are in contrast to the performance of alcoholic Korsakoff patients or those with idiopathic dementia who fail to encode conceptual or semantic properties (99-102).

The finding of relatively preserved semantic analysis suggests the possibility of teaching patients to utilize these abilities in everyday tasks. Patients could be taught the value of such mnemonics as clustering items on a grocery list into meaningful categories which are written down before shopping. Such skills applied to tasks that most neurologically intact individuals perform spontaneously could promote the efficiency of daily activities. Furthermore, preserved memory for concepts, indicated by head-injured patients' awareness of semantic relations among to-be-remembered stimuli, could be employed in conjunction with skill learning of new tasks. While the work of Schacter and Glisky indicates that amnesic patients can acquire new semantic knowledge, our investigations also suggest that some components of memory are still preserved after head injury. The integration of this intact fund of knowledge with the learning of new skills remains to be explored.

The literature reviewed in this chapter demonstrates that memory is extremely vulnerable to the effects of closed head injury and that such deficits impart a tremendous burden on patients and their families as well as a challenge to rehabilitation specialists. Hopefully, as knowledge focusing on preserved learning and memory advances in the field, so will our ability to substantially improve the quality and independent functioning of survivors.

ACKNOWLEDGMENTS

Preparation of this chapter and studies conducted in Galveston were supported by the Javits Neuroscience Investigator Award, NS-21889, and Grants #84-152 and #84-152A from The Moody Foundation of Galveston (HSL). We thank Liz Zindler for manuscript preparation.

REFERENCES

1. Brooks, N., Campsie, L., Symington, C., Beattie, A., and McKinlay, W. (1986). The five year outcome of severe blunt head injury: A relative's view. *J. Neurol. Neurosurg. Psychiatry 49*:764-770.
2. Levin, H.S., Benton, A.L., and Grossman, R.G. (1982). *Neurobehavioral Consequences of Closed Head Injury*. Oxford University Press, New York, pp. 1-279.
3. Oddy, M., Coughlan, T., Tyerman, A., and Jenkins, D. (1985). Social adjustment after closed head injury: A further follow-up seven years after injury. *J. Neurol. Neurosurg. Psychiatry 48*:564-568.
4. Parker, S.A., and Serrats, A.F. (1976). Memory of recovery after traumatic coma. *Acta Neurochir. 34*:71-77.
5. Van Zomeren, A.H., and Van Den Burg, W. (1985). Residual complaints of patients two years after severe head injury. *J. Neurol. Neurosurg. Psychiatry 48*: 21-28.
6. Brooks, N., McKinlay, W., Symington, C., Beattie, A., and Campsie, L. (1987). Return to work within the first seven years of severe head injury. *Brain Injury 1*:5-19.
7. Stuss, D.T., Ely, P., Hugenholtz, H., Richard, M.T., LaRochelle, S., Poirier, C.A., and Bell, I. (1985). Subtle neuropsychological deficits in patients with good recovery after closed head injury. *Neurosurgery 17*:41-47.
8. Levin, H.S., Mattis, S., Ruff, R.M. Eisenberg, H.M., Marshall, L.F., Tabaddor, K., High, Jr., W.M., and Frankowski, R.F. (1987). Neurobehavioral outcome following minor head injury: A three-center study. *J. Neurosurg. 66*:234-243.
9. McLean, A., Temkin, N.R., Dikmen, S., and Wyler, A.R. (1983). The behavioral sequelae of head injury. *J. Clin. Neuropsychol. 5*:361-376.
10. Gaidolfi, E., and Vignolo, L.A. (1980). Closed head injuries of school-age children: Neuropsychological sequelae in early adulthood. *Ital. J. Neurol. Sci. 1*:65-73.
11. Levin, H.S., Eisenberg, H.M., Wigg, N.R., and Kobayshi, K. (1982). Memory and intellectual ability after head injury in children and adolescents. *Neurosurgery 11*:668-673.
12. Levin, H.S., High, Jr., W.M., Ewing-Cobbs, L., Fletcher, J.M., Eisenberg, H.M., Miner, M.E., and Goldstein, F.C. (1988). Memory functioning during the first year after closed head injury in children and adolescents. *Neurosurgery 22*:1043-1052.
13. Dikmen, S., Temkin, N., McLean, A., Wyler, A., and Machamer, J. (1987). Memory and head injury severity. *J. Neurol. Neurosurg. Psychiatry 50*:1613-1618.
14. Teasdale, G., and Jennett, B. (1974). Assessment of coma and impaired consciousness: A practical scale. *Lancet 2*:81-84.
15. Fisher, C.M. (1982). Whiplash amnesia. *Neurology 32*:667-668.

16. Davidoff, G., Morris, J., Roth, E., and Bleiberg, J. (1985). Cognitive dysfunction and mild closed head injury in traumatic spinal cord injury. *Arch. Phys. Med. Rehabil. 66*:489-491.

17. Davidoff, G., Thomas, P., Berent, S., and Dijkers, M. (1986). Risk factors for closed head injury in acute traumatic spinal cord injury patients. *Arch. Phys. Med. Rehabil. 67*:653.

18. Buschke, H., and Fuld, P.A. (1974). Evaluating storage, retention, and retrieval in disordered memory and learning. *Neurology 24*:1019-1025.

19. Gronwall, D., and Wrightson, P. (1975). Cumulative effect of concussion. *Lancet 2*:992-997.

20. Adams, H.J., Graham, D.I., Scott, G., Parker, L.S., and Doyle, D. (1980). Brain damage in fatal non-missile head injury. *J. Clin. Pathol. 33*:1132-1145.

21. Gandy, S.E., Snow, R.B., Zimmerman, R.D., and Deck, M.D.F. (1984). Cranial nuclear magnetic resonance imaging in head trauma. *Ann. Neurol. 16*:254-257.

22. Han, J.S., Kaufman, B., and Alfidi, R.J. (1984). Head trauma evaluated by magnetic resonance imaging and computed tomography: A comparison. *Radiology 150*:71-77.

23. Jenkins, A., Teasdale, G., Hadley, M.D.M., MacPherson, P., and Rowan, J.O. (1986). Brain lesions detected by magnetic resonance imaging in mild and severe head injuries. *Lancet 2*:445-446.

24. Levin, H.S., Amparo, E., Eisenberg, H.M., Williams, D.H., High, Jr., W.M., McArdle, C.B., and Weiner, R.L. (1987). Magnetic resonance imaging and computerized tomography in relation to the neurobehavioral sequelae of mild and moderate head injuries. *J. Neurosurg. 66*:706-713.

25. Levin, H.S., Meyers, C.A., Grossman, R.G., and Sarwar, M. (1981). Ventricular enlargement after closed head injury. *Arch. Neurol. 38*:623-629.

26. Wilson, J.T.L., Wiedmann, K.D., Hadley, D.M., Condon, B., Teasdale, G., and Brooks, D.N. (1988). Early and late magnetic resonance imaging and neuropsychological outcome after head injury. *J. Neurol. Neurosurg. Psychiatry 51*: 391-396.

27. Langfitt, T.W., Obrist, W.D., Alavi, A., Grossman, R.I., Zimmerman, R., Jaggi, J., Uzzell, B., Reivich, M., and Patton, D.R. (1986). Computerized tomography, magnetic resonance imaging, and positron emission tomography in the study of brain trauma: Preliminary observations. *J. Neurosurg. 64*:760-767.

28. Alexandre, A., Colombo, F., Nertempi, P., and Benedetti, A. (1983). Cognitive outcome and early indices of severity of head injury. *J. Neurosurg. 59*:751-761.

29. Levin, H.S., Goldstein, F.C., High, Jr., W.M., and Eisenberg, H.M. (1988). Disproportionately severe memory deficit in relation to normal intellectual functioning after closed head injury. *J. Neurol. Neurosurg. Psychiatry 51*:1294-1301.

30. Levin, H.S., Grossman, R.G., Rose, J.E., and Teasdale, G. (1979). Long-term neuropsychological outcome of closed head injury. *J. Neurosurg. 50*:412-422.

31. Vilkki, J., Poropudas, K., and Servo, A. (1988). Memory disorder related to coma duration after head injury. *J. Neurol. Neurosurg. Psychiatry 51*:1452-1454.

32. Gronwall, D., and Wrightson, P. (1981). Memory and information processing capacity after closed head injury. *J. Neurol. Neurosurg. Psychiatry 44*:889-895.
33. Corkin, S.H., Hurt, R.W., Twitchell, T.E., Franklin, L.C., and Yin, R.K. (1987). Consequences of nonpenetrating and penetrating head injury: Retrograde amnesia, posttraumatic amnesia, and lasting effects on cognition. In *Neurobehavioral Recovery from Head Injury*. Edited by H.S. Levin, J. Grafman, and H.M. Eisenberg. Oxford University Press, New York, pp. 318-329.
34. Jennett, B., and Teasdale, G. (1981). *Management of Head Injuries*. F.A. Davis Company, Philadelphia.
35. Russell, W.R. (1971). *The Traumatic Amnesias*. Oxford University Press, New York.
36. Russell, W.R., and Smith, A. (1961). Post-traumatic amnesia in closed head injury. *Arch. Neurol. 5*:4-17.
37. Russell, W.R. (1932). Cerebral involvement in head injury. *Brain 55*:549-603.
38. Levin, H.S., and Eisenberg, H.M. (1987). Postconcussional syndrome. In *Current Therapy in Neurologic Disease-2*. Edited by R.T. Johnson. B.C. Decker, Inc., Philadelphia, pp. 193-196.
39. Levin, H.S., and Eisenberg, H.M. (1986). The relative durations of coma and posttraumatic amnesia after severe non-missile head injury: Findings from the pilot phase of the National Traumatic Coma Data Bank. In *Neural Trauma: Treatment, Monitoring, and Rehabilitation Issues*. Edited by M. Miner and K. Wagner. Butterworth Publishers, Inc., Stoneham, MA, pp. 89-97.
40. Gronwall, D., and Wrightson, P. (1980). Duration of post-traumatic amnesia after mild head injury. *J. Clin. Neuropsychol. 2*:51-60.
41. Levin, H.S., O'Donnell, V.M., and Grossman, R.G. (1979). The Galveston orientation and amnesia test: A practical scale to assess cognition after head injury. *J. Nerv. Ment. Dis. 167*:675-684.
42. Davidoff, G., Doljanac, R., Berent, S., Johnson, M.B., Thomas, P., Dijkers, M., and Klisz, D. (1988). Galveston orientation and amnesia test: Its utility in the determination of closed head injury in acute spinal cord injury patients. *Arch. Phys. Med. Rehabil. 69*:432-434.
43. Artiola, L., Fortuny, I., Briggs, M., Newcombe, F., Ratcliff, G., and Thomas, C. (1980). Measuring the duration of posttraumatic amnesia. *J. Neurol. Neurosurg. Psychiatry 43*:377-379.
44. Shores, E.A., Marosszeky, J.E., Sandanam, J., and Batchelor, J. (1986). Preliminary validation of a clinical scale for measuring the duration of post-traumatic amnesia. *Med. J. Aust. 144*:569-572.
45. High, Jr., W.M., Levin, H.S., and Gary, Jr., H.E. (In press). Recovery of orientation following closed-head injury. *J. Clin. Exp. Neuropsychol.*
46. Daniel, W.F., Crovitz, H.F., and Weiner, R.D. (1987). Neuropsychological aspects of disorientation. *Cortex 23*:169-187.
47. Levin, H.S., High, Jr., W.M., and Eisenberg, H.M. (1988). Learning and forgetting during posttraumatic amnesia in head injured patients. *J. Neurol. Neurosurg. Psychiatry 51*:14-20.

48. Parkin, A.J. (1982). Residual learning capability in organic amnesia. *Cortex 18*: 417-440.
49. Squire, L.R. (1986). Mechanisms of memory. *Science 232*:1612-1619.
50. Squire, L.R. (1987). *Memory and Brain*. Oxford University Press, New York, pp. 1-315.
51. Brooks, D.N., and Baddeley, A.D. (1976). What can amnesic patients learn? *Neuropsychologia 14*:111-122.
52. Cohen, N.J., and Squire, L.R. (1980). Preserved learning and retention of pattern analyzing skills in amnesia. Dissociation of knowing how and knowing that. *Science 210*:207-209.
53. Ewert, J., Levin, H.S., Watson, M.G., and Kalisky, Z. (1989). Procedural memory during posttraumatic amnesia in survivors of severe closed head injury: Implications for rehabilitation. *Arch. Neurol. 46*:911-16.
54. Russell, W.R., and Nathan, P.W. (1946). Traumatic amnesia. *Brain 69*:183-187.
55. Benson, D.F., and Geschwind, N. (1967). Shrinking retrograde amnesia. *J. Neurol. Neurosurg. Psychiatry 30*:539-544.
56. Crovitz, H.F., Horn, R.W., and Daniel, W.F. (1983). Interrelationships among retrograde amnesia, post-traumatic amnesia, and time since head injury: A retrospective study. *Cortex 19*:407-412.
57. Crovitz, H.F., and Daniel, W.F. (1987). Length of retrograde amnesia after head injury: A revised formula. *Cortex 23*:695-698.
58. Ribot, T. (1882). *Diseases of Memory: An Essay in the Positive Psychology*. Appleton, New York.
59. Cohen, N.J., and Squire, L.R. (1981). Retrograde amnesia and remote memory impairment. *Neuropsychologia 19*:337-356.
60. Marslen-Wilson, W.D., and Teuber, H.L. (1975). Memory for remote events in anterograde amnesia: Recognition of public figures from news photographs. *Neuropsychologia 13*:347-352.
61. Seltzer, B., and Benson, D.F. (1974). The temporal pattern of retrograde amnesia in Korsakoff's disease. *Neurology 24*:527-530.
62. Squire, L.R., Slater, P.C., and Chace, P.M. (1975). Retrograde amnesia: Temporal gradient in very long-term memory following electroconvulsive therapy. *Science 187*:77-79.
63. Levin, H.S., High, Jr., W.M., Meyers, C.A., Von Laufen, A., Hayden, M.E., and Eisenberg, H.M. (1985). Impairment of remote memory after closed head injury. *J. Neurol. Neurosurg. Psychiatry 48*:556-563.
64. Brooks, D.N. (1972). Memory and head injury. *J. Nerv. Ment. Dis. 155*:350-355.
65. Brooks, D.N. (1975). Long and short term memory in head injured patients. *Cortex 11*:329-340.
66. Brooks, D.N. (1976). Wechsler Memory Scale performance and its relationship to brain damage after severe closed head injury. *J. Neurol. Neurosurg. Psychiatry 39*:593-601.
67. Levin, H.S., and Peters, B.H. (1976). Neuropsychological testing following head injuries: Prosopagnosia without visual field defect. *Dis. Nerv. Syst. 37*:68-71.

68. Butters, N., and Cermak, L.S. (1980). *Alcoholic Korsakoff's Syndrome: An Information Processing Approach to Amnesia.* Academic Press, New York.
69. Wechsler, D. (1981). *WAIS-R Manual.* Psychological Corporation, New York.
70. Larsson, C., and Ronnberg, J. (1987). Memory disorders as a function of traumatic brain injury. *Scand. J. Rehab. Med. 19*:99-104.
71. Baddeley, A.D. (1986). *Working Memory.* Oxford University Press, Oxford.
72. Brown, J. (1958). Some tests of the decay theory of immediate memory. *Q. J. Exp. Psychol. 10*:12-21.
73. Peterson, L.R., and Peterson, M.J. (1959). Short-term retention of individual verbal items. *J. Exp. Psychol. 58*:193-198.
74. Kimura, D. (1963). Right temporal-lobe damage. *Arch. Neurol. 8*:264-271.
75. Milner, B. (1974). Sparing of language functions after early unilateral brain damage. *Neurosci. Res. Prog. Bull. 12*:213-217.
76. Milner, B. (1978). Clues to the cerebral organization of memory. In *Cerebral Correlates of Conscious Experience.* Edited by P.A. Buser and A. Rougeul-Busser. Elsevier North-Holland Biomedical Press, New York, pp. 139-153.
77. Goldstein, F.C., and Levin, H.S. (1988). Memory deficit after closed head injury. Presented at the Ninety-Sixth Annual Meeting of the American Psychological Association, Atlanta, GA.
78. Hannay, H.J., Levin, H.S., and Grossman, R.G. (1979). Impaired recognition memory after head injury. *Cortex 15*:269-283.
79. Tabaddor, K., Mattis, S., and Zazula, T. (1984). Cognitive sequelae and recovery course after moderate and severe head injury. *Neurosurgery 14*:701-708.
80. Wilson, B. (1984). Memory therapy in practice. In *Clinical Management of Memory Problems.* Edited by B.A. Wilson and N. Moffat. Aspen Systems Corporation, Rockville, MD, pp. 89-111.
81. Hasher, L., and Zacks, R.T. (1979). Automatic and effortful processes in memory. *J. Exp. Psychol. [Gen.] 108*:356-388.
82. Hasher, L., and Zacks, R.T. (1984). Automatic processing of fundamental information: The case of frequency of occurrence. *Am. Psychol. 39*:1372-1388.
83. Newman, R.P., Weingartner, H., Smallberg, S.A., and Calne, D.B. (1984). Effortful and automatic memory: Effects of dopamine. *Neurology 34*:805-807.
84. Roy-Byrne, P.P., Weingartner, H., Bierer, L.M., Thompson, R.M., and Post, R.M. (1986). Effortful and automatic cognitive processes in depression. *Arch. Gen. Psychiatry 43*:265-267.
85. Weingartner, H., Burns, S., Diebel, R., and Lewitt, P.A. (1984). Cognitive impairment in Parkinson's disease: Distinguishing between effortful and automatic cognitive processes. *Psychiatry Res. 11*:223-225.
86. Huppert, F.A., and Piercy, M. (1978). The role of trace strength in recency and frequency judgements by amnesic and control subjects. *Q. J. Exp. Psychol. 30*: 347-354.
87. Weingartner, H., Kaye, W., Smallberg, S., Cohen, R., Ebert, M.H., Gillin, J.C., and Gold, P. (1982). Determinants of memory failure in dementia. In *Alzheimer's Disease: A Review of Progress.* Edited by S. Corkin, K.L. Davis, J.H. Growdon, E., Usdin, and R.J. Wurtman. Raven Press, New York.

88. Levin, H.S., Goldstein, F.C., High, Jr., W.M., and Williams, D. (1988). Automatic and effortful processing after severe closed head injury. *Brain Cogn.* 7:283-297.

89. Hirst, W. (1982). The amnesic syndrome: Descriptions and explanations. *Psychol. Bull. 91*:435-460.

90. Levin, H.S., and Goldstein, F.C. (1986). Organization of verbal memory after severe closed-head injury. *J. Clin. Exp. Neuropsychol. 8*:643-656.

91. Levin, H.S., Handel, S.F., Goldman, A.M., Eisenberg, H.M., and Guinto, Jr., F.C. (1985). Magnetic resonance imaging after "diffuse" nonmissile head injury. *Arch. Neurol. 42*:963-968.

92. Schacter, D.L., and Glisky, E.L. (1986). Memory remediation: Restoration, alleviation, and the acquisition of domain-specific knowledge. In *Clinical Neuropsychology of Intervention.* Edited by B. Uzzell and Y. Gross. Martinus Nijhoff, Boston.

93. Glisky, E.L., and Schacter, D.L. (1988). Long-term retention of computer learning by patients with memory disorders. *Neuropsychologia 26*:173-178.

94. Glisky, E.L., and Schacter, D.L. (1989). Extending the limits of complex learning in organic amnesia: Computer training in a vocational domain. *Neuropsychologia 27*:107-120.

95. Tulving, E. (1983). *Elements of Episodic Memory.* Oxford University Press, New York.

96. Tulving, E. (1984). Relations among components and processes of memory. *Behav. Brain Sci. 7*:257-268.

97. Goldstein, F.C., Levin, H.S., and Boake, C. (1989). Conceptual encoding following severe closed head injury. *Cortex. 25*:541-554.

98. Goldstein, F.C., Levin, H.S., Boake, C., and Lohrey, J.H. (1990). Facilitation of memory performance through induced semantic processing in survivors of severe closed head injury. *J. Clin. Exp. Neuropsychol.*

99. Cushman, L.A., Como, P.G., Booth, H., and Caine, E.D. (1988). Cued recall and release from proactive interference in Alzheimer's disease. *J. Clin. Exp. Neuropsychol. 10*:685-692.

100. Freedman, M., and Cermak, L.S. (1986). Semantic encoding deficits in frontal lobe disease and amnesia. *Brain Cogn. 5*:108-114.

101. Squire, L.R. (1982). Comparisons between forms of amnesia: Some deficits are unique to Korsakoff's syndrome. *J. Exp. Psychol.: Learn. Mem. Cogn. 8*:560-571.

102. Weingartner, H., Kaye, W., Smallberg, S., Ebert, M.H., Gillin, J.C., and Sitram, N. (1981). Memory failures in progressive idiopathic dementia. *J. Abn. Psychol. 90*:187-196.

13

Transient Global Amnesia

John W. Miller
Washington University School of Medicine
St. Louis, Missouri

Ronald C. Petersen
and
Takehiko Yanagihara
Mayo Clinic and Mayo Foundation
Rochester, Minnesota

INTRODUCTION

Transient global amnesia (TGA) is a unique neurological condition. It is a frightening occurrence in which a previously healthy person abruptly loses the ability to form new memories. Despite the catastrophic appearance of this event, however, there is generally complete recovery within a few hours without apparent sequelae. Although TGA is universally recognized as an organic neurological syndrome, the exact site of the dysfunction in the nervous system is uncertain, and its pathophysiological mechanism is controversial.

Since TGA is not rare it is not surprising that the early literature contains many descriptions of spells of amnesia which may be instances of this syndrome (1-4). The first clear characterization of TGA, however, was by Morris Bender (5), who succinctly and accurately noted the essential features of this syndrome in 12 patients. It occurred in older people and consisted of the inability to form new memories for more than a few seconds (anterograde amnesia). This was accompanied by a loss of memory for recent events for a variable time prior to the onset (retrograde amnesia). Frequently the patients asked the same questions over and over, each time as if for the first time. Except for the memory deficit, the neurological examination was normal during the episode. The episode lasted for a few hours and was followed by complete recovery except for permanent amnesia of the episode. At the time, it was erroneously believed that this syndrome did not recur. This condition was later independently described and given its name by Fisher and Adams (6).

The adjective "global" refers to the fact that the disturbance affects memory for all modalities of information. These authors also described the first recurrent cases of this condition and noted that it commonly followed certain types of activity such as sexual intercourse, swimming, or showering (7).

CHARACTERISTICS OF THE SYNDROME
DEMOGRAPHIC FEATURES

The typical patient with transient global amnesia is a previously healthy middle-aged or elderly person. In a study of 277 patients who presented to the Mayo Clinic during the years 1964 through 1981 with a well-documented episode of transient global amnesia (8), we found a mean age of 63 years with a slight predominance of men (Fig. 1). Other series revealed almost identical age and sex distributions (9-11). The incidence of TGA for Rochester, Minnesota was 5.2 per 100,000 per year; among those 50 or older it was 23.5 per 100,000 per year (8).

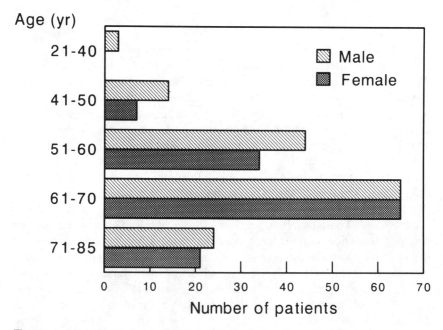

Figure 1   Distribution of age of first TGA episode. From Ref. 8.

ANTECEDENT EVENTS

An interesting clinical feature of TGA is that it often is preceded by certain events or activities (Fig. 2). Among these possible precipitating factors are sexual intercourse (7,8,10,12,13); swimming, bathing, or showering particularly in very hot or cold water (7,8,10,13,14); strenuous physical activity (8,10,15-20); intense pain (7,13); or unusual emotional stress or distress (8, 14,15,21,22). It is clear that this association between TGA and physical and emotional stress is not merely coincidental. In our study of 277 patients with 347 amnesic episodes (8), notable antecedant events simultaneous with the onset of TGA were reported in 33.4% (Fig. 2). Since this was a retrospective study there may have been other cases where precipitating factors were unreported.

Transient global amnesia has also occurred in patients undergoing laboratory procedures including three cases during coronary angiography (23,24), many cases after cerebral angiography (25-28), and single cases during a nasogastric tube insertion, a pulmonary function test, excretory urography, cystoscopy, and an exercise treadmill test (8). With the exception of the patients with cerebral angiography, the small number of cases and the possible con-

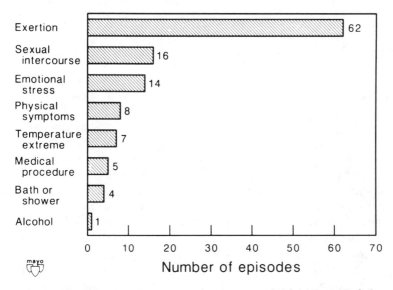

Figure 2   Activities or events occuring at onset of TGA. From Ref. 8.

comitant physical and emotional stress suggest that a direct causal association may not exist between these tests and TGA. TGA has also been reported after ingestion of various drugs including benzodiazepines (29,30), clioquinol (31), and digitoxin (32). The cases following clioquinol apparently were an acute encephalopathy rather than selective amnesia, and transient amnesia following benzodiazepine ingestion may have a different pathophysiological mechanism than that of typical TGA.

THE EPISODE

The essential feature of TGA is inability to form new memories. This is accompanied by a spotty, variable amnesia for events lasting for days, weeks, or even years prior to the episode. As a result the patient is intensely disoriented. Most patients ask questions about their surroundings, which seem unfamiliar, due to the retrograde amnesia. The answers are soon forgotten and the questions repeated. Other patients are silent and withdrawn but distressed. Invariably they are aware that something frightening is wrong but generally do not say that they have a memory problem. We are, however, aware of one patient, a neurologist, who was actually able to diagnose his problem during the episode. Despite this profound memory disturbance many patients carry out previously learned complex activities. For example, it is not uncommon for a patient to drive a car during an episode of amnesia. The retrograde amnesia gradually resolves but there is lasting amnesia for the episode itself. Headache, nausea, and vomiting during TGA have been reported by some patients (33), and we found such symptoms in 17% of episodes (8).

In our series (8), the mean duration of episodes was 6.2 h with 66% lasting 2 to 12 h. Other series had a similar duration (33,34). Neurological examination of patients during TGA typically revealed no abnormalities other than the memory deficit. For example, in our study, 21 of 23 patients who were examined during the amnesic episode had no abnormalities other than the characteristic memory deficit. Subtle abnormalities were noted in 2 patients during neurologic examination; one patient had a left Babinski sign while another had a very mild right hemiparesis. These deficits were not present the next day. The great majority of cases in the literature also had no neurological deficit other than the memory problem (7,9,10). Other small series (17,35-45), however, included patients with prominant new neurological signs and symptoms such as hemianopia, ataxia, or aphasia accompanying the amnesia. It has been argued (33) that cases of transient amnesia with significant accompanying neurological deficits should not be considered TGA. We strongly support this proposal since such cases of transient amnesia with other prominent neurological deficits may have different clinical characteristics, etiologies, and prognoses than TGA (35-37,46).

NEUROPSYCHOLOGICAL ASSESSMENT

Many studies have characterized in detail the memory deficit in patients during TGA (23,44,47-54). Studies of anterograde amnesia indicate that all types of memory, verbal and nonverbal, including visual, auditory, tactile, proprioceptive, and olfactory memories are impaired (23,44,47-50,52,54). During TGA, patients were able to recall information presented to them for up to 30 seconds, but no longer (48), corresponding to the period of immediate or short-term memory. In these cases, retrograde amnesia extended back as far as 20 or 30 years but was variable and incomplete (23,48,49,54). The retrograde amnesia has been noted to correlate with the severity of the anterograde amnesia, that is, at those times when the anterograde amnesia was subsiding, the period of retrograde amnesia was decreasing also (53). Following the end of anterograde amnesia, retrograde amnesia quickly improved but there remained a permanent amnesia of not only the spell, but of an average of 30 minutes prior to its onset, although precise delineation of the onset may be difficult (47). While the great majority of patients had no memory complaints shortly after the amnestic episode, mild deficits on formal psychometric testing can linger for days or weeks after the episode (18,48,50,51).

ASSOCIATED CONDITIONS

Many case reports and small series note an association of TGA with a variety of neurological, psychiatric, and medical conditions. TGA has been seen in migraine patients, often with typical headaches (7,8,10,11,13,20,22,39,55-60). It has been associated with recent or subsequent transient ischemic attack (TIA) or stroke as well (36-39,61). TGA also has been reported with hemorrhagic cerebrovascular disease (62-64). There are also a number of reports of TGA associated with primary or secondary cerebral neoplasms (8,65-69), as well as cases of transient amnesia resembling TGA but probably due to seizures in other patients with cerebral neoplasms (70,71). A variety of medical conditions, including aortic dissection (72), polycythemia rubra vera (73), and mitral valve prolapse (74,75) have also been seen with TGA.

Nevertheless, we found that most cases of TGA were not associated with significant neurological or medical conditions (8). Only 14% had a history of migraine, 6% prior or subsequent cerebral infarct, and 6% prior or subsequent TIA. An additional 2% had a history of unrelated seizure disorder and 3% of psychiatric disease. Only one of 277 had a cerebral neoplasm, a right posterior temporal astrocytoma. A history of cardiac disease was present in 23%, but only 5% had cardiovascular conditions with a significant risk of emboli. As for other cerebrovascular disease risk factors there was mild or moderate hypertension in 34%, hyperlipidemia in 5%, diabetes mellitus in 5%, and current cigarette use in 12%. Thus, although TGA has been seen in association with a variety of significant underlying medical and neurological conditions, most patients were in good health for age.

LABORATORY EVALUATION

There are several series of computed tomography studies in TGA. Ladurner and colleagues (40) reported that 7 of 16 patients had hypodense CT lesions but three actually had strokes with hemianopsia at the time of amnesia. Another study, with a more restricted definition of TGA, demonstrated prior cerebral infarction in 4 of 43 patients and a primary cerebral neoplasm in another (76). Other CT studies revealed infarcts in a minority of patients (10,37,61). We found cerebral infarcts in only 5 of 102 patients (8). Cerebral or brainstem atrophy was present in an additional 16 and another had a neoplasm.

Cerebral angiography has been performed in a number of TGA patients (8,33,35,36), showing significant occlusive disease in a minority of patients with no consistent pattern. Ultrasound examination revealed carotid plaques in 27% of TGA patients, a much lower incidence than in comparable patients with TIA or stroke (77).

Jaffe and Bender (78) first reported on EEG recordings in TGA in 1966. This was done during TGA in five patients; in four the EEG was entirely normal, while there was intermittent left temporal slowing in the fifth both during amnesia and in recordings days and months afterwards. Subsequently, however, there have been reports of spikes and sharp waves in interictal recordings of patients with TGA (41,43,79-83). These reports seemed to support the contention that TGA may be caused by an epileptic mechanism (7,13,84). In fact, the illustrations in these papers appear to actually show a variety of nonspecific findings which cannot at present be considered epileptogenic. As noted in the past (85) a number of these reports appear to show benign sporadic sleep spikes (small sharp spikes) which are common in normal populations and among patients without seizures (86-89). There have been other reports of genuine interictal epileptiform EEG abnormalities in patients with amnesia (71,90,91). The amnestic episodes in these reports, however, were atypical in that they were brief, repetitive, and responded to antiepileptic drugs.

To help clarify the relationship between TGA and epilepsy, we analyzed the EEG findings in 109 patients with 116 episodes of TGA (92). Electroencephalograms were obtained during 13 episodes: Eight were entirely normal and none showed seizure discharges or other epileptiform activity. The majority (61%) of tracings performed after TGA were also normal with mild or moderate nonfocal abnormalities in a minority. Epileptiform activity was found in interictal recordings of four patients. One had a seizure disorder which was apparently unrelated to TGA, while the other three patients had amnesia apparently due to seizures rather than TGA. These amnesic spells stopped with antiepileptic drugs. This epileptic amnesia probably represented brief partial seizures followed by a longer period of postical amnesia. The initial clinical ictal manifestations presumably were subtle, unnoticed, or unwitnessed. The lack of significant epileptiform EEG abnormalities in these 13 patients and the five patients of Jaffe and Bender (78) demonstrates that TGA does not have an epileptic mechanism. This is confirmed by other EEG studies in which a patient was recorded at the onset of TGA (93) and another recorded with sphenoidal electrodes during amnesia (94). Neither recording showed any abnormality.

PROGNOSIS

In our series of 277 patients (8), 23.8% had TGA recurrence with an average follow-up of 80 months. Four percent had more than three episodes. Among 104 patients with antecedent events, 16 patients (15.4%) experienced more than one episode. Since TGA could recur many years after the initial episode—the average time between episodes was 28.5 months in our series—a longer follow-up period would yield an even higher chance of multiple spells.

The risk of permanent long-term memory impairment following TGA is a matter of controversy. In most large series (8-10) permanent memory complaints were very uncommon, although formal neuropsychological testing was not systematically performed. A number of smaller series (36,45,61) reported lasting memory impairment in a third to one half of patients, as well as occasional patients with frank amnestic strokes (36). It should be noted, however, that these patients differed from those in most series in that most had risk factors for cerebrovascular disease and their episodes were often accompanied by major neurological deficits such as hemiparesis, visual field deficit, or even cortical blindness, implying cerebral ischemia or infarction of considerable magnitude.

Most patients with more typical TGA without significant neurologic deficits other than amnesia have complete recovery of memory on follow-up neuropsychological testing (52,53,95). One study of such patients (18), however, appeared to show persistent deficits in verbal IQ and verbal memory. Many of the patients in that study had only a few days or weeks of follow-up. More recent studies (50,51) have demonstrated that significant neuropsychological deficits could persist after subjective memory complaints have resolved but eventually recover completely over weeks to months. Thus, the available information indicates that the usual course for TGA episode without other significant accompanying neurological signs or symptoms is for eventual complete recovery.

The most important prognostic issue concerns the risk for subsequent cerebral infarction. Once again, the literature differs on this question, depending on how TGA is defined and the cases selected. Several authors have cited a significant risk for subsequent TIA and stroke (35,36,45,96). These series, in general, consisted of small number of patients who presumably were not randomly selected, and included many amnesic episodes with other significant neurological deficits such as hemianopia or hemiparesis. Numerous other studies, however, have reported on large series of patients with well-documented and rigidly defined TGA, making an effort to identify most or all cases seen at a particular institution or occurring in a particular population (8-11,37,97). Without exception, these series showed a low risk for subsequent TIA and stroke. As shown in Table 1, we found (8) the risk of stroke subsequent to TGA was approximately equal to that of normal populations of the same ages (98-102). This risk was very much lower than that expected subsequent to TIA (103). A similar result has been obtained in a prospective case control study of TGA in England by Hodges and Warlow (J.R. Hodges, personal communication).

Table 1   Outcome of patients with TGA

All patients	
No. of patients	277
Mean length of follow-up after initial episode	80 months
Known dead	23 (8.3%)
Dementia[a]	11 (4.0%)
Selective memory deficit on psychological testing	3
Patients with episodes in 1976-1981	
No. of patients	181
Mean length of follow-up after initial episode	74 months
Patients lost to follow-up prior to 3 years	1
Mortality in first 3 years (mortality rate per year)	4 (0.74%)
Patients with cerebral infarctions in first 3 years	3
Patients with TIAs and other transient neurologic signs and symptoms in first 3 years	8

[a]One patient had dementia prior to the initial episode.
Source: From Ref. 8.

DIFFERENTIAL DIAGNOSIS
AMNESIA DUE TO SEIZURES

Ordinarily, complex partial seizures should be easily distinguishable from TGA because of the presence of other signs or symptoms, such as abnormal motor activity or the loss of ability to respond. However, as we have noted (92) seizures may resemble TGA, presumably when a seizure with subtle or unwitnessed outward manifestations is followed by a prolonged postical memory disturbance. Because epileptic amnesia has clinical characterisitcs different from that of TGA, and because it may respond to antiepileptic drugs, it should not be mistaken for a form of TGA.

MIGRAINE

There is no question that migraine can produce an amnesic state. An example of this is the confusional state associated with migraine events in children (104-106), in which amnesia is accompanied by other cognitive deficits and neurological signs, as well as by bilateral EEG abnormalities. A similar state may also occur in adults.

CEREBROVASCULAR DISEASE

Thromboembolic mechanisms can also cause transient amnesia. Many cases of transient amnesia accompanied by other neurological deficits have been reported in patients with many risk factors for cerebrovascular disease with a high risk for subsequent cerebral infarction (35,36,61). These characteristics distinguish this syndrome from TGA.

ACUTE CONFUSIONAL STATE

A disorder which can present similarly to TGA is the acute confusional state or delirium (107-110). This is one of the most commonly encountered mental status disorders in a general hospital practice (111). Patients present with a primary disorder of attention and are often disoriented, anxious, restless, and may experience illusions and hallucinations. Often other cognitive functions including memory appear to be impaired as well, but this is secondary to disordered attention. There are many causes of this condition, including drug intoxication, and toxic or metabolic processes, but it can also arise from acute focal cerebral lesions, for example, infarcts in the right cerebral hemisphere (112-114). The primary distinction between the acute confusional state and TGA is the altered attention in the former leading to disorientation and agitation without a dramatic memory loss. In TGA, the hallmark is the loss of memory, with the patient being unable to store information, but other cognitive functions are relatively well preserved.

PSYCHOGENIC AMNESIA

TGA is clearly not due to a psychogenic mechanism because it exactly dupli-
cates the permanent memory deficit seen in patients with known lesions of
the central nervous system (e.g., Ref. 115). The nature of the memory disorder in psychogenic amnesia has been less well studied, but it has certain
distinguishing features. The patients tend to be inconsistent during testing,
do not exhibit a temporal gradient in retrograde amnesia, and frequently
complain of a loss of personal identity (3,7,115-117). These features are all
inconsistent with TGA. Nevertheless TGA is sometimes misdiagnosed as
psychogenic amnesia, and in cases with inadequate history it may be impossible to distinguish the two entities.

NEUROANATOMY OF TGA

One popular explanation of TGA is that it results from transient dysfunction of bilateral mesial temporal structures including the hippocampi (20,
21,43,44,53). Clinical cases have shown that static bilateral lesions produced
a persistent global amnesic state while unilateral lesions did not (115,118-124).
Careful examination of one patient demonstrated that bilateral selective CA1
hippocampal lesions could produce amnesia (125). Experimental work has
produced a similar memory disturbance in animals with bilateral lesions involving the hippocampi and amygdala (126), or the underlying white matter
(127).

Although the hypothesis that bilateral temporal dysfunction causes TGA
has been quite popular, it seems unlikely because TGA is not rare and characteristically has no other associated neurological deficits. Neither cerebrovascular disease nor migraine could be expected to cause dysfunction in two
separate cerebral sites without also affecting other neural systems, producing additional neurological signs or symptoms.

Therefore, TGA likely is the result of transient dysfunction at a single site.
One hypothesis could be that unilateral dysfunction in medial temporal structures, which cannot cause persistent global amnesia, could nevertheless produce a transient amnesia. Support for this view comes from reports of cases
where a strictly unilateral posterior cerebral artery infarction led to an amnesic state which then partially resolved (124,128,129). A unilateral temporal
abnormality has also been seen in a TGA patient with positron emission tomography (Raichle, personal communication cited in Ref. 8). This hypothesis,
however, is difficult to reconcile with the fact that global amnesia is generally
not seen after unilateral sodium amytal infusion to the carotid or posterior
cerebral artery (130,131) or temporal lobectomy if contralateral mesial temporal structures are normal (123,132,133). Alternatively it might be argued

that TGA could result from unilateral medial temporal ischemia if there is a pre-existing infarction or other static cerebral lesion on the other side. However, such lesions have not been found in neuroimaging studies nor in the only neuropathological examination of a case of TGA (8).

A more appealing explanation is that TGA results from dysfunction of medial diencephalic structures. It is well known that damage in these areas in many conditions including neoplasms and Korsakoff's syndrome can cause amnesia (134-139). Although it was initially proposed (134,137,138) that the mammillary bodies or their connections must be damaged to produce memory deficits, the work of Victor, Adams and Collins group (139) demonstrated that damage to the dorsal medial nuclei of the thalamus is required for a persistent memory deficit in alcoholic patients with Korsakoff's syndrome. Lesions involving the dorsal medial nucleus also caused significant memory impairment in primates (140-142). Dysfunction of diencephalic structures would be an attractive hypothesis since EEG and evoked potential recordings during TGA show no evidence of cortical dysfunction (92,94). In fact, there are a number of reports of persistent partial or global amnesia with discrete thalamic lesions involving the left dorsal medial nucleus from various causes including a stab wound of the basal forebrain (143,144), infarction (145,146), and hypertensive hemorrhage (83). Of particular interest is the case described by Gorelick et al. (146), where a patient who had two typical TGA episodes without other accompanying neurological deficits then had an amnesic stroke with persisting partial amnesia and only minor reflex asymmetry and sensory loss on neurological examination. Magnetic resonance imaging revealed a small infarction of the left thalamus involving the dorsal medial nucleus as well as the adjacent mammillothalamic tract and the anterior nuclear group of the thalamus on that side.

Although it is unclear at present which of these locations in the central nervous system is the typical or most common site responsible for TGA, these studies make it clear that simultaneous, bilateral dysfunction at distant sites may not be necessary. Future studies with improved neuroimaging techniques will undoubtedly clarify this issue.

MECHANISM OF TGA

Transient global amnesia is often felt to be a manifestation of migraine or cerebrovascular disease. There are a number of reports of TGA occurring in patients with a past history of migraine in which the episodes are accompanied by the typical headaches (8,22,60,147,148) suggesting a migrainous mechanism. Hodges and Warlow have found, in a case-controlled prospective study, that a history of migraine headaches was more common in the TGA group than in groups of control or TIA patients (J.R. Hodges, personal communication). It is likely that cerebrovascular disease is also reponsible for at least some cases of TGA. This is suggested by those reports of cases of TGA without other neurological defects in patients who were at high risk for embolic events (8,23), as well as the possible increased incidence of hypertension in TGA patients (8,37). Although it appears that some cases of TGA may be caused by these two mechanisms, it is not clear what causes the majority of typical cases, where global amnesia without other neurological signs or symptoms occurs in a previously healthy middle-aged or elderly person, and then resolves completely without subsequent stroke. While a migrainous mechanism would explain the good prognosis of this syndrome (22,33,148,149), it would not explain its age distribution or the low risk of recurrence. Furthermore, the various situations and activities which appear to bring on TGA in some cases are different from the typical precipitating factors for migraine. It is nevertheless possible that TGA could be caused by a unique process with clinical characteristics different from typical migraine but with a related pathophysiological mechanism (8,33). On the other hand, cerebrovascular disease would explain most of the clinical characteristics of TGA (36,37,73,150) except for its possible precipitating factors and the low probability of subsequent stroke as observed by us in the past (8) and more recently observed by Hodges and Warlow (J.R. Hodges, personal communication). Also, hypertensive cerebrovascular disease affecting small arteries is a mechanism which is consistent with the hypothesis that TGA results from dysfunction at a discrete thalamic site (146). Adequate information does not presently exist to distinguish among these possibilities.

PRACTICAL CONSIDERATIONS

Although its pathophysiological mechanism is a matter for speculation, there nevertheless are clear guidelines for the evaluation and treatment of TGA. The most important parts of the evaluation are the history and the neurological examination during or after the episode. This provides the most useful information for distinguishing TGA from other causes of transient amnesia. If the history is not consistent with the typical combination of anterograde and retrograde amnesia, the diagnosis should be questioned. If unusual motor activity occurs before or during this spell, if a large portion of the spell is unwitnessed, or if the spells are brief and repetitive, the possibility of epilepsy should be considered and an EEG should be a part of the evaluation. Because of the age of this population, many will have risk factors for cerebrovascular disease, but if these factors are numerous and other neurological deficits accompany the amnesia, cerebrovascular disease should be considered, and appropriate laboratory examination and prophylactic treatment should be followed.

However, in a patient with a typical, well-documented history without other neurological signs or symptoms, laboratory evaluation should be limited, and the prognosis is excellent. A general medical physical and laboratory examination should be performed and computerized tomography or magnetic resonance imaging of the head should be considered. If this evaluation is negative, no treatment is necessary but the patient should be advised that there is a possibility of recurrence but little risk of other subsequent neurological problems.

REFERENCES

1. Von Bechterew, W. (1900). Ueber periodische Anfälle retroactiver Amnesie. *Monatschrft. Psychiat. Neurol. 8*:353-358.
2. Moersch, F.P. (1924). Psychic manifestations in migraine. *Am. J. Psychiatry 80*:697-716.
3. Hauge, T. (1954). Catheter vertebral angiography. *Acta Radiol. 107(Suppl)*:1-219.
4. Kennedy, A., and Neville, J. (1957). Sudden loss of memory. *Br. Med. J.* 428-433.
5. Bender, M.B. (1956). Syndrome of isolated episode of confusion with amnesia. *J. Hillside Hosp. 5*:212-215.
6. Fisher, C.M., and Adams, R.D. (1958). Transient global amnesia. *Trans. Am. Neurol. Assoc. 83*:143-146.
7. Fisher, C.M., and Adams, R.D. (1964). Transient global amnesia. *Acta. Neurol. Scand. 40(Suppl 9)*:7-82.
8. Miller, J.W., Petersen, R.C., Metter, E.J., Millikan, C.H., and Yanagihara, T. (1987). Transient global amnesia: Clinical characteristics and prognosis. *Neurology 37*:733-737.
9. Nausieda, P.A., and Sherman, I.E. (1979). Long term prognosis in transient global amnesia. *JAMA 241*:392-393.
10. Shuping, J.R., Rollinson, R.D., and Toole, J.F. (1980). Transient global amnesia. *Ann. Neurol. 7*:281-285.
11. Hinge, H.H., Jensen, T.S., Kjaer, M., Marquardsen, J., and Olivarius, B.F. (1986). The prognosis of transient global amnesia. *Arch. Neurol. 43*:673-676.
12. Mayeux, R. (1979). Sexual intercourse and transient global amnesia. *N. Engl. J. Med. 300*:864.
13. Fisher, C.M. (1982). Transient global amnesia: precipitating activities and other observations. *Arch. Neurol. 39*:605-608.
14. Martin, E. (1970). Transient global amnesia: a report of eleven cases including five of amnesia at the seaside. *Irish J. Med. Sci. 3*:331-335.
15. Stevens, H., and Ammerman, B. (1974). Transient global amnesia. *Med. Ann. DC 43*:593-596.
16. Cortson, R., and Goodwin-Austen, R. (1982). Transient global amnesia in four brothers. *J. Neurol. Neurosurg. Psychiatry 45*:375-377.
17. Godlewski, S. (1968). Les épisodes amnésiqués (transient global amnesia). *Sem. Hôp. 44*:553-569.

18. Mazzucchi, A., Moretti, G., Caffarra, P., and Parma, M. (1980). Neuropsychological functions in the follow-up of transient global amnesia. *Brain 103*: 161-178.
19. Hogg, M., and Hull, P. (1980). Transient global amnesia and temporary memory loss. *Med. J. Australia 1*:558.
20. Heathfield, K., Croft, P., and Swash, M. (1973). The syndrome of transient global amnesia. *Brain 96*:729-736.
21. Bolwig, T. (1968). Transient global amnesia. *Acta Neurol. Scand. 44*:101-106.
22. Caplan, L.B., Chedru, F., Lehrmitte, F., and Mayman, C. (1981). Transient global amnesia and migraine. *Neurology 31*:1167-1170.
23. Shuttleworth, E.C., and Wise, G.R. (1973). Transient global amnesia due to arterial embolism. *Arch. Neurol. 29*:340-342.
24. Koehler, P.J., Endtz, L.J., and Den Bakker, P.B. (1986). Transient global amnesia after coronary angiography. *Clin. Cardiol. 9*:170-171.
25. Tribolet, N., Assal, G., and Oberson, R. (1975). Syndrome de Korsakoff et cécité corticale transitoiries aprés angiographie vertébrale. *Schweiz. Med. Wochenschr. 10*:1506-1509.
26. Wales, L., and Nov, A. (1981). Transient global amnesia: complications of cerebral angiography. *Am. J. Neuroradiol. 2*:275-277.
27. Cochran, J.W., Morrell, F., Huckman, M.S., and Cochran, E.J. (1982). Transient global amnesia after cerebral angiography: report of seven cases. *Arch. Neurol. 39*:593-594.
28. Reichter, R.E., Belt, T.G., and Stevens, J. (1986). Transient global amnesia: complication of arterial DSA. *Am. J. Neurorad. 8*:179-180.
29. Sandyk, R. (1985). Transient global amnesia induced by lorazepam. *Clin. Neuropharm. 8*:297-298.
30. Morris, H.H., and Estes, M.L. (1987). Traveler's amnesia: Transient global amnesia secondary to triazolam. *JAMA 258*:945-946.
31. Kaeser, H. (1984). Transient global amnesia due to clioquinol. *Acta Neurol. Scand. 70*(Suppl. 100):175-179.
32. Greenlee, J.E., Crampton, R.S., and Miller, T.Q. (1975). Transient global amnesia associated with cardiac arrhythmia and digitalis intoxication. *Stroke 6*:513-516.
33. Caplan, L.B. (1985). Transient global amnesia. In *Handbook of Clinical Neurology*, Vol. I (45), *Clinical Neuropsychology*. Edited by J. Fredericks. Elsevier, Amsterdam, pp. 205-218.
34. Rollinson, R.D. (1978). Transient global amnesia: a review of 213 cases from the literature. *Aust. NZ J. Med. 8*:547-549.
35. Jensen, T.S., and Olivarius, B.D.F. (1981). Transient global.amnesia—its clinical and pathophysiological basis and prognosis. *Acta Neurol. Scand. 63*:220-230.
36. Mathew, M.T., and Meyer, J.S. (1974). Pathogenesis and natural history of transient global amnesia. *Stroke 5*:303-311.
37. Kushner, M.J., and Hauser, W.A. (1985). Transient global amnesia: a case controlled study. *Ann. Neurol. 18*:684-691.
38. Halsey, J. (1967). Cerebral infarction with transient global amnesia. *Ala. J. Med. Sci.* 436-438.

39. Laplane, D., and Truelle, J. (1974). Le mécanisme de l'ictus amnésique. Nouv. Presse Méd. 3:721-725.
40. Ladurner, G., Skvarc, A., and Sager, D. (1982). Computed tomography and transient global amnesia. *Eur. Neurol. 21*:34-40.
41. Lou, H. (1968). Repeated episodes of transient global amnesia. *Acta Neurol. Scand. 44*:612-618.
42. Tolosa, E., and Gumnit, R. (1973). Isolated memory loss and transient global amnesia. *Neurology 23*:399-400.
43. Steinmetz, E., and Vroom, S. (1972). Transient global amnesia. *Neurology 22*: 1193-1200.
44. Ponsford, J., and Donnan, J.A. (1980). Transient global amnesia—A hippocampal phenomenon? *J. Neurol. Neurosurg. Psychiatry 43*:285-287.
45. Jensen, T.S., and Olivarius, B.D.F. (1980). Transient global amnesia as a manifestation of transient cerebral ischemia. *Acta Neurol. Scand. 61*:115-124.
46. Poser, C., and Ziegler, D. (1960). Temporary amnesia as a manifestation of cerebral vascular insufficiency. *Trans. Am. Neurol. Assoc.* 221-223.
47. Shuttleworth, E.L., and Morris, C.E. (1966). The transient global amnesia syndrome: A defect in the second stage of memory in man. *Arch. Neurol. 15*:515-520.
48. Caffarra, P., Moretti, G., Mazzucchi, A., and Parma, M. (1981). Neuropsychological testing during transient global amnesia episode and its follow-up. *Acta Neurol. Scand. 63*:44-50.
49. Gordon, B., and Martin, O.S.M. (1979). Transient global amnesia: An extensive case report. *J. Neurol. Neurosurg. Psychiatry 42*:572-575.
50. Regard, M., and Landis, T. (1984). Transient global amnesia: Neuropsychological dysfunction during attack and recovery in two "pure" cases. *J. Neurol. Neurosurg. Psychiatry 47*:668-672.
51. Stracciari, A., Rabucci, G.G., and Gallassi, R. (1987). Transient global amnesia: Neuropsychological study of a "pure" case. *J. Neurol. 234*:126-127.
52. Stracciari, A., and Morreale, A. (1987). Memory performances before and after transient global amnesia. *Stroke 18*:813-814.
53. Kritchevsky, N., Squire, L.R., and Zouzounis, J.A. (1988). Transient global amnesia: Characterization of anterograde and retrograde amnesia. *Neurology 38*:213-219.
54. Hodges, J.R., and Ward, C.D. (1989). Observations during transient global amnesia: A behavioral and neuropsychological study of five cases. *Brain 112*: 595-620.
55. Evans, J. (1966). Transient loss of memory, an organic syndrome. *Brain 89*: 539-548.
56. Whitty, C., and Zangwill, O. (1966). *Amnesia*. Butterworth, London.
57. Gilbert, J., and Benson, D. (1972). Transient global amnesia: Report of two cases with definite etiologies. *J. Nerv Ment. Dis. 154*:461-463.
58. Steinmetz, E., and Broom, F. (1972). Transient global amnesia. *Neurology 22*: 1193-1200.
59. Frank, G. (1976). Amnestische Episoden bei Migräne—Ein Beitrag zur Differential-diagnose der transienten globalen Amnesie. *Schweiz. Arch. Neurol. Neurochir. Psychiatr. 119*:253-274.

60. Olivarius, B., and Jensen, T. (1979). Transient global amnesia in migraine. *Headache 19*:335-338.

61. Cattaino, G., Querin, F., Pomes, A., and Piazza, P. (1984). Transient global amnesia. *Acta Neurol. Scand. 70*:385-390.

62. Landi, G., Giusti, M.C., and Guidotti, M. (1982). Transient global amnesia due to left temporal hemorrhage. *J. Neurol. Neurosurg. Psychiatry 456*:1062-1063.

63. Sandyk, R. (1984). Transient global amnesia: A presentation of subarachnoid hemorrhage. *J. Neurol. 231*:283-284.

64. Chatham, P.E., and Brillman, J. (1985). Transient global amnesia associated with bilateral subdural hematomas. *J. Neurosurg. 17*:971-973.

65. Aimard, G., Trillet, M., Perroudon, C., Tommasi, N., and Carrier, H. (1971). Ictus amnésique symptomatique d'un glioblastoma intéressant le trigone. *Rev. Neurol. 124*:392-396.

66. Hartley, T., Heilman, K., and Garcia-Bengochea, F. (1974). A case of global amnesia due to pituitary tumor. *Neurology 24*:998-1000.

67. Boudin, G., Pépin, R., Mikol, J., Haguenau, M., and Vernant, J. (1975). Gliome du systéme limbique postérior révélé par une amnésie globale transitoire. *Rev. Neurol. 131*:157-163.

68. Lisak, R., and Zimmerman, R. (1977). Transient global amnesia due to a dominant hemisphere tumor. *Arch. Neurol. 34*:317-318.

69. Findler, G., Feinsod, M., Lijovetzky, G., and Hadani, M. (1983). Transient global amnesia associated with a single metastasis in a nondominant hemisphere. *J. Neurosurg. 58*:303-305.

70. Shuping, J., Toole, J., and Alexander, E. (1980). Transient global amnesia due to glioma in a dominant hemisphere. *Neurology 30*:88-90.

71. Meador, K.J., Adams, R.J., and Flanigan, H.F. (1985). Transient global amnesia and meningioma. *Neurology 35*:769-771.

72. Rosenberg, G.A. (1979). Transient global amnesia with a dissecting aortic aneurysm. *Arch. Neurol. 36*:255.

73. Matias-Guiu, J., Masagué, I., and Codina, A. (1985). Transient global amnesia and high hematocrit levels. *J. Neurol. 232*:383-384.

74. Jackson, A.C., Boughner, D.R., Bolton, C.F., Hopkins, M., and Barnett, H.J.M. (1985). Transient global amnesia associated with mitral valve prolapse. *Neurology 35*(1):215.

75. Jackson, A.C. (1986). Neurological disorders associated with mitral valve prolapse. *Can. J. Neurosci. 13*:15-20.

76. Matias-Guiu, J., Colomer, R., Segura, A., and Codina, A. (1986). Cranial CT scan in transient global amnesia. *Acta Neurol. Scand. 73*:298-301.

77. Feuer, D., and Weinbeger, J. (1987). Extracranial carotid artery in patients with transient global amnesia: evaluation by real-time b-mode ultrasonography with duplex doppler flow. *Stroke 18*:951-953.

78. Jaffe, R., and Bender, M.B. (1966). EEG studies in the syndrome of isolated episodes of confusion with amnesia "transient global amnesia." *J. Neurol. Neurosurg. Psychaitry 29*:472-474.

79. Tharp, B.R. (1969). The electroencephalogram in transient global amnesia. *Electroenceph. Clin. Neurophysiol. 26*:96-99.

80. Greene, H.H., and Bennett, D.R. (1974). Transient global amnesia with a previously unreported EEG abnormality. *Electroenceph. Clin. Neurophysiol. 36*: 409-413.
81. Gilbert, G.J. (1978). Transient global amnesia: manifestation of medial temporal lobe epilepsy. *Clin. Electroenceph. 9*:147-152.
82. Rowan, A.J., and Protass, L.M. (1979). Transient global amnesia: clinical and electroencephalographic findings in 10 cases. *Neurology 29*:869-872.
83. Moonis, M., Jain, S., Prasad, K., Mishra, N.K., Goulatia, R.K., and Maheshwari, M.C. (1988). Left thalamic hypertensive hemorrhage presenting as transient global amnesia. *Acta Neurol. Scand. 77*:331-337.
84. Cantor, F.K. (1971). Transient global amnesia and temporal lobe seizures. *Neurology 21*:430-431.
85. Tharp, B.R. (1979). Letter to the editor: Transient global amnesia: manifestation of medial temporal lobe epilepsy. *Clin. Electroenceph. 10*:54-56.
86. Klass, D.W., and Westmoreland, B.F. (1985). Nonepileptogenic epileptiform electroencephalographic activity. *Ann. Neurol. 18*:627-635.
87. Reiher, J., and Klass, D.W. (1968). Two common EEG patterns of doubtful clinical significance. *Med. Clin. North Am. 52*:933-940.
88. White, J.C., Langston, J.W., and Pedley, T.A. (1977). Benign epileptiform transients of sleep. Clarification of the small sharp spike controversy. *Neurology 27*:1061-1068.
89. Lebel, M., Reiher, J., and Klass, D.W. (1977). Small sharp spikes (sss): Electroencephalographic characteristics and clinical significance. *Electroenceph. Clin. Neurophysiol. 43*:463.
90. Deisenhammer, E. (1981). Transient global amnesia as an epileptic manifestation. *J. Neurol. 225*:289-292.
91. Pritchard, P.B. III, Holstrom, L., and Roitzsch, J.C. (1984). Epileptic amnestic attacks: Differentiation from transient global amnesia and benefit from antiepileptic drugs. *Neurology 34*:161.
92. Miller, J.W., Yanagihara, T., Petersen, R.C., and Klass, D.W. (1987). Transient global amnesia and epilepsy: Electroencephalographic distinction. *Arch. Neurol. 44*:629-633.
93. Cole, A.J., Gloor, P., and Kaplan, R. (1987). Transient global amnesia: The electroencephalogram at onset. *Ann. Neurol. 22*:771-772.
94. Meador, K.J., Loring, D.W., King, D.W., and Nichols, F.J. (1988). The P3 evoked potential and transient global amnesia. *Arch. Neurol. 45*:465-467.
95. Matias-Guiu, J., and Codina, A. (1985). Neuropsychological functions in the follow-up with transient global amnesia. *J. Neurol. Neurosurg. Psychiatry 48*: 713-725.
96. Fogelholm, R., Kivalo, E., and Bergstrom, L. (1975). The transient global amnesia syndrome. *Eur. Neurol. 13*:72-84.
97. Colombo, A., and Scarpa, M. (1988). Transient global amnesia: pathogenesis and prognosis. *Eur. Neurol. 28*:111-114.
98. Alter, M., Christoferson, L., Resch, J., Meyers, G., and Ford, J. (1970). Cerebrovascular disease: Frequency and population selectivity in an upper midwestern community. *Stroke 1*:454-465.

99. Whisnant, J.P., Fitzgibbons, J.P., Kurland, L.T., and Sayre, G.P. (1971). Natural history of stroke in Rochester, Minnesota, 1945 through 1965. *Stroke* 2:11-22.

100. Matsumoto, N., Whisnant, J.P., Kurland, L.J., and Okazaki, H. (1973). Natural history of stroke in Rochester, Minnesota, 1955 through 1969: An extension of a previous study, 1945 through 1954. *Stroke 4*:20-20.

101. Hansen, B.S., and Marquardsen, J. (1977). Incidence of stroke in Frederiksberg, Denmark. *Stroke 8*:663-665.

102. Garraway, W.M., Whisnant, J.P., and Drury, I. (1983). The continuing decline in the incidence of stroke. *Mayo Clin. Proc. 58*:520-523.

103. Cartlidge, M.E.F., Whisnant, J.P., and Elveback, L.R. (1977). Carotid and vertebral-basilar transient cerebral ischemia attacks: a community study, Rochester, Minnesota. *Mayo Clin. Proc. 52*:117-120.

104. Gascon, G., and Barlow, C. (1970). Juvenile migraine presenting as an acute confusional state. *Pediatrics 45*:628-635.

105. Emery, E.S. III (1977). Acute confusional state in children with migraine. *Pediatrics 60*:110-114.

106. Ehyai, A., and Fenichel, G.M. (1978). The natural history of acute confusional migraine. *Arch. Neurol. 35*:368-369.

107. Lipowski, J.Z. (1987). Delirium (acute confusional state). *JAMA 258*:1789-1792.

108. Strub, R.L. (1982). Acute confusional state. In *Psychiatric Aspects of Neurologic Disease*, Vol II. Edited by D.F. Benson and D. Blumer. Grune and Stratton, New York.

109. Mesulam, M.M. (1985). Attention, confusional states, and neglect. In *Principles of Behavioral Neurology*. Edited by M.M. Mesulam. F.A. Davis, Philadelphia.

110. Morse, R.M., and Litin, E.M. (1971). The anatomy of a delirium. *Am. J. Psych. 128*:111-116.

111. Geschwind, N. (1982). Disorders of attention. *Philos. Trans. R. Soc. Lond. Biol. 298*:173-185.

112. Mesulam, M.M., Waxman, S.G., Geschwind, N., and Sabin, T.D. (1976). Acute confusional states with right middle cerebral artery infarctions. *J. Neurol. Neurosurg. Psychiatry 298*:173-185.

113. Mori, E., and Yamadori, A. (1987). Acute confusional state and acute agitated delirium. *Arch. Neurol. 44*:1139-1143.

114. Schmidley, J.W., and Messing, R.O. (1984). Agitated confusional states in patients with right hemisphere infarctions. *Stroke 15*:883-885.

115. Scoville, W., and Milner, B. (1957). Loss of recent memory after bilateral hippocampal lesions. *J. Neurol. Neurosurg. Psychiatry 20*:11-21.

116. American Psychiatric Association (1980). *Diagnostic and Statistical Manual of Mental Disorders*, 3rd ed. APA, Washington, DC.

117. Schacter, D.L., Wang, P.L., Tulving, E., and Freedman, M. (1982). Functional retrograde amnesia. A quantitative case study. *Neuropsychologia 20*:523-532.

118. Penfield, W., and Milner, B. (1958). Memory defect produced by bilateral lesion in the hippocampal region. *Arch. Neurol. Psych. 79*:475-497.

119. Rose, F.C., and Symonds, C.P. (1960). Persistent memory defect following encephalitis. *Brain 83*:195-212.

120. Victor, M., Angevine, J.B., Mancall, E.L., and Fisher, C.M. (1961). Memory loss with lesions of hippocampal formation. *Arch. Neurol. 5*:26-45.

121. Drachman, D.A., and Ommaya, A.K. (1964). Memory and the hippocampal complex. *Arch. Neurol. 10*:411-425.

122. DeJong, R.N., Itabashi, H.H., and Olson, J.R. (1969). "Pure" memory loss with hippocampal lesions: A case report. *Arch. Neurol. 20*:339-348.

123. Penfield, W., and Mathieson, G. (1974). Memory: autopsy findings and comments on the role of the hippocampus in experiential recall. *Arch. Neurol. 31*: 145-154.

124. Benson, D.F., Marsden, C.D., and Meadows, J.C. (1974). The amnesic syndrome of posterior cerebral artery occlusion. *Acta Neurol. Scand. 50*:133-145.

125. Zola-Morgan, S., Squire, L.R., and Amaral, D.G. (1986). Human amnesia and the medial temporal region: enduring memory impairment following a bilateral lesion limited to field CA₁ of the hippocampus. *J. Neurosci. 6*:2950-2967.

126. Mishkin, M., Spiegler, B.J., Saunders, R.C., and Malamut, B.L. (1982). An animal model of global amnesia. *Aging 19*:235-248.

127. Horel, J.A. (1978). The neuroanatomy of amnesia: a critique of the hippocampal memory hypothesis. *Brain 101*:403-445.

128. Geschwind, N., and Fusillo, M. (1966). Color-naming defects in association with alexia. *Arch. Neurol. 15*:137-146.

129. Mohr, J.P., Leicester, J., Stoddard, L.T., and Sidman, N. (1971). Right hemianopia with memory and color deficits in circumscribed left posterior cerebral artery territory infarction. *Neurology 21*:1104-1113.

130. Jack, C.R., Nichols, D.A., Sharbrough, F.W., Marsh, W.R., and Petersen, R.C. (1988). Selective posterior cerebral artery amytal test for evaluating memory function before surgery for temporal lobe seizure. *Radiology 168*:787-793.

131. Milner, B., Branch, C., and Rasmussen, T. (1962). Study of short-term memory after intracarotid injection of sodium amytal. *Trans. Am. Neurol. Assoc. 87*: 224-226.

132. Milner, B., and Penfield, W. (1955). The effect of hippocampal lesions on recent memory. *Trans. Am. Neurol. Assoc. 80*:42-48.

133. Dimsdale, H., Logue, V., and Piercy, M. (1964). A case of persisting impairment of recent memory following right temporal lobectomy. *Neuropsychologia 1*:287-298.

134. Gudden, H. (1891). Klinische und anatomische Beiträge zur Kenntniss der Multiplen Alkoholneuritis Nebenbemerkungen über die Regenerationsvorgange in peripheren Nervensystem. *Arch. Psychiatr. Nervenk. 28*:643-744.

135. Williams, M., and Pennybacker, J. (1954). Memory disturbance in third ventricle tumors. *J. Neurol. Neurosurg. Psychaitry 17*:115-123.

136. Delay, J., Brion, S., and Elissalde, B. (1958a). Corps mamillaires et syndrome de Korsakoff. Etude Anatomique de huit cas de syndrome de Korsakoff d'origine alcoolique sans alteration significative du cortex cerebral-I. Etude anatomio-clinique. *Presse Med. 66*:1849-1853.

137. Delay, J., Brion, S., and Elissalde, B. (1958b). Corps mamillaires et syndrome et Korsakoff. Etude Anatomique de huit cas de syndrome de Korsakoff d'origine alcoolique sans alteration significative du cortex cerebral-II. Tubercules mamillaires et mecanisme de la mémoire. *Presse Med. 66*:1865-1868.

138. Mair, W.G.P., Warrington, E.K., and Weiskrantz, L. (1979). Memory disorder in Korsakoff's psychosis, a neuropathological and neuropsychological investigation of two cases. *Brain 102*:749-783.

139. Victor, M., Adams, R.D., and Collins, G.H. (1971). *The Wernicke-Korsakoff Syndrome*. F.A. Davis, Philadelphia.

140. Aggleton, J.P., and Mishkin, M. (1983a). Visual recognition impairment following medial thalamic lesions in monkeys. *Neuropsychologia 21*:189-197.

141. Aggleton, J.P., and Mishkin, M. (1983b). Memory impairments following restricted medial thalamic lesions in monkeys. *Exp. Brain Res. 52*:199-209.

142. Zola-Morgan, S., and Squire, L.R. (1985). Amnesia in monkeys after lesions of the mediodorsal nucleus of the thalamus. *Ann. Neurol. 17*:558-564.

143. Teuber, H.-L., Milner, B., and Vaughn, H.G. (1968). Persistent anteriograde amnesia after stab wound of the basal brain. *Neuropsychologia 6*:267-282.

144. Squire, L.R., and Moore, R.Y. (1979). Dorsal thalamic lesion in a noted case of human memory dysfunction. *Ann. Neurol. 6*:503-506.

145. Speedie, L.J., and Heilman, K.M. (1982). Amnestic disturbance following infarction of the left dorsal medial nucleus of the thalamus. *Neuropsychologia 20*:597-604.

146. Gorelick, P.B., Amico, L.L., Ganellen, R., and Benevento, L.A. (1988). Transient global amnesia and thalamic infarction. *Neurology 38*:496-499.

147. Gilbert, J.J., and Benson, D.F. (1972). Transient global amnesia: report of two cases with definite etiologies. *J. Nerv. Ment. Dis. 154*:461-464.

148. Crowell, G.F., Stump, D.A., Biller, J., McHenry, L.C. Jr., and Toole, J.F. (1984). Transient global amnesia-migraine connection. *Arch. Neurol. 41*:75-79.

149. Olesen, J., and Jorgensen, M.B. (1986). Leao's spreading depression in the hippocampus explains transient global amnesia. *Acta Neurol. Scand. 73*:219-220.

150. Logan, W., and Sherman, D.G. (1983). Transient global amnesia. *Stroke 14*:1005-1007.

14

Memory Function and Epilepsy

Warren T. Blume
University Hospital
University of Western Ontario
London, Ontario, Canada

INTRODUCTION

Many patients with epilepsy complain of impaired memory. This usually involves difficulty in recall of recently acquired information, particularly after turning attention to a different matter. Some patients learn to compensate for this deficit by verbal rehearsal or by concentrating extra attention on particularly important material; others remain functionally and socially embarrassed by this handicap.

Mechanisms underlying this annoying side effect of epilepsy and its therapy are becoming increasingly well understood even though further advances are clearly needed. This chapter briefly reviews first the fundamental anatomical and physiological data relating to memory. A complete review of this topic is furnished by Aggleton (Chap. 3). From this, the significance of human electrophysiological data can be better appreciated.

Such information provides the framework for psychological studies comparing patients with epilepsy and controls. The effect of medical epilepsy management upon memory is included in this section.

The chapter concludes with brief observations on the disruptive effect the several types of epileptic seizures can have on memory.

EXPERIMENTAL AND LABORATORY STUDIES
ANATOMY

For many years the left and right hippocampal formations alone have been considered the structures effecting memory; however, newer data have modified this theory to suggest that profound global amnesia manifested by certain patients with bilateral temporal lobe pathology represents combined amygdalo-hippocampal lesions. The following reviews clinical and experimental findings which have developed these concepts.

Scoville (1) reported a series of 30 patients in whom he resected the medial temporal regions bilaterally in an effort to relieve schizophrenic symptoms (29 cases) and epilepsy (1 case). In most cases the amygdalae and surrounding pyriform cortices alone were resected and no memory loss was apparent. In 5 of the cases in whom the resections extended 5-6 cm from the temporal tips to include a portion of the anterior hippocampi, a moderately severe memory defect occurred. In 2 cases, one schizophrenic and one epileptic patient, the anterior two-thirds of both hippocampi and the underlying hippocampal gyri were removed. Both of these patients developed a profound, global, anterograde amnesia. Thus, it involved memory for experience of all the senses. Moreover, no new memories could be formed. The epileptic patient (HM) could no longer recognize the staff who attended him; nor could he remember directions around the hospital or everyday events. In contrast, his early memories were "vivid and intact."

Thus, the amnesia appeared to be proportionate to the extent of bilateral hippocampal removal. However, the associated bilateral amygdalae resections may also have contributed to the amnesia, as acknowledged by Scoville and Milner (2). Mishkin and Appenzeller (3) refer to a study of amnesics which suggested that memory loss might vary directly with the quantity of combined amygdala and hippocampal damage.

The hippocampus was further implicated in memory through Penfield's 90 patients who underwent unilateral temporal lobectomy for seizure control (4,5). Two of these became amnestic at surgery. In one patient a 4 cm left anterior temporal removal sparing the hippocampus and uncus 5 years earlier had no effect on memory. Because of persisting seizures, the left amygdala and hippocampus were then resected which resulted in a "generalized loss of recent memory." Preoperatively, this patient's EEGs had contained spike discharges arising from the left temporal region and a metrazol-induced seizure which may have arisen from the right temporal lobe. Further evidence of bitemporal dysfunction came from preoperative neuropsychological testing which showed deficits in both verbal and nonverbal memory, and impairment on the McGill Picture Anomaly Series. Subsequent neuropathological examination at autopsy several years later revealed an atrophic right (contralateral) hippocampus but a normal appearing right amygdala (5). Therefore global amnesia in this patient was associated with bilateral hippocampal and left amygdala loss.

The other patient suffered a permanent impairment of recent memory following a left anterior temporal lobectomy including uncus, hippocampus, and amygdala. Again, EEG abnormalities (interictal spikes) appeared over each temporal lobe preoperatively, but principally on left. Moreover, neuropsychological testing disclosed impairment on the Logical Memory Test and McGill Picture Anomaly Series reflecting left and right temporal dysfunction, respectively. Thus, although no pathological confirmation became available, tests of function—EEG and neuropsychological testing—suggested abnormalities of right temporal memory structures. Removal of the left temporal region thus deprived him of a memory system.

These clinical data suggest that bilateral damage to mesial temporal structures in humans will result in a severe memory loss which is: (1) global, in that it involves all the senses, (2) anterograde, in that formation of new memories is impaired, and (3) is permanent with little recovery.

Because hippocampal and amygdala lesions often coexist and a substantial anterior temporal lobectomy would remove the amygdala, most of the hippocampus, and a corresponding portion of neocortex; clinical data likely will not determine which of these structures mediates memory storage. Experimental data do shed some light upon this question.

Mishkin et al. (6) designed a graded amnesia model in monkeys who underwent unilateral or bilateral hippocampal and/or amygdala removals. Using a nonmatching-to-sample task, Mishkin's group found mild memory impairment following bilateral hippocampal (H) or bilateral amygdala (A) removal, moderate impairment when three of these structures (H + a or A + h) were removed, and considerable impairment when both amygdala and hippocampi were removed bilaterally (H + A). Aggleton reviews these data in Chapter 00.

These experimental results appear to find a parallel in patients who had developed amnesia after temporal lobe resections. A recognition test similar to the experimental one reveals a poorer memory in Scoville's patient with radical bilateral temporal lobe excision than in Penfield's unilateral lobectomy with an intact contralateral amygdala (5).

The hippocampus may play a greater role in learning spatial relations (3) as bilaterally amygdalectomized monkeys quickly learned a memory task of object location while bihippocampal-lesioned monkeys could not. Similarly, Smith and Milner [quoted by Mishkin and Appenzeller (3)] were able to correlate extent of hippocampal removal in humans with impairment of memory for object location.

Mishkin and Appenzeller (3) distinguish a second system of learning in which the critical element is stimulus-response repetition or "habit." In the monkey this is tested by asking the monkey to select which member of 20 pairs of objects contains a food reward. When presented with such 20 pairs once a day on successive days, bilaterally limbic-lesioned monkeys learned this task about as quickly as intact animals. A human parallel may be Milner's (7) finding that the patient (HM) with extensive bilateral temporal lobectomies learned mirror drawing (drawing while observing one's own hand in a mirror) almost at a normal rate even though he could not recall having done the task before. Corkin (8) also found that patient HM acquired motor skills such as rotary pursuit, bimanual tracking, and tapping tests normally indicating that mesial temporal structures are unnecessary for acquiring these skills.

PHYSIOLOGY: LONG-TERM POTENTIATION (LTP)

Hebb suggested in 1949 (9) that simultaneous discharge of pre- and postsynaptic neurones strengthen the synapse and postulated that this was the basic mechanism for memory storage. As long-term potentiation is a lasting increase in synaptic strength that depends on coincidence of transmitter release and postsynaptic depolarization, it appears to represent the synaptic plasticity postulated by Hebb. The following summarizes some aspects of LTP.

Strength of transmission at synapses in the hippocampus and neocortex increases with repetitive use such as with tetanic afferent stimulation (10,11). When this increase in synaptic efficiency lasts more than a few minutes, it is called long-term potentiation (LTP).

Nearly simultaneous presynaptic activation and sufficient postsynaptic depolarization are normally required to effect LTP. This coincidence of activity results in an influx of calcium ions into the (postsynaptic) dendritic spine mediated by voltage-dependent excitatory amino acid receptor channels of the N-methyl D aspartate (NMDA) type. Such channels allow calcium influx only in the presence of excitatory amino acid transmitter and depolarization. The calcium influx then initiates processes leading to a potentiation of the monosynaptic excitatory postsynaptic potential (EPSP) produced by activation of excitatory amino acid receptor channels of the non-NMDA type. The exact nature of such intradendritic processes are not yet known [see discussion by Smith (10)], but the intracellular calcium likely acts via protein kinases (see discussion below about protein kinase C and conditioning.)

Hippocampal LTP, first described by Bliss and Lomo (12) develops in the CA1 region about 3 seconds after high-frequency afferent tetanization and achieves maximum value after 15-20 seconds. It may last days or weeks, but convincing evidence of permanence is lacking (13). A weak afferent stimulus produces LTP lasting only a few minutes. Unlike posttetanic potentiation (PTP), LTP does not require high-frequency afferent activity, but can be induced by a single afferent volley.

LTP can be produced by the associative interaction of two excitatory inputs in which a weak input becomes potentiated only after a strong tetanus or more LTP is produced when two strong afferent inputs occur together. This effect may be explained by the facilitory effect of postsynaptic depolarization which would be greater under these conditions. For example, EPSPs evoked by single low-frequency afferent volleys can develop LTP when paired with postsynaptic depolarization. In contrast, postsynaptic hyperpolarization can block LTP. This cooperative interaction between simultaneously active afferent inputs to produce LTP is based on postsynaptic calcium influx through voltage dependent NMDA channels. Such cooperativeness between inputs occurs not only when their synaptic sites are close together; but also as far apart as basal and apical dendrites of CA1 if postsynaptic inhibition is blocked. Since depolarization is required for NMDA channel opening, associative action can occur as long as the multiple inputs are spatially close enough together for electrotonic spread of depolarization. Electrotonic spread would increase with postsynaptic inhibition blockage.

In addition to such cooperativity, input specificity is another characteristic of LTP. Thus, LTP is specific to those synapses that are active during the tetanus as calcium can only enter where NMDA channels are activated by transmitter molecules.

The property of cooperative interaction with LTP suggests that multimodal (vision + auditory) afferent stimuli including emotionally charged (? hypothalamic input) stimuli will more likely be remembered. The input specificity of LTP perhaps underlies the phenomenon of recognition memory (i.e., the distinction between novel and familiar objects).

Long-term potentiation depends for its development upon ongoing protein synthesis (11). Therefore any process which impedes protein synthesis might diminish memory capacity in humans. Agents that induce retrograde amnesia in animal models inhibit brain protein synthesis (14). Thus, in experimental animals, electroconvulsive shock induces retrograde amnesia and reduces brain protein synthesis. This applies particularly to experimentally induced status epilepticus, even in paralyzed and ventilated animals. One may speculate that repetitive seizures inhibit protein synthesis and LTP, leading to cognitive and memory deficits particularly in the immature brain (15).

In summary, LTP is a physiological phenomenon with specific mechanisms and properties which at least partially underlies the phenomenon of memory in humans and experimental animals.

Alkon (16) used pavlovian conditioning as a model of memory in the snail retina and rabbit hippocampus. The rabbit was taught to associate a tone (conditioned stimulus) with a puff of air to its eye (unconditioned stimulus) and the snail turbulent movement of a surface (unconditioned stimulus) with a flash of light (conditioned stimulus). A clear increase in membrane-localized protein kinase C (PKC) activity occurred in association with pavlovian conditioning of both CA1 pyramidal cells of the rabbit and photoreceptor cells of the snail. Receptivity of neurones to afferent stimuli was enhanced for at least several days by such migration of PKC from the cytoplasm to the membrane as the transmembrane flow of potassium ions is reduced. Movement of PKC occurs in response to an increase in intracellular calcium and a second messenger, diacylglycerol.

PKC movement to membranes from cytoplasm with conditioning appears principally in dendrites and involves many CA1 cells of the rabbit hippocampus. Alkon (16) suggests that this involves only portions of dendrites, but that extensive interaction between postsynaptic dendritic sites occurs which is critical for memory storage. Such local storage mechanisms would permit thousands of memories to be stored on a single neurone.

PATHOLOGICAL DATA

The mesial temporal structures bear the brunt of the epileptic assault upon the brain (17,18).

First described by Bouchet and Cazauvieilh (19), the most damaged regions in idiopathic generalized convulsive epilepsy are Ammon's horn of the hippocampus and the cerebellum. Within Ammon's horn, CA1 and CA3 are principally affected while CA2 is spared. Patchy, diffuse damage to the thalamus as well as a laminar-like damage through intermediate layers of the cerebral cortex are reviewed by Meldrum and Corsellis (17). Amygdala lesions are not uncommon (17).

Pathology of the partial epilepsies will depend heavily on the nature of the seizures as partial seizures are almost always based on a lesion. As epilepsy arising from the limbic portion(s) of the temporal lobe(s) is the most common type of partial seizure disorder, mesial temporal lobe lesions will be those most frequently found among the partial epileptic patients.

Finally, systemic, intracranial, or focal intracerebral injection of convulsants produces seizures and pathology primarily involving the limbic system (20). From this one could postulate that extratemporal-originating partial seizures may damage mesial temporal structures. Thus three types of seizures could impair memory: temporal, extratemporal, and generalized convulsive.

Additional evidence for the specificity of such memory deficits to side of temporal lobe lesion comes from a study by Borghesi and Blume (21), who found that type of principal memory deficit (verbal or nonverbal) correlated with side of temporal lobe seizure onset in 34 of 38 cases (89%).

HUMAN ELECTROPHYSIOLOGY AND MEMORY: STIMULATION STUDIES AND RECORDED SPONTANEOUS SEIZURES

Mechanisms for storage and retrieval of information can also be gleaned from effects of electrical stimulation of structures such as the hippocampus and effects of spontaneous discharges.

Halgren et al. (22) stimulated human mesial temporal structures bilaterally through implanted depth electrodes. Stimulation during either presentation (P) or recall (R) of material, such as a complex scene containing objects or people, impaired recall from 69% of total material without stimulation to 36% (P) and 46% (R) while stimulation during both P and R reduced recall to 16%. The authors concluded that mesial temporal structures contribute to both input processing and retrieval.

Moreover, stimulation of mesial temporal, including hippocampal, regions reportedly produces retrograde amnesia for material learned 1-2 hours previously [Kapur (23) quoting Shandurina and Kalyagina (24) and Shandurina, Kambarova and Kalyagina (25)].

By unilateral stimulation of the posterior part of the middle temporal gyrus 1.5 to 2.0 cm below the surface, Bickford et al. (26) produced amnesia in two patients for events up to several days prior with normal recall of more remote occurrences. A clear relationship was found between the duration of electrical stimulation and the span of amnesia as well as the time required for recovery. Amnesia was usually, but not always, associated with an after-discharge.

Similarly, Chapman et al. (27) obtained memory loss in two patients with bilateral hippocampal stimulation. In one, clouding of consciousness occurred while the other transiently lost memories for the previous two weeks. Unilateral hippocampal stimulation had no effect on retrograde memory, unlike the Bickford study. Health of the contralateral temporal lobe, stimulus parameters and extent of propagation of any afterdischarge might explain this difference, but assessment and comparison of these factors from their publications is difficult.

Conversely, Halgren et al. (28) found 5 hippocampal gyrus units which discharged at high rates (> 50 times background rate) during recall of certain recent memories; in other words, they fired between the posing of a question and its response.

The foregoing data provide further evidence of the mesial temporal lobe's function in the process of recall.

Ojemann (29) distinguished areas involved in short-term verbal memory (STVM) from those involved in language by stimulating several areas of the dominant (left) frontal-parietal-temporal cortex in humans at epilepsy surgery. Cortex was stimulated during object naming (i.e., input to STVM), during a distraction task (storage phase) and during recall. Stimulation of areas adjacent to the posterior language area (Wernicke's) at time of input or storage, impaired STVM while stimulation during output did not, suggesting that this area is involved in the storage phase of verbal memory. Evidence for a retrieval function of cortex adjacent to the anterior language area was less firm. Such findings suggest that more than mesial temporal structures are involved in memory. However, propagation of any stimulus-related afterdischarge to mesial temporal structures such as the hippocampus was not sought by simultaneous electrocorticography.

Implications of findings from stimulation studies in humans in elucidating normal memory mechanisms are limited by the abnormality of brain function in these patients, the considerable interindividual differences in results, the varying stimulus parameters and lack of afterdischarge monitoring in many instances (23).

Spontaneously occurring spike discharges in the hippocampal formation and the amygdala may also affect memory function. Rausch et al. (30) found that active bitemporal spiking from hippocampal and amygdala depth electrodes in humans correlated with a lower Wechsler Memory Scale Memory Quotient. Patients whose spikes were more restricted to the nondominant (right) temporal region scored higher on verbal memory tests. (Too few had left-maximum spikes for statistical analysis.) Similarly, Mirsky et al. (31) found lower memory scores in patients with bitemporal scalp-recorded epileptic foci than among those with unilateral abnormalities. Aarts et al. (32) found that 58% of patients with focal subclinical electrographic seizures had a cognitive impairment. Those arising from left hemisphere were associated with impaired verbal short-term memory while right hemisphere discharges impaired nonverbal memory.

Registration of presented material may be impaired during diffuse epileptiform discharges. Thus, Geller and Geller found that generalized spike-wave discharges occurring during presentation of material diminished accuracy of recall (33). Spike-wave bursts beginning immediately after presentation of material had the greatest effect on recall; recall varied inversely with burst length in the Geller and Geller study. Fifty percent of Aarts et al.'s (32) patients with generalized subclinical discharges demonstrated impaired memory. Such discharges occurring during presentation of material disrupted memory whereas those occurring only during recall had no significant effect. This effect also may be found with photic-induced spike waves (34). Thalamic dysfunction during generalized spike-wave discharges (35,36) may have impeded recall in these studies. In this sense, the mechanism of amnesia would be similar to that in Korsakoff's syndrome.

Amnesia associated with spontaneous or stimulated temporal lobe discharge suggests this lobe affects storage and retrieval of memories, but where are memories lodged? A limited answer is afforded by the fact that temporal lobe stimulation can also evoke several types of memory phenomena. In 1933, Penfied (37) stimulated the temporal neocortex of a conscious patient with intractable seizures and evoked a memory "flashback." Bickford et al. (26) evoked past experiences in an epileptic patient by stimulating a restricted portion of the left superior temporal gyrus. Weingarten et al. (38) elicited visual experiences of their epileptic patients' early lives by stimulating the right anterior pes hippocampi.

Penfield and Jasper (39) felt that such stimulation only produced specific recollections in patients who also had spontaneous electrical discharges in the temporal region and could occur from stimulation of either nondominant or dominant temporal lobe. However, Gloor et al. (40) doubt that this evocation of memories and other experiential phenomena is a property unique to epileptic cortex, but that it reflects a usual function of the temporal lobe to encode an individual's life experiences and to attach emotional significance to these events.

Gloor's group had investigated 29 patients with medically intractable temporal lobe epilepsy by stereotaxically implanted depth electrodes in the amygdala, hippocampus, hippocampal gyrus, and a restricted sector of temporal neocortex. Their method simultaneously sampled a greater number of structures than the earlier works. Various experiential phenomena occurred during spontaneous seizures or were evoked by electrical stimulation in 18 of the 29 patients. Some of these were memory flashbacks or illusions of familiarity (deja vu). Seizures or afterdischarges were confined to limbic structures in 37 instances, involved limbic and neocortex regions in 49 and involved the temporal neocortex alone in only 2. Of limbic structures, the amygdala was involved in seizures with experiential phenomena slightly more often than was the hippocampus and the hippocampal gyrus. This suggested to Gloor's group that the limbic system brings to conscious level percepts residing in or elaborated by the temporal neocortex. This relationship is supported by anatomical studies (41,42) showing that temporal neocortical areas subserving higher visual and auditory perceptions project primarily to temporal lobe limbic structures.

The illusion of having already experienced an event that is in fact new, deja vu, can occur spontaneously in a temporal lobe seizure or after electrical stimulation of the temporal lobe (40). Such phenomena occur more commonly with right temporal stimulation (43). In addition to Gloor et al. (40), Chapman et al. (27) and Weingarten et al. (38) obtained deja vu experiences by limbic stimulation.

CLINICAL DATA
INTRODUCTION

Several aspects of epileptic disorders could lead to a memory impairment. In a mentally handicapped patient, the memory deficit will form part of a general intellectual impairment. In those with higher intellectual abilities, focal epileptogenic lesions in structures mediating memory can produce verbal and/or nonverbal memory impairment. The most common example would be uni- or bilateral mesial temporal sclerosis in otherwise unhandicapped patients with complex partial seizures from febrile convulsions in infancy. A third circumstance would be the damaging effect of prolonged generalized convulsions on the mesial temporal regions with resulting memory impairment as discussed earlier. Finally, considerable anticonvulsant medication can disrupt memory.

The following studies concern (1) memory performance in patients with epilepsy and in controls (2) patients with temporal lobe epilepsy versus those with nontemporal epilepsy, and (3) effect of medication.

EPILEPSY PATIENTS COMPARED WITH NONEPILEPTIC CONTROLS

Loiseau et al. (44) found that 100 epileptic patients who were leading otherwise normal lives and who showed no clinical evidence of specific cerebral pathology performed less well than controls on the Wechsler Adult Intelligence Scale digit span test, the visual reproduction subtest of the Wechsler Memory Scale and the Rey List Learning Test. Subsequently, Loiseau et al. (45) studied a similar group using immediate verbal recall with Wechsler's memory span for digits, immediate visual recall using geometric figures from the Wechsler Memory Scale, 15 words from the Rey Memory Scale (46), and a short story containing the previously presented 15 words. Epileptic patients' memories were poorer than those of controls. Patients with primary generalized epilepsy had poorer memories than did temporal lobe epileptics who did not differ from controls. However, as all patients in this study had no other disability and lead virtually normal lives, the temporal lobe group unlikely represented most patients with temporal lobe epilepsy. Glowinski (47) also found poorer performance among epileptic patients than controls when delayed recall and recall with distraction were tested (see below).

Comparisons between patients with nontemporal epilepsy and controls have failed to find significant differences in memory (31,48,49). Thus, patients with nontemporal partial seizures do not have specific memory impairments (50).

Several aspects of the seizure history which one would expect to correlate with memory have not uniformly done so. Thus, Dodrill (51) and Delaney et al. (52) found no relationship between seizure frequency and memory. Only a history of status epilepticus was associated with poorer memory (51). These findings correlate with the lack of pathological changes in brief, experimentally induced seizures (53). Studies on the effect that duration of seizure disorder has on memory have not yielded consistent results. Although Delaney et al. (52) found worse memory among patients with a long history of epilepsy, Loiseau et al. (45) obtained no such correlation. A longitudinal study would best determine whether and under what conditions such a relationship exists.

Most data concerning memory loss among epileptic patients come from those with temporal lobe seizures, particularly in cases implicating medial temporal structures.

TEMPORAL LOBE VERSUS NONTEMPORAL EPILEPSY

One would expect that memory dysfunction would be more impaired among patients with temporal lobe epilepsy than among those with focal seizures from other lobes or from generalized seizures, but studies on this have often yielded only minor differences (31,49). There may be several possible reasons for this. The most likely is case selection: temporal and nontemporal cases cannot always be reliably distinguished and overlap may occur. Generalized seizure disorders may secondarily have temporal lobe dysfunction and lesions (see the discussion on pathology), and predominantly extratemporal partial seizure disorders may have coexisting temporal abnormalities. Moreover, mild but definite temporal lobe epilepsy can be unassociated with any measurable deficit. I am unaware of any studies of patients over time. Does memory deteriorate? Finally, medications such as phenytoin can impair memory (see the discussion on anticonvulsants). With these considerations, the following studies are reviewed.

Mirsky et al. (31) compared temporal lobe and primary generalized epilepsy as categorized by clinical and EEG criteria; the Wechsler Memory Scale was used. No difference between generalized and unilateral temporal epileptic patients was found; bitemporal patients scored lower than the other groups but the difference failed to attain statistical significance. Memory ability correlated inversely with duration of seizure disorder.

Glowinski (47) investigated memory function with the Wechsler Memory Scale (WMS) in severe unilateral temporal epileptics, those with generalized seizures, and normals. Unfortunately, the precise criteria used to categorize these patients was not stated. The only specific area of memory function differentiating the two groups was on immediate recall of narrative texts where temporal lobe patients performed less well. None of the other WMS subtests discriminated between these two groups. From immediate recall, both groups deteriorated to the same level on delayed recall and this deterioration with delay was greater among both epileptic groups than for normals. Distraction also diminished memory scores more among epileptic patients than among normals. No significant relationship was found between laterality of the temporal lobe epilepsy and relative verbal and nonverbal memory abilities.

Delaney et al. (52) compared memory function among three groups unilateral temporal and unilateral frontal epileptic patients and normals. The epileptic patients were classified according to clinical evaluation, EEG criteria over several recordings and neuroimaging. Only patients in whom abnormalities in these spheres were congruent to a single region were included. Such careful selection criteria enhance the validity of their findings. Verbal memory was examined by the logical memory subtest of the WMS and word lists. Nonverbal memory was studied by the visual reproduction subtest of the WMS and a recurring figures test. Left and right temporal lobe epilepsy patients both performed less well than frontal patients or controls on logical memory, with left slightly worse than right. Memory for word lists differed little among these groups except for free recall where left temporal patients had significantly poorer scores than all other groups. While immediate reproduction of Wechsler designs was good for all groups, the right temporal group was less able to reproduce designs after a 30 minute delay than other patients and controls. Left-right temporal memory differences were not apparent for immediate recall for verbal and nonverbal material but such differences did emerge on recall after a delay.

These authors doubted the specificity of relatively simple nonverbal tasks as they can be verbalized.

Ladavas et al. (54) similarly found no immediate memory difficulty in temporal or frontal cases but delayed memory was impaired in temporal but not frontal cases.

Berent et al. (55) used verbal paired associates and visual-graphic reproduction tasks to study memory in patients with focal and generalized seizures. Those with left hemisphere and with generalized seizures performed worse on a verbal task than those with right hemisphere foci. No significant differences among the groups appeared for nonverbal tasks.

LEFT VERSUS RIGHT TEMPORAL STUDIES

Milner (50) studies memory function by delayed recall for logical memory and associative learning subtests of the Wechsler Memory Scale among candidates for surgical relief of seizures. Preoperative verbal memory was worse for left (language dominant) temporal patients (mean number of items recalled = 12) than right temporal (14), right frontal (14), or left frontal (16). According to Milner (56,57), learning and recognition of verbal material is impaired whether it is aurally or visually presented and regardless of whether retention is measured by recognition, free recall, or rate of associative learning. Evidence for an opposite view is derived from several studies [see Walsh (58) for review] which indicate that patients with dominant temporal lesions have impaired verbal memory for all forms of auditory material (words, letters, numbers) but not for the same material presented visually.

Hermann et al. (59) also studied verbal learning ability and verbal memory among 30 temporal lobe epileptics who were candidates for surgical resection. Impaired immediate memory and retrieval of verbal material was found among left temporal patients, but not among right temporal patients and controls.

In contrast, nondominant or right temporal lesions impair recall of nonverbal material such as geometric figures, topographic details, faces and melodies (60). Thus these patients have difficulty in distinguishing recurrent from nonrecurrent nonsense patterns. Although they can discriminate pitch, they have difficulty analyzing melodic patterns (60). Verbal memory is intact.

Thus, using recall of the complex Rey-Osterrieth figure (61,62), Milner found a defective nonverbal memory in right temporal patients, but the left-right difference in such memory was less than for verbal memory. Memory was not significantly impaired among patients with frontal lobe epileptogenic lesions.

In contrast, Mayeux et al. (63) found no significant differences in memory between patients with generalized epilepsy and those with left or right temporal lobe attacks. Several tests were used: Wechsler Memory Scale, consonant trigram retention, prose recall, recall of the Rey-Osterrieth figure, and the Benton Visual Retention Test. Loiseau et al.'s (45) memory data also failed to distinguish among types of epilepsy.

Case selection likely accounts for differences in these studies from those of Milner. Milner's subjects were patients with longstanding atrophic lesions who were candidates for epilepsy surgery. Only patients with progressive lesions and large arteriovenous malformations were excluded. The Mayeux and Loiseau studies excluded patients with any neurological impairment other than temporal lobe epilepsy; their patients were not necessarily candidates for surgery. Therefore, Milner likely studied a more neurologically impaired population than did Mayeux and Loiseau.

The effect of epilepsy surgery on memory and the intracarotid amytal test for memory are covered by Smith (Chap. 00).

ANTICONVULSANTS AND MEMORY

The most common but least recognized adverse effects of anticonvulsant drugs on the nervous system are impairment of cognitive function and deterioration in behavior. Although the more intellectually active patients will notice such effects on concentration, mood and memory; others may be unaware of such subtle consequences, especially if they have taken anticonvulsant mediation for many years. In practice, such impairments are dose-related (64) and polytherapy compounds the impact.

While such cognitive difficulties are evident with toxic anticonvulsant levels, they are also present at levels within the "therapeutic range." In either situation, a dosage reduction may improve memory considerably. Thus, Thompson and Trimble (65) observed that patients with high anticonvulsant levels had greater memory impairment than those with low levels and that dosage reduction improved performance. Such difficulty was particularly evident on immediate and delayed recall of stories. Trimble and Thompson (66) later showed that recall of pictures was inversely related to dose.

Some of the studies reviewed below compare cognitive effects between drugs. While anticonvulsants may differ in their propensities to impair cognition, the factor of dose must always be considered. Thus, a highly effective medication for a certain seizure disorder of an individual patient will impair cognition, including memory, less than a less effective drug even if cognitive studies would favor the latter. For example, although primidone is usually associated with more cognitive side effects than carbamazepine, some patients will be more alert on primidone if it is more effective and the dose can be smaller.

Andrewes et al. (67) compared memory performance between carbamazepine and phenytoin among new referrals with epilepsy who were matched for age and intelligence and who were similar with respect to seizure type, frequency, and duration. Memory for series of digits, word lists, prose, and delayed picture recognition was studied. Memory performance for the group on carbamazepine exceeded that on phenytoin for all four memory tasks even though more patients on carbamazepine than phenytoin had serum levels within the therapeutic range.

Among previously untreated epileptics Butlin et al. (64) showed a decline in memory after 3 months on phenytoin while untreated controls and those treated with sodium valproate or carbamazepine showed little change. Memory improved among patients who were switched from phenytoin to carbamazepine. Those remaining on phenytoin showed no change when tested after the same three month period. Carbamazepine-treated patients who were switched to valproate and those who remained on carbamazepine showed no memory change after three months. Thus phenytoin, but not carbamazepine or sodium valproate, is associated with impaired memory in these patients.

Thompson and Trimble (68) found markedly improved memory performance in patients switched from various other anticonvulsant medications to carbamazepine, especially on tests of delayed recall. Slight improvement occurred among those whose dosages of same medications were simply lowered while no memory change appeared among those maintained on the same regime.

Why does phenytoin affect memory and other cognitive functions more than carbamazepine or valproate? Anticonvulsants may deplete serum and cerebrospinal fluid (CSF) folate (69) and folate-deficient patients have a higher incidence of impairment of cognitive function than nondeficient patients (70-72). Surprisingly Butlin et al. (73) found no differences in mean memory performance among patients taking phenytoin, carbamazepine, or valproate. However, memory performance and serum folate levels correlated significantly. Phenytoin-treated patients had lower folate levels, possibly accounting for its effect on memory in some other studies.

ICTAL MEMORY IMPAIRMENT

COMPLEX PARTIAL SEIZURES

As suggested by the effects of spontaneously recorded seizures and electrical stimulation on memory, prominent alterations of memory are commonly encountered clinically during complex partial seizures of temporal lobe origin.

Blumer and Walker (74) found incomplete recall of complex partial seizures (CPS) in 55 of 60 patients. Memory of the aura was usually retained possibly because any emotional component seems to imprint experiences more firmly into memory (40). Nonetheless, an aura can be forgotten if the CPS is prolonged or the seizure becomes secondarily generalized. Automatisms and other ictal behaviors are not retained, reflecting the anterograde amnesia of CPS. In fact, distinction between impaired consciousness and amnesia in complex partial seizures is often difficult. As reaction to at least some environmental stimuli is usually retained in CPS, it appears that consciousness is less often affected than is memory. Thus "complex" and "simple" may relate more often to memory than to consciousness.

A retrograde amnesia lasting minutes to a day may occur. An unfortunate student patient of mine would forget all that she had studied for 3 hours prior to her CPS. As the stress of examinations increased her seizure incidence, this retrograde amnesia greatly lowered her school performance.

Several reports (75-77) claim that epilepsy can present solely as episodic disturbances of memory but none of these contains an EEG-recorded temporal lobe seizure. Ictal descriptions in some reports more resemble transient global amnesia than epileptic attacks (75,76,78); attacks in the Gallassi report are scantly described.

The duration of postical amnesia is probably restricted to a few minutes. Although Miller et al. (79) carefully distinguish complex partial seizures from transient global amnesia, their data do not establish whether a lingering amnesia is indeed postictal. Blumer and Benson (80) claim that the postictal phase may last 1-2 hours, but present no data to show that the seizure has stopped. Indeed, temporal lobe seizures may persist for several hours (81-83). Moreover, Kaibara and Blume (84) found that the EEG reverts to its preictal state within 5 minutes in almost all cases of partial seizures.

Taken together, these data suggest that a lingering amnestic state in a patient with known complex partial seizures reflects continuing temporal lobe seizure activity.

GRAND MAL

Fortunately, many patients retain no recollection of a grand mal attack; only aftereffects such as a bitten tongue or incontinence serve as reminders. A retrograde amnesia of varying length occurs which may shrink postictally to seconds before the ictus. Length of postictal amnesia is difficult to assess because of the tendency to sleep. Multiple grand mal attacks (i.e., status epilepticus) can produce a considerable peri-ictal amnesia which may persist.

ABSENCE

Absence attacks can usually be clinically distinguished from complex partial seizures by their brevity and their suddeness of onset and termination. The intraictal impairment of consciousness produces anterograde amnesia for that period but this becomes significant for the patient only in those unusual instances of prolonged absence; 10 seconds or more. Hutt et al. (34) found impaired recall of digits presented up to 2 seconds prior to photically induced spike waves in 2 of 4 patients with such photic-sensitive absence.

CLINICAL IMPLICATIONS OF THESE STUDIES

Such memory impairments surrounding seizures, along with denial, account for the common underestimation of seizure frequency by epileptic patients. This underestimation is, in my experience, independent of the patient's intelligence and education. To obtain an adequate estimation of seizure frequency, an interview with a companion or relative is needed.

As a retrograde amnesia obliterates the trace of some auras, the lack of known warning does not exclude a simple partial onset for a complex partial seizure or for a secondarily generalized grand mal. Others' observations of behavior at seizure onset would aid in this distinction.

ACKNOWLEDGMENTS

I thank Dr. Jeannette McGlone for her review of the manuscript and provision of helpful references.

This work could not have been realized without the dedicated library research, organizational help and typing of Mrs. Maria Raffa.

REFERENCES

1. Scoville, W.B. (1954). The limbic lobe in man. *J. Neurosurg. 11*:64-66.
2. Scoville, W.B., and Milner, B. (1957). Loss of recent memory after bilateral hippocampal lesions. *J. Neurol. Neurosurg. Psychiatry 20*:11-21.
3. Mishkin, M., and Appenzeller, T. (1987). The anatomy of memory. *Sci. Am. 256*:80-89.
4. Penfield, W., and Milner, B. (1958). Memory deficit produced by bilateral lesions in the hippocampal zone. *Arch. Neurol. Psychiatry 79*:475-497.
5. Penfield, W., and Mathieson, G. (1974). An autopsy and a discussion of the role of the hippocampus in experimental recall. *Arch. Neurol. 31*:145-154.
6. Mishkin, M., Spiegler, B.J., Saunders, R.C., and Malamut, B.L. (1982). An animal model of global amnesia. In *Alzheimer's Disease: A Report of Progress*. Edited by S. Corkin et al. Raven Press, New York, pp. 235-247.
7. Milner, B. (1972). Disorders of learning and memory after temporal lobe lesions in man. *Clin. Neurosurg. 19*:421-446.
8. Corkin, S. (1968). Acquisition of motor skill after bilateral medial temporal-lobe excision. *Neuropsychologia 6*:255-264.
9. Hebb, D.O. (1949). *The Organization of Behavior*. John Wiley, New York.
10. Smith, S.J. (1987). Progress on LTP at hippocampal synapses: a post-synaptic Ca2 + trigger for memory storage? *Trends Neurosci. 10*:142-144.
11. Gustafsson, B., and Wigstrom, H. (1988). Physiological mechanisms underlying long-term potentiation. *Trends Neurosci. 11*:156-162.
12. Bliss, T.V.P., and Lomo, T. (1973). Long-lasting potentiation of synaptic transmission in the dentate area of the anaesthetised rabbit following stimulation of the perforant path. *J. Physiol. 232*:331-356.
13. deJonge, M., and Racine, R.J. (1985). The effects of repeated induction of long-term potentiation in the dentate gyrus. *Brain Res. 328*:181-185.
14. Dwyer, B.E., Wasterlain, C.G., Fujikawa, D.G., and Yamada, L. (1986). Brain protein metabolism in epilepsy. In *Advances in Neurology*, Vol. 44. Edited by A.V. Delgado-Escueta, A.A. Ward, Jr., D.M. Woodbury, and R.J. Porter. Raven Press, New York, pp. 903-918.

15. Chevrie, J.J., and Aicardi, J. (1972). Childhood epileptic encephalopathy with slow spike-waves. A statistical study of 80 cases. *Epilepsia 13*:259-271.

16. Alkon, D.L. (1989). Memory storage and neural systems. *Sci. Am. 261*:42-50.

17. Meldrum, B.S., and Corsellis, J.A.N. (1984). Epilepsy. In *Greenfield's Neuropathology*. Edited by H. Adams, J. Corsellis, and L.W. Duchen. pp. 921-950.

18. Margerison, J.H., and Corsellis, J.A.H. (1966). Epilepsy and the temporal lobes. *Brain 89*:499-530.

19. Bouchet, C., and Cazauvieilh, P. (1825). De l'epilepsie consideree dans ses rapports avec l'alienation mentale. *Archives generales de medecine (Paris) 9*:510-542.

20. Olney, J.W., Collins, R.C., and Sloviter, R.S. (1986). Excitotoxic mechanisms of epileptic brain damage. In *Advances in Neurology*, Vol. 44. Edited by A.V. Delgado-Escueta, A.A. Ward, Jr., D.M. Woodbury, and R.J. Porter. Raven Press, New York, pp. 857-877.

21. Borghesi, J.L., and Blume, W.T. (1986). Value of interictal scalp EEG in determining site of seizure origin. XXIst Canadian Congress of Neurological Sciences, London, Ontario, June 24-28.

22. Halgren, E., Wilson, C.L., and Stapleton, J.M. (1985). Human medial temporal-lobe stimulation disrupts both formation and retrieval of recent memories. *Brain Cogn. 4*:287-295.

23. Kapur, H. (1988). *Memory Disorders in Clinical Practice*. Butterworths, London, pp. 182-193.

24. Shandurina, A., and Kalyagina, G. (1979). Dynamics of mental functions in epileptics during electrical stimulation of deep brain structures. *Human Physiol. 5*:764-773.

25. Shandurina, A., Kambarova, D.K., and Kalyagina, G. (1982). Neuropsychological and neurophysiological analysis of different types of amnesia. *Human Physiol. 8*:350-366.

26. Bickford, R.G., Mulder, D.W., Dodge, H.W. Jr., Svien, H.J., and Rome, H.P. (1958). Changes in memory function produced by electrical stimulation of the temporal lobe in man. In *The Brain and Human Behavior*. Edited by H.C. Solomon, S. Cobb, and W. Penfield. Williams & Wilkins, Baltimore, pp. 227-243.

27. Chapman, L.F., Walter, R.D., Markham, C.H., Rand, R.W., and Crandall, P.H. (1967). Memory changes induced by stimulation of hippocampus or amygdala in epilepsy patients with implanted electrodes. *Trans. Am. Neurol. Ass. 92*: 50-56.

28. Halgren, E., Babb, T.L., and Crandall, P.H. (1978). Activity of human hippocampal formation and amygdala neurons during memory testing. *Electroenceph. Clin. Neurophysiol. 45*:585-601.

29. Ojemann, G.A. (1978). Organization of short-term verbal memory in language areas of human cortex: evidence from electrical stimulation. *Brain Language 5*:331-340.

30. Rausch, R., Lieb, J.P., and Crandall, P.H. (1978). Neuropsychologic correlates of depth spike activity in epileptic patients. *Arch. Neurol. 35*:699-705.

31. Mirsky, A., Primac, D., Ajmone Marsan, C., Rosvold, H., and Stevens, J. (1960). A comparison of the psychological test performance of patients with focal and nonfocal epilepsy. *Exp. Neurol. 2*:75-89.

32. Aarts, J.H.P., Binnie, C.D., Smit, A.M., and Wilkins, A.J. (1984). Selective cognitive impairment during focal and generalized epileptiform EEG activity. *Brain 107*:293-308.

33. Geller, M.R., and Geller, A. (1970). Brief amnestic effects of spike wave discharges. *Neurology 20*:380-381.

34. Hutt, S.J., Lee, D., and Ounsted, C. (1963). Digit memory and evoked discharges in four light-sensitive epileptic children. *Dev. Med. Child. Neurol. 5*:559-571.

35. Avoli, M., Gloor, P., Kostopoulos, G., and Gotman, J. (1983). An analysis of penicillin-induced generalized spike and wave discharges using simultaneous recordings of cortical and thalamic single neurons. *J. Neurophysiol. 50*:819-837.

36. Pellegrini, A., and Gloor, P. (1979). Effects of bilateral partial diencephalic lesions in cortical epileptic activity in generalized penicillin epilepsy in the cat. *Exp. Neurol. 66*:285-308.

37. Penfield, W. (1975). *The Mystery of the Mind. A Critical Study of Consciousness and the Human Brain.* Princeton University Press, Princeton.

38. Weingarten, S.M., Cherlow, D.G., and Halgren, E. (1977). Relationship of hallucinations to the depth structures of the temporal lobe. In *Neurosurgical Treatment in Psychiatry, Pain, and Epilepsy.* Edited by W.H. Sweet, S. Obrador and J.G. Martin-Rodriguez. University Park Press, Baltimore, pp. 553-568.

39. Penfield, W., and Jasper, H.H. (1954). *Epilepsy and the Functional Anatomy of the Human Brain.* Little, Brown and Co., Boston.

40. Gloor, P., Olivier, A., Quesney, L.F., Andermann, F., and Horowitz, S. (1982). The role of the limbic system in experiential phenomena of temporal lobe epilepsy. *Ann. Neurol. 12*:129-144.

41. Jones, E.G., and Powell, T.P.S. (1970). An anatomical study of converging sensory pathways within the cerebral cortex of the monkey. *Brain 93*:793-820.

42. Turner, B.H., Mishkin, M., and Knapp, M. (1980). Organization of the amygdalopetal projections from modality-specific cortical association areas in the monkey. *J. Comp. Neurol. 191*:515-543.

43. Penfield, W., and Roberts, L. (1959). *Speech and Brain Mechanisms.* Princeton University Press, Princeton, NJ.

44. Loiseau, P., Strube, E., Broustet, D., Battellochi, S., Gomeni, C., and Morselli, P.L. (1980). Evaluation of memory function in a population of epileptic patients and matched controls. *Acta Neurol. Scand. 80*(Suppl.)*62*:58-61.

45. Loiseau, P., Strube, E., Broustet, D., Battellochi, S., Gomeni, C., and Morselli, P.L. (1983). Learning impairment in epileptic patients. *Epilepsia 24*:183-192.

46. Rey, A. (1970). *L'examen clinique en psychologie.* Paris, Presses Universitaires de France.

47. Glowinski, H. (1973). Cognitive deficits in temporal lobe epilepsy; an investigation of memory functioning. *J. Nerv. Ment. Dis. 157*:129-137.

48. Scott, D., Moffatt, A., Matthews, A., and Ettlinger, G. (1967). The effect of epileptic discharges on learning and memory in patients. *Epilepsia 8*:188-194.

49. Stevens, J., Milstein, V., and Goldstein, S. (1972). Psychometric test performance in relation to the psychopathology of epilepsy. *Arch. Gen. Psychiatry 26*:532-538.

50. Milner, B. (1975). Psychological aspects of focal epilepsy and its neurosurgical management. In *Advances in Neurology,* Vol. 8. Edited by D.P. Purpura, J.K. Penry, and R.D. Walter. Raven Press, New York, pp. 299-321.

51. Dodrill, C.B. (1986). Correlates of generalized tonic-clonic seizures with intellectual, neuropsychological, emotional, and social function in patients with epilepsy. *Epilepsia 27*:399-411.

52. Delaney, R.C., Rosen, A.J., Mattson, R.H., and Novelly, R.A. (1980). Memory function in focal epilepsy: a comparison of nonsurgical unilateral temporal lobe and frontal lobe samples. *Cortex 16*:103-117.

53. Meldrum, B.S., and Brierley, J.B. (1973). Prolonged epileptic seizures in Primates. *Arch. Neurol. 28*:10-17.

54. Ladavas, E., Umilta, C., and Provinciali, L. (1979). Hemisphere-dependent cognitive performances in epileptic patients. *Epilepsia 20*:493-502.

55. Berent, S., Giordani, B., Sackellares, J.C., O'Leary, D., and Boll, T.J. (1983). Cerebrally lateralized epileptogenic foci and performance on a verbal and visual-graphic learning task. *Percept. Motor Skills 56*:991-1001.

56. Milner, B. (1958). Psychological defects produced by temporal lobe excision. *Res. Publ. Ass. Res. Nerv. Ment. Dis. 36*:244-257.

57. Milner, B. (1962). Laterality effects in audition. In *Interhemispheric Relations and Cerebral Dominance*. Edited by V.B. Mountcastle. Johns Hopkins Press, Baltimore.

58. Walsh, K.W. (1978). *Neuropsychology. A Clinical Approach*. Churchill Livingstone, London, pp. 169-201.

59. Hermann, B.P., Wyler, A.R., Richey, E.T., and Rea, J.M. (1987). Memory function and verbal learning ability in patients with complex partial seizures of temporal lobe origin. *Epilepsia 28*:547-554.

60. Milner, B. (1968). Visual recognition and recall after right temporal-lobe excision in man. *Neuropsychologia 6*:191-209.

61. Rey, A. (1942). L'examen psychologique dans les cas d'encephalopathie traumatique. *Arch. Psychol. 28*:No. 112.

62. Osterrieth, P. (1944). Le test de copie d'une figure complexe. *Arch. Psychol. 30*:206-356.

63. Mayeux, R., Brandt, J., Rosen, J., and Benson, D.F. (1980). Interictal memory and language impairment in temporal lobe epilepsy. *Neurology 30*:120-125.

64. Butlin, A.T., Danta, G., and Cook, M.L. (1984). Anticonvulsant effects on the memory performance of epileptics. *Clin. Exp. Neurol. 20*:27-35.

65. Thompson, P.J., and Trimble, M.R. (1983). Anticonvulsant serum levels: relationship to impairments of cognitive functioning. *J. Neurol. Neurosurg. Psychiatry 46*:227-233.

66. Trimble, M.R., and Thompson, P.J. (1984). Sodium valproate and cognitive function. *Epilepsia 25*(Suppl. 1):S60-S64.

67. Andrewes, D.G., Tomlinson, L., Elwes, R.D.C., and Reynolds, E.H. (1984). The influence of carbamazepine and phenytoin on memory and other aspects of cognitive function in new referrals with epilepsy. *Acta Neurol. Scand. 99*:23-30.

68. Thompson, P.J., and Trimble, M.R. (1981). Further studies on anticonvulsant drugs and seizures. *Acta Neurol. Scand. 89*:51-58.

69. Reynolds, E.H., Mattson, R.H., and Gallagher, B.B. (1972). Relationships between serum and cerebrospinal fluid anticonvulsant drug and folic acid concentrations in epileptic patients. *Neurology 22*:841-844.

70. Snaith, R.P., Mehta, S., and Raby, A.H. (1970). Serum folate and vitamin B12 in epileptics with and without mental illness. *Br. J. Psychiatry 116*:179-183.
71. Reynolds, E.H. (1979). Cerebrospinal fluid folate: clinical studies. In *Folic Acid in Neurology, Psychiatry, and Internal Medicine*. Edited by M. Botez and M. Reynolds. Raven Press, New York.
72. Trimble, M.R., Corbett, J., and Donaldson, D. (1980). Folic acid and mental symptoms in children with epilepsy. *J. Neurol. Neurosurg. Psychiatry 43*:1030-1034.
73. Butlin, A.T., Danta, G., and Cook, M.L. (1984). Anticonvulsant folic acid and memory dysfunction in epileptics. *Clin. Exp. Neurol. 20*:57-62.
74. Blumer, D., and Walker, A.E. (1969). Memory in temporal lobe epileptics. In *The Pathology of Memory*. Edited by G. Talland, and N. Waugh. Academic Press, New York, pp. 65-73.
75. Dugan, T.M., Nordgren, R.E., and O'Leary, P. (1981). Transient global amnesia associated with bradycardia and temporal lobe spikes. *Cortex 17*:633-638.
76. Pritchard, P.B., Holmstrom, V.L., Roitzsch, J.C., and Giacinto, J. (1985). Epileptic amnesic attacks: benefit from antiepileptic drugs. *Neurology 35*:1188-1189.
77. Gallassi, R., Morreale, A., Lorusso, S., Pazzaglia, P., and Lugaresi, E. (1988). Epilepsy presenting as memory disturbances. *Epilepsia 29*:624-629.
78. Mayeux, R., Alexander, M.P., Benson, D.F., Brandt, J., and Rosen, J. (1979). Poriomania. *Neurology 29*:1616-1619.
79. Miller, J.W., Yanagihara, T., Petersen, R.C., and Klass, D.W. (1987). Transient global amnesia and epilepsy. *Arch. Neurol. 44*:629-633.
80. Blumer, D., and Benson, D.F. (1982). Psychiatric manifestations of epilepsy. In *Psychiatric Aspects of Neurologic Disease*. Grune and Stratton, New York, pp. 25-48.
81. Lugaresi, E., Pazzaglia, P., and Tassinari, C.A. (1971). Differentiation of "Absence status and temporal lobe status." *Epilepsia 12*:77-87.
82. Mayeux, R., and Lueder, H. (1978). Complex partial status epilepticus. Case report and proposal for diagnostic criteria. *Neurology 28*:957-961.
83. McLachlan, R.S., and Blume, W.T. (1980). Isolated fear in complex partial status epilepticus. *Ann. Neurol. 8*:640-641.
84. Kaibara, M., and Blume, W.T. (1988). The postictal electroencephalogram. *Electroenceph. Clin. Neurophysiol. 70*:99-104.

15

Amnesia Associated With Temporal Lobectomy

Mary Lou Smith

Erindale College
University of Toronto
Mississauga, Ontario, Canada

INTRODUCTION

Our knowledge of the role played by the temporal lobes in memory has been derived largely from the study of patients who have undergone unilateral brain surgery for the relief of medically intractable epilepsy. Horsley (1) first demonstrated that excision of epileptogenic tissue would result in the cessation of seizure activity, and in present neurosurgical practice, more than 80% of all cortical excisions for the treatment of epilepsy are from the temporal lobes (2). Surgery is considered for individuals with complex partial seizures that have proved to be pharmacologically resistent and whose seizure focus can be reliably localized to the anterior temporal lobe in one hemisphere (3-6).

Studies of the outcome of temporal lobectomy have revealed that almost two-thirds of the patients have either no, or very few seizures at follow-up, and that an additional number of patients experience a significant reduction in the number of seizures (2,6-8). Neurological complications are rare and the mortality rates are low (9,10). From a psychological perspective, this population is an ideal one for study because the patients tend to be young (with an average age ranging from the mid-20s to mid-30s) and the operation produces a discrete, well-defined removal. For the most part, the epileptogenic lesions are static and atrophic, dating from birth or early life, although temporal lobectomies are also performed on patients with tumors; in the cases where the tumor is indolent, it has been reported that the cognitive effects of the surgery are similar to those seen with static lesions (11).

321

The typical temporal lobectomy always includes the anterior temporal neocortex, and, in some neurosurgical centers, the amygdala and varying amounts of the hippocampus and parahippocampal gyrus are also removed. The extent of excision from the hippocampal region is often individually tailored, either because of the presence of documented abnormality (12,13) or because of the risk of memory disturbance (13,14). As we shall see later, the appearance or the severity of memory deficits on certain tasks is dependent upon the degree of encroachment of the removal upon the hippocampal region. In those studies reviewed here that examined this factor, the patients had been subdivided into groups according to whether they had small or large hippocampal removals; such classification was based on the surgeon's drawings and report at the time of operation. The excision was considered small if the hippocampus had been either spared entirely or the removal had not exceeded the pes; large hippocampal excisions were those that extended beyond the pes into the body of the hippocampus and/or the parahippocampal gyrus.

With respect to cognitive function, the effects of a unilateral temporal lobectomy are specific. There is no lasting generalized loss in intellectual functioning, at least as measured by standardized tests of intelligence, although there is a transient lowering in IQ ratings seen in the immediate postoperative period. This finding is illustrated in Figure 1, which gives Full Scale IQ Ratings for a group of 116 patients with temporal lobe lesions who were seen for neuropsychological assessments prior to surgery, 14 days postoperatively, and again two or more years after the operation at the Montreal Neurological Institute (15). Before surgery, the intellectual ratings fall within the average range. For patients with either left or right temporal lobectomy, the immediate postoperative effect is a significant decline in Full Scale IQ, but over time, there is recovery to the preoperative level. It has been reported that at follow-up testing in some cases, the overall level of intelligence is significantly improved relative to the baseline obtained preoperatively, an effect presumed to be due to the relief of the widespread, noxious effects of an epileptic focus (16-18).

Against this background of normal intellectual functioning, the patient with a unilateral temporal lobe lesion nonetheless experiences difficulty in the realm of learning and memory. These deficits are often apparent preoperatively, but are exacerbated by the surgery (17,19-24). For the most part, the memory impairments are material-specific in nature as related to the hemisphere of the lesion. In patients with speech representation in the left hemisphere, a left temporal lobectomy results in impairments on tasks of verbal learning and verbal memory, whereas a right temporal lobectomy impairs performance on tasks in which the memoranda are difficult to verbalize. The few exceptions to the finding of material-specific memory disorders

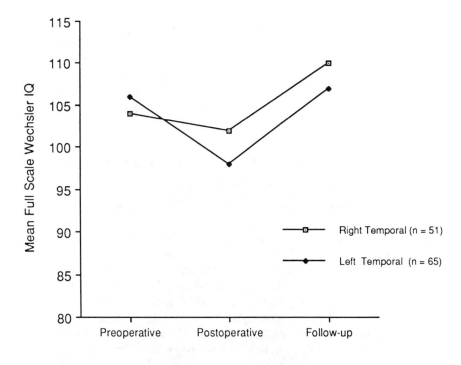

TIME OF TESTING

Figure 1 Graphs showing the Full-Scale Wechsler IQ ratings at three different times of testing. [Postoperative testing took place approximately two weeks after surgery; follow-up assessment was conducted two or more years after surgery.]

generally have been documented in studies in which the tasks contain memoranda that can be processed using either a verbal or a visual code (25-28).

Prevey et al. (29) have investigated metamemory, or knowledge about one's own memory functions, in unoperated patients with focal temporal lobe epilepsy. One of their experiments utilized the feeling of knowing procedure, in which the subjects were asked to predict whether they would be able to recognize the correct answers to general information questions when unable to recall that information. Relative to normal control subject, the seizure patients overestimated their abilities to recognize information presumably stored in long-term memory. A second study examined the patients' knowledge of their own short-term memory span by asking them to estimate the length of a list of words or geometric designs they would be able to recall or reproduce accurately. Their estimated spans were then compared with their actual memory spans. When compared with the control subjects, patients with a left temporal lobe focus tended to overestimate their spans for words, and those with a right temporal lobe focus tended to overestimate their spans for the designs. These results extend previous findings of deficits in memory performance associated with temporal lobe dysfunction to the individual's ability to introspect about his or her actual memory capacity. They also indicate that, even in the realm of metamemory, the memory deficits tend to be of material-specific nature.

THE EFFECT OF LEFT TEMPORAL LOBE LESIONS ON MEMORY

One of the first demonstrations (21) of a deficit in verbal memory in patients with lesions of the left, or dominant, temporal lobe was for the recall of the information contained in the short prose passages of the Logical Memory Subtest of the Wechsler Memory Scale (30). In this task, recall is obtained immediately after the patient has heard each story and again 90 minutes later, the deficit being particularly marked after the delay. The patients forget many of the important details of the stories, recalling sparse and fragmented versions. A similar defect is also seen on the verbal paired-associate learning task of the Wechsler Memory Scale (20,22). Because of the similarity in the results from these two tests, Milner (22) developed a composite score of delayed verbal memory, comprised of the mean number of items correctly recalled from the prose passages plus the number of word associates retained after a delay. Figure 2 shows the composite recall scores for essentially the same group of patients whose IQ ratings had been illustrated earlier (four patients were excluded because of incomplete memory testing). These data demonstrate that lesions in the left temporal lobe produce a postoperative decline in ability to retain verbal information.

Although the patients in whom the lesion invades the temporal lobe of the left hemisphere show some recovery of function over time, two or more years after surgery their verbal recall scores remain significantly depressed relative to their preoperative scores. This evidence for a residual impairment in verbal recall represents a specific cognitive defect, contrasting both with the recovery in general intelligence seen over the same time span, and with the normal verbal memory of patients with similar lesions in the right hemisphere, a finding also illustrated in Figure 2.

The role of the left temporal lobe in verbal memory has been demonstrated in many centers and with a variety of learning and memory tasks. Not only is the deficit apparent with information presented in the auditory modality (20-24,31); it is elicited also under conditions of visual presentation (22,32). The finding of the impairment has been extended to other story-learning tasks (33), and to learning and recalling lists of words (23,24,27,34-36), even when the words are drawn from a restricted number of categories. Similarly,

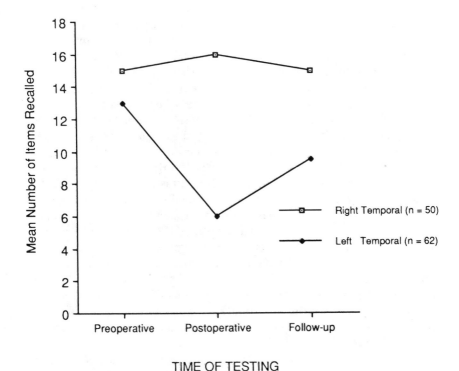

TIME OF TESTING

Figure 2 Graphs showing the mean number of items recalled on a verbal memory test as related to time of assessment. [Postoperative testing took place approximately two weeks after surgery; follow-up assessment was conducted two or more years after surgery.]

deficits are seen for the recall of the names of pictured objects (37-39) or the names of toy models of objects (40). The deficits are not specific to a particular method of testing, as they are found in recognition as well as recall paradigms (32,34).

It is true that the defect in verbal memory is not the only impairment exhibited by patients with lesions of the left temporal lobe. Mild impairments have also been noted on selected verbal subtests of the Wechsler Adult intelligence Scale (23,24), and on verbal perceptual tasks, such as identifying digits presented by dichotic listening techniques (41), and on speed reading comprehension tasks (22). Nonetheless, it has also been true that the difficulty in retaining verbal material is disproportionate to the deficits on these other types of tasks. For this reason, several investigations have been aimed at trying to uncover the mechanisms underlying the memory impairment.

Along this line, one approach has drawn on the work with normal subjects showing the interdependence of memory and other cognitive processes. For example, it has been demonstrated that the organization inherent in stimulus material influences the subsequent recall of that material (42,43), and furthermore, that when subjects impose their own organization on otherwise unorganized material, recall is also enhanced (44-46). Such findings have raised the question of whether the verbal memory impairment of patients with left temporal lobe lesions is associated with a corresponding impairment in cognitive organization. Several studies bearing on this question have yielded mixed results. For example, a reduction in clustering during recall of taxonomically organized (47,48) or of associatively organized words (49) has been found after left temporal lobectomy. In contrast, Incisa della Rocchetta (37) demonstrated that left temporal lobectomy does not impair the ability to sort pictures of objects into inappropriate taxonomic categories, although it does impair the ability to recall later the names of those pictures. Such patients also show the normal pattern of recalling more words from a taxonomically organized list than from a nonorganized list (47,49). The benefit derived from such organization was not sufficient to compensate for the verbal memory impairment; patients with left temporal lobe lesions still recalled fewer words from the taxonomically organized list than did normal control subjects, and also failed to improve their learning scores across trials at a normal level (47).

In the experiments mentioned above, the material to be remembered contained a preimposed organization. With a different kind of task, one that contained no inherent organization of the material but which made demands of the patients to impose subjective organization, Jaccarino-Hiatt (47) found that lists of unrelated words were sorted into fewer categories than were designs by patients with left temporal lobe lesions; the opposite pattern of results was seen in patients with right temporal lobe lesions, whereas normal control subjects sorted an equal number of categories for both types of stimuli. For the patient groups, however, no correlation was found between the number of categories sorted and the number of items later recalled. Thus, the evidence relating the verbal memory impairment to deficits in cognitive organization is inconclusive, and any such cognitive impairments are mild in comparison to the impoverished verbal recall associated with left temporal lobectomy.

The previously described experiments emphasized learning and retention in the realm of episodic memory, or memory for unique, specific, personally experienced events (50). Wilkins and Moscovitch (51) investigated the possibility that semantic memory, the system involving memory for general principles, facts, and associations (50), is also impaired after anterior temporal lobectomy. Two classification tasks were used, one in which patients were asked to classify common objects (represented by drawings or words) as larger or smaller than a chair, and the other requiring a decision as to whether objects were living or manmade. Patients with right temporal lobe lesions performed normally on both tasks, but those with left temporal lobe lesions were impaired on the living/manmade classification. The authors suggested that left temporal lobectomy disrupts the semantic memory systems that involve verbal or lexical representations. They also emphasized, however, that the observed semantic deficits appeared to be mild relative to the deficits in episodic memory seen in such patient groups.

Another aspect of cognitive functioning that has been investigated in relation to the verbal memory impairment is the type of emphasis given to the memoranda at the time of encoding. In normal subjects, orienting tasks involving semantic aspects of words result in better recall than do tasks that draw attention to phonemic or physical aspects (52). Rains (53) hypothesized that if defective encoding formed the basis of the deficit in verbal memory, then the recall and recognition performance of patients with left temporal lobe lesions should show a different relationship to the depth of processing than that seen in normal subjects. He used an incidental learning task adapted from Craik and Tulving (54), which varied the type of encoding performed on each word in a list and then tested the recall and recognition of the previously processed words. During presentation, each word was preceded by a question that emphasized either the semantic aspects, the phonemic aspects, or the physical structure of the word. The results indicated that left temporal lobectomy produced the expected verbal memory impairment, reflected in an overall lower level of recall and recognition of the words, but that the patients nonetheless showed the normal pattern of deriving benefit from semantic encoding. This finding suggested to Rains, and corroborated the point made earlier by Wilkins and Moscovitch (51), that impairment of the semantic memory system per se cannot account for the extent of the verbal memory impairment.

Despite showing a benefit of semantic encoding, the patients with left temporal lobe lesions in Rains' study showed no advantage in recall of phonemic over physical encoding. A similar deficit in the use of phonemic features to aid recall was obtained by Read (27; see also 55) on a variant of the Slamecka and Graf (56) word-generation task, in which subjects had to generate words on the basis of either semantic (e.g., a synonym—BIG: LARGE), or phonetic cues (e.g., a rhyme—RICE: NICE). Immediately after generating a list of words, patients with left temporal lobe lesions were impaired in recalling the rhymes, whereas an impairment for the recall of synonyms appeared only in a delayed recall (24 h) condition. Taken together, the results of Rains and Read provide evidence that the left temporal lobe is specialized for the encoding and/or utilization of phonemic information for subsequent recall of verbal material.

Recently, attention has once again been focused on the severe impairment in story recall evident in patients with left temporal lobe dysfunction. Their recall tends to be sparse, containing only a few details often not given in the order in which these facts had appeared in the original story. This poor quality of recall led Frisk (57) to ask whether the underlying basis of the impairment was an inability to integrate information contained in the sentences comprising the text. For this reason, she varied the textual continuity inherent in prose passages by using stories presented either in the normal fashion, or in a scrambled fashion, where the order of the sentences was randomized. Frisk hypothesized that if patients with left temporal lobe lesions did have a deficit in integration, their recall would be less severely affected by the scrambling manipulation than would that of normal subjects. The results indicated, however, that recall of scrambled text was poor for all groups, but that there was no interaction between group and type of story. On this basis, poor integration had to be ruled out as a major source contributing to the impairment in recall. One other feature of this experiment emphasized the severity of the verbal memory deficit; Frisk found that cuing recall with specific questions about the content of the story did not compensate totally for the inability of the left temporal lobe group to remember the details that they had heard.

Frisk then suggested that these patients may have difficulty with the initial assimilation of the content of stories due to a reduction in working memory capacity. Working memory is considered to be a limited-capacity system that carries out both processing and storage functions simultaneously (58,59). She tested this hypothesis by measuring working memory capacity with a span test modeled after that of Daneman and Carpenter (60). Subjects had to listen to a group of sentences and decide whether each was true or false; after hearing the entire group (ranging from two to seven sentences), they attempted to recall the final word from each sentence. The patients were tested at three times: preoperatively, 3 to 5 days postoperatively, and 14 to 17 days postoperatively. A transient decline in working memory capacity was found for patients with left temporal lobe excisions only when they were tested 3 to 5 days after surgery. These same patients did not differ from control subjects in the preoperative period nor 14 to 17 days postoperatively, even though their verbal memory deficits were evident on story-recall tasks at both these times.

Finally, Frisk examined the effects of left temporal lobectomy on one other variable that influences the initial processing of stories: the rate at which verbal material is processed. Rate of processing was manipulated by presenting words, sentences, or stories at slow, normal, and fast reading rates (2, 5, and 8 words per second, respectively). The subjects were required to make lexical decisions about the words, plausibility judgements to the sentences, and to respond true or false to statements based on information contained in the stories. If the impairment in story recall seen in patients with left temporal lobe lesions was secondary to an inability to process material at a normal rate, then their performance was expected to be deficient on these tasks when the information was presented at normal or fast rates. The results did not support this prediction; the left temporal-lobe group did not differ from normal control subjects or patients with unilateral frontal or right temporal lobe lesions.

Thus, attempts to delineate the factors underlying the impairment in verbal memory have yielded clues to the function of the left temporal lobe, but have left unanswered questions. The implications of a poor verbal memory for the person with left temporal lobe dysfunction are important, for the deficit often proves to be troublesome in everyday living. Milner (20) has described examples of difficulty experienced with a variety of activities, ranging from formal studies to handling the give and take of demanding conversation. Attempts to compensate for such impairments are often made with techniques such as keeping notes as reminders. Jones (61) demonstrated that patients with left temporal lobe lesions can use visual imagery to improve their performance on verbal paired-associate learning tasks, although not to normal levels.

THE EFFECT OF RIGHT TEMPORAL-LOBE LESIONS ON MEMORY

The verbal learning and verbal memory tasks described above, on which performance is so sensitive to the effects of left temporal lobectomy, are accomplished normally by patients with comparable lesions in the right hemisphere. The right, nondominant temporal lobe, like the left, is specialized in function for memory, but for memoranda that are not easily verbalized or coded into words. As was the case for the memory deficits characteristic of left temporal lobe lesions, the nonverbal memory impairments associated with temporal lobectomy on the right are not modality-specific, and have been demonstrated for information presented via the auditory (62), visual (63-65), and tactile senses (36,66).

Right temporal lobectomy impairs the recall of geometric designs as long as they do not lend themselves easily to the use of verbal mnemonics to aid recall (26,67,68). These deficits are evident even though the patients are able to copy the designs accurately and do not show distortions or neglect in their drawings. Furthermore, the impairment in memory for designs is not restricted to free recall by drawing, but is also seen when the task requires the subject to learn to recognize abstract figures that recur throughout a long list (63).

Abstract designs are not the only stimuli that can elicit the visual memory deficit associated with right temporal lobectomy. Faces also represent the kind of complex visual pattern resistent to accurate verbal coding. Milner (65) demonstrated that when patients with right anterior temporal lobe lesions are asked to study a set of photographs of faces and after a short delay are required to choose faces from among a larger array, they show pronounced failure of recognition.

Thus far, it has been emphasized that the memory functions of the right temporal lobe are specific for material that is essentially nonverbal in nature. The contribution of this area to visual memory has been emphasized in a different context by Jaccarino (38), in a study in which she presented line drawings of common objects, one at a time, in varying order over several trials. Immediately after the final trial, and again 24 hours later, the subjects were required to name from memory as many of the pictures as possible. In immediate recall, a mild impairment was evident for patients with left temporal lobe lesions, whereas, as expected, patients with right temporal lobe lesions performed as well as the normal control subjects. Twenty-four hours later, however, both groups of patients showed a marked deficit in recall. Jaccarino interpreted these results as emphasizing the duality of memory processing, the notion that in many circumstances, both a verbal and an imaginal code are used to mediate recall (69). In this instance she presumed that the verbal code was sufficient for the initial recall of the pictures, but that recall after a long delay has also an important visual component.

Further evidence of the role of the right temporal lobe in the recall of material that can be dually encoded is provided by the work of Jones-Gotman (70) and Jones-Gotman and Milner (71) on image-mediated verbal learning. Patients who have undergone right temporal lobectomy are indistinguishable from normal control subjects in learning lists of single words or word pairs when verbal mediational strategies are emphasized. In contrast, when visual imagery is used as a learning strategy, these same patients are impaired. They have no difficulty in generating appropriate images, and, in fact, in certain conditions showed normal recall immediately after learning the list, with the deficits emerging only after a delay (70). These findings suggest that the images became less accessible over time so that the critical fault lay in the re-evocation of the images from memory.

Beatty et al. (72) studied remote memory for visuospatial information in a patient who had undergone a radical right temporal lobectomy for treatment of a glioblastoma. Despite having deficits in several cognitive domains, including visual perception and anterograde memory, she did have access to previously acquired geographical knowledge. Although the clinical features of this patient may not be what are typically seen after right temporal lobectomy, Beatty and his colleagues interpret their findings as suggesting that the right temporal lobe is not required for the retrieval of remotely encoded spatial information. With respect to the retention of new spatial memories, however, there is convincing evidence to show that the structures of the right temporal lobe do contribute. Memory tasks with a spatial component have consistently been shown to elicit deficits after right temporal lobectomy. Thus, impairments are seen in maze learning, whether it be in the visual (65) or tactual modality (66), in the recall of simple position, again for information presented either visually (31) or tactually (36), in spatial conditional associative learning (73) and in the recall of the locations of small objects in a visually presented array (40,74). An important feature of these tasks is that either the very presence of a deficit or the degree of severity of the deficit is related to the extent to which the lesion encroaches upon the hippocampal region. The spatial memory deficit associated with lesions of the right temporal lobe will be discussed in more depth in the following section.

HIPPOCAMPAL CONTRIBUTIONS TO MEMORY

In 1957, Scoville and Milner (75) reported the now famous case of HM, a young man who had undergone bilateral medial temporal lobe removal for the relief of intractable seizures. The resection was said to have extended back 8 cm along the medial surface of both temporal lobes, destroying the amygdala, the uncus, and the anterior two-thirds of the hippocampus and the parahippocampal gyrus, but sparing the lateral neocortex. The surgery left HM with a severe, global anterograde amnesia, the characteristics of which have been extensively studied over the past 30 years (75-78).

The amnesia documented in HM focused attention on the contribution of the hippocampus to memory, and led to the question of whether the material-specific impairments observed after unilateral temporal lobectomy are contingent upon encroachment of the lesion into the hippocampal region. This possibility was first examined systematically by Corsi (31, reported also in 39,79), using formally similar verbal and nonverbal learning and memory tasks. One such set of tasks required the learning of supraspan sequences. The verbal version of these learning tasks was the Hebb (80) recurring digits test, for which Corsi devised a nonverbal analog, a block-tapping test, in which the subject must tap out a series of blocks, repeating exactly a sequence demonstrated by an examiner. In these tasks, each sequence exceeds by one digit or block, respectively, the subject's immediate memory span. Each task consists of 24 sequences in total, with the same sequence repeating every third trial (a feature of which the subject is not informed), while the intervening sequences occur only once. Under these conditions, normal subjects show learning of the recurrent sequence, while continuing to make errors on the nonrecurrent sequences (31,39,80,81).

Although unilateral temporal lobectomy did not impair immediate memory span for either the digit or block sequence, Corsi demonstrated a double dissociation in the effects of left and right temporal lobe lesions on the performance of these tasks, with deficits on the verbal version being seen only after left temporal lobectomy, and deficits on the nonverbal version seen only after right temporal lobectomy. More importantly, when he divided the patients into four groups based on the extent of hippocampal removal, he found that the degree of impairment was proportional to the size of the hippocampal lesion. Milner (39) subsequently demonstrated that these sequence-learning tasks can also be used to detect hippocampal dysfunction in patients tested preoperatively.

This relationship between the size of the hippocampal lesion and the severity of the memory deficit so clearly demonstrated by Corsi does not, however, hold true for all tests of memory. Performance on many of the tasks described earlier in the discussion of the memory disorders associated with left or right temporal lobectomy is not sensitive to the effects of hippocampal dysfunction. For certain tasks, a lesion of the lateral neocortex alone is sufficient to bring out the impairment, and that impairment is not exacerbated further by excision from the hippocampal region.

Examination of the tasks on which deficits are or are not contingent upon degree of medial temporal lobe damage does not yield a simple explanation of the particular contribution of the hippocampus to memory. Lateral neocortical lesions in the left temporal lobe are sufficient to produce the impairment in recall of stories (22,82), in the recall of words generated as rhymes (27, and cited in 55), and in the recall of the names of pictured (37) or real objects (40). Lateral right temporal lobe lesions impair performance on the recall of complex geometric designs (68), and on the recognition of faces (65), recurring nonsense figures (63), and unfamiliar tonal melodies (28). The hippocampus appears to contribute when the tasks require sequence learning (31) or when the material to be remembered lacks intrinsic structure (83), such as consonant trigrams (31), or a complex geometric design presented in a piecemeal fashion so that its organization is not apparent (67). Furthermore, hippocampal lesions have been associated with reduced primacy effects, both for lists of words (27) and lists of designs (26).

A number of possible explanations of the role of the hippocampus in memory have been proposed. One such view, put forth to explain the findings in both animal and human subjects, is that the hippocampus functions to reduce interference (31,70,71,84). This hypothesis is not satisfactory, however, in that a number of memory tasks which contain large series of stimuli and hence seem open to considerable interference effects have been shown not to be sensitive to hippocampal dysfunction (63,67). Another view has been that the hippocampus is necessary for the organization of unstructured material in memory, a suggestion that again can account for some (47,67), but not all findings (31,36,70). To date, there has not been one explanation that has been successful in accounting for all the results.

Milner (55) points out that the differential effects of left and right hippocampal lesions on verbal and visuospatial memory, and the diversity of tasks in which the hippocampus is implicated probably do not result from a particular specialization of the hippocampus per se, but are a reflection of the connections between the hippocampal structures and widespread areas of the ipsilateral neocortex (85-91). Thus, the hippocampal region may be part of a memory circuit involving a variety of cortical systems (77,92-96). By this view, for tasks on which a temporal neocortical lesion is sufficient to impair performance, additional damage to the hippocampal structures would not increase the severity of the impairment. If, however, successful performance on a task with a memory component requires a cortical area other than the temporal lobe, a deficit would be expected after damage to the hippocampal region because of the interruption of the critical memory circuit involving that part of the cortex.

One consistent finding with respect to the functions of the hippocampal region in the right hemisphere is that this area is implicated in spatial learning and spatial memory. This function was first noted in 1965, when Corkin (66) and Milner (65) published their papers on stylus maze-learning in the tactual and visual modalities, respectively. Patients with right temporal lobe lesions were impaired in learning the correct path through the maze relative to patients with left temporal lobe lesions or normal control subjects. When the right temporal lobe group was subdivided into those with little or no involvement of the hippocampus in the removal, and those with radical excisions of this structure, the results indicated that the impairment was contingent upon the inclusion of a large part of the hippocampus in the excision. As described earlier, Corsi (31) was able to demonstrate, using his recurring block-sequence task, an impairment in spatial learning that was dependent upon the extent of damage to the right hippocampal region. Performance on a spatial conditional associative learning task has also been demonstrated to be sensitive to extensive right hippocampal damage (73).

In his series of experiments, Corsi (31) also included a task requiring the memorization of the location of a dot positioned along an eight-inch line, and again found a deficit related to right hippocampal damage. Later, Rains (36) demonstrated a similar impairment in memory for simple position, but for spatial information derived from touch, instead of by vision. The similarity in the findings, like that seen in the Corkin (66) and Milner (65) studies on maze-learning, emphasizes that the important aspect of the task that is sensitive to the function of the right hippocampus is the spatial nature of the memoranda and not the modality of presentation.

Smith and Milner (40,74) examined the right hippocampal contribution to spatial memory using more complicated materials and with demands closer to those imposed in everyday life. Instead of requiring their subjects to remember the position of a single, meaningless stimulus like a dot on a line, they employed arrays of a real objects, in which not only the absolute location, but also the relative location of each object was important. The results from a series of experiments showed that patients with right temporal lobe lesions that included radical hippocampal excisions showed normal ability to recall the locations of objects immediately after viewing the array, but were impaired when recall was tested after a delay as short as four minutes. This contrast in performance suggests that despite a normal ability to encode location, the patients with large right hippocampal lesions are susceptible to rapid forgetting of that information.

Although the above results do suggest a contribution by the right hippocampal region specifically to the learning and recall of spatial memoranda, there are other findings that do not fit the notion of such a complete specialization. Impairments in the retrieval of visual information to mediate verbal recall have been found to be related to the extent of right hippocampal damage (40,70,71). As well, certain requirements of design learning and recall tasks have been demonstrated to elicit deficits in patients with radical right hippocampal lesions (26,67). For example, in a study examining both the learning of and memory for a list of abstract designs, Jones-Gotman (26) found that patients with either large or small hippocampal lesions were impaired in terms of the number of learning trials taken to reach criterion, but that the accuracy of the drawings reproduced across the learning trials was reduced only in the group with the large hippocampal excisions. Furthermore, Jones-Gotman (67) demonstrated that presenting a complex drawing for copy in a piecemeal form results in an impairment directly related to the extent of right hippocampal removal, whereas a similar design presented in an organized fashion yields a deficit that is not related to the size of the hippocampal lesion.

Attempting to assign a role specifically to the hippocampus is difficult because the lesions in the patients in whom these impairments have been demonstrated also include the amygdala, together with varying amounts of the parahippocampal gyrus and the anterior temporal neocortex. Whether such impairments would be found if the lesions were to be restricted to the hippocampus remains to be seen. There is considerable evidence from work in monkeys that the amygdala makes a significant contribution to memory (97,98), and that combined lesions of the amygdala and hippocampus are necessary to produce severe impairments on certain memory tasks (99). However, a recently reported clinicopathological case study has demonstrated that amnesia can result from a lesion confined to the hippocampus. Zola-Morgan et al. (100) extensively examined a patient, RB, who developed an anterograde amnesia after an ischemic episode. Five years after the onset of amnesia, RB died. Histological examination revealed a bilateral circumscribed lesion in the CA1 field of the hippocampus, with sparing of the other medial temporal lobe regions.

THE SODIUM AMYTAL TEST FOR MEMORY

Sodium amytal was first used as a method of investigating hemispheric function by Juhn Wada (101,102) in his studies of the mechanisms underlying the spread of epileptic discharge between the cerebral hemispheres in man. Intra-carotid injection of sodium amytal produces a transient loss of function in the ipsilateral hemisphere, a property that led to the appreciation of this method as a test for determining the lateralization of cerebral speech domi-nance. Injection of the dominant hemisphere results in a variety of aphasic symptoms, including speech arrest, dysnomia, comprehension deficits, and difficulty on verbal serial ordering tasks such as counting or reciting the days of the week, whereas injection of the nondominant hemisphere does not cause interference with speech (103-105).

A few years after the adoption of the sodium amytal procedure for assessing speech lateralization, it was realized that the procedure could also yield valu-able information regarding memory function. The need for a preoperative assessment of the risk of global memory deficit following unilateral temporal lobectomy became evident with the appearance of rare cases in which uni-lateral anterior temporal lobectomy (including the amygdala and hippocampus) produced a global and persistent amnesic syndrome. One such case, reported by Penfield and Milner in 1958 (106), was the patient PB, who underwent a two-stage removal from the left temporal region. During the first operation, the anterior 4 cm of the temporal lobe were excised, but the hippocampal region was left intact. The postoperative phase was marked by only a brief period of dysphasia. Five years later, because PB was still having seizures, a second operation was undertaken, in which the excision was extended to in-clude the uncus, amygdala, and hippocampus. This procedure was not fol-lowed by any aphasia, but there was a serious and generalized loss of recent memory, an anterograde amnesia that persisted for the remainder of PB's life.

To explain the appearance of this amnesia, Penfield and Milner hypothe-sized that there had been an additional, and possibly more extensive lesion in the hippocampal region in the right hemisphere. Essentially, then, the removal of the epileptogenic but still partially functioning hippocampus on the side of operation deprived the patient of hippocampal function bilaterally. Several years later, PB died of a pulmonary embolism, and this hypothesis was confirmed by the findings on autopsy (107). Examination of the brain indicated that approximately 22 mm of the left posterior hippocampus remained. On the right, the lateral neocortex and the amygdala appeared normal; in contrast, the right hippocampus was shrunken and histologic studies revealed dense gliosis in the pyramidal cell layer and to a lesser extent, in the dentate gyrus.

The findings in this, and a few other such cases, led Milner et al. (108) to use the technique of intracarotid injection of sodium amytal as a safeguard against the risk of severe memory loss after unilateral removal of the hippo-campus. The rationale of the test is as follows: the procedure allows the as-sessment of memory in patients temporarily deprived of the functions of most of one hemisphere by the action of the drug. Inactivation of one temporal lobe should not in itself provoke a generalized amnesia, so that a global memory loss is not expected after unilateral injection unless there is a hippocampal lesion in the opposite hemisphere. If there were such a lesion, a transient generalized memory disorder characteristic of the amnesia seen in patients with bilateral medial temporal-lobe damage should be seen (17,39). It is important to stress that the transient amnesia is expected to be a generalized one, and not be be of a material-specific nature. The critical test is one for anterograde amnesia, or failure to remember material presented while the functions of the hemisphere are inactivated by the amytal, not material present before the injection.

The assessment of memory using the intracarotid amytal procedure is limited by the short-acting nature of the drug, which necessitates the use of simple tests. There is no standardized protocol in existence, and the actual procedure used varied widely from center to center (39,109-114). At the Montreal Neurological Institute, where amytal memory testing was pioneered, the patient is presented with five items while under the effect of the drug: two line drawings of objects, a real object, a simple sentence, and a concrete word (see Refs. 14,17, and 39 for complete details of the test procedure). After the drug has worn off, and speech functions have returned to baseline levels (when the injection is made into the dominant hemisphere), the patient is first tested for recall of these items, and if necessary, for recognition using multiple-choice procedures. The time between the presentation of the stimuli and the memory test varies somewhat from case to case, but averages approximately 10 minutes. The criterion for significant memory impairment is taken as two or more errors of recognition.

In a retrospective study (115) of patients seen at the Montreal Neurological Hospital between 1979 and 1984, 116 cases with temporal lobe lesions were identified who had had sodium amytal tests of both hemispheres, and in whom the results of both tests were unambiguous. Of these cases, 59 had a clearly defined epileptic focus in the left temporal lobe, 37 had a right temporal lobe focus, and 20 had epileptic activity occurring independently in both temporal lobes. In patients with a clear, unilateral focus, injection of the hemisphere contralateral to the lesion was associated with a significantly higher failure rate (41%) than injection of the ipsilateral hemisphere (15%). This pattern of findings replicates the results reported earlier by Milner (17, 39) with a similar group of patients, and using an earlier form of the memory test that contained only three items. The data also demonstrated that when there was dysfunction in both temporal lobes, the side of injection had no significant bearing on the incidence of memory impairment. The incidence of anterograde amnesia after injection to the hemisphere ipsilateral to the planned operation was 50%, and after contralateral injection was 60%. Patients in whom there is evidence of bitemporal lobe dysfunction are especially at risk for memory loss after unilateral temporal lobectomy, and the results of amytal memory testing can be used by the surgeon as an indication of whether to spare the hippocampus and parahippocampal gyrus in the temporal lobe removal.

In recent years, the issue of the reliability of the sodium amytal technique as a test for memory has been raised. The reliability question came out of reports based on relatively small series of patients who had repeat sodium amytal tests; in certain cases the second test yielded different conclusions than had the first. Novelly (116) reported that 12 of 18 patients who failed the memory test after injection ipsilateral to the seizure focus were found not be have impaired memory when retested. Dinner et al. (117) found improvements in memory scores on retesting ranging from 9% to 66% in five patients.

Findings such as these led McGlone and MacDonald (118) to conduct two retrospective studies on the reliability of a sodium amytal procedure adapted from that of Milner (39). The first study examined alternate form reliability by evaluating the results from 13 patients who underwent the procedure more than one time (representing a total of 23 repeat injections). Changes in the conclusions drawn from the memory tests were made only in cases where the procedure had been repeated because of technical problems with the first injection, or where the patients had undergone functional deterioration over the period between the tests. Of 13 injections repeated to reinvestigate memory or speech, 12 yielded the same outcome as that obtained from the first test.

McGlone and McDonald's second study was conducted to follow-up Dinner et al.'s (117) suggestion that the improvement in memory scores seen with the repeat test in their series may have been due to a practice effect. McGlone and McDonald found that in a group of 70 patients who had received sodium amytal tests of both hemispheres, there was no evidence of a practice effect or of transfer of learning, when performance for the side tested first was compared with that for the side tested second. Thus, McGlone and MacDonald's findings suggest that the sodium amytal technique is a reliable test for memory when examined from the perspective of alternate forms and test-retest criteria.

A new approach to memory testing with sodium amytal has recently been developed at the Mayo Clinic by Jack et al. (119). Instead of injecting the sodium amytal into the internal carotid artery, this group introduces the drug into the posterior cerebral artery. The rationale for their approach lies in the nature of the blood supply to the medial temporal lobe region. Only the amygdala, uncus, and the anteriormost portion of the hippocampus receive their arterial supply via the internal carotid artery, while the majority of the hippocampal formation and the parahippocampal gyrus is fed from the posterior cerebral artery. Thus, selective injection of sodium amytal into the posterior cerebral artery selectively anesthetizes the medial temporal region, unlike injection into the internal carotid, which anesthetizes much of the lateral aspect of the hemisphere, but only the anterior part of the hippocampus. Injection into the posterior cerebral artery does not produce any aphasic symptoms or alterations in mental status, thereby circumventing the problems of interpretation that may arise from these symptoms which are often associated with the traditional internal carotid approach. Jack et al. suggest that their technique may be more useful than the traditional internal carotid approach due to this combination of anatomic, functional, and practical reasons.

Rausch (120) surveyed participants about the validity and utility of the memory test in a workshop on the sodium amytal procedure at a conference on the surgical treatment of epilepsy. No cases of persistent amnesia after temporal lobectomy were reported among patients who had "passed" the memory test. One case was described who had "failed" and became amnesic after undergoing a selective amygdalohippocampectomy. However, one center reported that two patients who had "failed" subsequently underwent temporal lobectomy and did not develop amnesia. A major problem in evaluating such results is the failure to use a standardized memory test and a lack of consensus on the criteria to define a pass or a failure.

CONCLUSIONS

In 1900 Bekhterev (121) reported on a case of severe memory impairment; on autopsy, the brain of this patient was found to have bilateral abnormalities in the uncus, hippocampus, and adjoining medial temporal cortex. This was the first evidence that the temporal lobes have a specialized role in memory. Since the 1950s, the specific contributions of the temporal lobes to memory has been rigorously investigated in patients undergoing surgery for epilepsy.

The reader will appreciate that the title "Amnesia associated with temporal lobectomy" is accurate only in a relative sense. Patients with unilateral temporal-lobe lesions do have "amnesia," but their memory disorders are not global, and their nature (verbal or nonverbal) is governed by the specialization of the lesioned hemisphere. These memory impairments are mild in comparison to many of the amnesias seen as a consequence of the neuropsychiatric disorders described elsewhere in this volume. Nonetheless, the study of the memory disorders associated with temporal lobectomy has uncovered much of the function of the temporal neocortex and the medial temporal structures in memory. These investigations have also highlighted the interactive nature of the hippocampus with widespread areas of the neocortex in memory processing. The sodium amytal procedure for testing memory, devised as a clinical instrument to avoid amnesia after unilateral removal of the temporal lobe and the hippocampal region, has provided corroborating evidence of the importance of these anatomical structures for memory.

ACKNOWLEDGMENTS

The author acknowledges the support of an operating grant from the Natural Sciences and Engineering Research Council. Barbara Gilstrap kindly helped in the preparation of the manuscript.

REFERENCES

1. Horsley, V. (1986). Brain surgery. *Br. Med. J. 2*:670-675.
2. Engle, J. Jr. (Ed.) (1987). *Surgical Treatment of the Epilepsies*. Raven Press, New York.
3. Andermann, F. (1987). Identification of candidates for surgical treatment of epilepsy. In *Surgical Treatment of the Epilepsies*. Edited by J. Engel Jr. Raven Press, New York, pp. 51-70.
4. Gumnit, R.J. (1987). Postscript: Who should be referred for surgery? In *Surgical Treatment of the Epilepsies*. Edited by J. Engel Jr. Raven Press, New York, pp. 71-74.
5. McNaughton, F.L., and Rasmussen, T. (1975). Criteria for the selection of patients for neurosurgical treatment. In *Advances in Neurology*, Vol. 8, *Neurosurgical Measurement of the Epilepsies*. Edited by D.P. Purpura, J.K. Penry, and R.D. Walter. Raven Press, New York, pp. 37-48.
6. Ojemann, G.A. (1987). Surgical therapy for medically intractable epilepsy. *J. Neurosurg. 66*:489-499.
7. Penfield, W., and Baldwin, M. (1952). Temporal lobe seizures and the technique of subtotal temporal lobectomy. *Ann. Surg. 136*:625-634.
8. Spencer, D.D. (1987). Postscript: Should there be a surgical treatment of choice, and if so, how should it be determined? In *Surgical Treatment of the Epilepsies*. Edited by J. Engel Jr. Raven Press, New York, pp. 477-484.
9. Rasmussen, T. (1979). Cortical resection for medically refractory focal epilepsy: Results, lessons and questions. In *Functional Neurosurgery*. Edited by T. Rasmussen and R. Marino. Raven Press, New York, pp. 253-269.
10. Van Buren, J.M. (1987). Complications of surgical procedures in the diagnosis and treatment of epilepsy. In *Surgical Treatment of the Epilepsies*. Edited by J. Engel, Jr. Raven Press, New York, pp. 465-475.
11. Cavazzuti, V., Winston, K., Baker, R., and Welch, K. (1980). Psychological changes following surgery for tumors in the temporal lobe. *J. Neurosurg. 53*: 618-626.
12. Crandall, P.H. (1987). Cortical resections. In *Surgical Treatment of the Epilepsies*. Edited by J. Engel, Jr., Raven Press, New York, pp. 377-404.
13. Olivier, A. (1987). Commentary: Cortical resections. In *Surgical Treatment of the Epilepsies*. Edited by J. Engel, Jr. Raven Press, New York, pp. 405-418.

14. Jones-Gotman, M. (1987). Psychological evaluation: Testing hippocampal function. In *Surgical Treatment of the Epilepsies*. Edited by J. Engel, Jr. Raven Press, New York, pp. 203-211, 1987.
15. Smith, M.L., and Milner, B. (1984). Residual memory deficits after unilateral cerebral excision. Paper presented at the annual meeting of the International Neuropsychology Symposium, Beaune.
16. Blakemore, C.B., Ettlinger, G., and Falconer, M.A. (1966). Cognitive abilities in relation to frequency of seizures and neuropathology of the temporal lobes in man. *J. Neurol. Neurosurg. Psychiatry 29*:268-272.
17. Milner, B. (1975). Psychological aspects of focal epilepsy and its neurosurgical management. In *Advances in Neurology*, Vol. 8. Edited by D.P. Purpura, J.K. Penry, and R.D. Walter. Raven Press, New York, pp. 299-321.
18. Novelly, R.A., Augustine, E.A., Mattson, R.H., Glaser, G.H., Williamson, P.D., Spencer, D.D., and Spencer, S.S. (1984). Selective memory improvement and impairment in temporal lobectomy for epilepsy. *Ann. Neurol. 15*:64-67.
19. Fedio, P., and Mirsky, A.F. (1969). Selective intellectual deficits in children with temporal-lobe or centrencephalic epilepsy. *Neuropsychologia 7*:276-300.
20. Meyer, V., and Yates, A.J. (1955). Intellectual changes following temporal lobectomy for psychomotor epilepsy. *J. Neurol. Neurosurg. Psychiatry 18*:44-52.
21. Milner, B. (1958). Psychological defects produced by temporal lobe excision. *Assoc. Nerv. Ment. Disorders 36*:244-257.
22. Milner, B. (1967). Brain mechanisms suggested by studies of the temporal lobes. In *Brain Mechanisms Underlying Speech and Language*. Edited by F.D. Darley. Grune and Stratton, New York, pp. 122-145.
23. Ivnik, R.J., Sharbrough, F.W., and Laws, E.R. Jr. (1987). Effects of anterior temporal lobectomy on cognitive function. *J. Clin. Psychol. 43*:128-137.
24. Ivnik, R.J., Sharbrough, F.W., and Laws, E.R. Jr. (1988). Anterior temporal lobectomy for the control of partial complex seizures: Information for counseling patients. *Mayo Clin. Proc. 63*:783-793.
25. Eskenazi, B., Cain, W.S., Novelly, R.A., and Mattson, R. (1986). Odor perception in temporal lobe epilepsy patients with and without temporal lobectomy. *Neuropsychologia 24*:553-562.
26. Jones-Gotman, M. (1986a). Memory for designs: The hippocampal contribution. *Neuropsychologia 24*:193-203.
27. Read, D.E. (1981). Effects of medial temporal-lobe lesions on intermediate memory in man. Unpublished Ph.D. thesis, McGill University, Montreal.
28. Zatorre, R. (1985). Discrimination and recognition of tonal melodies after unilateral cerebral excisions. *Neuropsychologia 23*:31-41.
29. Prevey, M.L., Delaney, R.C., and Mattson, R.H. (1988). Metamemory in temporal-lobe epilepsy: Self-monitoring of memory functions. *Brain Cognition 7*: 298-311.
30. Wechsler, D. (1945). A standardized memory scale for clinical use. *J. Psychol. 19*:87-95.
31. Corsi, P. (1972). Human memory and the medial temporal region of the brain. Unpublished Ph.D. thesis, McGill University, Montreal.

32. Milner, B., and Kimura, D. (1964). Dissociable visual learning defects after unilateral temporal lobectomy in man. Paper presented at the annual meeting of the Eastern Psychological Association, Philadelphia.
33. Frisk, V., and Milner, B. (1985). Retention of verbal information in scrambled and unscrambled texts by patients with unilateral cerebral lesions. Paper presented at the annual meeting of the Canadian Psychological Association, Halifax.
34. Dennis, M., Farrell, K., Hoffman, H.J., Hendrick, E.B., Becker, L.E., and Murphy, E.G. (1988). Recognition memory of item, associative, and serial-order information after temporal lobectomy for seizure disorder. *Neuropsychologia* 26:53-65.
35. Herman, B.P., Wyler, A.R., Richey, E.T., and Rea, J.M. (1987). Memory function and verbal learning ability in patients with complex partial seizures of temporal lobe origin. *Epilepsia* 28:547-554.
36. Rains, G.D. (1987). Incidental verbal memory as a function of depth of encoding in patients with temporal-lobe lesions. *J. Clin. Exp. Neuropsychol.* 9:18.
37. Incisa della Rocchetta, I. (1986). Classification and recall of pictures after unilateral frontal or temporal lobectomy. *Cortex* 22:189-211.
38. Jaccarino, G. (1975). Dual encoding in memory: Evidence from temporal-lobe lesions in man. Unpublished M.A. thesis, McGill University, Montreal.
39. Milner, B. (1987). Clues to the cerebral organization of memory. In *Cerebral Correlates of Conscious Experience*. Edited by P. Buser and A.L. Rougeul-Buser. Elsevier, Amsterdam, pp. 139-153.
40. Smith, M.L., and Milner, B. (1981). The role of the right hippocampus in the recall of spatial location. *Neuropsychologia* 19:781-793.
41. Kimura, D. (1961). Some effects of temporal-lobe damage on auditory perception. *Can. J. Psychol.* 15:156-165.
42. Bousfield, W.A. (1953). The occurrence of clustering in recall of randomly arranged associates. *J. Gen. Psychol.* 49:229-240.
43. Marshall, G.R. (1967). Stimulus characteristics contributing to organization in free recall. *J. Verbal Learn. Verbal Behav.* 6:364-374.
44. Mandler, G. (1967). Organization and memory. In *The Psychology of Learning and Motivation*, Vol. 1. Edited by K.W. Spence and J.T. Spence. Academic Press, New York, pp. 327-372.
45. Mandler, G. (1970). Words, lists and categories: An experimental view of organized memory. In *Studies in Thought and Language*. Edited by J.L. Cowan. University of Arizona Press, Tucson, pp., 99-131.
46. Tulving, E. (1962). Subjective organization in free recall of "unrelated" words. *Psychol. Rev.* 69:344-354.
47. Jaccarino-Hiatt, G. (1978). Impairment of cognitive organization in patients with temporal-lobe lesions. Unpublished Ph.D. thesis, McGill University, Montreal.
48. Moscovitch, M. (1976). Verbal and spatial clustering in the free recall of drawings following left or right temporal lobectomy: Evidence for dual encoding. Paper presented at the annual meeting of the Canadian Psychological Association, Toronto.
49. Weingartner, H. (1968). Verbal learning in patients with temporal lobe lesions. *J. Verbal Learn. Verbal Behav.* 7:520-526.

50. Tulving, E. (1972). Episodic and semantic memory. In *Organization and Memory*. Edited by E. Tulving and W. Donaldson. Academic Press, New York, pp. 381-403.

51. Wilkins, B., and Moscovitch, M. (1978). Selective impairment of semantic memory after temporal lobectomy. *Neuropsychologia 16*:73-79.

52. Craik, F.I.M., and Lockhart, R.S. (1972). Levels of processing: a framework for memory research. *J. Verbal Learn. Verbal Behav. 11*:671-684.

53. Rains, G.D. (1987). Incidental verbal memory as a function of depth of encoding in patients with temporal-lobe lesions. *J. Clin. Exp. Neuropsychol. 9*:18.

54. Craik, F.I.M., and Tulving, E. (1975). Depth of processing and the retention of words in episodic memory. *J. Exp. Psychol. Gen. 104*:268-294.

55. Milner, B. (1975). Psychological aspects of focal epilepsy and its neurosurgical management. In *Advances in Neurology*, Vol. 8. Edited by D.P. Purpura, J.K. Penry, and R.D. Walter, Raven Press, New York, pp. 299-321.

56. Slamecka, N.J., and Graf, P. (1978). The generation effect: Delineation of a phenomenon. *J. Exp. Psychol. Human Learn. Memory 4*:592-604.

57. Frisk, V. (1988). Comprehension and recall of stories following left temporal lobectomy. Unpublished Ph.D. thesis, McGill University, Montreal.

58. Baddeley, A.D. (1986). *Working Memory*. Oxford University Press, New York.

59. Just, M.A., and Carpenter, P.A. (1980). A theory of reading: From eye fixations to comprehension. *Psychol. Rev. 87*:329-354.

60. Daneman, M., and Carpenter, P.A. (1980). Individual differences in working memory and reading. *J. Verbal Learn. Verbal Behav. 19*:450-466.

61. Jones, M.K. (1974). Imagery as a mnemonic aid after left temporal lobectomy: Contrast between material-specific and generalized memory disorders. *Neuropsychologia 12*:21-30.

62. Shankweiler, D. (1966). Defects in recognition and reproduction of familiar tunes after unilateral temporal lobectomy. Presented at the annual meeting of the Eastern Psychological Association, New York.

63. Kimura, D. (1963). Right temporal lobe damage. *Arch. Neurol. 8*:264-271.

64. Milner, B. (1965). Visually-guided maze-learning in man: Effects of bilateral hippocampal, bilateral frontal, and unilateral cerebral lesions. *Neuropsychologia 3*:317-338.

65. Milner, B. (1968). Visual recognition and recall after right temporal-lobe excision in man. *Neuropsychologia 6*:191-209.

66. Corkin, S. (1965). Tactually-guided maze-learning in man: Effects of unilateral cortical excisions and bilateral hippocampal lesions. *Neuropsychologia 3*:339-351.

67. Jones-Gotman, M. (1986). Right hippocampal excision impairs learning and recall of a list of abstract designs. *Neuropsychologia 24*:659-670.

68. Taylor, L.B. (1969). Localization of cerebral lesions by psychological testing. *Clin. Neurosurg. 16*:269-287.

69. Paivio, A. (1971). *Imagery and Verbal Processes*. Holt, Rinehart and Winston, New York.

70. Jones-Gotman, M. (1979). Incidental learning of image-mediated or pronounced words after right temporal lobectomy. *Cortex 15*:187-197.

71. Jones-Gotman, M., and Milner, B. (1978). Right temporal-lobe contribution to image-mediated verbal learning. *Neuropsychologia 16*:61-71.
72. Beatty, W.W., MacInnes, W.D., Porphyres, H.S., Troster, A.I., and Cermak, L.S. (1988). Preserved topographical memory following right temporal lobectomy. *Brain Cogn. 8*:67-76.
73. Petrides, M. (1985). Deficits on conditional associative-learning tasks after frontal- and temporal-lobe lesions in man. *Neuropsychologia 23*:601-614.
74. Smith, M.L., and Milner, B. (1989). Right hippocampal impairment in the recall of location: Encoding deficit or rapid forgetting? *Neuropsychologia 27*:71-82.
75. Scoville, W.B., and Milner, B. (1957). Loss of recent memory after bilateral hippocampal lesions. *J. Neurol. Neurosurg. Psychiatry 20*:11-21.
76. Corkin, S. (1984). Lasting consequences of bilateral medial temporal lobectomy: Clinical course and experimental findings in H.M. *Sem. Neurol. 4*:249-259.
77. Milner, B. (1959). The memory defect in bilateral hippocampal lesions. *Psychiatric Res. Rep. 11*:43-58.
78. Milner, B., Corkin, S., and Teuber, H.L. (1968). Further analyses of the hippocampal amnesic syndrome: 14-year follow-up study of H.M. *Neuropsychologia 6*:215-234.
79. Milner, B. (1974). Hemispheric specialization: Scope and Limits. In *The Neurosciences: Third Study Program*. Edited by F.O. Schmitt and F.G. Worden. MIT Press, Boston, pp. 75-89.
80. Hebb, D.O. (1961). Distinctive features of learning in the higher animal. In *Brain Mechanisms and Learning*. Edited by J.F. Delafresnaye. Oxford University Press, London, pp. 37-51.
81. Melton, A.W. (1963). Implications of short-term memory for a general theory of memory. *J. Verbal Learn. Verbal Behav. 2*:1-21.
82. Ojemann, G., and Dodrill, C. (1985). Verbal memory deficits after left temporal lobectomy for epilepsy. *J. Neurosurg. 62*:101-107.
83. Milner, B. (1980). Complementary functional specializations of the human cerebral hemispheres. In *Nerve Cells, Transmitters and Behavior*. Edited by R. Levi-Montalcini. Pontificia Academia Scientiarum, Vatican City, pp. 601-625.
84. Jarrard, L.E. (1975). Role of interference in retention by rats with hippocampal lesions. *J. Comp. Physiol. Psychol. 89*:400-408.
85. Pandya, D.N., Van Hoesen, G.W., and Mesulam, M.M. (1981). Efferent connections of the cingulate gyrus in the rhesus monkey. *Exp. Brain Res. 42*:319-330.
86. Seltzer, B., and Pandya, N. (1976). Some cortical projections to the parahippocampal area in the rhesus monkey. *Exp. Neurol. 50*:146-160.
87. Seltzer, B., and Van Hoesen, G.W. (1979). A direct inferior parietal lobule projection to the presubiculum in the rhesus monkey. *Brain Res. 179*:157-161.
88. Van Hoesen, G.W. (1982). The parahippocampal gyrus: New observations regarding its cortical connections in the monkey. *Trends Neurosci. 5*:345-350.
89. Van Hoesen, G.W., and Pandya, D.N. (1975a). Some connections of the entorhinal (area 28) and perihinal (area 35) cortices of the rhesus monkey. I. Temporal lobe afferents. *Brain Res. 95*:1-24.

90. Van Hoesen, G.W., Pandya, D.N., and Butters, N. (1975). Some connections of the entorhinal (area 28) and perirhinal (area 35) cortices of the rhesus monkey. II. Frontal lobe afferents. *Brain Res.* *95*:25-38.
91. Van Hoesen, G.W., and Pandya, D.N. (1976b). Some connections of the entorhinal (area 28) and perirhinal (area 35) cortices of the rhesus monkey. III. Efferent connections. *Brain Res.* *95*:39-59.
92. Hirsh, R. (1974). The hippocampus and contextual retrieval of information from memory: A theory. *Behav. Biol.* *12*:421-444.
93. Mishkin, M. (1982). A memory system in the monkey. *Phil. Trans. Roy. Soc. London B298*:85-95.
94. O'Keefe, J., and Nadel, L. (1978). *The Hippocampus as a Cognitive Map.* Clarendon Press, Oxford.
95. Petrides, M., and Milner, B. (1982). Deficits on subject-ordered tasks after frontal- and temporal-lobe lesions in man. *Neuropsychologia 20*:249-262.
96. Squire, L.R., Cohen, N.J., and Nadel, L. (1984). The medial temporal region and memory consolidation: A new hypothesis. In *Memory Consolidation.* Edited by H. Weingartner and E. Parker. Lawrence Erlbaum Associates, Hillsdale, NJ, pp. 185-206.
97. Spiegler, B.J., and Mishkin, M. (1981). Evidence for the sequential participation of inferior temporal cortex and amygdala in the acquisition of stimulus-reward associations. *Behav. Brain Res. 3*:303-317.
98. Saunders, R.C., Murray, E.A., and Mishkin, M. (1984). Further evidence that amygdala and hippocampus contribute equally to visual recognition. *Neuropsychologia 22*:785-796.
99. Mishkin, M. (1978). Memory in monkeys severely impaired by combined but not by separate removal of amygdala and hippocampus. *Nature (London) 273*:297-298.
100. Zola-Morgan, S., Squire, L.R., and Amaral, D.G. (1986). Human amnesia and the medial temporal region: Enduring memory impairment following a bilateral lesion limited to field CA1 of the hippocampus. *J. Neurosci. 6*:2950-2967.
101. Wada, J. (1949). A new method for the determination of the side of cerebral speech dominance. A preliminary report on the intracarotid injection of sodium amytal in man. *Igaku to Seibutsugaku (Med. Biol.) 14*:221-222 (Japanese).
102. Wada, J. (1951). An experimental study on the neural mechanism of the spread of epileptic impulse. *Folia Psychiatrica Japonica 4*:289-301.
103. Milner, B., Branch, C., and Rasmussen, T. (1964). Observations on cerebral dominance. In *Ciba Foundation Symposium on Disorders of Language.* Edited by A.V.S. DeReuck and M. O'Connor. J. and A. Churchill, London, pp. 200-214.
104. Rasmussen, T., and Milner, B. (1975). Clinical and surgical studies of the cerebral speech areas in man. In *Cerebral Localization.* Edited by K.J. Zulch, O. Creutzfeldt, and G.C. Galbraith. Springer-Verlag, Berlin, pp. 238-257.
105. Wada, J., and Rasmussen, T. (1960). Intracarotid injection of sodium amytal for the lateralization of cerebral speech dominance: Experimental and clinical observations. *J. Neurosurg. 17*:266-282.

106. Penfield, W., and Milner, B. (1958). Memory deficit produced by bilateral lesions in the hippocampal zone. *Arch. Neurol. Psychiatry 79*:475-497.
107. Penfield, W., and Mathieson, G. (1974). An autopsy and a discussion of the role of the hippocampus in experiential recall. *Arch. Neurol. 31*:145-154.
108. Milner, B., Branch, C., and Rasmussen, T. (1962). Study of short-term memory after intracarotid injection of sodium amytal. *Trans. Am. Neurol. Assoc. 87*: 224-226.
109. Blume, W.T., Grabow, J.D., Darley, F.L., and Aronson, A.E. (1973). Intracarotid amobarbital test of language and memory before temporal lobectomy for seizure control. *Neurology 23*:812-819.
110. Fedio, P., and Weinberg, L.K. (1971). Dysnomia and impairment of verbal memory following intracarotid injection of sodium amytal. *Brain Res. 31*: 159-168.
111. Klove, H., Grabow, J.D., and Trites, R.L. (1969). Evaluation of memory functions with intracarotid sodium amytal. *Trans. Am. Neurol. Assoc. 94*:76-80.
112. Klove, H., Trites, R.L., and Grabow, J.D. (1970). Intracarotid sodium amytal for evaluating memory function. *Electroenceph. Clin. Neurophysiol. 28*:418-419.
113. Mateer, C.A., and Dodrill, C.B. (1983). Neuropsychological and linguistic correlates of atypical language lateralization: Evidence from sodium amytal studies. *Human Neurobiol. 2*:135-142.
114. Rausch, R., Fedio, P., Ary, C.M., Engell, J. Jr., and Crandall, P.H. (1984). Resumption of behavior following intracarotid sodium amobarbital injection. *Ann. Neurol. 15*:31-35.
115. Smith, M.L., and Milner, B. (1985). Carotid amytal studies of memory function. Paper presented at the annual meeting of the International Neuropsychology Society, San Diego.
116. Novelly, R.A. (1987). Relationship of intracarotid amytal procedure to clinical and neurosurgical variables in epilepsy surgery. *J. Clin. Exp. Neuropsychol. 9*:33.
117. Dinner, D.S., Luders, H., Morris, H.H. III, Wyllie, E., and Kramer, R.E. (1987). Validity of intracarotid sodium amobarbital (Wada test) for evaluation of memory function. *Neurology 37S*:142.
118. McGlone, J., and MacDonald, B.H. (1989). Reliability of the sodium amobarbital test for memory. *J. Epilepsy 2*:31-39.
119. Jack, C.R., Nichols, D.A., Sharbrough, F.W., Marsh, W.R., and Petersen, R.C. (1988). Selective posterior cerebral artery amytal test for evaluating memory function before surgery for temporal lobe seizures. *Radiology 168*:787-793.
120. Rausch, R. (1987). Psychological evaluation. In *Surgical Treatment of the Epilepsies.* Edited by J. Engel Jr. Raven Press, New York, pp. 181-195.
121. Bekhterev, V.M. (1900). Demonstration eines Gehirns mit Zerstorung der vorderen und inneren Theile der Hirnrinde beider Schlafenlappen. *Neurologisches Zentralblatt 19*:990-991.

16

Memory Functions in Normal Aging

Fergus I.M. Craik

University of Toronto
Toronto, Ontario, Canada

INTRODUCTION

The belief that memory performance declines from young to older adulthood is virtually universal in our society. This belief, based on subjective estimates and personal observations, is generally well supported by experimental studies of age differences in memory (1-5), yet clinical investigators typically experience great difficulty in relating subjective reports of memory impairments to performance on standardized tests (6). Part of this problem may stem from the greater incidence of depression in older people, and from the observation that ratings of depression correlate with reports of memory failures (7,8). Undoubtedly, a further source of the difficulty is the unreliability and lack of validity of current methods of assessing memory at the level of individual patients. The present chapter reviews the evidence for memory changes as a function of normal aging; for the most part, the studies reported are drawn from the literature in the areas of cognitive psychology and neuropsychology, but attempts will also be made to relate theories and findings to the practical business of clinical assessment.

Experimental studies in cognitive aging typically contrast a group of young adults in their late teens and 20s with a group of older adults aged 60-80, although it is becoming more common to divide older participants into "young-old" (60-75) and "old-old" (75-90) subgroups. The methodology is thus cross-sectional rather than longitudinal, and this factor can sometimes make interpretations difficult. For example, are the observed differences between the groups genuinely attributable to the processes of aging, or are they partly or wholly a function of group differences in education, recent practice in taking tests, health, social and intellectual activities, general intelligence, motivation, and other variables? Much has been written on these severe methodological problems (9,10) but there is no space to deal with them in the present chapter. Experiments attempt to control for some of these confounding variables by matching samples on health, level of education, and verbal intelligence but it may still be advisable to interpret the findings with caution.

The most striking feature of the experimental literature is that age differences in memory performance are very large in certain tasks but much smaller or nonexistent in other tasks. For example, age differences are consistently found in tasks requiring unaided recall of recently presented word lists or text passages (1,11) and in working memory tasks (12,13), but age-related differences in performance are much less in digit span tasks (1,4) and in memory for well-learned general knowledge (14,15). A major concern of the experimental psychology literature has been to provide a theoretical framework that gives a satisfactory account of these apparently discrepant findings.

In the 1960s and early 1970s, the dominant model of memory was one in which incoming information was first registered in the appropriate sensory memory store, was then transferred by the processes of attention to a limited-capacity short-term store, and finally transferred again by rehearsal and learning processes to a large and relatively permanent long-term store (16). From the observation that differences in digit span were slight it seemed possible that age differences were minimal in the sensory and short-term stores, but were substantial in the acquisition and retrieval operations associated with the long-term store (1,4). However, as described more fully later, there *are* large age-related decrements in working memory, which apparently involves the short-term store; further, age differences in long-term storage tasks can be greatly reduced under certain conditions (1). The stores model does not appear to fit the facts too well.

Other possible theoretical schemes include the levels of processing approach of Craik and Lockhart (17) and the memory systems approach advocated by Tulving (18) and others. Craik and Lockhart suggested that incoming stimuli were processed to different levels or depths depending on the task requirements and the subject's goals; initial levels of analysis were concerned with sensory information, whereas deeper levels involved phonemic and then semantic-associative analyses. It was postulated that memory was essentially the byproduct of those analyses carried out, with deeper analyses being associated with longer-lasting memory traces. In this framework, an age-related decrement in memory performance should presumably mean that older people process events less deeply for some reason. There is some evidence to support this contention (1,19), but the evidence has also been disputed (20) so at the very least the proposal remains controversial. Tulving (18) distinguishes three major memory systems—procedural, semantic, and episodic—and suggests that the systems are embedded concentrically, so that procedural memory is the most general (and most primitive), semantic memory is a subset of procedural, and episodic memory (the most highly evolved system) is a subset of semantic memory. Procedural memory is concerned with learned habits, both motor and cognitive; semantic memory is more representational, but deals with general knowledge and facts; finally, episodic memory is the system that deals with specific events, specified with respect to time and place of occurrence. With regard to aging, older people typically complain that they forget specific instances and happenings, whereas their memory for learned procedures remains good. It is therefore tempting to speculate that the most recent system in evolutionary terms—episodic memory—is also the most vulnerable to various insults, including those associated with normal aging, and that the oldest—procedural memory—is the least vulnerable (21). However, this appealing idea is also not free from criticism. Semantic memory should show slight age decrements, yet one of the most common complaints of older people is that they experience difficulty in remembering names, and even specific words from time to time. Clearly such information must be retrieved from semantic memory.

My own view is that memory can best be understood in terms of the various *processes* involved in remembering, and that age differences reflect changes in the kinds of processes that older people can perform (2,19,22). The analysis is thus in terms of inefficiency of functions and processes rather than in terms of damage or loss of structures. The suggestion is that successful acquisition or encoding entails processing events meaningfully and distinctively in relation to existing knowledge, and that successful retrieval involves reinstating the same pattern of mental activity that occurred at the time of encoding. A further idea is that "appropriate" mental processes (e.g., semantic processing at the time of encoding, and reinstatement of the same mental operations at the time of retrieval) are partly initiated by the subject himself or herself and partly induced by some aspect of the external environment. For example, the question "What is the object used for?" will encourage thinking about the object (and thus encoding it in memory) in semantic terms. Similarly, representing an item for recognition in its original context will help to reinstate the original patern of mental operations and thereby enhance retrieval. I have suggested (22) that older people have particular difficulty in carrying out self-initiated mental operations, and that they therefore are more dependent on the external environment to support adequate encoding and retrieval processes. Conversely, older people will be at the greatest relative disadvantage when the environment does not support the appropriate processes.

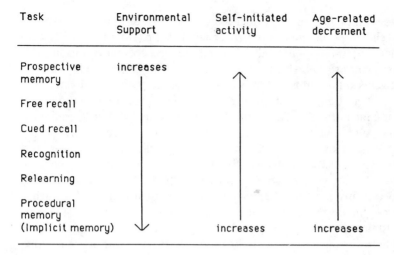

Task	Environmental Support	Self-initiated activity	Age-related decrement
Prospective memory	increases		
Free recall			
Cued recall			
Recognition			
Relearning			
Procedural memory (Implicit memory)		increases	increases

Figure 1   Memory tasks showing differential effects of aging.

Figure 1 shows different retrieval paradigms used often in experimental studies of aging. A task such as free recall (e.g., in which a list of 20 unrelated words must be recalled without hints or cues) affords relatively slight environmental support and the subject must necessarily "self-initiate" the appropriate operations; by the present view, age differences should be large. In recognition, on the other hand, the stimulus word or picture is re-presented, environmental support is therefore greater, and age differences should be smaller. The next sections review current findings from this perspective.

AGE DIFFERENCES IN SHORT-TERM MEMORY FUNCTIONING

The term "short-term memory" has unfortunately been used in a number of different senses, and these differences in usage have led to confusion and apparent contradictions in the literature. "Short-term" has been used both to describe a time interval (from 5 seconds to hours or days!) and also to refer to a separate memory storage system. I will argue that there is a useful distinction to be drawn between memory for material that has just been presented, or just been retrieved, and is still in the subject's conscious awareness ("in mind"), and material that has left conscious awareness from seconds ago to years ago) and therefore must be retrieved. These types of retention were referred to as 'primary memory' and 'secondary memory' by William James, and the terms are still in current use. The point is that primary memory (PM) and secondary memory (SM) do seem to have quite different principles of operation (23), whereas encoding and retrieval operations for material that has been dropped from conscious awareness seem to follow the same principles of operation, regardless of whether the retention interval is minutes, hours, or years. I therefore doubt the usefulness of such terms as 'recent memory,' 'long-term memory,' and 'tertiary memory' if they are meant to imply separate memory systems that obey different rules.

AGE DIFFERENCES IN PRIMARY MEMORY

Primary memory has been indexed by the recency effect in free recall; the superior recall of the last few words presented in a list of unrelated words. Digit span, the longest list of random digits that a person can repeat back immediately after presentation, is also an approximate measure of PM. Neither of these measures shows much change across the adult lifespan (1), although digit span does show slight declines (24). The virtual absence of an effect of aging on PM echoes a similar absence of effect in amnesic patients. For example, Baddeley and Warrington (25) showed that amnesic patients have both normal recency effects and normal digit spans. This relative invulnerability of digit span to either aging or most forms of brain damage has two important implications: First it provides good confirmatory evidence for the validity of the PM/SM distinction and, second, it means that whereas digit span is an easily administered clinical test it is essentially useless as an index of general memory functioning.

Age-related differences in *speed* of retrieval of material from PM are typically found, although even in this case the age differences are relatively slight compared with the differences in retrieval latency observed in SM tasks (26). Another apparent exception to the conclusion that age differences in PM are slight or nonexistent is provided by reports that *backward* digit span does decline with age (1). It does seem to be the case that when a short-term memory task requires the subject to manipulate and reorganize the material, age differences appear. Such tasks are better classified as working memory tasks, however.

AGE DIFFERENCES IN WORKING MEMORY

"Working memory" is a term introduced by Baddeley and Hitch (27) to describe tasks in which subjects must both hold information in mind and also carry out some computation or some decision-making activity on that information or on other incoming information. An example of a working memory (WM) task is one in which subjects are given a series of unrelated words to hold in mind, and are then presented with a sentence whose truth they must verify (e.g., "Elephants are not usually bigger than mice"); finally, they recall the word series. There is now good evidence that normal aging affects both the speed and the accuracy with which WM tasks can be carried out (28,29). A simple example is provided by Craik (30) who asked young and older adults to rearrange a list of unrelated words mentally and to say them back in alphabetical order; there were substantial age-related differences in this "alpha span" task although no such differences were found between the same groups of subjects in forward digit span. In another WM technique, a series of sentences is presented to subjects who must verify the truth of each sentence and also hold the last word of each sentence in mind, finally reproducing the series of last words. Substantial age-related differences have been found in this task (12,31). There is good agreement, then, that normal aging does affect the efficiency of WM functioning; in turn, this age-related loss is likely to be reflected in age decrements in other functions that depend on WM. Such functions include encoding for SM, problem solving and complex decision making.

DIVIDED ATTENTION TASKS

Working memory tasks typically require subjects to divide their attention between two sets of material or between information held in mind and further incoming information. Several studies have shown that older people are more adversely affected than are younger people by the necessity to divide attention on tasks of this type. One example is the dichotic listening task in which subjects hear two short series of numbers presented simultaneously, one series to each ear; the task is simply to repeat back the numbers. Older people are no worse than their younger counterparts if they attend especially to one ear and reproduce these numbers first; however, they are considerably poorer at reproducing the unattended series (1). Interestingly, some recent studies (12,32) have found that older people are not differentially penalized when a second subtask is introduced in working memory situations. One possible solution to the puzzle is that age differences in divided attention appear when both subtasks require on-line processing (like driving a car and carrying on a conversation), but that age-related differences are reduced when one subtask involves relatively passive storage of the material.

AGE DIFFERENCES IN LONG-TERM OR SECONDARY MEMORY

AGE DIFFERENCES IN RECALL AND RECOGNITION

Once an experienced event or newly learned material has been dropped from the mind, it must be retrieved from secondary memory; what are the major factors underlying successful memory performance in such cases? It was suggested earlier that older people show deficits in both encoding (acquisition) and retrieval unless these memory operations are adequately "supported" by aspects of the environment. Thus, age differences should be greatest under conditions in which subjects must "self-initiate" appropriate encoding and retrieval operations, and least under conditions in which appropriate operations are guided and supported by the task, by instructions, or by the physical or mental context.

In laboratory tasks, it is well documented that age differences are large in free recall, somewhat less in cued recall, and less again in recognition (1-4). To give one example, Craik and McDowd (33) had younger and older subjects recall and recognize word lists while they were performing a 4-choice reaction-time (RT) task. The RT task was straightforward; one of four lights appeared, the subject pressed a key under the light, the key press extinguished the light but immediately caused another light to appear. The task was thus continuous; it was used to assess the amount of processing resources left over from the primary task of recalling or recognizing. Subjects were presented with lists of cues and words such as 'part of the body—ELBOW.' In the recall task they were given the cues in a scrambled order and had to recall the words; in the recognition task, the original words were mixed with new distractor items. By manipulating list lengths and the difficulty of distractors, the recognition task was made more difficult than the recall task.

The results are shown in Figure 2. Although in this case recall was easier, there was a reliable age decrement in that task, whereas the older group's performance was slightly superior in recognition. The greater retrieval demands associated with cued recall led to relatively poorer performance in the older group (see Fig. 1). The lower panel of Figure 2 shows the average choice RT. The figure shows that older subjects' RTs are considerably longer, especially while performing the recall task; this result was interpreted as showing that the older group had a smaller pool of "processing resources" left free from the memory task and that this was especially true of recall. That is, recall demands more processing resources than does recognition, and since normal aging is associated with a reduction in processing resources, older people are especially penalized in recall, which necessitates a greater amount of self-initiated activity.

The implication of these results is therefore that whereas at first sight it seems reasonable to suggest that age decrements increase simply as the task increases in difficulty (34), the true state of affairs is more complicated. In an influential article, Hasher and Zacks (35) suggested that age decrements increase as the task becomes more "effortful" and this formulation is closer to the one endorsed here, although I would specify the mental effort more particularly as effort associated with self-initiated operations. A further point is that the age-related deficit in recall found in studies using word lists

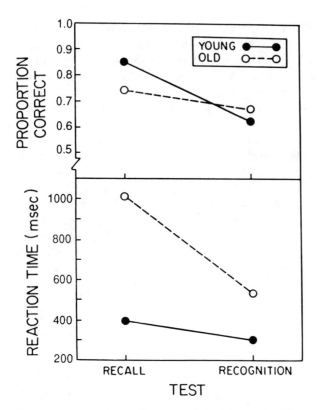

Figure 2 Proportions of items recalled and recognized (top panel), and mean reaction times on the secondary task (bottom panel) for young and old subjects. From Ref. 33.

has also been found with other materials; with passages of text (11,29), with drawings, pictures, and objects (36,37). It therefore does not seem reasonable to argue that age deficits observed in laboratory tasks are attributable to the use of artificial or unfamiliar materials.

The present analysis suggests that age differences in longer-term retention should be greatest when both encoding and retrieval operations are relatively unsuppported by the task itself or by the environment, and least when encoding and retrieval *are* supported in this way. A number of recent studies support this suggestion. For example, Waddell and Rogoff (38) presented a set of 30 miniature items (cars, furniture, animals, etc.) either on a model panorama made up of roads, buildings, hills and trees, or in featureless cubicles; the task was to remember the spatial position of each item in both cases. The subjects were middle-aged (mean = 46 years) and older (mean = 71 years) women; the cubicle condition performance levels were 73% and 36%, respectively, and in the panorama condition (which presumably afforded greater levels of environmental support) the corresponding scores were 75% and 72%. That is, the older group performed as well as the younger group under conditions of greater environmental support. A similar result has been reported by Sharps and Gollin (37). In their study, younger (mean = 20.5 years) and older (mean = 74.9 years) participants attempted to remember 40 common objects which were presented under various conditions. In the two extreme conditions the objects were presented earlier as a list (i.e., one after another for 5 s each) or in the context of a room, with each object placed in an arbitrary location for the participant to inspect for 5 s while being led on a tour round the room. In the list condition, younger and older participants recalled 18.0 and 9.3 objects, respectively, whereas in the room condition recall levels were 22.7 and 20.7, respectively. The first age difference was highly significant statistically but the second difference was not. Again, greater degrees of environmental support differentially enhanced the performance of older subjects.

To summarize, the present suggestions (discussed more fully in 2,22,30) are that deeper and more elaborate encoding operations, also specific retrieval operations, are more difficult for older people to carry out in a self-initiated manner, although if such operations are guided and supported by the environment they *can* be performed by older participants. Speculatively, these difficulties with self-initiated operations can be characterized as stemming from a reduction with age of the processing resources necessary to orchestrate and execute encoding and retrieval operations. As I see it, the reduction in processing resources has a biological basis, although this suggestion is also clearly speculative at this stage.

One line of evidence supporting the notion of decreased processing resources in older people comes from the finding (22) that young subjects learning and retrieving material under conditions of divided attention perform like older subjects working under conditions of full attention. The argument is that the second task in the divided attention paradigm requires some processing resources, thereby depleting the pool of resources from which the primary task may draw. Younger 'divided attention' subjects are rendered functionally old by the withdrawal of processing resources. It should also be mentioned, however, that Huppert (3) uses the same evidence to suggest that older people have as great a pool of processing resources as their younger counterparts, but that older people simply have more competing demands on their attention; that is, they are more inclined to be thinking of family, work, social, and leisure activities. A third possibility is that the pool of resources does not decrease with age but that mental operations themselves require more 'mental energy' to manage and execute as a person grows older. Further work is obviously required to clarify these different conceptual accounts.

AGE DIFFERENCES IN EXPLICIT AND IMPLICIT
MEMORY TASKS

The recall and recognition tasks discussed in the previous section have been termed "explicit memory" tasks since typically subjects are consciously aware of the requirement to learn and remember the material in question. However, memory may also be assessed in other less obvious ways and these "implicit memory" tasks (39,40) have stimulated much recent research since they give very different patterns of results from those obtained using more traditional explicit tasks. In particular, amnesics and other patients with memory disorders who show large losses on tests of explicit memory often show little impairment on implicit memory tasks. Such tasks include word fragment completion (39), stem completion (40), and perceptual identification (41). Many studies have now shown that if a word (e.g., MARKET) has been studied recently, subjects are more successful in completing a word fragment (e.g., --RK-T) or a word stem (e.g., MAR__) presented later; they are also more successful in identifying the word itself flashed very briefly on a tachistoscope. It should be stressed that subjects in these implicit memory tasks are typically unaware that they are trying to remember words from the previously presented list, they are simply attempting to complete or identify the word. The point is that prior experience can affect later performance in the absence of conscious knowledge or conscious recollection of the original episode (41). Moreover, such implicit memory or "priming" effects appear to be relatively invulnerable to conditions associated with gross impairments in explicit memory functions (40).

Does normal aging affect performance on implicit memory tasks? I have argued that the effect of aging should be small or nonexistent (22), since implicit memory tasks are very well supported by their local environment. That is, subjects are not asked whether a word was on the original list, they are simply asked to complete the fragment or identify the briefly presented word. Evidence is now mounting to support this position. In the lexical decision task, subjects have to decide as rapidly as possible whether a string of letters forms a real word; decision times are speeded when the word has been seen recently. Moscovitch (42) has shown that this type of repetition priming effect is as great in older as in younger subjects. Priming effects also appear with repetition of semantic categories, although the effects are short-lived. Byrd (43) tested younger and older people in a paradigm requiring a decision about category membership; the stimulus slide "fruit-cherry" would elicit a positive decision and "fruit-tiger" a negative decision. Byrd showed that if the same category was repeated after a short lag, but with a different exemplar (e.g., "fruit-apple"), positive decision times were speeded—and to the same extent in younger and older subjects.

Light and her colleagues (44,45) have also demonstrated an age invariance in implicit memory. In one study, Light and Singh (45) found no reliable age differences in either stem completion or perceptual identification although age differences were found in free recall, cued recall, and recognition. They argue against the environmental support idea on the grounds that a recognition memory test, in which the complete word is re-presented, presumably affords greater support to mental operations than does stem completion, in which only the first three letters are presented. However, the point can be made that the functional requirements of the tasks are very different; in recognition, the question being asked is "was this word on the list presented some time ago?"; that is, it is necessary to recollect the original episode. In stem completion, on the other hand, the subject is not asked anything about the original event, he or she must simply attempt to complete the word in any legitimate way. Whereas I argue that the priming and implicit memory results lend weight to the notion of environmental support, it should be acknowledged that others (3,45) argue persuasively that the data confirm a multiple memory systems approach, with age differences appearing in explicit but not implicit memory tasks.

The work on implicit memory is probably of greater interest to theorists than to practitioners at the present stage. However, the finding that performance on implicit memory tasks is unaffected by the process of normal aging may have important implications for work on memory rehabilitation. Techniques are being investigated at present (46) to capitalize on these laboratory findings.

AGE DIFFERENCES IN MEMORY FOR SOURCE

It has been shown that amnesic patients can sometimes remember facts but forget where or when they learned the facts (47). That is, they show a greater deficit in episodic than in semantic memory. One possible reason for the inability to remember the source of retained information is that the patients in question may fail to integrate focal events with their contexts of occurrence. Burke and Light (20) suggest that one effect of normal aging is a reduction in the efficiency of such contextual integration. If true, this factor could underlie much of the observed memory deficit in older people, since even a good reinstatement of the context would be less helpful to them if the context and the focal event were less fully integrated.

McIntyre and Craik (48) reported a study of "source amnesia" in normal elderly people. They found that older subjects showed substantially greater forgetting of where and when they had learned new facts, even though the facts themselves were remembered reasonably well. In further work, Craik and his colleagues have shown that variations in the ability to remember source within an elderly group were related to measures of frontal lobe functioning. The suggestion is that one of the functions of the frontal lobes is to facilitate the integration of focal events and their contexts of occurrence; if the frontal lobes are more vulnerable than other parts of the brain to the effects of normal aging (49), then this relationship between subclinical frontal impairment and source amnesia would be expected. More generally, the role of context in remembering, and age differences in this respect, is a topic likely to generate much interesting research in the next few years.

AGE DIFFERENCES IN PROSPECTIVE MEMORY

The term "prospective memory" has been used to refer to situations in which the person must remember to carry out some task in the future. Many everyday situations are obviously of this kind; remembering to call a friend tomorrow or to go to the store on the way home from work. Since such prospective memory tasks (or "remembering to remember") often involve few cues to remind the person what he or she was supposed to do, large age differences would be expected. That is, prospective memory tasks typically have poor environmental support (Fig. 1). To date little work has been done on this important topic, but Cockburn and Smith (50) found age differences on two prospective memory tasks included in the Rivermead Behavioral Memory Test. The tasks consisted of remembering to ask later for a hidden belonging, and remembering to make a further appointment at the end of the session. It should also be mentioned that Moscovitch (42) found that older people were *better* at remembering to telephone the laboratory at various predesignated times, possibly because the task was more important or more salient to them. Clearly, future experiments will have to separate out social and motivational factors from underlying abilities in order to assess the effects of aging on prospective memory.

VERY LONG-TERM MEMORY
AND GENERAL KNOWLEDGE

AGE DIFFERENCES IN REMOTE MEMORY

Older people often remark that whereas their memory for recent events is quite poor, their memory for events of their youth is excellent. This idea can be extended to the suggestion that since early memories become progressively more salient in the elderly person's thinking, he or she will show a progressive tendency to live in the past. Are these impressions backed by research findings?

There are a number of obvious objections to accepting the anecdotal evidence too readily. One is that the episodes remembered from 50 or 60 years ago are highly selected and often emotional in tone (first day at school, a birthday party, death of a pet); clearly it is not reasonable to compare such memories with memories for everyday events (where you parked your car yesterday, what you ate for lunch on Monday). Second, such personally important memories have typically been retrieved and recounted on many previous occasions; they are not really being retrieved from 50 years ago, but from last week when the tale was last told. Third, despite the older person's certainty about the facts and events remembered, the recollected events may be seriously distorted from the original happenings. A fourth, more theoretical, point is the suggestion by Cermak (51) that such memories acquire the characteristics of family folk tales and are therefore better classified as part of the person's general knowledge; that is, they take on the characteristics of semantic memory rather than episodic memory.

The experimental literature on remote memory has been reviewed by Erber (52) and Poon (4). In general, the studies show that memory declines as the events become more remote; that is, when the salience of events is controlled, there is no evidence for superior recollection of early events. Nonetheless, memory for early personal experiences does remain high into the 60s and 70s, especially for knowledge acquired over some time, like names and faces of high school colleagues (53) and memory for the street plan of a town in which one used to live (54). Memory for specific events that occurred many years ago remains a difficult topic to investigate.

AGE DIFFERENCES IN THE RETENTION OF KNOWLEDGE

In general, it seems that *knowledge* is retained well by older people, although whether the better retention of knowledge than of specific events reflects retrieval from two distinct memory systems (semantic and episodic memory) remains a matter of debate (2,21). Several studies have reported an increase in vocabulary and general knowledge from youth to middle age, and stability or a slight decline from middle age to older adulthood (14,15,34). One important factor may be the extent to which various kinds of knowledge are actually used by the older person (15); the supposition is that continued use would prolong the retention, or at least the retrievability, of specific types of information. Charness's studies of chess and bridge skills (55,56) show that older players retain their skill, although they may respond more slowly. Another factor may be the extent to which knowledge is explicit or is implicit (procedural) as in many motor skills; the evidence previously reviewed under this heading suggests that procedural knowledge should be relatively invulnerable to the effects of aging.

As with episodic memory, the type of operation required to perform a particular task may strongly influence the result observed. For example, it is known that older people perform less well than their younger counterparts on tests of generating words beginning with a given letter (34) and in remembering names (57). Such self-initiated processes may again show greater age-related losses than do tasks involving greater degrees of environmental support. This suggestion is supported by Schaie's (58) study showing greater age decrements in a word production task than in a vocabulary test in which possible synonyms were presented.

AGE DIFFERENCES IN METAMEMORY

Finally in this section, recent work on "metamemory" should be mentioned briefly. Metamemory refers to a person's knowledge of his or her own mnemonic capabilities—what kinds of strategies will be most effective, which events will and which will not be recalled later and so on. This topic is still very much under investigation but it is perhaps a fair interim conclusion to say that age changes in the knowledge aspects of metamemory appear to be relatively slight (59).

MODULATING VARIABLES AND UNDERLYING CAUSES

This brief section is appended to give a fuller picture of memory changes with age, and of the various factors that must be taken into account before an adequate scientific formulation of age differences in cognition can be produced.

VARIABLES AFFECTING THE RELATIONS BETWEEN AGING AND MEMORY PERFORMANCE

When an older and a younger group are compared with a view to studying their ability to learn and remember, the groups inevitably differ in more respects than in their mean ages. Typically the two groups had different educational experiences, and often their social backgrounds are different. The groups may also differ in their average state of health, their daily activity levels, the recency of their involvement in formal education, their verbal intelligence, and their motivation to perform well on laboratory tasks. The resulting methodological difficulties have received much attention (9,10), and researchers make efforts to match their samples on at least some of the confounding variables. One reassuring aspect of many of the experiments discussed in the present chapter is that *interactions* are often the result of interest, rather than a simple old-young difference. For example, if the two age groups do not differ on a digit span test but do differ on an alpha span test (30), it is difficult to attribute the result to cohort differences or to differences in health or motivation.

Some factors clearly do modify the results obtained, however. For example, Dixon and his colleagues (60) have shown different patterns relating age to text recall as a function of verbal intelligence. Specifically, older subjects of high verbal intelligence showed no age-related decrement in the ability to recall high-level propositions from a text, although the decrement appeared for low-level propositions. Subjects of lower verbal intelligence showed an equivalent age-related decrement at all levels of propositions. Other studies have shown different patterns of aging effects as a function of daily activity levels (61); as expected, active older people perform more like their younger counterparts. In general, there is increasing awareness in the research community that the confounding effects of age differences in health (62), lifestyle, and in the incidence of depression (5) must be dealt with seriously before a valid picture of age changes in memory can emerge.

RELATIONS TO ABNORMAL AGING

Another important question, still to be resolved satisfactorily, is whether normal aging is associated with memory deficits that are less severe but qualitatively similar to the deficits seen in conditions such as Alzheimer's disease. Researchers have pointed out similarities between the effects of normal aging and those associated with focal right hemisphere damage (63) and with frontal damage (49), but a satisfactory resolution of the problem awaits the development of more sophisticated diagnostic instruments, both in the domain of neuropsychology and in the domain of brain imaging techniques.

The concept of "age-associated memory impairment" has recently been proposed by an NIMH workgroup (64). Crook and his colleagues have suggested diagnostic criteria and treatment strategies (65) for the condition, which describes healthy people over 50 years of age who are not demented but who have experienced a gradual decline in memory abilities. If the memory problems associated with normal aging can be alleviated by drugs or other organic therapies, it is clearly important to know about it. However, there is a potential danger in labelling a normal condition as a medical syndrome (see also Ref. 3). The danger stems from an undue reliance on organic as opposed to psychological and social-environmental manipulations. There are clearly ethical, political, and commercial considerations here, that must be disentangled from the evolving scientific evidence.

UNDERLYING BIOLOGICAL CHANGES WITH AGE

Normal aging is associated with a number of changes in brain structure and function, but the relations between these changes and cognitive performance are still not well worked out. It is generally accepted that a certain amount of cerebral atrophy accompanies the aging process, there is also neuronal loss, a decrease in cerebral blood flow, and an increase in neurofibrillary tangles and plaques (see Refs 3-5, 66 for reviews). The linkage between these changes and age-related changes in memory functions is quite speculative at present, however.

Some of the brain regions that may be possible sites for such linkages include the hippocampus (66) and the prefrontal cortex (49,66). Diffuse damage to frontal cortex appears to be one strong candidate in light of recent notions linking this region to episodic memory (67), and evidence for source amnesia in older people (48). Other influential hypotheses include age-related changes in the cholinergic system; Drachman and Leavitt (68) have demonstrated very similar patterns of memory dysfunction in elderly people and in young subjects who have been given anticholinergic drugs. Mishkin and his colleagues (69) have carried out an extensive experimental program to reveal two distinct memory systems in animals; one dealing with learned habits and the other with specific memories. Clearly these systems are very similar to the implicit and explicit memory systems described by Schacter (40) and others, and it would therefore be expected that aging is associated with greater damage to the explicit 'memory' system, rather than to the 'habit' system.

Recently, a number of investigators have suggested that glucose metabolism may be disrupted in the aging brain (70-72). I personally find this an attractive hypothesis since it links well to the psychological notion of processing resources—the 'mental energy' postulated to enable encoding and retrieval processes to be executed effectively. A decline in cerebral energy in frontal regions might also underlie the declining efficiency of the planning or executive functions of working memory—this dysfunction in turn could lead to decrements in encoding, retrieval, and strategy use. To end on a more optimistic note, there is growing evidence for the maintenance of neural plasticity into old age (73). This line of work is also theoretically attractive since is points to the continued role of the environment in maintaining cognitive functions. Active involvement in social and intellectual pursuits still seems to be an excellent antidote to the effects of aging on memory and other cognitive abilities.

SUMMARY AND CONCLUSIONS

The present chapter has presented recent evidence from experimental psychology and neuropsychology on the changes in memory that accompany normal aging. The most striking conclusion is that such age-related changes are much larger in some tasks than in others; age decrements are typically large in free recall and in working memory, but are typically slight or nonexistent in primary memory, in recognition memory, and in tasks involving well-learned knowledge. Various theoretical schemes have been suggested to account for this pattern of differential changes. One possibility is that performance on different tasks is mediated by different brain structures, and that these structures (e.g., memory stores or memory systems) are differentially vulnerable to the effects of aging. A somewhat different line of explanation, more favored by the present writer, is that different memory tasks vary in the necessity to employ "self-initiated" mental operations, and that older people have relatively greater problems with tasks requiring such operations. Tasks such as recognition memory are relatively well supported by the external environment and thus show slight age decrements, whereas tasks such as free recall require a substantial amount of self-initiated activity and are therefore associated with larger age differences in performance.

The factors that cause or modify age-related changes in memory functioning are still not well understood. It seems likely that biological factors play a major role here, with changes in blood flow, in neuronal structure, and in the organization of neuroanatomical and neuropharmacological systems all playing a part. The discipline of 'cognitive neuroscience' is in its infancy, but holds great promise for the future. It is also likely that social and intellectual factors play a role in mediating the observed changes. It seems probable, in fact, that continued social and intellectual activity can do much to counteract the underlying biological changes.

For practitioners, a good final message might be to pay some attention to psychological findings and theories—especially as they relate to the types of diagnostic tests used to assess memory dysfunction. Recent work has made it clearer that an adequate test battery must assess a variety of different memory functions; memory can no longer be thought of as one monolithic entity. All of us, getting older ourselves, may wait hopefully for a wonder drug that will eliminate our growing difficulties with remembering. Meanwhile we may perhaps draw some comfort from the evidence on neural plasticity in the older brain, and on the strategies we can adopt to increase environmental support for memory processes.

REFERENCES

1. Craik, F.I.M. (1977). Age differences in human memory. In *Handbook of the Psychology of Aging*. Edited by J.E. Birren and K.W. Schaie. Van Nostrand Reinhold, New York, pp. 384-420.
2. Craik, F.I.M. (1984). Age differences in remembering. In *Neuropsychology of Memory*. Edited by L.R. Squire and N. Butters. Guilford Press, New York, pp. 3-12.
3. Huppert, F.A. (1989). Age-related changes in memory: Learning and remembering new information. In *Handbook of Neuropsychology*. Edited by F. Boller and J. Grafman. Elsevier, Amsterdam.

4. Poon, L.W. (1985). Differences in human memory with aging: Nature, causes, and clinical implications. In *Handbook of the Psychology of Aging*, 2nd ed. Edited by J.E. Birren and K.W. Schaie. van Nostrand Reinhold, New York, pp. 427-462.

5. Poon, L.W., Editor (1986). *Handbook for Clinical Memory Assessment of Older Adults*. American Psychological Association, Washington, D.C.

6. Sunderland, A., Watts, K., Baddeley, A.D., and Harris, J.E. (1986). Subjective memory assessment and test performance in elderly adults. *J. Geront. 41*:376-384.

7. Kahn, R.L., Zavit, S.H., Hilbert, N.M., and Niederhe, G. (1975). Memory complaint and impairment in the aged. *Arch. Gen. Psychiat. 32*:1569-1573.

8. Thompson, L.W. Editor (1986). Assessing the effects of depression. In *Handbook for Clinical Memory Assessment of Older Adults*. Edited by L.W. Poon. American Psychological Association, Washington, D.C., pp. 197-267.

9. Nesselroade, J.R., and Labouvie, E.W. (1985). Experimental design in research on aging. In *Handbook of the Psychology of Aging*, 2nd ed. Edited by J.E. Birren and K.W. Schaie. Van Nostrand Reinhold, New York, pp. 35-60.

10. Schaie, K.W., and Hertzog, C. (1985). Measurement in the psychology of adulthood and aging. In *Handbook of the Psychology of Aging*, 2nd ed. Edited by J.E. Birren and K.W. Schaie. Van Nostrand Reinhold, New York, pp. 61-92.

11. Hultsch, D.F., and Dixon, R.A. (1984). Text processing in adulthood. In *Life Span Development and Behavior*, Vol. 6. Edited by P.B. Baltes and O.G. Brim, Jr. Academic Press, New York, pp. 77-108.

12. Craik, F.I.M., Morris, R.G., and Gick, M.L. (1989). Adult age differences in working memory. In *Neuropsychological Impairments of Short-term Memory*. Edited by G. Vallar and T. Shallice. Cambridge University Press, Cambridge.

13. Dobbs, A.R., and Rule, B.G. (1989). Adult age differences in working memory. *Psychol. Aging 4*:500-503.

14. Perlmutter, M. (1978). What is memory aging the aging of? *Dev. Psychol. 14*:330-345.

15. Lachman, J.L., and Lachman, R. (1980). Age and the actualization of world knowledge. In *New Directions in Memory and Aging*. Edited by L.W. Poon, J.L. Fozard, L.S. Cermak, D. Arenberg, and L.W. Thompson. Lawrence Erlbaum Associates, Hillsdale, NJ, pp. 285-311.

16. Murdock, B.B. Jr. (1967). Recent developments in short-term memory. *Br. J. Psychol. 58*:421-433.

17. Craik, F.I.M., and Lockhart, R.S. (1972). Levels of processing: A framework for memory research. *J. Verb. Learn. Verb. Behav. 11*:671-684.

18. Tulving, E. (1983). *Elements of Episodic Memory*. Oxford University Press, New York.

19. Craik, F.I.M., and Simon, E. (1980). Age differences in memory: The roles of attention and depth of processing. In *New Directions in Memory and Aging*. Edited by L.W. Poon, J.L. Fozard, L.S. Cermak, D. Arenberg, and L.W. Thompson. Lawrence Erlbaum Associates, Hillsdale, NJ, pp. 95-112.

20. Burke, D.M., and Light, L.L. (1981). Memory and aging: The role of retrieval processes. *Psychol. Bull. 90*:513-546.

21. Mitchell, D.B. (1989). How many memory systems? Evidence from aging. *J. Exp. Psychol. Learn Mem. Cogn. 15*:31-49.
22. Craik, F.I.M. (1983). On the transfer of information from temporary to permanent memory. *Phil. Trans. R. Soc. Lond. 302*:341-359.
23. Craik, F.I.M., and Levy, B.A. (1976). The concept of primary memory. In *Handbook of Learning and Cognitive Processes*. Edited by W.K. Estes. Lawrence Erlbaum Associates, Hillsdale, NJ, pp. 133-175.
24. Parkinson, S.R. (1982). Performance deficits in short-term memory tasks: A comparison of amnesic Korsakoff patients and the aged. In *Human Memory and Amnesia*. Edited by L.S. Cermak. Lawrence Erlbaum Associates, Hillsdale, NJ, pp. 77-96.
25. Baddeley, A.D., and Warrington, E.K. (1970). Amnesia and the distinction between long- and short-term memory. *J. Verb. Learn. Verb. Behav. 9*:176-189.
26. Waugh, N.C., Thomas, J.C., and Fozard, J.L. (1978). Retrieval time from different memory stores. *J. Gerontol. 3*:718-724.
27. Baddeley, A.D., and Hitch, G. (1974). Working memory. In *The Psychology of Learning and Motivation*, Vol. 8. Edited by G.H. Bower. Academic Press, New York, pp. 47-89.
28. Wright, R.E. (1981). Aging, divided attention, and processing capacity. *J. Gerontol. 36*:605-614.
29. Light, L.L., and Anderson, P.A. (1985). Working-memory capacity, age, and memory for discourse. *J. Gerontol. 40*:737-747.
30. Craik, F.I.M. (1986). A functional account of age differences in memory. In *Human Memory and Cognitive Capabilities: Mechanisms and Performances*. Edited by F. Klix and H. Hagendorf. Elsevier, Amsterdam, pp. 409-422.
31. Wingfield, A., Stine, E.A.L., Lahar, C.J., and Aberdeen, J.S. (1988). Does the capacity of working memory change with age? *Exp. Aging Res. 14*:103-107.
32. Baddeley, A.D., Logie, R., Bressi, S., Della Sala, S., and Spinnler, H. (1986). Dementia and working memory. *Q. J. Exp. Psychol. 38*:603-618.
33. Craik, F.I.M., and McDowd, J.M. (1987). Age differences in recall and recognition. *J. Exp. Psychol. Learn. Mem. Cogn. 13*:474-479.
34. Salthouse, T.A. (1982). *Adult Cognition: An Experimental Psychology of Human Aging*. Springer Verlag, New York.
35. Hasher, L., and Zacks, R.T. (1979). Automatic and effortful processes in memory. *J. Exp. Psychol. Gen. 108*:356-388.
36. Rissenberg, M., and Glanzer, M. (1986). Picture superiority in free recall: The effects of normal aging and primary degenerative dementia. *J. Gerontol. 41*: 64-71.
37. Sharps, M.J., and Gollin, E.S. (1988). Aging and free recall for objects located in space. *J. Gerontol. 43*:P8-11.
38. Waddell, K.J., and Rogoff, B. (1981). Effects of contextual organization on spatial memory of middle-aged and older women. *Develop. Psychol. 17*:878-885.
39. Tulving, E., Schacter, D.L., and Stark, H. (1982). Priming effects in word-fragment completion are independent of recognition memory. *J. Exp. Psychol. Learn. Mem. Cogn. 8*:336-342.

40. Schacter, D.L. (1987). Implicit Memory: History and current status. *J. Exp. Psychol. Learn. Mem. Cog. 13*:501-518.
41. Jacoby, L.L. (1983). Remembering the data: Analyzing interactive processes in reading. *J. Verb. Learn. Verb. Behav. 22*:485-508.
42. Moscovitch, M. (1982). A neuropsychological approach to perception and memory in normal and pathological aging. In *Aging and Cognitive Processes*. Edited by F.I.M. Craik and S. Trehub. Plenum Press, New York, pp. 55-78.
43. Byrd, M. (1984). Age differences in the retrieval of information from semantic memory. *Exp. Aging Res. 10*:29-33.
44. Light, L.L., Singh, A., and Capps, J.L. (1986). The dissociation of memory and awareness in young and older adults. *J. Clin. Exp. Neuropsychol. 8*:62-74.
45. Light, L.L., and Singh, A. (1987). Implicit and explicit memory in young and older adults. *J. Exp. Psychol. Learn. Mem. Cogn. 13*:531-541.
46. Glisky, E.L., Schacter, D.L., and Tulving, E. (1986). Computer learning by memory-impaired patients: Acquisition and retention of complex knowledge. *Neuropsychologia 24*:313-328.
47. Schacter, D.L., Harbluk, J.L., and McLachlan, D.R. (1984). Retrieval without recollection: An experimental analysis of source amnesia. *J. Verb. Learn. Verb. Behav. 23*:593-611.
48. McIntyre, J.S., and Craik, F.I.M. (1987). Age differences in memory for item and source information. *Canad. J. Psychol. 41*:175-192.
49. Albert, M.S., and Kaplan, E.G. (1980). Organic implications of neuropsychological deficits in the elderly. In *New Directions in Memory and Aging*. Edited by L.W. Poon, J.L. Fozard, L.S. Cermak, D. Arenberg, and L.W. Thompson. Lawrence Erlbaum Associates, Hillsdale, NJ, pp. 403-432.
50. Cockburn, J., and Smith, P.T. (1988). Effects of age and intelligence on everyday memory tasks. In *Practical Aspects of Memory: Current Research and Issues*. Edited by M.M. Gruneberg, P.E. Morris, and R.N. Sykes. Wiley, Chichester, pp. 132-136.
51. Cermak, L.S. (1984). The episodic/semantic distinction in amnesia. In *The Neuropsychology of Memory*. Edited by L.R. Squire and N. Butters. Guilford Press, New York, pp. 55-62.
52. Erber, J.T. (1981). Remote memory and age: a review. *Exp. Aging Res. 7*:189-199.
53. Bahrick, H.P., Bahrick, P.O., and Wittlinger, R.P. (1975). Fifty years of memory for names and faces: A cross-sectional approach. *J. Exp. Psychol. Gen. 104*:54-75.
54. Bahrick, H.P. (1979). Maintenance of knowledge: Questions about memory we forgot to ask. *J. Exp. Psychol. Gen. 108*:296-308.
55. Charness, N. (1981). Aging and skilled problem solving. *J. Exp. Psychol. Gen. 110*:21-38.
56. Charness, N. (1983). Age, skill, and bridge bidding: A chronometric analysis. *J. Verb. Learn. Verb. Behav. 22*:406-416.
57. Obler, L.K., and Albert, M.L. (1985). Language skills across adulthood. In *Handbook of the Psychology of Aging*, 2nd ed. Edited by J.E. Birren and K.W. Schaie. Van Nostrand Reinhold, New York, pp. 463-473.

58. Schaie, K.W. (1980). Cognitive development in aging. In *Language and Communication in the Elderly: Clinical, Therapeutic and Experimental Issues.* Edited by L.K. Obler and M.L. Albert. Lexington Books, Lexington, MA, pp. 152-165.
59. Hultsch, D.F., Hertzog, C., and Dixon, R.A. (1987). Age differences in meta-memory: Resolving the inconsistencies. *Canad. J. Psychol. 41*:193-208.
60. Dixon, R.A., Hultsch, D.F., Simon, E.W., and von Eye, A. (1984). Verbal ability and text structure effects on adult age differences in text recall. *J. Verb. Learn. Verb. Behav. 23*:569-578.
61. Craik, F.I.M., Byrd, M., and Swanson, J.M. (1987). Patterns of memory loss in three elderly samples. *Psychol. Aging. 2*:79-86.
62. Siegler, I.C., and Costa, P.T. Jr. (1985). Health behavior relationships. In *Handbook of the Psychology of Aging*, 2nd ed. Edited by J.E. Birren and K.W. Schaie. Van Nostrand Reinhold, New York, pp. 144-166.
63. Zarit, S.H., Eiler, J., and Hassinger, M. (1985). Clinical assessment. In *Handbook of the Psychology of Aging*, 2nd ed. Edited by J.E. Birren and K.W. Schaie. Van Nostrand Reinhold, New York, pp. 725-754.
64. Crook, T.H., Bartus, R.T., Ferris, S.H., Whitehouse, P., Cohen, G.D., and Gershon, S. (1986). Age-associated memory impairment. Proposed diagnostic criteria and measurement of clinical change—Report of a National Institute of Mental Health work group. *Dev. Neuropsychol. 24*:261-276.
65. Crook, T.H. (1989). Assessment of drug efficacy in age-associated memory impairment. In *Alzheimers Disease.* Compiled by R.J. Wurtman, S. Corkin, J.H. Growdon, and E. Ritter-Walker. Center for Brain Sciences and Metabolism Charitable Trust, Cambridge, MA, pp. 339-350.
66. Squire, L.R. (1987). *Memory and Brain.* Oxford University Press, New York.
67. Tulving, E., Risberg, J., and Ingvar, D.H. (1988). Regional cerebral blood flow and episodic memory retrieval. Presented at the Psychonomic Society Annual Meeting, Chicago.
68. Drachman, D.A., and Leavitt, J. (1974). Human memory and the cholinergic system: A relationship to aging? *Arch. Neurol. 30*:113-121.
69. Mishkin, M., Malamut, B., Bachevalier, J. (1984). Memories and habits: Two neural systems. In *Neurobiology of Learning and Memory.* Edited by G. Lynch, J.L. McGaugh, and N.M. Weinberger. Guilford Press, New York, pp. 65-77.
70. Smith, C.B. (1984). Aging and changes in cerebral energy metabolism. *Trends Neurosci. 7*:203-208.
71. Riege, W.H., Metter, E.J., Kuhl, D.E., and Phelps, M.E. (1985). Brain glucose metabolism and memory function: Age decreases in factor scores. *J. Gerontol. 40*:459-467.
72. Gold, P.E. (1987). Sweet memories. *Am. Sci. 75*:151-155.
73. Black, J.E., Greenough, W.T., Anderson, B.J., and Isaacs, K.R. (1987). Environment and the aging brain. *Can. J. Psychol. 41*:111-130.

17

Memory Disorders in Degenerative Neurological Diseases

Richard J. Caselli
and
Takehiko Yanagihara
Mayo Clinic and Mayo Foundation
Rochester, Minnesota

Memory derives from physiologic plasticity of the central nervous system and can be modeled at many levels of the neuraxis from brainstem to cerebrum (1-4). Underlying neurophysiologic properties of plastic neural circuits may be distinct in different types of memory processes. As described in patient HM (5,6), and subsequently shown in patients with Alzheimer's disease (7), loss of mesial temporal structures may preclude learning new facts but not a new motor skill. Degenerative neurological diseases which involve specific anatomic structures may be expected to cause specific types of memory impairment.

DEGENERATIVE DISEASES OF THE BASAL GANGLIA
ANATOMIC CONSIDERATIONS

The basal ganglia provide a crucial interface between the limbic system, the mesocorticolimbic dopaminergic system, and the somatic motor system (Fig. 1). Cortical input to the basal ganglia enters the striatum and output from the basal ganglia exits the pallidum. Cortical projections to the striatum can be divided into neocortical and allocortical projections (8). The neocortical projection to the neostriatum (caudate and putamen) is topographically organized (9). Similarly, the allocortical projection (hippocampus and piriform cortex) is topographically distinct in its striatal termination which is collectively called the ventral striatum. The ventral striatum comprises roughly

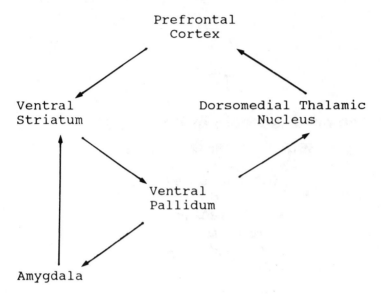

Figure 1 Neural pathways in the limbic, striatopallidal, and mesocorticolimbic dopaminergic system.

40% of the volume of the striatum (10), and includes the nucleus accumbens and a portion of the substantia innominata (8,11-14). There is topographic heterogeneity in the distribution of dopamine, acetylcholine, and neuropeptides throughout the striatum (15,16).

Dopaminergic input from the pars compacta of the substantia nigra preferentially innervates the dorsal striatum, whereas dopaminergic input from the ventral tegmental area preferentially innervates the ventral striatum (8, 10). The ventral tegmental area gives rise to the mesolimbic dopaminergic system which ascends within the medial forebrain bundle and innervates the ventral striatum and septal nuclei; and to the mesocortical dopaminergic system which innervates the prefrontal and orbitofrontal cortex (9,10). The area of prefrontal cortex receiving input from the mesocortical dopaminergic system in turn innervates the ventral striatum, topographically overlapping with the mesolimbic dopaminergic input (9,17).

Cortical input to the ventral striatum includes the hippocampus, piriform (entorhinal and perirhinal) cortices, amygdala, anterior cingulate, temporal pole, medial orbitofrontal cortex, and superior and inferior temporal gyri (8,18). The input to the ventral striatum therefore derives mainly from the limbic system. The limbic system has two major cortical outflows: a direct system independent of the basal ganglia, represented by the postcommissural fornix and an indirect system through the basal ganglia (13), represented by the precommissural fornix which projects to the nucleus accumbens, part of the ventral striatum. The ventral striatum therefore is an indirect limbic outflow target innervated by the mesocorticolimbic dopaminergic system.

The output of the ventral striatum is to the ventral pallidum (8,19) including lateral and medial segments. The pallidal segments extend below the anterior commissure into an area not previously included in pallidal anatomy, the substantia innominata, which contains the cholinergic basal forebrain nuclei including the nucleus basalis of Meynert. It is unclear whether the basal forebrain is an intrinsic pallidal structure or not (11,19).

The dorsal striatum innervates the dorsal pallidum, which in turn innervates the substantia nigra and the subthalamic nucleus (19). The ventral pallidum also innervates the substantia nigra and subthalamic nucleus, but additionally innervates the dorsomedial nucleus of the thalamus, anterior cingulate cortex, amygdala, lateral habenula, hypothalamus, ventral tegmental area, and other midbrain tegmental sites (19). The dorsomedial nucleus of the thalamus projects heavily upon the prefrontal cortex (20). Analogous to the motor loop which exists for the extrapyramidal motor system, consisting of projections from motor cortex to striatum to globus pallidus to thalamic ventralis anterior and ventralis lateralis nuclei to supplementary motor cortex and back to motor cortex, so too has a "cognitive loop" been described in which the limbic system has at least two separable circuits: prefrontal cortex to ventral striatum to ventral pallidum to thalamic dorsomedial nucleus and back to prefrontal cortex; and amygdala to ventral striatum to ventral pallidum and back to amygdala (12-14,19) (Fig. 2).

There are many links then between the limbic system and the basal ganglia, and disruption of these links may occur in various degenerative diseases. The main lesion in Parkinson's disease involves mesencephalic dopaminergic systems. Though the movement disorder derives from degeneration of the pars compacta of the substantia nigra (21) thereby causing dopaminergic denervation of the motor loop, dopamine depletion also occurs in the ventral tegmental area (17), thereby causing dopaminergic denervation of the previously outlined "cognitive loops." The roles of these cognitive loops in normal human memory are currently unknown. In rats (22) and monkeys (23), dopaminergic denervation of the prefrontal cortex impairs learning and retention of a delayed alternation task, probably due to increased distractibility and inattention rather than to any specific memory deficit per se (22). A second potentially significant lesion in Parkinson's disease is degeneration of the nucleus basalis of Meynert and reduction of cortical choline acetyltransferase activity (24-28). The role of the cholinergic system in memory has been extensively investigated (29,30) and underscores another point of possible cognitive vulnerability in Parkinson's disease. Finally, degeneration of other

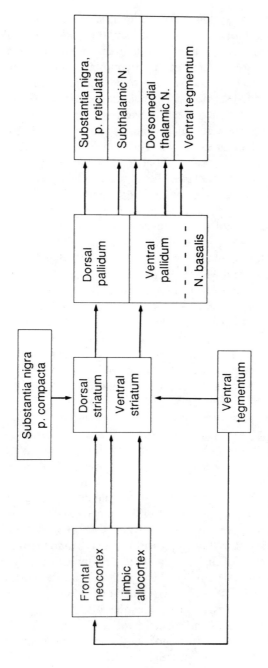

Figure 2 Frontostriatal "cognitive" loop.

neurochemical projection systems including the serotoninergic raphe nuclei (28) and the noradrenergic locus ceruleus (31) have also been considered as contributory factors in parkinsonian dementia.

Huntington's disease causes severe dementia, including memory loss. The most salient lesion underlying the memory impairment of Huntington's disease is not known, although both anatomic and physiologic indices of caudate damage correlate with neuropsychological decline (32,33). Degeneration of medium-sized spiny neurons in the striatum, the projection neurons which innervate the pallidum and the pars compacta of the substantia nigra, are lost early (34,35), and loss of striatal cells may involve the "cognitive loops." Also cortical neuronal degeneration and cytoarchitectural disarrangement are potential contributors to the cognitive decline (34).

Cognitive impairment in patients with "subcortical dementia" (36) including both Huntington's (37) and Parkinson's (38) disease, has been likened to that seen in patients with frontal lobe damage. All parts of the frontal lobes project to the striatum (9), and the latter is either destroyed in Huntington's or dopaminergically denervated in Parkinson's disease. Hence, there is some anatomical support for the clinical inference that cognitive impairments of these degenerative basal ganglia diseases reflect frontal lobe dysfunction.

CLINICAL OBSERVATIONS

THE CONCEPT OF "SUBCORTICAL DEMENTIA"

Mnemonic dysfunction is central to the concept of dementia and seldom occurs as an isolated cognitive deficit in degenerative conditions. Separation of "subcortical dementia" and "cortical dementia" (36) reflects the purportedly distinct constellation of cognitive deficits seen in degenerative diseases which predominantly affect basal ganglia from that seen in cortical dementia represented by Alzheimer's disease. There are qualitative differences in the memory disturbances which are central to both types of dementia. In subcortical dementia, patients are described as "forgetful" in that they have difficulty retrieving successfully learned material (36,39) in contrast to "amnestic" patients with cortical dementia who have difficulty learning new material (39). A second distinction is that patients with subcortical dementia do not exhibit agnosia, apraxia, and aphasia as patients with cortical dementias do (36,39-42). The central distinction postulated between the two dementias is that subcortical dementia results from disordered executive control of structurally intact cortical network/cognitive systems, whereas cortical dementia results directly from the structural disruption of cortical networks/cognitive systems (36,39). This is an oversimplification, and the validity of the distinction between these two types of dementia has been questioned on both clinical and pathological grounds (43). However, it is useful to consider what specific cognitive correlates may result in cortical and subcortical degenerative processes in view of the intriguing and intimate anatomical relationships between basal ganglia and limbic structures.

PARKINSON'S DISEASE

Degenerative forms of parkinsonism include idiopathic Parkinson's disease, familial Parkinson's disease, Parkinson's disease with additional pathologic features of Alzheimer's disease, and the parkinsonism-amyotrophic lateral sclerosis-dementia complex of Guam. The pathologic features of Alzheimer's disease including neurofibrillary tangle formation and cholinergic depletion are prominent in the latter two conditions (24-27,30,44-46) and different types of cognitive deficits might therefore be expected. Since it is not possible to reliably identify a parkinsonian patient who simultaneously has the pathologic features of Alzheimer's disease without autopsy (30,44), and since the Alzheimer type pathology is prevalent in patients with Parkinson's disease with dementia (24,25,30,44,45), it is difficult to conclusively ascribe any demonstrated cognitive deficits in patients with Parkinson's disease to dopaminergic depletion specifically. Furthermore, antiparkinsonian drugs are fraught with cognitive side effects (47). Therefore, attempts to attribute observed cognitive deficits to selective dopaminergic depletion must be viewed with those limitations in mind.

Idiopathic Parkinson's Disease. By one account, approximately one-third of patients with Parkinson's disease are demented (48) but many of them are affected only mildly. Cognitive impairment in patients with Parkinson's disease has been ascribed to "bradyphrenia" or "slowing of thought" in a manner analogous to bradykinesia (49), although the precise neuropsychological nature and mechanism of bradyphrenia is unclear. Bradyphrenia is impairment of "attention-shifting," "set-shifting," or "the inability to generate plans," all of which are reminiscent of Baddeley's central executive in the working memory model (50), and all of which have been attributed to frontal lobe or fronto-striatal dysfunction consequent to dopaminergic denervation (51-53). Impairment of the central executive would be expected to impair performances in many test paradigms, though such impaired performances may not specifically reflect structural or physiological disruption of another cognitive substrate.

Declarative memory functions have been reported to be impaired in patients with Parkinson's disease. Supraspan memory test paradigms including immediate recall of paired associated words and nonverbal visual material have demonstrated impaired "free recall" but preserved "recognition memory" suggesting a retrieval deficit rather than an encoding deficit (54). One explanation for the observed results is that parkinsonian patients are disproportionately impaired on more "effortful" tasks, i.e., those placing greater demands on selective attention and concentration, consistent with the frontral lobe hypothesis (55). Although dopaminergic agonists have been shown in normal subjects to selectively enhance performance on "difficult" tasks (56), it has also been shown in parkinsonian patients that there is a "state-dependent" effect of dopaminergic levels on learning. Patients will be more impaired on a learning paradigm if the plasma dopamine level is either decreased or increased between the time of original learning and the time of subsequent memory retrieval (57).

Impairment of temporal contextual memory in new learning paradigms, i.e., impaired recency discrimination, has been shown to be a relatively specific qualitative feature of the memory impairment of parkinsonian patients (53). Remote memory may be impaired in Parkinson's disease with a temporal gradient of severity reflecting greater impairment for more recent decades. Remote memory reflecting "dating capacity" or temporal context appears to be more impaired than recall of event content (58). This is reminiscent of the amnestic syndrome following focal basal forebrain lesions described by Damasio et al. in which there is failure of "temporal tagging" of remote events due to the inability to compute co-occurrence of separate stimuli (59).

Nondeclarative memory has received less attention, but one recent study showed that nondemented parkinsonian patients performed normally on motor learning and lexical priming paradigms, but demented parkinsonian patients were impaired on both (60). Patients with Alzheimer's disease by comparison performed poorly only on the lexical priming task suggesting that parkinsonian dementia is not identical to, but might share some pathological substrates with Alzheimer's disease (60). The authors postulated that the corticostriatal system was necessary for motor skill learning and the neocortical association areas were necessary for storage of semantic knowledge (60).

Familial Parkinson's Disease. The presence of dementia and memory impairment has been documented among patients with familial Parkinson's disease, although no qualitatively unique aspects of memory disturbance have yet been described (61-63). While dementia can result from coexisting Alzheimer's disease, Heston found 12 familial parkinsonian probands with dementia whose brains were accompanied by insufficient quantities of senile plaques and neurofibrillary tangles to conclude the coexistence of Parkinson's and Alzheimer's disease (62). Rosenberg et al. more recently described a kindred of clinically diagnosed dominantly inherited parkinsonism dementia with unusual neuropathological findings different from those of typical idiopathic Parkinson's disease (63), where the substantia nigra was pale but devoid of Lewy bodies and the striatum and pallidum showed neuronal loss and gliosis. Eosinophilic amyloid plaques which were distinct from Alzheimer plaques were scattered throughout subcortical and cortical grey matter regions (63). Both reports show that dementia occurs in parkinsonism without coexistent Alzheimer's disease.

Parkinson's Disease with coexistent Alzheimer's Pathology. Morphological (30,44,45) and neurochemical (24-26,28) abnormalities consistent with Alzheimer's disease are common in demented patients with Parkinson's disease. While there is insufficient neuropsychological data to infer a specific type of memory disturbance among neuropathologically verified cases, a general cognitive profile has been provided by Boller et al. (44). Patients without dementia have psychomotor slowing, while patients with mild dementia additionally have mild disorientation and impaired memory for recent events. Patients with severe dementia have a labile affect, mild inattentiveness, mild difficulty with naming and language comprehension, severe disorientation and constructional apraxia, moderately impaired immediate and remote memory, and severely impaired new learning and recent memory (44). Important to note, however, was the absence, even in severely demented patients, or anosognosia, frank aphasia, and ideomotor apraxia which are usually prominent in Alzheimer's disease (44).

Parkinsonism-Amyotrophic Lateral Sclerosis-Dementia Complex of Guam. The neuropathological abnormalities of Alzheimer's disease are prominent (46) but Lewy bodies are seen in only 8% of cases. Nonetheless, the cognitive profile reportedly does not resemble typical Alzheimer's disease, most notably because of the relative absence of aphasia, apraxia, and agnosia. Memory deficits are prominent within the context of dementia (46).

HUNTINGTON'S DISEASE

Dementia, including memory impairment, is a consistent, inheritable feature of patients with Huntington's disease. Lieberman et al. found that 90% of patients with Huntington's disease were demented at a mean age of 48.3 years and the dementia preceded the motor disorder in 24%, while 32% of patients with Parkinson's disease were demented at a mean age of 70.4 years and the dementia preceded the motor disorder in 3.6% (48). Although Huntington's disease may affect the cerebral cortex and other nonstriatal brain regions (34), the bulk of abnormality invariably is in the neostriatum (64). Neurochemically, selective depletion of enkephalin-containing neurons and the NMDA subtype of glutamate receptor may occur in the striatum of presymptomatic gene carriers (65). Some neuropsychological investigations of subjects at risk for carrying the Huntington's disease gene have suggested that statistically significant intellectual decline antedates actual "clinical onset" (66,67), though other studies have not supported this contention (68).

Among various cognitive functions which may ultimately fail, memory impairment occurs early (69,70). Butters et al. found that logical memory and associative learning are particularly vulnerable (69). Impairment at all stages of memory processing, including registration, encoding, and retrieval has been noted (71) and both anterograde and retrograde memory are affected (72). Despite difficulty in learning new material, the material can be retained to a greater extent than in patients with Alzheimer's disease, once it is learned (71,72). The failure of memory retrieval, including impairment of verbal fluency (69,73) in Huntington's disease, is postulated to arise from either an inefficiency of encoding in which information is stored in a non-contextual fashion (71,74), or from a "generalized inability to initiate systematic retrieval of stored information" (72) reminiscent of Baddeley's central executive function (50). Retrieval performance deteriorates rapidly with increasing the time interval between stimulus presentation and the retrieval task (71). Patients do not benefit from high imagry words, increase of the time allotted to learn words, or rehearsal (74,75), and they show no release from proactive interference (75). Frontal lobe/frontostriatal dysfunction manifests as inconsistent retrieval of previously acquired information and as the inability to benefit from contextual cues either at a categorical level or as a recognition task (71). As the dementia advances, the inability to register new material (e.g., digit span) interferes more prominently (69,70).

With regard to remote memory function, Beatty et al. demonstrated that patients with Huntington's disease had impaired recall of remote events but the severity of impairment did not follow a temporal gradient (72). These patients were as impaired for recalling events in the most recent past decade as they were for events five decades old (72). Since the events learned five decades earlier were learned before the clinical onset of Huntington's disease, these events were presumably encoded properly and hence the failure of recall reflects a retrieval problem (72).

Heindel et al. recently demonstrated that patients with Huntington's disease were impaired on a rotary-pursuit task reflecting motor skill learning but not on a lexical priming test (60), while patients with Alzheimer's disease were impaired on a lexical priming test but not on a rotary-pursuit task (60). The double dissociation between patients with Huntington's and Alzheimer's disease was thought to reflect the impairment of different neuroanatomic systems between these diseases in that motor skill learning was mediated by a corticostriatal pathway and lexical priming was executed by the neocortical association areas involved in the storage of semantic knowledge (60).

PROGRESSIVE SUPRANUCLEAR PALSY (STEELE- RICHARDSON-OLSZEWSKI DISEASE)

Progressive supranuclear palsy (PSP) was the model for "subcortical dementia" conceptualized by Albert et al. (36). Implicit in this category of disorders is a homogeneity of clinical expression among the member diseases

(42,76). Relevant clinical observations of memory impairment have been discussed for Parkinson's and Huntington's disease, two examples of "subcortical dementia." Although the absence of aphasia, apraxia, and agnosia is used to distinguish subcortical from cortical dementia (42), such deficits are occasionally observed in neuropathologically confirmed cases of PSP (77). Biochemical studies of brains with PSP have revealed marked reduction of neostriatal (excluding nucleus accumbens) dopamine, homovanillic acid, and dopamine receptors, though the decrease was less than that observed in Parkinson's disease (77,78). Mesencephalic dopamine levels are likewise depressed and there is neurofibrillary degeneration in the substantia nigra (77, 78). Kish et al. observed normal *choline acetyltransferase* activities even in the presence of severe dementia (77) and considered the dopaminergic deficit in the caudate nucleus and paraolfactory cortex (mesocortical dopaminergic projection) to be a plausible anatomical substrate for dementia. However, Ruberg et al. observed cholinergic deficit in the frontal cortex, neostriatum and ventral striatum, and regarded this as a cause of dementia in PSP (78). Positron emission tomographic studies of patients with PSP have demonstrated frontal hypometabolism (79,80). While frontal lobe/frontostriatal dysfunction may be a cause of dementia in PSP, underlying biochemical contributions have not been well established.

DIFFUSE LEWY BODY DISEASE

This rare disorder, usually diagnosed at autopsy, is characterized by Lewy bodies in the substantia nigra, locus ceruleus, periaqueductal grey, pontine raphe nuclei, mammillary bodies, and other subcortical and hypothalamic nuclei as well as in the deeper layers of neocortex, including the hippocampi (81,82). There is less cortical neurofibrillary degeneration than in Alzheimer's disease (82). Clinically these patients exhibit dementia with or without a parkinsonian extrapyramidal movement disorder (81,82). Memory loss is prominent but aphasia, apraxia, and agnosia have been observed only rarely (83).

WILSON'S DISEASE
(HEPATOLENTICULAR DEGENERATION)

Wilson's disease initially manifests as hepatic disease in 40% of patients, neurologic disease as an extrapyramidal motor disorder in 40% and psychiatric disease including psychotic behavior in 20% (84). Neuropathological abnormalities are most striking in the basal ganglia, particularly in the putamen, but copper deposition occurs widely in the brain. Intellect usually remains unaffected. Two important considerations in interpreting the data regarding memory impairment in patients with Wilson's disease are the possible coexistence of hepatic encephalopathy and the separation of motor and cognitive impairment. Patients without clincially significant neurologic manifestations sometimes show evidence of impairment on tests sensitive to motor speed and dexterity (85,86). Patients with clinically significant neurologic manifestations may show evidence of mild memory impairment (86,87). Even in these instances, however, actual scores on neuropsychologic testing may be in the normal range, making it difficult to infer any significant cognitive defect. However, some improvement in general intelligence and memory may be observed if individual patients under treatment are followed for a prolonged period (87).

OTHER DEGENERATIVE DISORDERS OF BASAL GANGLIA

Multiple system atrophy including Shy-Drager syndrome (88) and striatonigral degeneration in adults and Hallervorden-Spatz disease in children may be accompanied by dementia, though there is little data available specifically in regard to the qualitative nature of the memory disorder.

DEGENERATIVE DISEASES OF THE CEREBELLUM

ANATOMIC AND PHYSIOLOGIC CONSIDERATIONS

Cerebellar brainstem circuits have been studied in animals to define the actual cellular networks of simple adaptive behavioral responses (1-4). The vestibulo-ocular reflex, which corrects conjugate ocular deviation to maintain gaze fixation on a visual target during head movement, represents a simple model of motor learning and is subserved by the brainstem and cerebellum, particularly cerebellar flocculus (4). A conditioned eyelid blink behavior is another example of motor learning and the critical structure is the nucleus interpositus of the cerebellum. There are many conceptual models which attempt to epitomize the fundamental role of the cerebellum, but all emphasize the ability of the cerebellum to monitor the dynamic condition of muscle activity and limb geometry and to modify intentional movements with this learned information (89). Despite the role of the cerebellum in motor learning, however, clinical observations of degenerative diseases involving the cerebellum have focused on impairment of declarative memory, an indication for extracerebellar pathology.

CLINICAL OBSERVATIONS

OLIVOPONTOCEREBELLAR ATROPHY

There are five different types of olivopontocerebellar atrophy (OPCA), but cognitive impairment has been described only in types III, IV, and V (90,91). In type IV OPCA, pathologic alterations include cerebellar, inferior olivary, and pontine atrophy, and neuronal loss and degeneration of the nucleus basalis of Meynert with resultant cortical cholinergic deficiency of similar severity to Alzheimer's disease (92). However, even patients with moderate to severe ataxia retain the ability to care for themselves and show only mild to moderate impairment on tests of memory and frontal lobe function (90).

OTHER DISEASES AFFECTING THE CEREBELLUM

There are a large number of degenerative diseases with prominent cerebellar involvement and dementia of varying severity. However, there are little specific cognitive data regarding the types of memory impairment exhibited by these patients. Recessively inherited ataxias with severe dementia include those of infantile or early childhood onset (e.g., ataxia-telangiectasia, Marinesco-Sjoegren syndrome, Troyer syndrome, Behr disease) (91). Recessively inherited ataxias with mild dementia include those of middle childhood onset (e.g., Friedreich disease, abetalipoproteinemia) (91). Dominantly inherited ataxias with severe dementia usually begin during adulthood and include familial spastic ataxia and familial ataxia with photomyoclonus and lipomas (91). Dominantly inherited ataxias producing mild dementia include the olivopontocerebellar atrophies.

DEGENERATIVE DISEASES OF THE CEREBRAL CORTEX
ANATOMIC CONSIDERATIONS

Alzheimer's disease represents "cortical dementia" and is the most common cause of dementia (93-95). The cerebral cortex is cytoarchitecturally heterogenous and cortical degenerative diseases including Alzheimer's disease are expected to cause specific types of cognitive impairments which reflect the functional specialization of the differentially affected cortical regions (96). None are truly diffuse though some components of all cognitive systems may be involved in Alzheimer's disease and there may be no surviving functional networks in the terminal stages of this illness despite preservation of certain cytoarchitectural regions.

The cortical mantle can be divided into five major cytoarchitectural subdivisions; corticoid (basal forebrain), allocortical (hippocampal formation, piriform cortex), paralimbic (orbitofrontal, temporopolar, parahippocampal, and cingulate cortices), homotypical association (unimodal and polymodal sensory and motor association cortices) and idiotypic (primary sensory and motor cortices) cortical regions (97,98). Cortical connections are characterized by increasing convergence of information originating in primary sensory regions which project to successively higher order cortical association areas, those in turn projecting to parahippocampal regions, and finally to the hippocampus and amygdala; and many of these connections are reciprocal (98,

99). Different degenerative diseases will affect topographic and cytoarchitectural brain regions.

Alzheimer's disease has a distinct and evolving topographical pattern. Early stages may be difficult to distinguish from age-matched controls (100). Middle pathological stages consistently demonstrate that the most severe changes occur in mesial temporal corticoid and allocortical structures, including medial portions of the amygdala, hippocampus, entorhinal cortex, and subicular regions (93,100-104); followed by posterior cingulate gyrus and superior parietal lobule (100,101). Less severe abnormalities occur in inferior parietal lobule and lateral temporal neocortical regions (inferior and middle temporal gyri); mild changes occur in the superior temporal gyrus and frontal lobes; and no pathological alterations occur in primary sensorimotor regions (pre- and postcentral gyri, striate cortex, and Heschl's gyri) (99-101). Late stage pathology is characterized by cytoarchitectural disruption paralleling the middle stage topography, but with commensurately more severe involvement of previously mildly affected regions (100,101). Hyman et al. have shown that neuropathological severity increases as cytoarchitectural complexity diminishes from primary auditory cortex to succeeding primary, secondary, and tertiary auditory association cortices (99). Brun and Gustafson inferred a possible relationship between cortical sites of pathological sparing, early ontogenetic development and lack of nonspecific subcortical excitatory input (100). Histopathological changes include neurofibrillary tangles, senile amyloid plaques, granulovacuolar degeneration of the hippocampus and in more severely affected regions and more advanced stages, spongiform degeneration of the neutrophil (93,100,101). Wolozin et al. have developed a monoclonal antibody which distinguishes Alzheimer brain tissue from normal age-matched controls (105) and appears to identify neurons destined for neurofibrillary degeneration (106). Subcortical projection systems are also involved, and the cholinergic lesion resulting from severe degeneration of the basal forebrain nuclei (particularly the nucleus basalis of Meynert) has received the most attention (93,96,107-115). Aminergic projection systems (28,116-119) and neuropeptide systems (particularly somatostatin) (120) are likewise involved, though perhaps to a lesser degree than the cholinergic system.

CLINICAL OBSERVATIONS

COGNITIVE SYSTEMS AND NEURAL NETWORKS

Dividing mentation into functionally discrete "cognitive systems" creates arbitrary boundaries but simplifies analysis of the complex behavioral disorders which cortical lesions produce. For example, prosopagnosia (inability to distinguish familiar from unfamiliar faces) is a modality specific visual memory disturbance which Damasio et al. have defined as "the result of defective contextual evocation for stimuli belonging to a visually 'ambiguous' category" (121). The qualitative distinction between prosopagnosia and cortical blindness results from the different anatomical substrates underlying the two. Cortical blindness results from destruction of primary visual cortex, while prosopagnosia results from destruction of visual association cortex (121). Though both disorders reflect dysfunction within the same cognitive system, they result from lesions placed in very different parts of the visual "neural network." Therefore, patients with degenerative diseases of the cerebral cortex will exhibit dysfunction within certain cognitive systems but the qualitative nature of their deficits will reflect the differential location of their lesions within the respective neural networks of each cognitive system.

ALZHEIMER'S DISEASE

Two prominent categories of memory disturbances result from the anatomical distribution of pathology. The first category of memory disturbances reflects faulty associative processing within specific cognitive systems at the level of association cortex, analogous to (and including), the illustrative example of prosopagnosia. The agnosias, apraxias, and aphasias belong to this first category. The second category, amnesia, results from disruption of the hippocampal system which all sensory systems share for new learning and memory retrieval (122,123). Frontal lobe damage also affects memory by impairment of strategy planning (58).

Associative Cognitive Disturbances. Agnosia has been defined by Damasio and Eslinger as "a modality-specific impairment of the ability to recognize previously known stimuli (or stimuli for which regular learning would normally have occurred), occurring in the absence of disturbances of perception, intellect, or language as the result of acquired cerebral damage" (40). However, agnosia has been regarded as a hallmark of Alzheimer's disease despite the presence of other cognitive impairments (124). The frequently encountered difficulty of demented patients in recognizing their friends, relatives and possessions is reminiscent of prosopagnosia (121) and the ease with which demented patients become lost, even in a familiar neighborhood, is reminiscent of atopographagnosia (125). Agnosialike disturbances include anosognosia (denial of the existence of bodily defect) (126) and reduplicative paramnesia (Capgras syndrome), a rare disorder in which the patient correctly identifies familiar people and places but believes them to be imposters (127). Ideomotor apraxia may be regarded as the motor analog of agnosia or, as Heilman and Rothi state, "agnosia for gesture" (128). Limb transitive movements appear to be especially vulnerable in Alzheimer's disease (129).

Aphasia is often recognized even at an early stage in patients with Alzheimer's disease. The most salient aspect of the language disturbance is progressive impairment of lexical accession including both retrieval and comprehension with relative preservation of syntactic processing (96,130-132). There is progressive disruption of semantic knowledge characterized by the inability to distinguish subordinate and specific members of a supraordinate category (96,130-132). When attempting to name a specific item (e.g., wrench), the patient may offer either the supraordinate category title (e.g., tool), or an incorrect subordinate member of the same category that is a semantic paraphasia (e.g., pliers). As the dementia progresses, naming and the ability to comprehend specific names becomes progressively more impaired and speech becomes progressively more paraphasic resembling a Wernicke-type aphasia (96).

Amnesia. Impairment of the declarative memory system is the earliest sign and most severe manifestation of Alzheimer's disease (41,93,96). Primary memory is impaired as shown by tests of digit and word span, particularly when coupled with a distractor task (Brown-Peterson paradigm), reflecting either a primary attentional disturbance or a frontal lobe disturbance as in Baddeley's central executive model (57,133-135). Additional signs of frontal lobe dysfunction including perseveration and impaired verbal and design fluency often are seen in later stages of the dementia. Primary and secondary memory disturbances often are concurrent, but reflect independent processes which may sometimes be dissociated (135). Conversely, impaired primary memory may impede secondary memory function both in anterograde and retrograde compartments (58,136).

Impairment of secondary memory, particularly episodic and explicit aspects, is the usual heralding sign of Alzheimer's disease. The neuropathological changes dissect the afferent and efferent connectivity of the hippocampus, and this is likely the anatomic basis of the amnesic syndrome (96, 102). Amnesia implies a disturbance of episodic memory, relatively confined to the anterograde compartment during the early stages (96), but clearly invading the remote memory compartment as well in later stages (58,72). Impairment at a categorical or generic level usually occurs in later stages and clinically approaches the agnosic disturbances alluded to above (96). The remote memory compartment appears to possess a gradient effect so that the earliest memories are the least affected, with progressively more severe impairment as the retrograde interval shortens (58,72). Beatty et al. have suggested that the gradient effect reflects a primary failure of remote memory retrieval and cannot be explained by a failure of anterograde encoding of recent past events (72). Patients derive far less benefit from retrieval aids such as recognition cues than patients with "subcortical dementia." Damasio refers to a failure of "autobiographical update memory" as a central component of Alzheimer's dementia (96) in which there is a disturbance in the ability to encode and recall new personally experienced events. The amnestic disturbance precludes the normally occurring "continuous update of fundamental autobiographical data" thereby interfering with the "interpretation of ongoing percepts and the evocations they trigger" (96). In short, failure of autobiographic update memory degrades the resolution of conscious thought.

Within the nondeclarative memory system, patients with Alzheimer's disease have been shown to perform normally on tests of motor memory (7,60), but are impaired on a lexical priming paradigm (60). Presumably the latter observation reflects the known pathological alteration of neuroanatomical substrates subserving semantic knowledge (60), whereas the former reflects the relative preservation of motor and somatosensory cortices, basal ganglia, thalamus, and cerebellum (7,60).

As reviewed here, Alzheimer's disease disrupts all aspects of the declarative memory system including primary and secondary memory, episodic and semantic memory, and anterograde and retrograde memory, reflecting the widespread involvement of associative and limbic cortices. Aphasia, agnosia, and apraxia representing associative cortical dysfunction, and the qualitative and quantitative differences in amnesic syndromes distinguish Alzheimer's disease from subcortical degenerative diseases such as Huntington's and Parkinson's disease and from circumscribed amnesic disorders resulting from bilateral hippocampal or medial thalamic (e.g. Korsakoff's syndrome) damage.

FOCAL CORTICAL DEGENERATIVE DISEASES

Several degenerative diseases of the cerebral cortex may produce localized or asymmetric atrophy, and cognitive dysfunction reflects the anatomical distribution of the atrophic process, despite histopathological differences. Clinicopathological entities whose interrelationships have yet to be conclusively determined include Pick's disease (137), frontal lobe type dementia (138,139), hereditary dysphasic dementia (140), progressive aphasia (141), and focal spongiform degeneration (142). Frontal lobe type dementia and Pick's disease have been postulated to represent pathological variants of a single clinical process whose main distinguishing feature is the presence or absence of Pick bodies (143). Patients with these disorders develop memory impairment but alteration of personality and social behavior may be prominent in early stages, more so than patients with Alzheimer's disease (139,143). Graff-Radford et al. have shown that neuropathologically confirmed Pick's disease can be clinically indistinguishable from primary progressive aphasia (144), and hereditary dysphasic dementia and focal spongiform degeneration have also been shown to underlie specific cases of progressive aphasia (140, 142).

Although aphasia has been the most frequently reported cognitive disorder within the context of focal cortical degeneration, apraxia and spatial perceptual disorders have occasionally been reported as well, though the neuropathological substrate is not as well defined (145). Alajouanine's description of Maurice Ravel's progressive amusia in addition to aphasia (146) is also suggestive of a progressive focal cortical degenerative syndrome quite unlike Alzheimer's disease, though the exact etiology in this case remains unknown. The main point of clinical distinction between any of the "focal degenerations" and Alzheimer's disease is the early appearance and persistence of a cognitive disturbance other than memory, most commonly progressive aphasia. No clinical parameter is absolute, however, and pathologically confirmed Alzheimer's disease has occasionally presented as progressive aphasia (147) or as a progressive apraxia-spatial perceptual disturbance (148).

Computed tomography and magnetic resonance imaging demonstrate asymmetric atrophy, usually of the frontal and temporal lobes (140-142,144,149), and physiologic imaging including positron emission tomography (150) and single photon emission tomography reveals corresponding reduction in metabolism and blood flow in the affected regions.

The quality of the aphasic disturbance in some patients closely resembles the breakdown in semantic knowledge described in patients with Alzheimer's disease (151) and in this regard must be considered an associative memory disturbance. These patients also perform quite poorly on more conventional tests of verbal learning and memory, though it is difficult to distinguish the language component from a true verbal amnesic disturbance. Patients with isolated progressive aphasia perform normally on tests of nonverbal memory, presumably mediated by the relatively unaffected nondominant hemisphere (151). Patients with supervening dementia, however, perform poorly on both verbal and nonverbal memory tasks.

SUMMARY

Memory derives from plasticity of central nervous system networks and can therefore be compromised at some level by essentially any neurodegenerative condition. In most instances memory impairment in degenerative disease occurs within the broader context of dementia. Subcortical degenerative processes produce cognitive impairment which is consistently severe in Huntington's disease, but may be mild or severe in Parkinson's disease, and in some instances there may be no discernible cognitive impairment. Cortical degenerative diseases usually produce the most severe cognitive disturbances in general and memory disturbances in specific. The memory disturbance in patients with "subcortical dementia" reflects in large part dysfunction of the frontostriatal systems. In "cortical dementia," particularly Alzheimer's disease, amnesia results from the neuropathological dissection of paralimbic and limbic structures, although there is also widespread dysfunction of neurochemical projection systems, especially the cholinergic system, and this may contribute to some of the cognitive deficits particularly in early stages. Despite the severity and consistency of the amnesic disturbance in Alzheimer's disease, it is the associative cognitive disturbances (aphasia, agnosia, apraxia) which serve as clinically important discriminators between subcortical and cortical degenerative dementias. Focal cortical degenerative diseases may present a relatively isolated cognitive disturbance, most commonly aphasia, and this helps to distinguish them from other cortical as well as subcortical degenerative illnesses. In advanced cases, however, cognitive dysfunction can be more widespread making clinical distinction from other dementing illnesses difficult.

REFERENCES

1. Lisberger, S.G. (1988). The neural basis for motor-learning in the vestibular-ocular reflex in monkeys. *Trends Neurosci. 11*:147-152.
2. Lisberger, S.G. (1988). The neural basis for the learning of simple motor skills. *Science 242*:728-735.
3. Lisberger, S.G., and Pavelko, T.A. (1988). Brain stem neurons in modified pathways for motor learning in the primate vestibulo-ocular reflex. *Science 242*:771-773.
4. Thompson, R.E. (1986). The neurobiology of learning and memory. *Science 233*:941-947.
5. Milner, B. (1962). Les troubles de la memoire accompagnant des lesions hippocampiques bilaterales. *Centre National de la Recherche Scientifique, Paris*:257-272.
6. Corkin, S. (1968). Acquisition of motor skill after bilateral medial temporal-lobe excision. *Neuropsychologia 6*:255-265.
7. Eslinger, P.J., and Damasio, A.R. (1986). Preserved motor learning in Alzheimer's disease: Implications for anatomy and behavior. *J. Neurosci. 6*:3006-3009.
8. Heimer, L., and Wilson, R.D. (1975). The subcortical projections of the allocortex: Similarities in the neural associations of the hippocampus, the piriform cortex, and the neocortex. In *Golgi Centennial Symposium Proceedings*. Edited by M. Santini. Raven Press, New York, pp. 177-193.
9 Iversen, S.D. (1984). Behavioral aspects of the cortico-subcortical interaction with special reference to frontostriatal relations. In *Cortical Integration*. Edited by F. Reinoso-Suarez and C. Ajmone-Marsan. Raven Press, New York, pp. 237-254.
10. Domesick, V.B. (1988). Neuroanatomical organization of dopamine neurons in the ventral tegmental area. In *Annals of the New York Academy of Sciences*, Vol. 537, *The Mesocorticolimbic Dopamine System*. Edited by P.W. Kalivas and C.B. Nemeroff. New York Academy of Sciences, New York, pp. 10-26.

11. Nauta, W.J.H. (1979). A proposed conceptual reorganization of the basal ganglia and telencephalon. *Neuroscience 4*:1875-1881.
12. Nauta, W.J.H. (1986). Circuitous connections linking cerebral cortex, limbic system, and corpus striatum. In *The Limbic System: Functional Organization and Clinical Disorders*. Edited by B.K. Doane and K.E. Livingston. Raven Press, New York, pp. 43-54.
13. Nauta, W.J.H. (1986). A simplified perspective on the basal ganglia and their relation to the limbic system. In *The Limbic System: Functional Organization and Clinical Disorders*. Edited by B.K. Doane and K.E. Livingston. Raven Press, New York, pp. 67-77.
14. Nauta, W.J.H. (1986). The relationship of the basal ganglia to the limbic system. In *Handbook of Clinical Neurology*, Vol. 5 (49), *Extrapyramidal Disorders*. Edited by P.J. Vinken, G.W. Bruyn, and H.L. Klawans. Elsevier, Amsterdam, pp. 19-31.
15. Graybiel, A.M. (1984). Modular patterning in the development of the striatum. In *Cortical Integration*. Edited by F. Reinoso-Suarez and C. Ajmone-Marsan. Raven Press, New York, pp. 223-235.
16. Penney, J.B., and Young, A.B. (1986). Striatal inhomogeneities and basal ganglia function. *Movement Dis. 1*:3-15.
17. Javoy-Agid, F., and Agid, Y. (1980). Is the mesocortical dopaminergic system involved in Parkinson disease? *Neurology 30*:1326-1330.
18. Alexander, G.E., DeLong, M.R., and Strick, P.L. (1986). Parallel organization of functionally segregated circuits linking basal ganglia and cortex. *Ann. Rev. Neurosci. 9*:357-381.
19. Haber, S.N., Groenewegen, H.J., Grove, E.A., and Nauta, W.J.H. (1985). Efferent connections of the ventral pallidum: Evidence of a dual striato pallido-fugal pathway. *J. Comp. Neurol. 235*:322-335.
20. Jones, E.G. (1985). *The Thalamus*. Plenum Press, New York, pp. 649-671.
21. Bernheimer, H., Birkmayer, W., Hornykiewicz, O., Jellinger, K., and Seitelberger, F. (1973). Brain dopamine and the syndromes of Parkinson and Huntinton. Clinical, morphological, and neurochemical correlations. *J. Neurol. Sci. 20*:415-455.
22. Simon, H., and LeMoal, M. (1988). Mesencephalic dopaminergic neurons: role in the general economy of the brain. In *Annals of the New York Academy of Sciences*, Vol. 537, *The Mesocroticolimbic Dopamine System*. Edited by P.W. Kalivas and C.B. Nemeroff. New York Academy of Sciences, New York, pp. 330-338.
23. Browzowski, T.J., Brown, R.M., Rosvold, H.E., and Goldman, P.S. (1979). Cognitive deficit caused by regional depletion of dopamine in the prefrontal cortex of rhesus monkey. *Science 205*:929-932.
24. Ruberg, M., Ploska, A., Javoy-Agid, F., and Agid, Y. (1982). Muscarinic binding and choline acetyltransferase activity in parkinsonian subjects with reference to dementia. *Brain Res. 232*:129-139.
25. Dubois, B., Ruberg, M., Javoy-Agid, F., Ploska, A., and Agid, Y. (1983). A subcorticocortical cholinergic system is affected in Parkinson's disease. *Brain Res. 288*:213-218.

26. Hornykiewicz, O., and Kish, S.J. (1984). Neurochemical basis of dementia in Parkinson's disease. *Can. J. Neurol. Sci. 11*:185-190.

27. Dubois, B., Danze, F., Pillon, B., Cusimano, G., Lhermitte, F., and Agid, Y. (1987). Cholinergic dependent cognitive deficits in Parkinson's disease. *Ann. Neurol. 22*:26-30.

28. D'Amato, R.J., Zweig, R.M., Whitehouse, P.J., Wenk, G.L., Singer, H.S., Mayeux, R., Price, D.L., and Snyder, S.H. (1987). Aminergic systems in Alzheimer's disease and Parkinson's disease. *Ann. Neurol. 22*:229-236.

29. Coyle, J.T., Price, D.L., and DeLong, M.R. (1983). Alzheimer's disease: A disorder of cortical cholinergic innervation. *Science 219*:1184-1190.

30. Hakin, A.M., and Mathieson, G. (1979). Dementia in Parkinson's disease: A neuropathological study. *Neurology 29*:1209-1214.

31. Cash, R., Dennis, T., L'Heureux, R., Raisman, R., Javoy-Agid, F., and Scatton, B. (1987). Parkinson's disease and dementia: Norepinephrine and dopamine in locus ceruleus. Neurology 37:42-46.

32. Caine, E.D., and Fisher, J.D. (1985). Dementia in Huntington's disease. In *Handbook of Clinical Neurology*, Vol. 2 (46), *Neurobehavioral Disorders*. Edited by J.A.M. Frederiks. Elsevier, Amsterdam, pp. 305-310.

33. Berent, S., Giordani, B., Lehtinen, S., Markel, D., Penney, J.B., Buchtel, H.A., Starosta-Rubinstein, S., Hichwa, R., and Young, A.B. (1988). Positron emission tomographic scan investigations of Huntington's disease: Cerebral metabolic correlates of cognitive function. *Ann. Neurol. 23*:541-546.

34. Bruyn, G.W., Bots, G.T.A.M., and Dom, R. (1979). Huntington's chorea: Current neuropathological status. In *Advances in Neurology*, Vol. 23, *Huntington's Disease*. Edited by T.N. Chase, N.S. Wexler, and A. Barbeau. Raven Press, New York, pp. 83-93.

35. Young, A.B., Greenamyre, J.T., Hollingsworth, A., Albin, R., D'Amato, C., Shoulson, I., and Penney, J.B. (1988). NMDA receptor losses in putamen from patients with Huntington's disease. *Science 241*:981-983.

36. Albert, M.L., Feldman, R.G., and Willis, A.L. (1974). The 'subcortical dementia' of progressive supranuclear palsy. *J. Neurol. Neurosurg. Psychiatry 37*:121-130.

37. Brouwers, P., Cox, C., Martin, A., Chase, T., and Fedio, P. (1984). Differential perceptual spatial impairment in Huntington's and Alzheimer's dementias. *Arch. Neurol. 41*:1073-1076.

38. Taylor, A.E., Saint-Cyr, J.A., and Lang, A.E. (1986). Frontal lobe dysfunction in Parkinson's disease. *Brain 109*:845-883.

39. Cummings, J.L., and Benson, D.F. (1984). Subcortical dementia: review of an emerging concept. *Arch. Neurol. 41*:874-879.

40. Damasio, A.R., and Eslinger, P. (1986). The agnosias. In *Diseases of the Nervous System: Clinical Neurobiology*. Edited by A.K. Asbury, G.M. McKhann, and W.I. McDonald. W.B. Saunders, Philadelphia, pp. 839-847.

41. Cummings, J.L. (1982). Cortical dementias. In *Psychiatric Aspects of Neurologic Disease*, Vol. II. Edited by D.F. Benson and D. Blumer. Grune and Stratton, New York, pp. 93-121.

42. Freedman, M., and Albert, M.L. (1985). Subcortical dementia. In *Handbook of Clinical Neurology*, Vol. 2, *Neurobehavioral Disorders*. Edited by J.A.M. Frederiks. Elsevier, Amsterdam, pp. 311-316.
43. Whitehouse, P.J. (1986). The concept of subcortical and cortical dementia: another look. *Ann. Neurol. 19*:1-6.
44. Boller, F., Mizutani, T., Roessmann, U., and Gambetti, P. (1980). Parkinson disease, dementia, and Alzheimer disease: Clinicopathological correlations. *Ann. Neurol. 7*:329-335.
45. Ball, M.J. (1984). The morphological basis of dementia in Parkinson's disease. *Can. J. Neurol. Sci. 11*:180-184.
46. Chen, K.M., and Chase, T.N. (1986). Parkinsonism-dementia. In *Handbook of Clinical Neurology*, Vol. 3, *Movement Disorders*. Edited by H.L. Klawans. Elsevier, Amsterdam, pp. 167-182.
47. Parkes, J.D. (1981). Adverse effects of antiparkinsonian drugs. *Drugs 21*:341-352.
48. Lieberman, A., Dziatolowski, M., Neophytides, A., Kupersmith, M., Aleksic, S., Serby, M., Korein, J., and Goldstein, M. (1979). Dementias of Huntington's and Parkinson's disease. In *Advances in Neurology*, Vol. 23, *Huntington's Disease*. Edited by T.N. Chase, N.S. Wexler, and A. Barbeau. Raven Press, New York, pp. 273-280.
49. Naville, F. (1922). Etudes sur les complications et les sequelles mentales de l'encephalite epidemique. La bradyphrenie. *Encephale 17*:336-369.
50. Baddeley, A. (1988). Cognitive psychology and human memory. *Trends Neurosci. 11*:176-181.
51. Taylor, A.E., Saint-Cyr, J.A., and Lang, A.E. (1986). Frontal lobe dysfunction in Parkinson's disease. The cortical focus of neostriatal outflow. *Brain 109*: 845-883.
52. Morris, R.G., Downes, J.J., Sahakian, B.J., Evenden, J.L., Heald, A., and Robbins, T.W. (1988). Planning and spatial working memory in Parkinson's disease. *J. Neurol. Neurosurg. Psych. 51*:757-766.
53. Sagar, H.J., Sullivan, E.V., Gabrieli, J.D.E., Corkin, S., and Growdon, J.H. (1988). Temporal ordering and short-term memory deficits in Parkinson's disease. *Brain 111*:525-539.
54. Brown, R.G. and Marsden, C.D. (1987). Neuropsychology and cognitive function in Parkinson's disease. In *Movement Disorders*, Vol. Two. Edited by C.D. Marsden and S. Fahn. Butterworths, London, pp. 99-123.
55. Hasher, L., and Zacks, R.T. (1979). Automatic and effortful processes in memory. *J. Exp. Psychol. 108*:356-388.
56. Newman, R.P., Weingartner, H., Smallberg, S.A., and Calne, D.B. (1984). Effortful and automatic memory effects of dopamine. *Neurology 34*:805-807.
57. Huber, S.J., Schulman, H.G., Paulson, G.W., and Shuttleworth, E.C. (1987). Fluctuations in plasma dopamine level impair memory in Parkinson's disease. *Neurology 37*:1371-1375.
58. Sagar, H.J., Cohen, N.J., Sullivan, E.V., Corkin, S., and Growden, J.H. (1988). Remote memory function in Alzheimer's disease and Parkinson's disease. *Brain 111*:185-206.

59. Damasio, A.R., Graff-Radford, N.R., Eslinger, P.J., Damasio, H., and Kassell, N. (1985). Amnesia following basal forebrain lesions. *Arch. Neurol.* 42:263-271.

60. Heindel, W.C., Salmon, D.P., Shults, C.W., Walicke, P.A., and Butters, N. (1989). Neuropsychological evidence for multiple memory systems: a comparison of Alzheimer's, Huntington's, and Parkinson's disease patients. *J. Neurosci.* 9:582-587.

61. Mjones, H. (1949). Paralysis agitans: a clinical and genetic study. *Acta Psychiatr. Scand.* 52(Suppl):1-130.

62. Heston, L.L. (1980). Dementia associated with Parkinson's disease: a genetic study. *J. Neurol. Neurosurg. Psychiatry* 43:846-848.

63. Rosenberg, R.N., Green, J.B., White, C.L. III, Sparkman, D.R., DeArmond, S.J., and Kepes, J.J. (1989). Dominantly inherited dementia and parkinsonism with non-Alzheimer amyloid plaques: a new neurogenetic disorder. *Ann. Neurol.* 25:152-158.

64. Vonsattel, J.P., Myers, R.H., Stevens, T.J.l, Ferrante, R.J., Bird, E.D., and Richardson, E.P. Jr. (1985). Neuropathological classification of Huntington's disease. *J. Neuropathol. Exp. Neurol.* 44:559-577.

65. Albin, R.L., Young, A.B., Markel, D.S., Reiner, A., Anderson, K.D., Handelin, B., Tourtellotte, W., and Penney, J.B. (1989). N-methyl-D-aspartate receptor and enkephalin abnormalities in a case of presymptomatic Huntington's disease. *Neurology* 39(Suppl):423.

66. Lyle, O.E., and Gottesmann, I.I. (1979). Subtle cognitive deficits as 15- to 20-year precursors of Huntington's disease. In *Advances in Neurology*, Vol. 23, *Huntington's Disease*. Edited by T.N. Chase, N.S. Wexler, and A. Barbeau. Raven Press, New York, pp. 227-238.

67. Fedio, P., Cox, C.S., Neophytides, A., Canal-Frederick, G., and Chase, T.N. (1979). Neuropsychological profile of Huntington's disease: patients and those at risk. In *Advances in Neurology*, Vol. 23, *Huntington's Disease*. Edited by T.N. Chase, N.S. Wexler, and A. Barbeau. Raven Press, New York, pp. 239-255.

68. Wexler, N.S. (1979). Perceptual-motor, cognitive, and emotional characteristics of persons at risk for Huntington's disease. In *Advances in Neurology*, Vol. 23, *Huntington's Disease*. Edited by T.N. Chase, N.S. Wexler, and A. Barbeau. Raven Press, New York, pp. 257-271.

69. Butters, N., Sax, D., Montgomery, K., and Tarlow, S. (1978). Comparison of the neuropsychological deficits associated with early and advanced Huntington's disease. *Arch Neurol.* 35:585-589.

70. Fisher, J.M., Kennedy, J.L., Cain, E.D., and Shoulson, I. (1983). In *The Dementias*. Edited by R. Mayeux and W.G. Rosen. Raven Press, New York, pp. 229-238.

71. Caine, E.D., Ebert, M.H., and Weingartner, H. (1977). An outline for the analysis of dementia. *Neurology* 27:1087-1092.

72. Beatty, W.W., Salmon, D.P., Butters, N., Heindel, W.C., and Granholm, E.L. (1988). Retrograde amnesia in patients with Alzheimer's or Huntington's disease. *Neurobiol. Aging* 9:181-186.

73. Butters, N., Granholm, E., Salmon, D.P., and Grant, I. (1987). Episodic and semantic memory: a comparison of amnestic and demented patients. *J. Clin. Exp. Neuropsychol.* 9:479-497.

74. Weingartner, H., Cain, E.D., and Ebert, M.H. (1979). Encoding processes, learning, and recall in Huntington's disease. In *Advances in Neurology*, Vol. 23, *Huntington's Disease.* Edited by T.N. Chase, N.S. Wexler, and A. Barbeau. Raven Press, New York, pp. 215-226.

75. Butters, N., Albert, M.S., and Sax, D. (1979). Investigations of the memory disorders of patients with Huntington's disease. In *Advances in Neurology*, Vol. 23, *Huntington's Disease.* Edited by T.N. Chase, N.S. Wexler, and A. Barbeau. Raven Press, New York, pp. 201-213.

76. Benson, D.F. (1982). The treatable dementias. In *Psychiatric Aspects of Neurologic Disease*, Vol. 2. Edited by D.F. Benson and D. Blumer. Grune and Stratton, New York, pp. 123-148.

77. Kish, S.J., Chang, L.J., Mirchandani, L., Shannak, K., and Hornykiewicz, O. (1985). Progressive supranuclear palsy: relationship between extrapyramidal disturbances, dementia, and brain neurotransmitter markers. *Ann. Neurol. 18*:530-536.

78. Ruberg, M., Javoy-Agid, F., Hirsch, E., Scatton, B., LHeureux, R., Hauw, J.J., Duyckaerts, C., Gray, F., Morel-Maroger, A., Rascol, A., Serdaru, M., and Agid, Y. (1985). Dopaminergic and cholinergic lesions in progressive supranuclear palsy. *Ann. Neurol. 18*:523-529.

79. D'Antona, R., Baron, J.C., Samson, Y., Serdaru, M., Viader, F., Agid, Y., and Cambier, J. (1985). Subcortical dementia: frontal cortex hypometabolism detected by positron tomography in patients with progressive supranuclear palsy. *Brain 108*:785-799.

80. Goffinet, A.M., DeVolder, A.G., Gillain, C., Rectem, D., Bol, A., Michel, C., Cogneau, M., Labar, D., and Laterre, C. (1989). Positron tomography demonstrates frontal lobe hypometabolism in progressive supranuclear palsy. *Ann. Neurol. 25*:131-139.

81. Okazaki, H., Lipkin, L.E., and Aronson, S.M. (1961). Diffuse intracytoplasmic ganglionic inclusions (Lewy type) associated with progressive dementia and quadriparesis in flexion. *J. Neuropathol. Exp. Neurol. 20*:237-244.

82. Burkhardt, C.R., Filley, C.M., Kleinschmidt-Demaster, B.K., de la Monte, S., Norenberg, M.D., and Schneck, S.A. (1988). Diffuse Lewy body disease and progressive dementia. *Neurology 38*:1520-1528.

83. Itoh, T., Momma, Y., and Ogasawara, N. (1982). An electron microscopic study of atypical presenile dementia with numerous Lewy bodies in the cerebral cortex. *Folia Psychiatrica et Neurologica Japonica 36*:99-106.

84. Scheinberg, I.H., and Sternlieb, I. (1984). In *Major Problems in Internal Medicine*, Vol. 23, *Wilson's Disease.* W.B. Saunders Company, Philadelphia, pp. 64-92.

85. Tarter, R.E., Switala, J., Carra, J., Edwards, N., and Van Thiel, D.H. (1987). Neuropsychological impairment associated with hepatolenticular degeneration (Wilson's disease) in the absence of overt encephalopathy. *Int. J. Neurosci. 37*: 67-71.

86. Medalia, A., Isaacs-Glaberman, K., and Scheinberg, H. (1988). Neuropsychological impairment in Wilson's disease. *Arch. Neurol. 45*:502-504.
87. Goldstein, N.P., Ewert, J.C., Randall, R.V., and Gross, J.B. (1968). Psychiatric aspects of Wilson's disease (hepatolenticular degeneration): Results of psychometric tests during long-term therapy. *Am. J. Psychiat. 124*:1555-1561.
88. Shy, G.M., and Drager, G.A. (1960). A neurological syndrome associated with orthostatic hypotension. *A.M.A. Arch. Neurol. 2*:511-527.
89. Llinas, R.R. (1987). Electrophysiology of the cerebellar networks. In *Handbook of Physiology, The Nervous System II*. Edited by V.B. Mountcastle. American Physiological Society, Bethesda, pp. 831-876.
90. Kish, S.J., El-Awar, M., Schut, L., Leach, L., Oscar-Berman, M., and Freedman, M. (1988). Cognitive deficits in olivopontocerebellar atrophy: Implications for the cholinergic hypothesis of Alzheimer's dementia. *Ann. Neurol. 24*:200-206.
91. Gilman, S., Bloedel, J.R., Lechtenberg, R. (1981). *Disorders of the Cerebellum*. F.A. Davis, Philadelphia, pp. 231-262.
92. Kish, S.J., Currier, R.D., Scut, L., Perry, T.L., and Morito, C.L. (1987). Brain choline acetylcholinesterase reduction in dominantly inherited olivopontocerebellar atrophy. *Ann. Neurol. 21*:272-275.
93. Terry, R., and Katzman, R. (1983). Senile dementia of the Alzheimer type: defining a disease. In *The Neurology of Aging*. Edited by R. Katzman and R.D. Terry. F.A. Davis, Philadelphia, pp. 51-84.
94. Kokmen, E., Offord, K.P., and Okazaki, H. (1987). A clinical and autopsy study of dementia in Olmsted County, Minnesota, 1980-1981. *Neurology 37*: 426-430.
95. Schoenberg, B.S., Kokmen, E., and Okazaki, H. (1987). Alzheimer's disease and other dementing illnesses in a defined United States population: incidence rates and clinical features. *Ann. Neurol. 22*:724-729.
96. Van Hoesen, G.W., and Damasio, A.R. (1987). Neural correlates of cognitive impairment in Alzheimer's disease. In *Handbook of Physiology, The Nervous System*. Edited by V.B. Mountcastle. American Physiological Society, Bethesda, pp. 871-198.
97. Mesulam, M.M., and Mufson, E.J. (1982). Insula of the old word monkey. I: Architectonics in the insulo-orbito-temporal component of the paralimbic brain. *J. Comp. Neurol. 212*:1-22.
98. Mesulam, M.M. (1985). Patterns in behavioral neuroanatomy: association areas, the limbic system, and hemispheric specialization. In *Principles of Behavioral Neurology*. Edited by M.M. Mesulam. F.A. Davis Co., Philadelphia, pp. 1-70.
99. Hyman, B.T., Maskey, K.P., Van Hoesen, G.W., and Damasio, A.R. (1988). The auditory system in Alzheimer's disease: hierarchical pattern of pathology. *Neurology 38(Suppl. 1)*:133.
100. Brun, A., and Guftafson, L. (1976). Distribution of cerebral degeneration in Alzheimer's disease. *Arch. Psychiat. Nervenkr. 223*:15-33.
101. Brun, A., and Englund, E. (1981). Regional pattern of degeneration in Alzheimer's disease: neuronal loss and histopathological grading. *Histopathology 5*: 549-564.

102. Hyman, B.T., Van Hoesen, G.W., Kromer, L.J., and Damasio, A.R. (1986). Perforant pathway changes and the memory impairment of Alzheimer's disease. *Ann. Neurol. 20*:472-481.

103. Hyman, B.T., Van Hoesen, G.W., Damasio, A.R., and Barnes, C.L. (1984). Alzheimer's disease: cell-specific pathology isolates the hippocampal formation. *Science 225*:1168-1170.

104. Hyman, B.T., Kromer, L.J., Van Hoesen, G.W., and Damasio, A.R. (1988). Disruption of amygdala hippocampal connections demonstrated by Alz-50 immunohistochemistry in Alzheimer's disease. *Neurology 38(Suppl. 1)*:319.

105. Wolozin, B.L., Pruchnicki, A., Dickson, D.W., and Davies, P. (1986). A neuronal antigen in the brains of Alzheimer patients. *Science 232*:648-650.

106. Hyman, B.T., Van Hoesen, G.W., Wolozin, B.L., Davies, P., Kromer, K.J., and Damasio, A.R. (1988). Alz-50 antibody recognized Alzheimer-related neuronal changes. *Ann. Neurol. 23*:371-379.

107. Holman, B.L., Gibson, R.E., Hill, T.C., Eckelman, W.C., Albert, M., and Reba, R.C. (1985). Muscarinic acetylcholine receptors in Alzheimer's disease. In vivo imaging with iodine 123-labeled 3-quniuclidinyl-4-iodobenzilate and emission tomography. *JAMA 254*:3063-3066.

108. Mesulam, M.M., Geula, C., and Moran, M.A. (1987). Anatomy of cholinesterase inhibition in Alzheimer's disease: effect of physostigmine and tetrahydroaminoacridine on plaques and tangles. *Ann. Neurol. 22*:683-691.

109. Mesulam, M.M., and Moran, M.A. (1987). Cholinesterases within neurofibrillary tangles related to age and Alzheimer's disease. *Ann. Neurol. 22*:223-228.

110. Mesulam, M.M., Mufson, E.J., and Rogers, J. (1987). Age-related shrinkage of cortically projecting cholinergic neurons: a selective effect. *Ann. Neurol. 22*:31-36.

111. Hansen, L.A., DeTeresa, R., Davies, P., and Terry, R.D. (1988). Neocortical morphometry, lesion counts, and acetyltransferase levels in the age spectrum of Alzheimer's disease. *Neurology 38*:48-54.

112. Mouradian, M.M., Mohr, E., Williams, J.A., and Chase, T.N. (1988). No response to high-dose muscarinic agonist therapy in Alzheimer's disease. *Neurology 38*:606-608.

113. Mesulam, M.M. (1988). Acetylcholinesterase-rich pyramidal neurons in the human neocortex and hippocampus. *Ann. Neurol. 24*:765-773.

114. Whitehouse, P.J., Price, D.L., Struble, R.G., Clark, A.W., Coyle, J.T., and DeLong, M.R. (1982). Alzheimer's disease and senile dementia—loss of neurons in the basal forebrain. *Science 215*:1237-1239.

115. Perry, E.K., Tomlinson, B.E., Blessed, G., Bergmann, K., Gibson, P.H., and Perry, R.H. (1978). Correlation of cholinergic abnormalities with senile plaques and mental test scores in senile dementia. *Br. Med. J. 2*:1457-1459.

116. Bondaref, W., Mountjoy, C.Q., and Roth, M. (1982). Loss of neurons of origin of the adrenergic projection to the cerebral cortex (nucleus locus ceruleus) in senile dementia. *Neurology 32*:164-168.

117. Zweig, R.m., Ross, C.A., Hedreen, J.C., Steele, C., Cardillo, J.E., Whitehouse, P.J., Folstein, M.F., and Price, D.L. (1988). The neuropathology of aminergic nuclei in Alzheimer's disease. *Ann. Neurol. 24*:233-242.

118. Burke, W.J., Chung, H.D., Huang, J.S., Huang, S.S., Haring, J.H., Strong, R., Marshall, G.L., and Joh, T.H. (1988). Evidence for retrograde degeneration of epinephrine neurons in Alzheimer's disease. *Ann. Neurol.* *24*:532-536.
119. Sparks, D.L., DeKosky, S.T., and Markesbery, W.R. (1988). Alzheimer's disease: aminergic-cholinergic alterations in the hypothalamus. *Arch. Neurol.* *45*:994-999.
120. Beal, M.F. and Martin, J.B. (1986). Neuropeptides in neurological disease. *Ann. Neurol.* *20*:547-565.
121. Damasio, A.R., Damasio, H., and Van Hoesen, G.W. (1982). Prosopagnosia: anatomic basis and behavioral mechanisms. *Neurology* *32*:331-341.
122. Zola-Morgan, S., Squire, L.R., and Amaral, D.G. (1986). Human amnesia and the medial temporal region: enduring memory impairment following a bilateral lesion limited to field CA1 of the hippocampus. *J. Neurosci.* *6*:2950-2967.
123. Damasio, A.R., Eslinger, P.J., Damasio, H., Van Hoesen, G.W., and Cornell, S. (1985). Multimodal amnesic syndrome following bilateral temporal and basal forebrain damage. *Arch Neurol.* *42*:252-259.
124. McKhann, G., Drachman, D., Folstein, M., Katzman, R., Price, D., and Stadlan, E. (1984). Clinical diagnosis of Alzheimer's disease: report of the NINCDS-ADRDA Work Group under the auspices of Department of Health and Human Services Task Force on Alzheimer's disease. *Neurology* *34*:939-944.
125. Landis, T., Cummings, J.L., Benson, D.E., and Palmer, E.P. (1986). Loss of topographic familiarity: an environmental agnosia. *Arch. Neurol.* *43*:132-136.
126. Joynt, R.J., and Shoulson, I. (1985). Dementia. In *Clinical Neuropsychology*, 2nd Ed. Edited by K.M. Heilman and E.Valenstein. Oxford University Press, New York, pp. 453-479.
127. Pick, A. (1903). On reduplicative paramnesia. *Brain* *26*:260-267.
128. Heilman, K.M., and Rothi, L.J.G. (1985). Apraxia. In *Clinical Neuropsychology*, 2nd Ed. Edited by K.M. Heilman and E. Valenstein. Oxford University Press, New York, pp. 131-150.
129. Rapcsak, S.Z., Croswell, S.C., and Rubens, A.B. (1989). Apraxia in Alzheimer's disease. *Neurology* *39*:664-668.
130. Warrington, E.K. (1975). The selective impairment of semantic memory. *Q. J. Exp. Psychol.* *27*:635-657.
131. Schwartz, M.F., Marin, O.S.M., and Saffran, E.M. (1979). Dissociations of language function in dementia: a case study. *Brain Lang.* *7*:277-306.
132. Martin, A., and Fedio, P. (1983). Word production and comprehension in Alzheimer's disease: the breakdown of semantic knowledge. *Brain Lang.* *19*:124-141.
133. Morris, R.G., and Kopelman, M.D. (1986). The memory deficits in Alzheimer-type dementia: a review. *Exp. Psychol.* *38A*:575-602.
134. Freed, D.M., Corkin, S., Growdon, J.H., and Nissen, M.J. (1989). Selective attention in Alzheimer's disease: characterizing cognitive subgroups of patients. *Neuropsychologia* *27*:325-339.

135. Becker, J.T. (1988). Working memory and secondary memory deficits in Alzheimer's disease. *J. Clin. Exp. Neuropsychol. 10*:739-753.

136. Wilson, R.S., Bacon, L.D., Fox, J.H., and Kaszniak, A.W. (1983). Primary memory in dementia of the Alzheimer type. *J. Clin. Neuropsychol. 5*:337-344.

137. Pick, A. (1892). On the relation between aphasia and senile atrophy of the brain. In *Neurological Classics in Modern Translation*. Edited by D.A. Rottenberg and F.H. Hochberg. Hafner Press, New York, pp. 35-40.

138. Brun, A. (1987). Frontal lobe degeneration of non-Alzheimer type. I. Neuropathology. *Arch. Gerontol. Geriatr. 6*:193-208.

139. Gustafson, L. (1987). Frontal lobe degeneration of non-Alzheimer type. II. Clinical picture and differential diagnosis. *Arch. Gerontol. Geriatr. 6*:209-223.

140. Morris, J.C., Cole, M., Banker, B.Q., and Wright, D. (1984). Hereditary dysphasic dementia and the Pick-Alzheimer spectrum. *Ann. Neurol. 16*:455-466.

141. Mesulam, M.M. (1982). Slowly progressive aphasia without generalized dementia. *Ann. Neurol. 11*:592-598.

142. Kirshner, H.S., Tanridag, O., Thurman, L., and Whetsell, W.O. (1987). Progressive aphasia without dementia: two cases with focal spongiform degeneration. *Ann. Neurol. 22*:527-532.

143. Neary, D., Snowden, J.S., Northen, B., and Goulding, P. (1988). Dementia of frontal lobe type. *J. Neurol. Neurosurg. Psychiatry 51*:353-361.

144. Graff-Radford, N.R., Damasio, A.R., Hyman, B.T., Hart, M.N., Tranel, D., Damasio, H., Van Hoesen, G.W., and Rezai, K. (1990). Progressive aphasia in a patient with Pick's disease: a neuropsychological, radiologic, and anatomic study. *Neurology 40*:620-626.

145. DeRenzi, E. (1986). Slowly progressive visual agnosia or apraxia without dementia. *Cortex 22*:171-180.

146. Alajouanine, T. (1948). Aphasia and artistic realization. *Brain 71*:229-241.

147. Pogacar, S., and Williams, R.S. (1984). Alzheimer's disease as slowly progressive aphasia. *RI Med. J. 67*:181-185.

148. Crystal, H.A., Horoupian, D.S., Katzman, R. and Jotkowitz, S. (1982). Biopsyproved Alzheimer's disease presenting as a right parietal lobe syndrome. *Ann. Neurol. 12*:186-188.

149. Knopman, D.S., Christensen, K.J., Schut, L.J., Harbaugh, R.E., Reeder, T., Ngo, T., and Frey, W. (1989). The spectrum of imaging and neuropsychological findings in Pick's disease. *Neurology 39*:362-368.

150. Kamo, H., McGeer, P.L., Harrop, R., McGeer, E.G., Calne, D.B., Martin, W.R.W., and Pate, B.D. (1987). Positron emission tomography in Pick's disease. *Neurology 37*:439-445.

151. Basso, A., Capitani, E., and Laiacona, M. (1988). Progressive language impairment without dementia: a case with isolated category specific semantic defect. *J. Neurol. Neurosurg. Psychiatry 51*:1201-1207.

18

Memory Disorders
in Encephalitides, Encephalopathies,
and Demyelinating Diseases

Takehiko Yanagihara

Mayo Clinic and Mayo Foundation
Rochester, Minnesota

Memory disorders can occur in a variety of conditions such as infectious diseases of the central nervous sytem, various encephalopathies causing acute and subacute confusional states, and demyelinating diseases represented by multiple sclerosis. While memory impairments occur as a part of dementia in many instances, relatively pure memory disorders without a disturbance of sensorium or other cognitive functions can occur occasionally. While the pathophysiologic mechanism is different, amnesia associated with electroconvulsive therapy will be discussed here as well.

MEMORY DISORDERS ASSOCIATED WITH INFECTIOUS DISEASES OF THE CENTRAL NERVOUS SYSTEM

Patients with acute viral or bacterial meningoencephalitis often suffer from clouding of sensorium, and dementia may result if it is a chronic infectious process. Among them, herpes simplex encephalitis is known to cause selective memory impairment as neurologic sequelae and Creutzfeldt-Jakob disease (CJD) and acquired immunodeficiency syndrome (AIDS) may manifest with memory impairment as a part of dementia. Progressive multifocal leukoencephalopathy occurs in patients with lymphoma or while on immunosuppressive therapy and, more recently has been reported in patients with AIDS (1). Chronic bacterial infection also may cause altered mental states (2). Tuberculous meningitis has been known to cause a sustained period of memory impairment and even prolonged retrograde amnesia during recovery (3). Progressive dementia may be a prominent clinical feature in cryptococcal meningoencephalitis (2,4,5). In this section, herpes simplex encephalitis, CJD, and AIDS will be reviewed in more detail.

HERPES SIMPLEX ENCEPHALITIS

Herpes simplex type 1 virus can cause encephalitis by invading the temporal lobes and basal forebrain region. Cases described earlier as acute inclusion body encephalitis or acute necrotizing encephalitis had destructive lesions in the same areas and probably had the same etiology. While a reduced level of consciousness ranging from confusion to coma as well as focal neurological signs occurs in the acute phase (6), anterograde and retrograde amnesia may be prominent after recovery, and clinical manifestations of some patients are reminiscent of Korsakoff's syndrome (6-15). Detailed neuropsychologic examinations have been carried out in a few patients (10,11,14,15). While neuropathologic examinations were not carried out in these patients, the extent of damage shown by cranial computerized tomography in one patient (15) was similar to what had been observed in others at autopsy (6,7,9,12,13), showing destruction of the temporal lobes including hippocampal formation and amygdala, basal forebrain region, mammillary bodies, septal area, orbitofrontal cortex, and cingulate cortex. The thalamus and hypothalamus also may be affected (9,12).

Starr and Phillips (10) described a patient who suffered from disorientation, confabulation, and impaired learning upon recovering from coma. A pneumoencephalogram showed bilateral dilatation of the temporal horn of the lateral ventricles. The patient had a verbal IQ of above 135 and performance IQ of 110 but his memory quotient was only 89. His immediate recall was intact, but delayed recall was severely impaired. Memory function for motor tasks and remote memory were relatively well retained. Another patient described by Cermak, on two occasions (11,14), probably had destructive lesions in both temporal lobes and the left frontal region judging from pneumoencephalographic findings and brain scan. This patient had a verbal IQ of 130 and performance IQ of 133, but his memory quotient was 84. While immediate recall was intact and he performed well on the distraction task, he was unable to consolidate new information into long-term memory. He also had considerable retrograde amnesia. A subsequent study (14) revealed that he had no episodic memory for any events in his life, but his recollection was retrieved from a pool of general knowledge about himself, semantic memory. A detailed neuropsychological analysis of the patient described by Damasio et al. (15) again demonstrated anterograde and retrograde amnesia, where both episodic and semantic memory were affected in anterograde amnesia and episodic memory alone in retrograde amnesia. Thus, relatively pure amnesia may occur following herpes simplex encephalitis, although more extensive residual neurlogic deficits are more common.

CREUTZFELDT-JAKOB DISEASE

Creutzfeldt-Jakob disease is a progressive neurologic disorder in which dementia is a prominent feature. Other neurologic deficits may include aphasia, agnosia, and apraxia as well as pyramidal, extrapyramidal, cerebellar, and visual signs. Dementia, myoclonus, and characteristic EEG conform a triad of the disease (16-18). Death occurs within a few months in most instances. This is a transmissable disease, but the etiologic agent is still debated. While prominent dementia may make memory impairment inconspicuous, a memory disorder may be noted at an early stage of the illness and may become a prominent feature among patients with a protracted clinical course (19). This tends to occur more often in familial cases and in patients with onset at a younger age. In such patients, differentiation from Alzheimer's disease or amyotrophic lateral sclerosis with dementia may be difficult.

ACQUIRED IMMUNODEFICIENCY SYNDROME (AIDS)

Acquired immunodeficiency syndrome is caused by systemic infection with human immunodeficiency virus (HIV) type 1. The neurologic manifestation known as AIDS dementia complex occurs in high frequency in the advanced stage of the disease and is characterized by cognitive, behavioral, and motor dysfunction (20). Histopathologic abnormalities are prominent in the subcortical structures consisting of clusters of foamy macrophages, multinucleated cells, and rarefaction of the white matter but with relative sparing of the gray matter (21). HIV has been demonstrated in foamy macrophages and multinucleated cells in the brain and in cerebrospinal fluid (22,23). The neurologic symptom complex may occur together with signs and symptoms of a systematic infection, but also may occur as a presenting or sole manifestation of HIV-1 infection (24). Initially, it manifests with subtle cognitive changes, malaise, and lethargy but progressive dementia ensues within weeks to months. Impaired memory for recent events, lack of concentration and psychomotor slowing are the most common early behavioral manifestations (20). Confusion, disorientation, apathy, and social withdrawal are also common. In the advanced stage, patients develop global cognitive dysfunction and psychomotor slowing leading to an akinetic state. The profile resembles "subcortical dementia" in some respects (20).

Neuropsychological evaluation has disclosed abnormal cognitive function in more than half of patients with AIDS or AIDs-related complex without apparent dementia and even in HIV seropositive patients without any clinical symptoms (25). Notable neuropsychological abnormalities included slowing of information processing, mild impairment of abstract reasoning, and mild difficulty in learning. In another investigation, impairment of motor control, rapid sequential problem solving, visuospatial problem solving, spontaneity, and visual memory were observed in patients with early and advanced AIDS (26). However, no difference in neuropsychological testing has been observed by others between asymptomatic HIV seropositive and seronegative individuals (27). While forgetfulness is a common complaint in patients with early and advanced AIDS (20,26) and memory impairment has been detected on neuropsychological examination (25,26), further investigations are necessary to elucidate the nature of memory disorders associated with AIDS. Improvement of memory encoding and retrieval as well as attention and learning have been reported in patients with AIDS after treatment with zidovudine (AZT) and a similar trend was found in patients with AIDS-related complex (28).

LIMBIC ENCEPHALITIS

The term "limbic encephalitis" has been applied to patients having profound memory loss and neuronal degeneration in the hippocampus without evidence of a bacterial or viral infection of the central nervous system. Systemic malignancy, usually small cell carcinoma of the lung, is found in some patients and this disease may be paraneoplastic in nature. In 1968 Corsellis et al. described three such patients and reviewed other patients reported in the literature (29). An acute or subacute onset of profound amnesia occurred in these patients which was accompanied by seizure, confusion, and focal neurologic abnormalities. The patients were unable to encode new information and retrograde amnesia of several years was also present. At autopsy, there was no evidence of neoplastic cell infiltration in the central nervous system. However, extensive neuronal degeneration was present not only in the hippocampal pyramidal cells but also in other areas of the limbic system. Delsedime et al. reported a patient with small cell carcinoma of the lung who experienced complete loss of recent memory for 2 months but subsequently recovered (30). At autopsy several months later, there was no evidence of neuronal damage in the limbic system. The pathophysiologic mechanism for the amnesia is uncertain in this patient.

MEMORY DISORDERS ASSOCIATED WITH ENCEPHALOPATHIES

Several categories of neurologic disorders can be grouped as encephalopathies. While many patients manifest with acute confusion and disorientation, there are some instances where a memory disorder becomes predominant and others where dementia is a prominent feature.

ACUTE CONFUSIONAL STATE

This condition includes a variety of metabolic and toxic encephalopathies and is also called "delirium." This syndrome involves altered attention and consequently is not a memory disorder. The etiologic factors can be grouped into primary cerebral disorders such as infection, trauma, stroke, neoplasm, and epilepsy; systemic disorders including metabolic diseases, cardiopulmonary diseases, and collagen-vascular diseases; toxic states caused by therapeutic drugs, illicit drugs, alcohol, industrial toxic agents, and natural poisons; and withdrawal from alcohol and drugs (31). Individual offending chemicals and drugs have been described elsewhere (32). Elderly people are particularly susceptible to anticholinergic, sedative-hypnotic, and antihypertensive drugs (33). Delirium also occurs after major surgeries, particularly among elderly patients (34). Patients manifest with impaired attention and cognitive functions, while illusion and hallucinations occur in some. Memory function is globally affected but it is usually secondary to impaired attention span (31). However, metabolic and toxic disorders do not always manifest with acute or chronic confusional state and amnestic episodes may be a prominent clinical feature in some instances such as seen in patients with episodic hypoglycemia secondary to insulinoma.

ALCOHOLIC BLACKOUT

Amnesia for events occurring while under the influence of alcohol may be experienced by patients without loss of consciousness (35). During the amnesic period, which may last for hours to days, patients may become involved in altercations, social misconduct, or crimes and may travel far distances. Behavior during the amnesic period generally is not different from their usual behavior under alcoholic intoxication. Amnesia may occur abruptly with complete anterograde amnesia or may be fragmentary with subsequent partial recovery of memory of that period. When alcohol abusers were studied experimentally, those who had experienced alcoholic blackouts had an impairment of delayed recall with preserved immediate and remote recall when compared with those who had not experienced alcoholic blackouts (36). While this suggests memory impairment at the consolidation, this may not apply to memory dysfunction associated with alcoholic intoxication in general. Experimental aspects of the effect of alcohol on memory have been discussed in detail by Lawlor et al. (Chap. 5).

AMNESIA CAUSED BY BENZODIAZEPINES

Benzodiazepines are known to cause amnesia and have been used to induce experimental amnesia. This subject has been reviewed by Lawlor et al. (Chap. 5). A benzodiazepine drug which has drawn attention recently is triazolam (37,38). During the amnesic episode, patients are alert and show normal behavior; however, they subsequently are not able to recall recent events (anterograde amnesia). While the term "transient global amnesia" has been used to describe these episodes (38), the behavior is more reminiscent of alcoholic blackout, except for absence of intoxication, than the behavior observed during episodes of transient global amnesia as detailed by Miller et al. (Chap. 13).

COGNITIVE IMPAIRMENT CAUSED BY ANTIHYPERTENSIVE DRUGS

Loss of concentration and forgetfulness are complaints we hear from time to time from patients who take beta-adrenergic antagonists (propranolol, atenolol, etc.) or alpha-methyldopa. Impairment of both immediate and delayed recall has been observed in neuropsychological testing among hypertensive patients and normal volunteers who were on these medications (39-41). However, a recent review of the literature failed to substantiate specific memory impairment (42). Reduced alertness and attention which affected immediate recall could be the cause of such incidents of memory impairment.

COGNITIVE IMPAIRMENT CAUSED BY ANTICONVULSANTS

Anticonvulsants and memory have been reviewed in more detail by Blume (Chap. 15) and a recent review of this subject is also available (43). In clinical practice, we encounter patients who complain of forgetfulness or hazy memory while on phenytoin or phenobarbital, even at therapeutic plasma concentrations. Phenobarbital affects immediate recall and learning (44,45), while phenytoin affects concentration and decision-making speed as well as delayed recall (46). Cognitive dysfunction rarely occurs at a therapeutic concentration of carbamazepine (47). While no neuropsychological impairment has been noted with low therapeutic concentration of carbamazepine, errors in paired associated learning have been observed with carbamazepine over 8.0 mg/L (48). Valproic acid usually does not affect cognitive functions at therapeutic concentration, but slowing of decision making ability has been observed (49).

MEMORY DISORDERS ASSOCIATED WITH MULTIPLE SCLEROSIS

While dementia is a common outcome in a rapidly progressive or malignant form of demyelinating disease, it is encountered only occasionally in patients with the relapsing-remitting or chronic progressive form of multiple sclerosis (MS). The prevalence of clinically apparent cognitive and psychiatric

impairments has been estimated to be less than 3% (50) but it has been estimated by others to occur in 25% of patients later in the course of the disease
(51). Memory impairment usually occurs as a part of dementia but may also
occur without dementia and occasionally is the sole manifestation of MS.
Recent advances in neuropsychologic methodologies have facilitated analysis
of cognitive dysfunctions associated with MS as reviewed recently (52,53).
However, the investigations before the advent of magnetic resonance imaging
(MRI) often lack accurate anatomical correlations.

Neuropsychological abnormalities can be detected in 17.5% (54) to 72%
(55) of patients and tend to be present in patients having MS for many years
and those with the chronic progressive form. However, abnormalities can
be detected even in patients with short clinical histories (36), the relapsing-
remitting form (55), or minimal neurologic deficits (54,57). Memory impairment has often been detected neuropsychologically as a part of global cognitive dysfunction (55,57,58), but it may be a prominent neuropsychological
feature without major generalized cognitive impairments (59,60).

An impairment of memory and learning in patients with MS involves both
anterograde and retrograde memory for both verbal and nonverbal materials.
There has been general agreement that attention is not affected in MS (52,54),
but there are some exceptions (58,61). Van den Burg et al. (54) considered
the initial learning phase of the memory task to be the key deficit. Litvan et
al. (60) demonstrated impairment of information processing by the Paced
Auditory Serial Addition Test and suggested that a deficit in working memory
contributed to impairment of long-term memory. Beatty et al. (62) also observed impairment of rapid information processing with the Symbol-Digit
Modality Test and verbal fluency. Litvan et al. (63) later concluded that the
verbal memory deficit in MS was primarily caused by a deficit in working
memory where the limitation in working memory capacity interfered with
the encoding process.

Impairment in delayed recall and recognition has been observed commonly
in patients with MS (54,57,59,62-66). Patients who did poorly on delayed
recall still could perform well on delayed recognition and this observation
has led to the notion that memory deficit in MS affects retrieval of stored
information rather than acquisition (52,53). More recent publications also
support this notion (54,57,62). However, statistically significant impairment
of delayed recognition also existed in these studies and impairment of delayed recall still could be due to a defect in encoding processes in addition to
the retrieval processes. Accelerated forgetting also has been demonstrated in
patients with mild disability (54), and a significant impairment of remote memory without temporal gradient over five decades has been demonstrated (62).

The pattern of memory loss with predominant retrieval failure, the presence
of conceptual-reasoning disturbance with relatively preserved intellect, and

the absence of language disturbance have led Rao (52) to propose that cognitive and memory impairments in MS are consistent with subcortical dementia (67). The concept of subcortical dementia has been discussed by Caselli and Yanagihara. (Chap. 17). This notion has also been supported in more recent observations (62,68). Furthermore, a couple of investigations comparing cognitive dysfunctions seen in patients with MS and Huntington's disease (57) and another seen in patients with MS and Alzheimer's disease (58) have demonstrated similarities in cognitive impairments between patients with MS and Huntington's disease (57) and differences in the degree and pattern of mental impairment between patients with MS and Alzheimer's disease (58). However, even the patients with Huntington's disease differed from the patients with MS in having poorer performance in verbal and story recognition, immediate and delayed visual recall, and the use of written language (57). Beatty et al. (62) also observed naming difficulties in patients with MS which is more commonly observed in patients with cortical dementia.

Magnetic resonance imaging can provide the anatomic bases to neuropsychologically observed cognitive dysfunctions in patients with MS but information is still limited at the present time. While Litvan et al. did not find significant correlation between the number of plaques and impairment of working memory (63), Huber et al. observed a correlation between the degree of corpus callosum atrophy and intellectual impairment (68). Callanan et al. found a correlation between MRI total lesion score (number and size) and impairment of auditory attention and abstracting ability (61), and Franklin et al. observed a correlation between the bihemispheric MRI lesion score (number and size) and impairment of cognitive functions detected by neuropsychological screening batteries (65). More recently, Rao et al. observed a correlation between total lesion area and impairment of recent memory, abstract/conceptual reasoning, language, and visuospatial skills, and a correlation between size of the corpus callosum and speed of information processing (66).

In summary, some neuropsychological impairment, particularly in memory, may be present in many patients with MS even without obvious neurologic deficits. While attention is not affected commonly, memory appears to be affected at multiple steps from information processing for encoding to retrieval of stored information. Although the profile is reminiscent of subcortical dementia, MS lesions can disconnect any neural pathways in the white matter and cause variation in the severity and type of memory impairment which may be difficult to fit into a defined type of cognitive or memory impairment such as cortical or subcortical dementia.

MEMORY DISORDER ASSOCIATED WITH
ELECTROCONVULSIVE THERAPY

Memory impairment is a prominent side effect of electroconvulsive therapy (ECT). A deficit in recent memory can be produced by electric stimulation of the depth of the middle temporal lobe (69) or stimulation of the anterior temporal cortex (70), while retrograde amnesia can be produced by stimulation of the posterior temporoparietal cortex (70). These observations may relate to the amnesia associated with ECT. A comparison of bilateral, dominant unilateral, and nondominant unilateral ECT has shown no difference in the effectiveness for treatment of depression (71). On the other hand, memory impairment was more selective in that verbal learning was impaired after ECT to the dominant hemisphere and nonverbal learning after ECT to the nondominant hemisphere, while bilateral ECT resulted in an intermediate pattern of memory impairment. Impairment of verbal memory may persist for up to three months after ECT to the dominant hemisphere (71).

Detailed studies of memory impairment after ECT have been carried out in a series of investigations by Squire et al. (72-76). Memory testing 6 to 10 hours after the fifth standard bilateral or nondominant unilateral ECT showed greater impairment in delayed recall of a story and geometric figure after bilateral ECT, while delayed recall of the story was not affected after unilateral ECT. There was significant retrograde amnesia one hour after the fifth bilateral ECT extending from 1 to 3 years prior to ECT, while nondominant unilateral ECT resulted in no deficit of remote memory. Impairment of remote memory after bilateral ECT was largely gone 1 to 2 weeks after completion of ECT (75).

Memory function was also measured 6 to 9 months after bilateral or nondominant unilateral ECT (73). While no abnormality in delayed recall or remote memory was detected on neuropsychological examination, patients who had received bilateral ECT complained of a subjective feeling of memory impairment. In a subsequent study, Squire et al. found 67% of patients rated their memory to be not as good as before bilateral ECT, while only 27% of patients complained of recent memory and remote memory impairment after nondominant unilateral ECT (75). They suggested that the observed discrepancy between subjective and objective assessment could be due to the presence of genuine memory impairment which could not be detected by objective assessment or due to their increased expectation of memory problems after ECT. Anterograde and retrograde memory impairments were further examined 3 years after bilateral ECT by subjective assessment (76). There were persistent defects in the perception of their memory function in about half of the patients. Memory defects 3 years after ECT consisted of retrograde amnesia for 6 months and anterograde amnesia for 2 months, while retrograde amnesia was 2 years when examined 7 months after ECT and anterograde amnesia was 3 months in duration. Their survey also indicated that patients with depression reported difficulties in recalling the events occurring in the previous 5 months (median) even without receiving ECT. Therefore, a long-term memory impairment after ECT may be interpreted as showing persistent anterograde amnesia for a median of 2 months because of a lack of memory establishment during that period (76). Although their studies showed good recovery of memory function after ECT, residual memory deficits would be more profound if patients received more intensive ECT (77, 78).

SUMMARY

Memory disorders can occur in patients with infectious diseases of the central nervous system, various encephalopathies, and multiple sclerosis. While memory impairment is often a part of more extensive cognitive dysfunction, it may be a very prominent feature, particularly in patients who suffered from herpes simplex encephalitis. This is also true for patients with limbic encephalitis and those after electroconvulsive therapy. Unique amnestic episodes are known to occur after heavy alcohol consumption (alcoholic blackout) and use of benzodiazepines.

While memory impairment is observed in patients with acute confusional state, it occurs as the result of impaired attention. Memory impairment seen in patients taking antihypertensive or anticonvulsive medications is mostly caused by impaired attention and concentration. For patients with sequelae of herpes simplex encephalitis, patients with limbic encephalitis, and perhaps patients after receiving electroconvulsive therapy, functional impairment or structural damage in the temporal lobe, particularly hippocampus and amygdala, results in anterograde amnesia and, conceivably, retrograde amnesia with more selective impairment of episodic memory than semantic memory in some instances. Memory and other neuropsychological impairments may be present in many patients with multiple sclerosis even in the absence of neurologic deficits. While attention is usually spared, memory impairment appears to encompass multiple memory steps from information processing for encoding to retrieval of stored information. For patients with multiple sclerosis and AIDS, the concept of subcortical dementia has been introduced to characterize their memory and other cognitive dysfunctions. However, further investigations are needed for accurate characterization of memory and other cognitive dysfunctions in these disorders.

REFERENCES

1. Krupp, L.B., Lipton, R.B., Swerdlow, M.L., Leeds, N.E., and ILena, J. (1985). Progressive multifocal leukoencephalopathy: Clinical and radiographic features. *Ann. Neurol. 17*:344-349.
2. Anderson, N.E., and Willoughby, E.W. (1987). Chronic meningitis without predisposing illness—a review of 83 cases. *Q. J. Med. 63*:283-295.
3. Williams, M., and Smith, H.V. (1954). Mental disturbances in tuberculous meningitis. *J. Neurol. Neurosurg. Psychiatry 17*:173-182.

4. Stockstill, M.T., and Kauffman, C.A. (1983). Comparison of cryptococcal and tuberculous meningitis. *Arch. Neurol. 40*:81-85.

5. Steiner, I., Polacheck, I., and Melamed, E. (1984). Dementia and myoclonus in a case of cryptococcal encephalitis. *Arch. Neurol. 41*:216-217.

6. Drachman, D.A., and Adams, R.D. (1962). Herpes simplex and acute inclusion-body encephalitis. *Arch. Neurol. 7*:61-79.

7. Conrad, K., and Ule, G. (1951). Ein Fall von Korsakow-Psychose mit anatomischem Befund und Klinischen Betrachtungen. *Deutsche Z. f. Nervenheilkunde 165*:430-445.

8. Rose, F.C., and Symonds, C.P. (1960). Persistent memory defect following encephalitis. *Brain 83*:195-212.

9. Friedman, H.M., and Allen, N. (1969). Chronic effects of complete limbic lobe destruction in man. *Neurology 19*:679-690.

10. Starr, R., and Phillips, L. (1970). Verbal and motor memory in the amnestic syndrome. *Neuropsychologia 8*:75-88.

11. Cermak, L.S. (1976). The encoding capacity of a patient with amnesia due to encephalitis. *Neuropsychologia 14*:311-326.

12. Hierons, R., Janota, I., and Corsellis, J.A.N. (1978). The late effects of necrotizing encephalitis of the temporal lobes and limbic areas: a clinico-pathological study of 10 cases. *Psychol. Med. 8*:21-42.

13. Barbizet, J., Duizabo, Ph., and Poirier, J. (1978). Étude anatomo-clinique d'un cas d'encéphalite amnésiante d'origine herpétique. *Rev. Neurol. 134*:241-253.

14. Cermak, L.S., and O'Connor, M. (1983). The anterograde and retrograde retrieval ability of a patient with amnesia due to encephalitis. *Neuropsychologia 21*:213-234.

15. Damasio, A.R., Eslinger, P.J., Damasio, H., Van Hoesen, G.W., and Cornell, S. (1985). Multimodal amnesic syndrome following bilateral temporal and basal forebrain damage. *Arch. Neurol. 42*:252-259.

16. Roos, R., Gajdusek, D.C., and Gibbs, C.J., Jr. (1973). The clinical characteristics of transmissible Creutzfeldt-Jakob disease. *Brain 96*:1-20.

17. Brown, P., Cathala, F., Sadowsky, D., and Gajdusek, D.C. (1979). Creutzfeldt-Jakob disease in France: II. Clinical characteristics of 124 consecutive verified cases during the decade 1968-1977. *Ann. Neurol. 6*:430-437.

18. Brown, P., Cathala, F., Castaigne, P., and Gajdusek, D.C. (1986). Creutzfeldt-Jakob disease: Clinical analysis of a consecutive series of 230 neuropathologically verified cases. *Ann. Neurol. 20*:597-602.

19. Brown, P., Rodgers-Johnson, P., Cathala, F., Gibbs, C.J., Jr., and Gajdusek, D.C. (1984). Creutzfeldt-Jakob disease of long duration: Clinicopathological characteristics, transmissibility, and differential diagnosis. *Ann. Neurol. 16*: 295-304.

20. Navia, B.A., Jordan, B.D., and Price, R.W. (1986). The AIDS dementia complex. I. Clinical features. *Ann. Neurol. 19*:517-524.

21. Navia, B.A., Cho, E.-S., Petito, C.K., and Price, R.W. (1986). The AIDS dementia complex. II. Neuropathology. *Ann. Neurol. 19*:525-535.

22. Price, R.W., Brew, B., Sidtis, J., Rosenblum, M., Scheck, A.C., and Clearly, P. (1988). The brain in AIDS: Central nervous system HIV-1 infection and AIDS dementia complex. *Science 239*:586-592.

23. Ho, D.D., Rota, T.R., Schooley, R.T., Kaplan, J.C., Allan, J.D., Groopman, J.E., Resnick, L., Felsenstein, D., Andrews, C.A., and Hirsch, M.S. (1985). Isolation of HTLV-III from cerebrospinal fluid and neural tissues of patients with neurologic syndromes related to the acquired immunodeficiency syndrome. *N. Engl. J. Med. 313*:1493-1497.

24. Navia, B.A., and Price, R.W. (1987). The acquired immunodeficiency syndrome dementia complex as the presenting or sole manifestation of human immunodeficiency virus infection. *Arch. Neurol. 44*:65-69.

25. Grant, I., Atkinson, J.H., Hesselink, J.R., Kennedy, C.J., Richman, D.D., Spector, S.A., and McCutchan, J.A. (1987). Evidence for early central nervous system involvement in the acquired immunodeficiency syndrome (AIDS) and other human immunodeficiency virus (HIV) infections. *Ann. Int. Med. 107*:828-836.

26. Tross, S., Price, R.W., Navia, B., Thaler, H.T., Gold, J., Hirsch, D.A., and Sidtis, J.J. (1988). Neuropsychological characterization of the AIDS dementia complex: a preliminary report. *AIDS 2*:81-88.

27. Goethe, K.E., Mitchell, J.E., Marshall, D.W., Brey, R.L., Cahill, W.T., Leger, D., Hoy, L.J., and Boswell, R.N. (1989). Neuropsychological and neurological function of human immunodeficiency virus seropositive asymptomatic individuals. *Arch. Neurol. 46*:129-133.

28. Schmitt, F.A., Bigley, J.W., Mckinnis, R., Logue, P.E., Evans, R.W., Drucker, J.L., and the AZT Collaborative Working Group (1988). Neuropsychological outcome of zidovudine (AZT) treatment of patients with AIDS and AIDS-related complex. *N. Engl. J. Med. 319*:1573-1578.

29. Corsellis, J.A.N., Goldberg, G.J., and Norton, A.R. (1968). "Limbic encephalitis" and its association with carcinoma. *Brain 91*:481-496.

30. Delsedime, M., Cantello, R., Durelli, L., Gilli, M., Giordana, M.T., and Riccio, A. (1984). A syndrome resembling limbic encephalitis, associated with bronchial carcinoma, but without neuropathological abnormality: a case report. *J. Neurol 231*:165-166.

31. Lipowski, Z.J. (1987). Delirium (acute confusional states). *JAMA 258*:1789-1792.

32. Yanagihara, T. (1982). Toxic disorders of the nervous system. In *Clinical Medicine*, Vol. 11. Edited by J.A. Spittel, Jr. Harper and Row, Philadelphia, pp. 1-30.

33. Larson, E.B., Kukull, W.A., Buchner, D., and Reifler, B.V. (1987). Adverse drug reactions associated with global cognitive impairment in elderly persons. *Ann. Int. Med. 107*:169-173.

34. Morse, R.M., and Litin, E.M. (1971). The anatomy of a delirium. *Am. J. Psychiatry 128*:111-116.

35. Goodwin, D.W., Crane, J.B., and Guze, S.B. (1969). Phenomenological aspects of the alcoholic "blackout." *Br. J. Psychiatry 115*:1033-1038.

36. Goodwin, D.W., Othmer, E., Halikas, J.A., and Freemon, F. (1970). Loss of short term memory as a predictor of the alcholic "blackout." *Nature 227*:201-202.

37. Shader, R.I., and Greenblatt, D.J. (1983). Triazolam and anterograde amnesia: All is not well in the Z-zone. *J. Clin. Psychopharmacol. 3*:273.

38. Morris, H.H., III, and Estes, M.L. (1987). Traveler's amnesia. Transient global amnesia secondary to triazolam. *JAMA 258*:945-946.

39. Solomon, S., Hotchkiss, E., Saravay, S.M., Bayer, C., Ramsey, P., and Blum, R.S. (1983). Impairment of memory function by antihypertensive medication. *Arch. Gen. Psychiatry 40*:1109-1112.

40. Lichter, I., Richardson, P.J., and Wyke, M.A. (1986). Differential effects of atenolol and enalapril on memory during treatment for essential hypertension. *Br. J. Clin. Pharmacol. 21*:641-645.

41. Frcka, G., and Lader, M. (1988). Psychotropic effects of repeated doses of enalapril, propranolol and atenolol in normal subjects. *Br. J. Clin. Pharamcol. 25*:67-73.

42. Dimsdale, J.E., Newton, R.P., and Joist, T. (1989). Neuropsychological side effects of β-blockers. *Arch. Int. Med. 149*:514-525.

43. Trimble, M.R. (1987). Anticonvulsant drugs and cognitive function: a review of the literature. *Epilepsia 28 (Suppl. 3)*:S37-S45.

44. MacLeod, C.M., Dekaban, A.S., and Hunt, E. (1978). Memory impairment in epileptic patients: selective effects of phenobarbital concentration. *Science 202*: 1102-1104.

45. Vining, E.P.G., Mellits, E.D., Dorsen, M.M., Cataldo, M.F., Quaskey, S.A., Spielberg, S.P., and Freeman, J.M. (1987). Psychologic and behavioral effects of antiepileptic drugs in children: a double-blind comparison between phenobarbital and valproic acid. *Pediatrics 80*:165-174.

46. Thompson, P., Huppert, F.A., and Trimble, M. (1981). Phenytoin and cognitive function: effects on normal volunteers and implications for epilepsy. *Br. J. Clin. Psychol. 20*:155-162.

47. Duche, B., Louiset, P., Demotes-Mainard, J., and Loiseau, P. (1987). Encéphalopathie subaigue. Réaction idiosyncrasique à la carbamazépine? *Rev. Neurol. 143*:211-213.

48. O'Dougherty, M., Wright, F.S., Cox, S., and Walson, P. (1987). Carbamazepine plasma concentration. Relationship to cognitive impairment. *Arch. Neurol. 44*:863-867.

49. Thompson, P.J., and Trimble, M.R. (1981). Sodium valproate and cognitive functioning in normal volunteers. *Br. J. Clin. Pharamcol. 12*:819-824.

50. Kurtzke, J.F., Beebe, G.W., Nagler, B., Auth, T.L., Kurland, L.T., and Nefzger, M.D. (1972). Studies on the natural history of multiple sclerosis. 6. Clinical and laboratory findings at first diagnosis. *Acta Neurol. Scand. 48*:19-46.

51. Kahana, E., Leibowitz, U., and Alter, M. (1971). Cerebral multiple scleroiss. *Neurology 21*:1179-1185.

52. Rao, S.M. (1986). Neuropsychology of multiple sclerosis: a critical review. *J. Clin. Exp. Neuropsychol. 8*:503-542.

53. Petersen, R.C., and Kokmen, E. (1989). Cognitive and psychiatric abnormalities in multiple sclerosis. *Mayo Clin. Proc. 64*:657-663.

54. Van den Burg, W., van Zomeren, A.H., Minderhoud, J.M., Prange, A.J.A., and Meijer, N.S.A. (1987). Cognitive impairment in patients with multiple sclerosis and mild physical disability. *Arch. Neurol. 44*:494-501.

55. Heaton, R.K., Nelson, L.M., Thompson, D.S., Burks, J.S., and Franklin, G.M.
     (1985). Neuropsychological findings in relapsing-remitting and chronic-progres-
     sive multiple sclerosis. *J. Consult. Clin. Psychol. 53*:103-110.
56. Lyon-Caen, O., Jouvent, R., Hauser, S., Chaunu, M.-P., Benoit, N., Widlöcher,
     D., and Lhermitte, F. (1986). Cognitive function in recent-onset demyelinating
     diseases. *Arch. Neurol. 43*:1138-1141.
57. Caine, E.D., Banford, K.A., Schiffer, R.B., Shoulson, I., and Levy, S. (1986).
     A controlled neuropsychological comparison of Huntington's disease and mult-
     iple sclerosis. *Arch. Neurol. 43*:249-254.
58. Filley, C.M., Heaton, R.K., Nelson, L.M., Burks, J.S., and Franklin, G.M.
     (1989). A comparison of dementia in Alzheimer's disease and multiple sclerosis.
     Arch. Neurol. 46:157-161.
59. Beatty, P.A., and Gange, J.J. (1977). Neuropsychological aspects of multiple
     sclerosis. *J. Nerv. Ment. Dis. 164*:42-50.
60. Litvan, I., Grafman, J., Vendrell, P., and Martinez, J.M. (1988). Slowed infor-
     mation processing in multiple sclerosis. *Arch. Neurol. 45*:281-285.
61. Callanan, M.M., Logsdail, S.J., Ron, M.A., and Warrington, E.K. (1989).
     Cognitive impairment in patients with clinically isolated lesions of the type seen
     in multiple sclerosis. A psychometric and MRI study. *Brain 112*:361-374.
62. Beatty, W.W., Goodkin, D.E., Monson, N., Beatty, P.A., and Hertsgaard, D.
     (1988). Anterograde and retrograde amnesia in patients with chronic progres-
     sive multiple sclerosis. *Arch. Neurol. 45*:611-619.
63. Litvan, I., Grafman, J., Vendrell, P., Martinez, J.M., Jungué, C., Vendrell,
     J.M., and Barraquer-Bordas, L. (1988). Multiple memory deficits in patients
     with multiple sclerosis. Exploring the working memory system. *Arch. Neurol.
     45*:607-610.
64. Rao, S.M., Hammeke, T.A., McQuillen, M.P., Khatri, B.O., and Lloyd, D.
     (1984). Memory disturbance in chronic progressive multiple sclerosis. *Arch.
     Neurol. 41*:625-631.
65. Franklin, G.M., Heaton, R.K., Nelson, L.M., Filley, C.M., and Seibert, C.
     (1988). Correlation of neuropsychological and MRI findings in chronic/pro-
     gressive multiple sclerosis. *Neurology 38*:1826-1829.
66. Rao, S.M., Leo, G.J., Haughton, V.M., St. Aubin-Faubert, P., and Bernardin,
     L. (1989). Correlation of magnetic resonance imaging with neuropsychological
     testing in multiple sclerosis. *Neurology 39*:161-166.
67. Albert, M.L., Feldman, R.G., and Willis, A.L. (1974). The 'subcortical demen-
     tia' of progressive supranuclear palsy. *J. Neurol. Neurosurg. Psychiatry 37*:121-
     130.
68. Huber, S.J., Paulson, G.W., Shuttleworth, E.C., Chakeres, D., Clapp, L.E.,
     Pakalnis, A., Weiss, K., and Rammohan, K. (1987). Magnetic resonance imaging
     correlates of dementia in multiple sclerosis. *Arch. Neurol. 44*:732-736.
69. Bickford, R.G., Mulder, D.W., Dodge, H.W., Jr., Svien, H.J., and Rome, H.P.
     (1958). Changes in memory function produced by electrical stimulation of the
     temporal lobe in man. *Res. Publ. Ass. Nerv. Ment. Dis. 36*:227-243.
70. Fedio, P., and van Buren, J.M. (1974). Memory deficits during electrical stimu-
     lation of the speech cortex in conscious man. *Brain Lang. 1*:29-42.

71. Halliday, A.M., Davison, K., Browne, M.W., and Kreeger, L.C. (1968). A comparison of the effects on depression and memory of bilateral E.C.T. and unilateral E.C.T. to the dominant and non-dominant hemispheres. *Br. J. Psychiatry* *114*:997-1012.

72. Squire, L.R., Slater, P.C., and Chase, P.M. (1975). Retrograde amnesia: temporal gradient in very long term memory following electroconvulsive therapy. *Science 187*:77-79.   ˙

73. Squire, L.R., and Chase, P.M. (1975). Memory functions six to nine months after electroconvulsive therapy. *Arch. Gen. Psychiatry 32*:1557-1564.

74. Squire, L.R., Slater, P.C., and Chase, P.M. (1976). Anterograde amnesia following electroconvulsive therapy: no evidence for state-dependent learning. *Behav. Biol. 17*:31-41.

75. Squire, L.R. (1977). ECT and memory loss. *Am. J. Psychiatry 134*:997-1001.

76. Squire, L.R., and Slater, P.C. (1983). Electroconvulsive therapy and complaints of memory dysfunction: a prospective three-year follow-up study. *Br. J. Psychiatry 142*:1-8.

77. Stengel, E. (1951). Intensive E.C.T. *J. Ment. Sci. 97*:139-142.

78. Goldman, H., Gomer, F.E., and Templer, D.I. (1972). Long-term effects of electroconvulsive therapy upon memory and perceptual-motor performance. *J. Clin. Psychol. 28*:32-34.

19

Memory Disorders Associated with Brain Tumors, Hydrocephalus, and Neurosurgical Procedures

Takehiko Yanagihara

Mayo Clinic and Mayo Foundation
Rochester, Minnesota

Memory impairments can occur in association with various types of brain tumors. While they are often associated with reduced mental alertness and dementia, they can occur in relatively pure forms. Dementia is also known to occur in patients with communicating hydrocephalus, particularly those with normal pressure hydrocephalus. However, pure memory impairments have been observed in rare instances. Memory impairments have also been reported following certain neurosurgical procedures.

MEMORY DISORDERS ASSOCIATED WITH BRAIN TUMORS

Although not encountered frequently, memory impairments have been recognized for many years to occur in some patients with brain tumors. Knapp (1) observed mental disturbances ranging from somnolence, confusion, and disorientation to coma in 58 of 64 autopsy cases of brain tumors in 1906, but amnesia was not specifically mentioned other than being listed among other mental symptoms. Knapp compared his collection of patients with an earlier work by Schuster (2), who noted 2 of 352 patients to have mental symptoms similar to Korsakoff's syndrome. Upon reviewing 538 patients with intracranial tumors which were verified at the time of neurosurgical procedures, Busch noted impaired memory in 258 patients, particularly in 30 of 47 patients with frontal gliomas and 28 of 43 patients with gliomas situated around the third ventricle (3). He also noted impaired memory in 31 of 36 patients with meningiomas in the anterior cerebral convexities and all 5 patients with intraventricular meningiomas. Those earlier reviews pointed out that pure memory impairments were rare but could occur in association with other neuropsychiatric symptoms. The review by Busch suggested higher frequency of memory impairments in patients with frontal and intraventricular neoplasms (3). His observation was subsequently substantiated by Delay et al. (4), who demonstrated a close association between memory impairments and brain tumors in the third ventricle among 56 patients with Korsakoff's syndrome associated with brain tumors whom they found in the literature. Memory impairments have also been recognized in patients with thalamic tumors (5). With the technological advances in cranial computerized tomography, magnetic resonance imaging, and stereotactic brain biopsy techniques, brain tumors are diagnosed in much earlier stages and clinicopathologic correlations tend to be established by those imaging techniques. This section reviews brain tumors in the region of the third ventricle, thalamus, and other areas of the brain separately and analyze anatomical correlations for memory impairments.

TUMORS IN THE REGION OF THE THIRD VENTRICLE

Williams and Pennybacker found 26 patients with memory impairment and other mental symptoms by psychological screening of 180 patients with intracranial lesions (6). Fifteen patients had deep midline tumors with significant memory impairments of Korsakoff's syndrome. Delay et al. identified 35 patients with Korsakoff's syndrome in the literature who were found to have tumors filling the third ventricle or invading the floor of the third ventricle (4). All those patients had memory impairment, disorientation, and confabulation. Twenty of 35 patients were found to have craniopharyngiomas and 5 patients had gliomas.

CRANIOPHARYNGIOMA

Patients with craniopharyngiomas often manifest with headaches, visual disturbances, and hypopituitarism. Memory impairments were found in 15 of 100 patients by Love and Marshall (7) among other mental dysfunction such as confusion and slow mentation, whereas 15 of 32 patients with craniopharyngiomas studied by Williams and Pennybacker had memory impairments (6). While all of their patients with memory impairments had tumors invading the floor and the wall of the third ventricle, a memory impairment was not found in 11 patients with a chiasmal syndrome where tumors extended anteriorly compressing the optic chiasm.

Patients with craniopharyngiomas characteristically manifest with difficulty in retaining new information and retrieving memory for past experiences, and may have distortion and fractionation of recent memory (6). Memory impairments markedly improve or disappear after successful surgery (6,8,9) or improve after aspiration of cystic fluid from a craniopharyngioma (6,9). However, improvement does not occur after ventricular drainage alone to reduce intracranial pressure (6). Detailed psychological testing has been carried out in a patient before and after aspiration of cystic fluid (9). The patient had a full-scale IQ of 117 with normal digit span. However, he had impairment of learning and pronounced impairment of delayed recall after 24 hours for both verbal and nonverbal materials. Recall of past events was also significantly impaired. Three days after aspiration of cystic fluid, his delayed recall and remote memory returned to normal.

Grünthal described one of the earliest autopsy cases of craniopharyngioma with Korsakoff's syndrome (10), where he observed destruction of the mammillary bodies by the tumor tissue. Destruction and degeneration of the mammillary bodies have been further identified at autopsy in the patients described by Benedek and Juba (11), Wagner (12), and Delay et al. (4). Benedek and Juba also observed degeneration of the mammillothalamic tracts and the anterior nuclei of the thalamus (13), while Delay et al. observed destruction of the fornix (4). Thus, memory impairment or Korsakoff's syndrome associated with craniopharyngiomas appears to be caused by destruction and degeneration of the mammillary bodies and their afferent and efferent pathways when the tumors grow posteriorly toward the interpeduncular fossa, as often encountered in adult patients (8).

PITUITARY ADENOMA

In contrast to craniopharyngiomas, memory and other mental symptoms are encountered only rarely in patients with pituitary adenomas. White and Cobb identified four patients with pituitary adenomas and memory impairments in the literature (13) and Delay et al. found only two patients in the literature who had pituitary adenomas and Korsakoff's syndrome (4). The scarcity of memory impairment probably is due to the fact that pituitary adenomas tend to grow more anteriorly than craniopharyngiomas. White and Cobb noted prominent memory impairment in 3 of 5 patients with mental symptoms (13). Memory loss was mainly for recent events and one patient also had marked confabulation. White and Cobb concluded that the extension of pituitary adenomas upward and backward was responsible for the amnestic-confabulatory syndrome. Pituitary adenomas may also extend into the middle cerebral fossa. This was likely the cause of persistent memory impairment in one patient reported by Hartley et al. (14), where the tumor extended posteriorly under the left temporal lobe.

GLIOMAS

A variety of gliomas can occur in the vicinity of the third ventricle, but it is rare to cause amnesia or Korsakoff's syndrome as a sole clinical manifestation. Delay et al. identified three patients with spongioblastomas and two patients with unspecified gliomas in the literature who manifested with Korsakoff's syndrome (4). Lhermitte et al. reported a patient with glioblastoma multiforme of the third ventricle (15). She had impairment of recent memory, confabulation, and hallucinations and was found to have the tumor filling the third ventricle, infiltrating the floor of the third ventricle and the mammillary bodies and extending into the cerebral peduncles.

OTHER TUMORS

Foerster and Gagel described a patient with a cyst in the third ventricle (16). He had progressive headache, visual disturbance, and slow mentation with forgetfulness and disorientation for three years. An ependymal cyst was removed from the third ventricle by surgery and he recovered. A colloid cyst is a characteristic tumor in the third ventricle and the patients manifest with episodic headaches and other signs of increased intracranial pressure such as nausea, vomiting, blurred vision, and even loss of consciousness (17). They may show a lack of concentration and confusion but memory impairments do not occur as a prominent symptom.

THALAMIC TUMORS

Patients with tumors in the thalamus may develop memory impairments. Smyth and Stern observed that gliomas occurring in the medial part of the thalamus tended to manifest with progressive dementia early, while those occurring in the lateral part of the thalamus tended to cause hemiparesis (5). Three of their four patients showed severe memory impairment, particularly of recent memory, and a lack of attention and concentration. Autopsies showed gliomas in the medial thalamus bilaterally or on the left side. One of 3 patients Delay et al. reported had a giant cell spongioblastoma invading both thalami (4). The patient manifested with impairment of recent memory but good recall of old events. He underwent surgery for attempted removal of a tumor from the third ventricle but died soon after surgery. At autopsy, the medial half of each thalamus was destroyed by the tumor, while the anterior nucleus on the right side was replaced by the tumor and that on the left side was compressed. The left fornix was invaded by the tumor and the mammillothalamic tract was not identifiable. However, both mammillary bodies were spared.

McEntee et al. reported a patient who suffered a sudden loss of memory (18). He had severe impairment of recent memory and learning as well as considerable difficulties in recall of remote events. At autopsy he was found to have a metastatic bronchogenic carcinoma to the posterior part of the third ventricle forming a large midline mass invading the medial aspect of the thalamus bilaterally. The dorsomedial nucleus was largely destroyed and the centrum medianum, the medial pulvinar and the habenular nucleus as well as the stria medullaris were also affected. However, the mammillary body and the anterior thalamus were spared. A patient reported by Ziegler et al. also suffered a sudden loss of memory (19). He was found to have severe impairment of recent memory and some impairment of memory for past events. A tumor was found in the right temporo parieto-occipital region on cranial CT scan three months later, and surgery revealed glioblastoma multiforme. At autopsy, five months later he was found to have a large tumor infiltrating the thalamus bilaterally but more on the right side.

Thus, the tumors in the medial thalamus including the dorsomedial nucleus can cause severe impairment of recent memory and learning as well as considerable impairment of remote memory. Destruction of the anterior nucleus of the thalamus may be contributory. While many patients have bilateral thalamic involvement, unilateral thalamic tumors may also cause memory impairment.

TUMORS IN THE FRONTOSEPTAL REGION

Memory disorders have been observed in patients with brain tumors in the frontal lobe and/or septal region. While forgetfulness and memory loss in many patients could be secondary to inattention, a lack of concentration and/or perseveration, some patients manifest with memory impairments without such difficulties. Delay et al. identified 15 patients with brain tumors in the frontal or septal region among 56 patients with Korsakoff's syndrome in their review (4). The tumors often occurred bilaterally and were frequently gliomas. Two patients described by Sprofkin and Sciarra (20) and a patient observed by Delay et al. (4) belong to this group. All of them had glioblastoma multiforme or malignant astrocytoma and manifested with impairment of recent memory and confabulation. Two of them also had impairment of remote memory. At autopsy a patient had a tumor in the center of the frontal region occupying the septum pellucidum, fornices, corpus callosum, caudate nuclei, and thalami (20). Another patient had a midline tumor infiltrating the rostrum of the corpus callosum, septum pellucidum, and fornices (20). The third patient had a tumor involving the corpus callosum, fornices, and caudate nuclei (4).

TUMORS IN OTHER BRAIN REGIONS

Aimard et al. described a patient with progressive impairment of anterograde memory who was found to have glioblastoma multiforme destroying the anterior fornices and anterior thalamic nuclei and spreading along the wall of the third ventricle posteriorly to the pineal region (21). The mammillary body and hippocampus were not affected.

Another patient reported by Boudin et al. (22) experienced an episode suggestive of transient global amnesia and subsequent progressive memory impairment and disorientation. At autopsy 8 months after the transient episode, he was found to have a glioblastoma bilaterally invading the body of the fornix, the thalamus from the anterior nucleus to the pulvinar, the posterior pillar of the fornix, the hippocampus, and the splenium of the corpus callosum.

Heilman and Sypert reported a patient with impairment of recent memory who was found to have a spongioblastoma arising from the hippocampal commissure or the pineal body and destroying the posterior fornix bilaterally (23).

Shimauchi et al. recently described a patient with impairment of recent memory (24). Magnetic resonance imaging revealed a neoplasm in the right medial temporal lobe extending to both hippocampal formation symmetrically and infiltrating the body of the fornix bilaterally. A glioblastoma multiforme was found at surgery.

ANATOMICAL CONSIDERATION FOR MEMORY IMPAIRMENTS

The anatomy of memory has been discussed extensively in Chapter 3. Memory impairments can occur in patients with brain tumors at various locations but often are a component of dementia or caused by inattention and a lack of concentration. However, the cases reviewed in this chapter clearly demonstrate that memory impairments affecting recent memory and producing Korsakoff's syndrome have been encountered in patients with brain tumors and that those tumors usually affected the midline structures. The mammillary bodies are often affected in patients with memory impairment associated with craniopharyngiomas and other types of tumors in the third ventricle. Destruction of the fornices and the anterior thalamic nuclei are also contributory. When memory impairments occurred in patients with thalamic tumors, the dorsomedial nucleus and other medial thalamic nuclei are often invaded and usually on both sides. The septum and the fornix are often affected in patients with memory impairments associated with tumors in the anterior cerebrum, while the posterior pillar of the fornix and the hippocampal formation are often invaded in patients with tumors in the posterior cerebrum. However, destruction of those structures does not always cause memory impairment, as shown in a tumor destroying both fornices (25). A well-recognized anatomical pathway for memory circuit originates from the hippocampus and passes through the mammillary body, the anterior nucleus of the thalamus and the cingulate gyrus. Neoplasms invading those structures as well as the interconnecting pathways including the fornix, the mammillothalamic tract and the thalamocortical projection to the cingulate gyrus can disrupt this memory circuit and may cause memory impairment. The second memory circuit originates from the amygdalohippocampal complex and passes through the dorsomedial nucleus of the thalamus to the prefrontal cortex. Destruction of those gray matter structures as well as the interconnecting pathways by invading neoplasms may also cause memory impairment. The information obtained in this review was not sufficient to determine whether destruction of the corpus callosum was responsible for memory impairment in some patients. However, memory impairment is not a common problem after corpus callosectomy (26) and it is unlikely that invasion of the corpus callosum itself by a tumor causes severe memory impairment.

TRANSIENT GLOBAL AMNESIA ASSOCIATED WITH BRAIN TUMORS

Transient global amnesia (TGA) is a reversible neurologic event in which a patient suddenly loses the ability to form new memories without other neurologic signs. The clinical characteristics and possible pathophysiologic mechanisms of TGA have been discussed in Chapter 13. Including a patient with malignant astrocytoma briefly described in our series (27), several patients with TGA have been observed to have brain tumors (14,22,28-32). An additional patient with glioblastoma multiforme has been reported to have experienced TGA (33). However, this patient lost her own identity during her multiple amnesic episodes and the pathophysiologic mechanism may be different from TGA. Among 8 patients, 3 had glioblastoma multiforme or malignant astrocytomas, 2 had meningiomas, and 1 each had pituitary adenoma, metastatic transitional cell carcinoma from the bladder, and a tumor of unidentified origin. The hippocampus, temporal lobe, or thalamus on the dominant or left side was invaded in 4 patients, including a patient with a pituitary adenoma and another with a meningioma (14,28,29-31), while the temporal lobe on the nondominant side was involved in 2 patients (27,30). One patient had extensive involvement of the thalamus and the hippocampus bilaterally (22) and another patient had a meningioma in the right parietal region (32).

The pathophysiologic mechanism of transient amnesic episodes in those patients remains uncertain, but partial complex seizures are a likely explanation in some patients. Focal spike and sharp wave activities were found on electroencephalographic examination in 2 patients (28,31), while a patient was subsequently observed to have partial complex seizure (14) and another patient experienced grand mal seizure later on (29). Direct pressure or invasion of the structures in memory circuits by the neoplastic processes also is another possibility, particularly for those who subsequently developed persistent memory impairments (14,22,27-29). While the patient with a large meningioma in the parietal region (32) might have had seizure, the relationship between his TGA episode and the meningioma is uncertain.

MEMORY DISORDERS ASSOCIATED WITH HYDROCEPHALUS

Normal pressure hydrocephalus (NPH) (34,35) can manifest with dementia, gait disturbance, and incontinence in adults. Other forms of hydrocephalus can also occur in adults. When Hogan and Woolsey analyzed 50 patients with hydrocephalus of adult onsets, including 4 of their own in 1966 (36), they found 24% to be secondary to subarachnoid hemorrhage, 22% to be caused by aqueductal stenosis and 22% to be idiopathic. Fifty-eight (58%) percent of patients had dementia, either alone or among other symptoms. While forgetfulness and memory loss have been described frequently in adult patients with hydrocephalus, they are mostly caused by impairment of alertness and attention or as a component of dementia.

NORMAL PRESSURE HYDROCEPHALUS

Since the original description by Hakim and Adams (34) and Adams et al. (35) in 1965, a large number of patients with NPH have been reported in the literature. The cardinal symptom complex consists of dementia, gait disturbance, and incontinence. Several diagnostic procedures have shown the presence of communicating hydrocephalus but the cerebrospinal fluid pressure is not increased (less than 180 mm H_2O). While many patients belong to the idiopathic form without known causes, some patients have antecedent neurologic events which are responsible for malabsorption or circulation of cerebrospinal fluid. They include subarachnoid hemorrhage (37-40), head injury (40,41), and meningitis (40). However, the cerebrospinal fluid pressure may be elevated in communicating hydrocephalus with known causes.

Mental dysfunction may be a prominent symptom and may develop insidiously or rapidly (42,43). Mild forgetfulness or mild impairment of recent memory often occurs early along with apathy and psychomotor retardation. Abulia and akinetic mutism are seen in advanced cases. While impairment of recent memory and delayed recall have been noted on examination, patients usually have inattention and a lack of concentration (35). However, Theander and Granholm (39) reported 4 patients with Korsakoff's syndrome with impairment of recent memory, disorientation, and confabulation following subarachnoid hemorrhage. While Korsakoff's syndrome can occur following subarachnoid hemorrhage, particularly from a ruptured aneurysm in the anterior communicating artery (see Chap. 10), Korsakoff's syndrome in the patients described by Theander and Granholm was likely caused by hydrocephalus in view of the presence of severe hydrocephalus and marked improvement of mental dysfunction in three of them following shunt procedures.

Comprehensive neuropsychological testing of patients with NPH has not been reported frequently, partly because of the difficulties in execution of such testing for patients with advanced symptoms. Comparison of neuropsychological testing before and after shunting procedures by Thomsen et al. showed most significant postoperative improvement in continuous reaction time and lesser improvement in visuospatial learning (44), supporting the notion that impaired attention is often the primary cause of memory dysfunction in NPH. Mental dysfunction including memory impairment often improves after a ventriculoperitoneal or ventriculoatrial shunt. However, neuropsychological improvement (40%) after surgery is not as dramatic as overall neurological functional improvement (73%) (44). Better surgical outcomes have been predicted for patients with known causes for NPH (42,44,45), for patients with short histories (44,46) and for patients who developed gait disturbances before the onset of dementia (46,47).

The clinical and radiological findings consistent with NPH have been observed in association with cerebrovascular disease. Earnest et al. described two hypertensive patients with failing memory, dementia, gait disturbance, and incontinence as well as parkinsonian symptom complex (48). One patient improved after a ventriculoperitoneal shunt. At autopsy both patients were found to have multiple cystic infarcts in the basal ganglia, dentate nucleus, and white matter of the cerebral and cerebellar hemisphere. While they had concentric hypertrophy of small parenchymal arteries, no abnormality was found in the leptomeninges or the arachnoid villi, as having been observed at autopsy of a patient with NPH (49), and no fibrosis was found in the basilar arachnoid membranes. Koto et al. reported a patient who presented with a similar clinical and laboratory profile and improved significantly after a ventriculopleural shunt (50). At autopsy he also had multiple lacunae in the basal ganglia, thalamus and periventricular white matter. While multiple infarcts or lacunae can cause dementia (see Chap. 10), and urinary incontinence and gait disturbance can occur in patients with multi-infarct dementia (51), definite improvement of the mental state in the above-mentioned patients after shunting procedures (48,50) suggested that the clinical features of NPH were causally related to hypertensive cerebrovascular disease. Clinical and laboratory findings consistent with NPH have also occurred in patients who had parkinsonian symptom complex with dementia (see Chap. 17). All three patients reported by Sypert et al. showed prompt improvement of dementia and extrapyramidal signs after a ventriculoatrial or ventriculomastoid shunt (52). At autopsy, in one patient who had had subarachnoid hemorrhage, a dense adhesive arachnoiditis was found in the basilar cistern and the aqueduct was stenosed, but no parenchymal abnormality was found in the extrapyramidal system or cerebral hemispheres (52). The causal relationship between NPH and parkinsonian symptom complex with dementia is suggestive but not yet firmly established.

OTHER FORMS OF HYDROCEPHALUS AND RELATED DISORDERS

Memory impairment, dementia, gait disturbance, and incontinence can occur in noncommunicating (or obstructive) hydrocephalus, and akinetic mutism may develop in advanced cases (53). One patient described by Adams et al. (35) in their paper on NPH had a tumor in the third ventricle. The same symptom complex may also be caused by intrinsic or extrinsic tumors in the brainstem (53) or aqueductal stenosis (54,55).

Korsakoff's syndrome has been observed in a patient with a cyst of the septum pellucidum (56). The patient had severe impairment of recent memory and confabulation. While she did not have hydrocephalus, a large cyst of the cavum septi pellucidi was found at surgery, which flattened and displaced the fornices. She became asymptomatic postoperatively.

Giroud et al. reported two patients who experienced transient global amnesia and then were found to have communicating hydrocephalus (57). One patient developed an amnesic episode during a rugby football game and another patient experienced four amnesic episodes. They were asymptomatic otherwise. The causal relation between transient global amnesia and hydrocephalus remains undetermined.

MEMORY DISORDERS ASSOCIATED WITH NEUROSURGICAL PROCEDURES

There are a few neurosurgical procedures which are known to cause memory impairments. The most widely known is temporal lobectomy for management of intractable epilepsy or a brain tumor (see Chap. 15). Also well known is Korsakoff's syndrome in some patients after surgical repair of an aneurysm in the anterior communicating artery (see Chap. 10). Other neurosurgical procedures which may cause memory impairments will be reviewed in this section.

FORNICOTOMY

Bilateral fornical section has been carried out in an attempt to control epilepsy or to facilitate removal of a tumor from the third ventricle. While Garcia-Bengochea et al. found no neuropsychiatric sequelae in 12 patients following bilateral fornical section (58), Hassler and Riechert reported a patient who underwent bilateral fornical section in two stages for treatment of temporal lobe epilepsy and developed amnesia and disorientation (59). Another patient reported by Sweet et al. also developed severe loss of memory and some retrograde amnesia after bilateral fornical section for removal of a colloid cyst (60). Amnesia has not been observed after unilateral fornical section (59,61). Presence or absence of amnesia after bilateral fornical section may depend on the presence or absence of an alternate memory circuit.

COMMISSUROTOMY AND CORPUS CALLOSOTOMY

Commissurotomy and corpus callosotomy have been used for treatment of intractable epilepsy and removal of a tumor from the third ventricle. Commissurotomy involves division of the entire corpus callosum, the underlying hippocampal commissure, the fornix on one side and the anterior commissure. Corpus callosotomy involves division of the entire corpus callosum and the underlying hippocampal commissure. After corpus callosotomy, patients may develop an acute disconnection syndrome consisting of apraxia of the left limbs, mutism, apathy, and confusion (62). In order to minimize the acute disconnection syndrome, section of the anterior two third of the corpus callosum has also been performed (63,64). Some patients complain of memory problems postoperatively but these usually are not substantiated by objective examinations and memory impairment has not been reported as an adverse effect of complete corpus callosotomy (62), anterior corpus callosotomy (64), or even commissurotomy (61). Zaidel and Sperry reported 10 patients who were found to have memory quotients 15 or more points below their intelligent quotients, indicating selective memory impairment (65). However, Clark and Geffen recently reviewed memory impairment associated with corpus callosotomy and commissurotomy and concluded that persistent impairment of recent memory tended to occur only in cases with concurrent extracallosal surgery beyond section of the corpus callosum, particularly after sectioning of the fornix (26).

OTHER NEUROSURGICAL PROCEDURES

A transient Korsakoff-like state lasting for a few days has been observed immediately after bilateral cingulectomy for treatment of severe obsessional states or intractable aggressive outbursts (66). The condition was characterized by disorientation for time and by the difficulty in distinguishing between the mental events and the actual happenings in the external world. While patients appeared to be confabulating their recent experiences, the events actually had occurred earlier prior to surgery. The fundamental element appears to be a failure to organize previously remembered events in the correct temporal sequence.

Memory impairment has been observed after bilateral stereotactic surgery to the dorsomedial nucleus of the thalamus for treatment of schizophrenia, psychoneurosis, and other psychiatric disorders (67). The memory quotient declined 10 points after surgery on the Wechsler Memory Scale. While there was general decline of all subsets, orientation, personal and current information, and associative learning were particularly affected, suggesting a deficit in the acquisition of new materials and the recall of old learned materials. The memory deficits existed for only two months or less after surgery.

CONCLUSION

Impairment of recent memory and Korsakoff's syndrome have been encountered in patients with brain tumors, particularly tumors in the third ventricle. The most commonly reported are craniopharyngiomas, followed by gliomas. Survey of the cases described in the literature indicated that invasion or compression of the components of memory circuits, usually on both sides, including the hippocampus, fornix, mammillary body, anterior nucleus of the thalamus, dorsomedial nucleus of the thalamus, and septal region is responsible for memory impairments. Memory impairments associated with brain tumors are often accompanied by dementia and impaired alertness. In patients with NPH or obstructive hydrocephalus, the main cognitive impairments are also reduced attention and dementia. However, memory impairments may be prominent and even Korsakoff's syndrome has been observed in patients with NPH. Memory impairments are also observed after certain neurosurgical procedures which disrupt the structural components of memory circuits bilaterally including the fornix and dorsomedial nucleus of the thalamus. Memory impairments and Korsakoff's syndrome may therefore ensue, if the structural components of memory circuits are affected.

REFERENCES

1. Knapp, P.C. (1906). The mental symptoms of cerebral tumour. *Brain 29*:35-56.
2. Schuster, P. (1902). *Psychische Störungen by Hirntumoren: Klinische and Statistische Betrachtungen*. Ferdinand Enke, Stuttgart.
3. Busch, E. (1940. Psychical symptoms in neurosurgical disease. *Acta Psychiatrica et Neurologica 15*:257-290.
4. Delay, J., Brion, S., and Derouesné, C. (1964). Syndrome de Korsakoff et étiologie tumorale. Étude anatomo-clinique de trois observations. *Rev. Neurol. 111*:97-133.
5. Smyth, G.E., and Stern, K. (1938). Tumours of the thalamus—a clinico-pathological study. *Brain 61*:339-374.
6. Williams, M., and Pennybacker, J. (1954). Memory disturbances in third ventricle tumours. *J. Neurol. Neurosurg. Psychiatry 17*:115-123.

7. Love, J.G., and Marshall, T.M. (1950). Craniopharyngiomas (pituitary adamantinomas). *Surg. Gynecol. Obstet. 90*:591-601.
8. Kahn, E.A., and Crosby, E.C. (1972). Korsakoff's syndrome associated with surgical lesions involving the mamillary bodies. *Neurology 22*:117-125.
9. Ignelzi, R.J., and Squire, L.R. (1976). Recovery from anterograde and retrograde amnesia after percutaneous drainage of a cystic craniopharyngioma. *J. Neurol. Neurosurg. Psychiatry 39*:1231-1235.
10. Grünthal, E. (1939). Ueber das Corpus mamillare und den Korsakowschen Symptomenkomplex. *Conf. Neurol. 2*:64-95.
11. Benedek, L., and Juba, A. (1941). Korsakow-Syndrom bei den Geschwulsten des Zwischenhirns. *Arch. Psychiat. Nervenkr. 114*:366-376.
12. Wagner, W. (1942). Zum Problem affektiver Veränderungen bei Störungen im Bereich des Zwischenhirns, dargestellt an den klinischen und autoptischen Befunden von drei Craniopharyngeomen. *Deutsche Ztschr. Nervenh. 154*:1-18.
13. White, J.C., and Cobb, S. (1955). Psychological changes associated with giant pituitary neoplasms. *Arch. Neurol. Psychiatry 74*:383-396.
14. Hartley, T.C., Heilman, K.M., and Garcia-Bengochea, F. (1974). A case of a transient global amnesia due to a pituitary tumor. *Neurology 24*:998-1000.
15. Lhermitte, J., Doussinet, and de Ajuriaguerra. (1937). Une observation de la forme korsakowinne des tumeurs du 3^{e}ventricle. *Rev. Neurol. 68*:709-711.
16. Foerster, C., and Gagel, O. (1933). Ein Fall von Ependymcyste des III. Ventrikels. Ein Beitrag zur Frage der Beziehungen psychischer Storungen zum Hirnstamm. *Z. Ges. Neurol. Psychiat. 149*:312-344.
17. Poppen, J.L., Reyes, V., and Horrax, G. (1953). Colloid cysts of the third ventricle. Report of seven cases. *J. Neurosurg. 10*:242-263.
18. McEntee, W.J., Biber, M.P., Perl, D.P., and Benson, D.F. (1976). Diencephalic amnesia: a reappraisal. *J. Neurol. Neurosurg. Psychiatry 39*:436-441.
19. Ziegler, D.K., Kaufman, A., and Marshall, H.E. (1977). Abrupt memory loss associated with thalamic tumor. *Arch. Neurol. 34*:545-548.
20. Sprofkin, B.E., and Sciarra, D. (1952). Korsakoff's psychosis associated with cerebral tumors. *Neurology 2*:427-434.
21. Aimard, G., Trillet, M., Perroudon, C., Tommasi, M., and Carrier, H. (1971). Ictus amnésique d'un glioblastome interéssant le trigone. *Rev. Neurol. 124*: 392-396.
22. Boudin, G., Pépin, B., Mikol, J., Haguenau, M., and Vernant, J.Cl. (1975). Gliome du système limbique postérieur, révélé par une amnésie globale transitoire. *Rev. Neurol. 131*:157-163.
23. Heilman, K.M., and Sypert, G.W. (1977). Korsakoff's syndrome resulting from bilateral fornix lesions. *Neurology 27*:490-493.
24. Shimauchi, M., Wakisaka, S., and Kinoshita, K. (1989). Amnesia due to bilateral hippocampal glioblastoma. MRI finding. *Neuroradiology 31*:430-432.
25. Woolsey, R.M., and Nelson, J.S. (1975). Asymptomatic destruction of the fornix in man. *Arch. Neurol. 32*:566-568.
26. Clark, C.R., and Geffen, G.M. (1989). Corpus callosum surgery and recent memory. A review. *Brain 112*:165-175.
27. Miller, J.W., Petersen, R.C., Metter, E.J., Millikan, C.H., and Yanagihara, T. (1987). Transient global amnesia: clinical characteristics and prognosis. *Neurology 37*:733-737.

28. Lisak, R.P., and Zimmerman, R.A. (1977). Transient global amnesia due to a dominant hemisphere tumor. *Arch. Neurol. 34*:317-318.

29. Shuping, J.R., Toole, J.F., and Alexander, E. Jr. (1980). Transient global amnesia due to glioma in the dominant hemisphere. *Neurology 30*:88-90.

30. Findler, G., Feinsod, M., Lijovetzky, G., and Hadani, M. (1983). Transient global amnesia associated with a single metastasis in the non-dominant hemisphere. *J. Neurosurg. 58*:303-305.

31. Meador, K.J., Adams, R.J., and Flanigin, H.F. (1985). Transient global amnesia and meningioma. *Neurology 35*:769-771.

32. Collins, M.P., and Freeman, J.W. (1986). Meningioma and transient global amnesia: another report. *Neurology 36*:594.

33. Ross, R.T. (1983). Transient tumor attacks. *Arch. Neurol. 40*:633-636.

34. Hakim, S., and Adams, R.D. (1965). The special clinical problem of symptomatic hydrocephalus with normal cerebrospinal fluid pressure. Observations on cerebrospinal fluid hydrodynamics. *J. Neurol. Sci. 2*:307-327.

35. Adams, R.D., Fisher, C.M., Hakim, S., Ojemann, R.G., and Sweet, W.H. (1965). Symptomatic occult hydrocephalus with "normal" cerebrospinal-fluid pressure. *N. Engl. J. Med. 273*:117-126.

36. Hogan, P.A., and Woolsey, R.M. (1966). Hydrocephalus in the adult. *JAMA 198*:524-528.

37. Foltz, E.L., and Ward, A.A., Jr. (1956). Communicating hydrocephalus from subarachnoid bleeding. *J. Neurosurg. 13*:546-566.

38. Galera, R., and Greitz, T. (1970). Hydrocephalus in the adult secondary to the rupture of intracranial arterial aneurysms. *J. Neurosurg. 32*:634-641.

39. Theander, S., and Granholm, L. (1967). Sequelae after spontaneous subarachnoid hemorrhage, with special reference to hydrocephalus and Korsakoff's syndrome. *Acta Neurol. Scand. 43*:479-488.

40. Hill, M.E., Lougheed, W.M., and Barnett, H.J.M. (1967). A treatable form of dementia due to normal pressure communicating hydrocephalus. *Can. Med. Assoc. J. 97*:1309-1320.

41. Lewin, W. (1968). Preliminary observations on external hydrocephalus after severe head injury. *Br. J. Surg. 55*:747-751.

42. Ojemann, R.G., Fisher, C.M., Adams, R.D., Sweet, W.H., and New, P.F.J. (1969). Further experience with the syndrome of "normal" pressure hydrocephalus. *J. Neurosurg. 31*:279-294.

43. Benson, D.F., LeMay, M., Patten, D.H., and Rubens, A.B. (1970). Diagnosis of normal-pressure hydrocephalus. *N. Engl. J. Med. 283*:609-615.

44. Thomsen, A.M., Børgesen, S.E., Bruhn, P., and Gjerris, F. (1986). Prognosis of dementia in normal-pressure hydrocephalus after a shunt operation. *Ann. Neurol. 20*:304-310.

45. Stein, S.C., and Langfitt, T.W. (1974). Normal-pressure hydrocephalus. Predicting the results of cerebrospinal fluid shunting. *J. Neurosurg. 41*:463-470.

46. Petersen, R.C., Mokri, B., and Law, E.R., Jr. (1985). Surgical treatment of idiopathic hydrocephalus in elderly patients. *Neurology 35*:307-311.

47. Graff-Radford, N.R., and Godersky, J.C. (1986). Normal-pressure hydrocephalus. Onset of gait abnormality before dementia predicts good surgical outcome. *Arch. Neurol. 43*:940-942.

48. Earnest, M.P., Fahn, S., Karp, J.H., and Rowland, L.P. (1974). Normal pressure hydrocephalus and hypertensive cerebrovascular disease. *Arch. Neurol. 31*: 262-266.

49. Deland, F.H., James, A.E., Jr., Ladd, D.J., and Konigsmark, B.W. (1972). Normal pressure hydrocephalus: a histologic study. *Am. J. Clin. Pathol. 58*: 58-63.

50. Koto, A., Rosenberg, G., Zingesser, L.H., Horoupian, D., and Katzman, R. (1977). Syndrome of normal pressure hydrocephalus: possible relation to hypertensive and arteriosclerotic vasculopathy. *J. Neurol. Neurosurg. Psychiatry 40*: 73-79.

51. Kotsoris, H., Barclay, L.L., Kheyfets, S., Hulyalkar, A., and Dougherty, J. (1987). Urinary and gait disturbances as markers for early multi-infarct dementia. *Stroke 18*:138-141.

52. Sypert, G.W., Leffman, H., and Ojemann, G.A. (1973). Occult normal pressure hydrocephalus manifested by parkinsonism-dementia complex. *Neurology 23*:234-238.

53. Messert, B., Henke, T.K., and Langheim, W. (1966). Syndrome of akinetic mutism associated with obstructive hydrocephalus. *Neurology 16*:635-649.

54. Wilkinson, H.A., LeMay, M., and Drew, J.H. (1966). Adult aqueductal stenosis. *Arch. Neurol. 15*:643-648.

55. Little, J.R., Houser, O.W., and MacCarty, C.S. (1975). Clinical manifestations of aqueductal stenosis in adult. *J. Neurosurg. 43*:546-552.

56. Gil Neciga, E., Gil Peralta, A., Polaina, M., Sureda, F., and Bautista, J. (1989). Cyst of the septum pellucidum and Korsakoff's psychosis. *Eur. Neurol. 29*:99-101.

57. Giroud, M., Guard, O., and Dumas, R. (1987). Transient global amnesia associated with hydrocephalus. Report of two cases. *J. Neurol. 235*:118-119.

58. Garcia Bengochea, F., de la Torre, O., Esquivel, O., Vieta, R., and Fernandez, C. (1954). The section of the fornix in the surgical treatment of certain epilepsies. *Trans. Am. Neurol. Assoc. 79*:176-178:1954.

59. Hassler, R., and Riechert, T. (1957). Über einen Fall von doppelseitiger Fornicotomie bei sogenannter temporaler Epilepsie. *Acta Neurochir. 5*:330-340.

60. Sweet, W.H., Talland, F.A., and Ervin, F.R. (1959). Loss of recent memory following section of fornix. *Trans. Am. Neurol. Assoc. 84*:76-82.

61. Van Wagenen, W.P., and Herren, R.Y. (1940). Surgical division of commissural pathways in the corpus callosum. Relation to spread of an epileptic attack. *Arch. Neurol. Psychiatry 44*:740-759.

62. Wilson, D.H., Reeves, A.G., and Gazzaniga, M.S. (1982). "Central" commissurotomy for intractable generalized epilepy: series two. *Neurology 32*:687-697.

63. Gordon, H.W., Bogen, J.E., and Sperry, R.W. (1971). Absence of deconnexion syndrome in two patients with partial section of the neocommissures. *Brain 94*:327-336.

64. Purves, S.J., Wada, J.A., Woodhurst, W.B., Moyes, P.D., Strauss, E., Kosaka, B., and Li, D. (1988). Results of anterior corpus callosum section in 24 patients with medically intractable seizures. *Neurology 38*:1194-1201.
65. Zaidel, D., and Sperry, R.W. (1974). Memory impairment after commissurotomy in man. *Brain. 97*:263-272.
66. Whitty, C.W.M., and Lewin, W. (1960). A Korsakoff syndrome in the post-cingulectomy confusional state. *Brain 83*:648-653.
67. Orchinik, C.W. (1960). Some psychological aspects of circumscribed lesions of the diencephalon. *Conf. Neurol. 20*:292-310.

20

Psychogenic Amnesias

Christopher J. Mace
and
Michael R. Trimble

The National Hospital for Neurology and Neurosurgery
London, England

INTRODUCTION

The term "psychogenic amnesia" has recently been granted the status of an independent psychiatric diagnosis within the classification of DSM-III (1) and DSM-III-R (2). In DSM-III-R it is now also cited as a criterion of post-traumatic stress disorder. "Psychogenic amnesia" is recommended as a diagnostic label for cases where there is "an episode of sudden inability to recall important personal information that is too extensive to be explained by ordinary forgetfulness." It represents a variety of "dissociative disorder," to be diagnosed once other dissociative disorders, and organic mental disorder have been excluded. However, this designation appears too restrictive to the present writers, in failing to acknowledge that apparently psychogenic memory loss can be chronic as well as episodic in its course, or that other forms of memory apart from that for important personal information may be so affected. For the purposes of this chapter, therefore, "psychogenic amnesia" will refer to amnesias of pathological severity that appear to lack an adequate neurological basis, and where memory impairment is a dominant rather than an incidental clinical feature.

The term "functional amnesia" has been taken to be equivalent to psychogenic amnesia by some, following a commonly made but misguided equation between the terms "functional" and "psychological." In general, as Trimble has pointed out elsewhere (3), the term "functional," in embracing a range of connotations that have ranged from physiological (as opposed to structural) change through to the importance of willful motivation, has become meaningless and should be dropped from medical discussion or used only in its original, physiological sense. Nevertheless, when "functional amnesia" is used as a convenient way of denoting any amnesia occurring in the course of a "functional disorder," it inevitably acquires a wider scope than the concept of psychogenic amnesia that has just been proposed [cf. the usage of Kahn (4)]. Although amnesias can be evident in such primary disorders as schizophrenia, and so be labelled by some as "functional," it is rare for the amnesia, often very marked with respect to the content of earlier psychotic experiences, to dominate the clinical picture. In general, memory deficits have greater clinical salience in the syndromes that have been selected for further discussion here.

AMNESIA AND "PSYCHOGENESIS"

Before the clinical features of psychogenic amnesias are surveyed, some reservations concerning the notion of psychogenesis and its usefulness in discriminating between disorders must be expressed. The difficulties surrounding usage of "psychogenesis" have been discussed by Sir Aubrey Lewis (5) who, thinking the word to be trapped between too many different uses, concluded it was effectively left with none. Whether or not his criticism was correct, it is salutary to remind ourselves of the possibly conflicting associations of "psychogenesis" that Lewis referred to, viz: "psychogenic" as as the product of psychological operations; "psychogenic" as the result of stresses in the social environment; and "psychogenic" as nonorganic. Each of these senses offers a different perspective by which the robustness of the concept of "psychogenic" amnesia may be tested, and they will each be examined briefly here.

AMNESIA AS THE PRODUCT OF
PSYCHOLOGICAL MECHANISMS

There are many psychological theories of memory, usually based upon the positing of distinct "stores" and processes of deposition and retrieval. They are reviewed elsewhere in this volume, and although they can sometimes suggest reasons why amnesias should affect particular abilities and not others, they are not always helpful in practice. Indeed, they often seem to reflect a restricted clinical base, for example, the study of individuals with the relatively rare Korsakoff syndrome. In any case, theories of the fractionation of human memory, although they may be capable of explaining the selective amnesic effects of some localized structural insults, have been divorced for some time from attempts to explain how amnesias might arise entirely through psychological means. For this, psychology has had little progress to report for nearly a century: the concepts of dissociation and repression, which originally arose alongside rather different physiological models of memory to our own, are still widely looked to as the most appropriate explanatory paradigms.

"Dissociation" refers to the idea that parts of consciousness become reversibly detached from a whole, making their contents temporarily inaccessible to others. As developed by Janet, dissociation was a characteristic mechanism of hysteria, by which a reversible regrouping of "the systems of ideas and functions that constitute personality" occurred (6). A shift in the basis of personal control results, and Janet's implication of the whole field of mental operations in dissociation led him to give much attention to the coexistence of discrete "alternate" states (7). These still resemble modern descriptions of "multiple personality." Although dissociation may lead to amnesia for specific, interrelated contents of consciousness, it can arise through purely external interventions. In the last century, a structural weakness of the brain was held to predispose to its occurrence following trauma or hypnosis. Dissociation is still commonly cited as a recognized effect of hypnosis, and indeed attempts have spradically been made to link "hypnotizability" with predisposing brain states (8,9). Nevertheless, in some influential recent attempts to revive the notion of dissociation, it has been promoted as a purely psychological cause of memory failure. Nemiah has argued that, as a dynamic mechanism operating within the field of consciousness, dissociation represents a fundamental mode of ego functioning that could complement concepts of unconscious defences (10). Hilgard had promoted a "neodissociationist" theory, based upon experiments with hypnotic phenomena, in which dissociation allows a "hidden observer" to remain apart from a field of conscious operations, with hypnosis serving to make its observations accessible (11).

"Repression," as used by analytic thinkers from Freud onward, bears superficial resemblances to dissociation. It has been a mechanism whereby some conscious contents may not only become detached from others, but are actively removed from a putative center of operations to an "unconscious" repository. Paradoxically, the repressed items, once isolated, fail to lose their emotive power with the passage of time, and their return to consciousness remains a continuing possibility (12). The operation of repression is thought of as being universal, and as being activated psychodynamically by conflict between the content of the repressed material and an individual's motivational state. Therefore, as repression has been thought to influence the pattern of an individual's free recall, it has been assumed that the pattern of a repression-induced amnesia would itself point to his or her hidden motivations in the course of analytic investigation (13). No one is exempt from the operation of repression, with the universality of infantile amnesia being cited as support for this. On the other hand, individuals appear to differ in their capacity to exhibit phenomena which have been attributed to repression such as amnesia, or other hysterical symptoms. The question of why such differences in repressive capacity arise is unanswered by classical psychoanalytic theory, although Schilder's interesting attempt to link different degrees of repression with lesions at different sites in the central nervous system (i.e., his concept of "organic repression"), appears to have represented one attempt to do so (14).

The most significant attempt outside the tradition of dynamic psychology to link the occurrence of amnesia with specific psychological changes is possibly the linking of ability to recall with changes in mood. Several investigations by Lishman and colleagues (15,16) have suggested that whereas there can be considerable facility in recalling past unpleasant events during a depressive episode, recall for pleasant events is at the same time impaired. To account for this, it has been suggested that recall is state dependent with respect to mood. It is an intriguing possibility, but also one that raises a question as to whether intermediate physiological variables might not have a determining role within such an interaction. More recently, Lishman has speculated that the anatomical overlap between structures critical for memory, namely the mammillary bodies and the hippocampus, and limbic circuits implicated in emotional regulation might explain why the registration of new memory traces at least should vary with affective state (17).

AMNESIA AS A SITUATIONAL RESPONSE

Amnesia may also be recognized as "psychogenic" when there is prima facie evidence that its onset coincided with stressful precipitants, and that memory was lost for those events. There appear to be several situations in which such memory loss is commonly reported, notably following violent crime or during military conflict, and where a diagnosis of psychogenic amnesia (or perhaps of posttraumatic stress disorder) will be considered. It must not be forgotten that in the former case particularly, questions of legal culpability and fitness to withstand cross-examination might also contribute to the amnesiac's behavior. Even where the clinical presentation is strongly suggestive of psychogenic amnesia, it is wise not to assume that the most evident situational precipitants are necessarily the determining ones, as the following case history illustrates:

Case history 1
Mr. A.B. was a marine soldier on active service at the time of referral. A severe amnesia was coincident with a minor head injury sustained during

a road accident, after which he had an anterograde amnesia of about 4 hours. However, he could no longer recall the nature of his occupation, recognize family and close friends (despite experiencing different degrees of "being comfortable" with these individuals), and had also apparently lost familiarity with weapons with whose use he was familiar. His personal history was virtually blank with the exception of a very few isolated, trivial, incidents, but once reminders were given of facts he previously knew, he had no problems with their further retention. Detailed cognitive testing had confirmed the density of his personal retrograde amnesia, as well as the considerable difficulty he encountered in recalling famous figures from the past, while there was no evidence of impaired ability in the learning of new verbal and nonverbal material. His procedural memory and performance on a test for recognition of famous faces recovered in advance of a steady recovery of his personal memory over the next month. This was probably aided by several interviews, one under sodium amytal. As soon as he learned the nature of his predicament he repeatedly expressed a concern to return to his unit, and the only ambivalence that was expressed by him concerned a current relationship rather than his potentially dangerous career. All other investigations were negative, and his amnesia was judged to have been "non-organic."

Psychogenic amnesia can have considerable forensic significance, making it highly important that its natural history is understood. However, there is again a paucity of reference literature. In a good review, Schachter reports how testimony has been professionally presented to a court to the effect that an accused man could not have commited a crime he confessed to because he should have forgotten it (18). Reports are most readily available for the incidence of subsequent amnesia among murderers, which has been variously reported as between 23% (19) and 65% (20) with a majority in the region of 30%. However, Fenton has remarked how, on the basis of considerable personal experience, professions even of "epileptic" amnesia can subside once a criminal develops greater intimacy with his interviewer (21), and one should perhaps be mindful of the limitations of research methods in this area.

An issue that is keenly examined in forensic discussion is whether amnesia arises as the involuntary result of unconscious mechanisms, or whether it is simply simulated. This question can be extremely difficult to resolve in practice. A "confession" is not necessarily proof of malingering, and as Schacter (18) points out, even when tests holding some promise of distinguishing between involuntary and voluntary failures of recall are discovered and circulated, they might quickly be assimilated by the knowing simulator determined to better his performance.

Regardless of the legal interest that encourages tight distinctions when culpability is at issue, there appears in practice to be a continuum extending between cases of involuntary and voluntary failures of recall, with all positions thereon having an equal right to be classed as "psychogenic." Less judicial concern attaches to other factors that contribute to amnesia, such as the ingestion of alcohol and drugs, which have a strictly limited bearing on issues of criminal responsibility if they are knowingly self-administered, but which of course blur the entire question of psychogenesis. In examining factors that predisposed to amnesia among 19 men accused of violent crimes, Taylor and Kopelman (22) concluded that there were three chief sources of amnesia: (1) the pharmacological effects of alcohol; (2) a psychotic mental state; (3) psychological defences against recognizing an unplanned outburst of violence against someone with whom there had been an intense emotional involvement. They were not necessarily exclusive of each other.

It is not unknown also, however, for minor crimes such as shoplifting to be committed by women who fail to recollect incidents prior to their arrest, and who have been drinking and consuming significant quantities of minor tranquilizers such as benzodiazepines shortly beforehand. Whether or not the criminal action might be linked to disinhibitive effects of these drugs, their ability to impair anterograde memory has been well documented in independent studies (23). The association is perhaps not surprising, given the concentration of benzodiazepine receptors that is present in the hippocampal area (24).

An area of confusion both legal and clinical remains the epileptic automatism, more commonly implicated in alibis for criminal actions than successfully proven, and which is associated with subsequent, usually total, amnesia for any acts performed as a consequence (25). Although a true automatism is in no ordinary sense "psychogenic," British law still confusingly dictates that, if criminal acts are committed in its course, a defendant can only expect a "not guilty" plea to be respected if they are also willing to admit to "insanity."

ORGANICITY VERSUS PSYCHOGENESIS IN AMNESIA

The concept of psychogenic amnesia may also be developed through comparison with organically determined amnesias. This assumes that a clear basis exists for the explanation of memory disorders in terms of neurological change, and of course some well defined syndromes such as Korsakoff's psychosis have been successfully linked to a fairly consistent set of localized structural abnormalities. In cases where pathology is more varied and diffuse, for instance as a result of closed head injury, the pathogenesis of subsequent disruptions to memory and other cognitive functions is necessarily more elusive. In fact the task of disentangling distinct "organic" and "psychogenic" components of amnesia even when there is an evident organic precipitant can be surprisingly difficult.

To pursue the example of head injury, it is well-recognized that an initial anterograde posttraumatic amnesia bears some relation to the extent of tissue injury and subsequent prognosis. However, other symptoms commonly supervene, notably headache, dizziness, emotional lability, irritability, fatigue, and difficulties with memory and concentration, comprising what is commonly termed a postconcussion syndrome (26). This appears to bear less relation to the extent of brain damage, and its persistence to reflect personality and situational variables to a greater extent. As time elapses in the course of recovery from a closed head injury, therefore, psychological factors assume increasing importance in determining a patient's overall disability, including their ability to remember, while precise allocation of deficits to organic or psychogenic mechanisms at any one point remains hazardous.

Lishman has made an intriguing additional point (17) that close observation of the pattern of recovery from some traumatically induced retrograde amnesia reveals it has proceeded not according to an orderly sequence dictated by the recency of the lost material, but by the sporadic recovery of isolated memories that then prompt others through associative linkages. This is taken to be the manner of recovery from psychogenic amnesias, raising further doubts about their mutual exclusivity.

In practice, the presence of prior injury, a not uncommon antecedent of amnesias that are subsequently deemed nonorganic in character, can complicate the course of medical investigation considerably.

Case History 2
Mr. B.C. was admitted for assessment at the expense of a foreign government four years after receiving a sporting injury to the head, following which he had lost consciousness for 10 minutes. He was of apparently good premorbid personality with no prior psychiatric history. Within a further week he was complaining of headaches, depressed mood, and impairment of memory and concentration that were so severe as to preclude his return to work following the injury. Many hospital admissions and investigations followed during which he also had psychiatric treatment, including ECT, with only partial benefit. He had more recently developed spasmodic facial movements and a persistent tremor of one leg. Clinical examination and formal psychometry evidenced difficulties in sustaining attention, in memory for past events, and in new learning. His globally poor test scores were thought compatible with dementia, yet the patient had no difficulty in learning ward routines, and was able to travel by the London Underground unaccompanied. Expert opinion held his neurological symptoms to be inconsistent with any known pattern of organically determined pathology, although he had probably suffered a measure of vestibular damage. Investigations suggested that familial, occupational,

and compensation motives had contributed to his invalidism. His dementia and physical symptoms were all finally judged to have been nonorganic
in origin, after nearly four years of continual, conscientious, and costly
evaluation.

A further situation where memory impairment follows a physical insult,
and a controlled insult at that, but where the pathogenesis of amnesia can
be surprisingly difficult to identify, occurs following the administration of
electroconvulsive therapy. Although this indubitably has an independent
amnesic effect, the patients receiving ECT (= ECS) are likely to be severely
depressed and to exhibit some memory difficulties as a consequence of this
also. Cronholm and Ottoson (27), who paid attention to the profile of memory deficits, linked retrograde amnesia to the impact of ECT, and difficulties
with new learning to depressive symptomatology. Squire had confirmed the
impact of ECT on retrograde memory, and mapped the longitudinal process
of recovery from amnesia by which a residual 6 month retrograde and a 2
month anterograde amnesia was typically found 3 years after treatment with
(bilateral) ECT (28). This long-term loss was no worse among patients who
actively complained of memory difficulties when compared with those who
did not. Nevertheless, when the current performance of 26 "people who
complain" was examined in a study of Freeman et al. (29), 11 individuals
were singled out as having large test deficits in common. In 4, alternative
organic causes (alcohol, medication) were held responsible; in 3, depression,
while in a further 4 no specific explanation, either organic or psychogenic,
could be offered.

PSYCHOGENESIS AND THE SYNDROMES
OF AMNESIA

The notion of psychogenesis may prove to be a less useful way of distinguishing between amnesic syndromes than it first promised to be. Whether or not
its face validity is as strong as first appears, the question remains: do the
syndromes commonly thought of as psychogenic nevertheless remain distinctive in their clinical characteristics? Past writers have been pessimistic on this
point: a classic paper of Kennedy and Neville (30) looked at pathogenesis in
74 patients who had presented with sudden loss of memory. After excluding
13 who in their opinion were malingering or psychotic, they judged that 43%
of the remainder were explicable in terms of psychogenesis alone; 16% to
organic pathology with no evidence of psychogenesis; while 41% had features consistent with both organic and psychogenetic explanations. Their
study emphasized that there was no appreciable difference between the presentation of those cases of brief memory loss that were judged organic and
those that were thought to be psychogenic.

Since the time of that study, an important newcomer has appeared at this diagnostic borderland: transient global amnesia. It is recognized to be an "organic" syndrome, despite a dearth of knowledge concerning its pathology, because clinical findings follow a consistent pattern which is thought incompatible with the features of a "psychogenic" amnesia (31). Thus patients are typically males in the sixth and seventh decades who usually have a single attack of memory loss of several hours' duration. They are fully aware of this during the episode, and suffer no loss of identity or impairment of other psychological or motor functions. The amnesia is both retrograde, and affects learning for new material, prompting the patient to repeatedly request reminders from those around him for essential factual information during the episode. The retrograde amnesia progressively resolves, leaving a residual amnesia for a short period immediately prior to the episode, and for the episode itself. When repeated attacks have occurred, they have been associated with the onset of lasting intellectual deficits. As with any other form of amnesia, the presence of a past psychiatric history, or evidence of accompanying precipitants or gains, can still provoke suspicion of a psychogenic origin. Nevertheless, this syndrome, which can follow a vascular episode or an epileptic paroxysm, is well established as being "organic" in type.

Both Lewis (32) and Zangwill (33) have had to conclude that there is no presentation of amnesia, however bizarre, that could not have an organic causation. However, this does not preclude there being particular forms of memory disturbance that might be thought of as typically "nonorganic" by virtue of their clinical associations, on the same basis as transient global amnesia is taken to be "organic." Although the discrimination of a set of amnesias as "psychogenic" may be more a matter of convention than of conviction, the rest of this chapter will be devoted to a discussion of several syndromes that fall within the working definition of "psychogenic amnesia" proposed at the outset.

THE CLINICAL VARIETIES OF PSYCHOGENIC AMNESIA

A pragmatic if not entirely uncontroversial set of diagnoses that would subsume "psychogenic amnesia" are listed in Table 1. In general, those toward the bottom of the list are more chronic than those at its head. Some syndromes are marked there with asterisks if amnesia is not consistently present (PTSD, histrionic personality disorder) or if the nosological validity of the syndrome has been a subject of continual doubt (multiple personality disorder, Ganser syndrome). The allocation of a case to one or other diagnosis in the list is largely a question of the presence of auxiliary features, for example, wandering (psychogenic fugue); depression (depressive dementia); intrusions (PTSD);

Table 1 List of the
Psychogenic Amnesias (In
Approximate Order of
Chronicity)

Situational amnesia
Posttraumatic stress syndrome[a]
Ganser's syndrome[b]
Psychogenic fugue
Hysterical dementia or dysmnesia
Depressive dementia
Multiple personality disorder[b]
Histrionic personality disorder[a]

[a]Amnesia is commonly but not invariably present.
[b]The nosological validity of these syndromes is least certain.

and so forth. However, cases may differ radically from one another in other respects also, such as the specific character of the memory loss, and the chronicity of the symptoms. These variables each deserve further attention in their own right.

Some disorders appear to be regularly associated with particular defects in memory, for instance depressive dementia with impairment of new learning, or psychogenic fugue with an initial retrograde, possibly global, amnesia which is classically followed by residual amnesia for the period of wandering following recovery from the initial amnesia. Others, notably those that have been termed "hysterical" here, can exhibit a considerable range of forms. Indeed, nomenclature such as that adopted by DSM-III-R (2) for the discussion of psychogenic amnesia respects a set of clinical distinctions introduced by Janet when attempting to discuss the variety of amnesias encountered in hysteria (34). These include "general" amnesia (a lifelong retrograde loss); "localized" amnesia (a circumscribed episodic loss); "selective" amnesia (a loss restricted to material that is systematically linked by association); and "continuous" amnesia (an inability to recall experienced events that has continued up to the time of examination).

As indicated in the introduction, insufficient attention has been paid too to the variability of the time course of these disorders. Differences in duration are likely to be of considerable significance for questions of pathogenesis and treatment, as well as diagnosis. Kopelman has proffered a tentative if incomplete classification of psychogenic amnesia that highlighted a division between impairments that were discretely episodic and those that were sustained, a primary distinction he makes also in classifying "organic" amnesias

(35). It is important to recognize, however, that while some disorders are characteristically protracted (depressive dementia has been known to persist for years if untreated) and others brief (such as that to be described here as situational amnesia) yet others are highly variable in their course. The initial disruption of memory for identity in psychogenic fugue, for instance, may persist for a matter of hours only, or, as in the case to be described, for many many years. In the notes that follow, the disorders associated with relatively brief amnesia will be examined first.

SITUATIONAL AMNESIA

This term recommends itself for brief memory failures of apparently psychological origin given the caveats already made concerning the term "psychogenic amnesia," the DSM-III-R designation under which most cases would fall. It explicitly emphasizes the second of the three connotations of "psychogenic" that were discussed earlier. It is the most common variety of "psychogenic amnesia" encountered in practice, is seen at all ages, and need not necessarily be associated with other forms of psychopathology. Thus, "situational amnesia" refers here to short-lived memory impairment that is linked to a particular situation of emotional significance for the individual through the timing of the amnesia and its effects. Most commonly, its onset and offset encompass an event that is perceived as traumatic, and memory may be lost either for all events within a given period, or, occasionally, for a group of memories that are thematically linked.

Considerable uncertainty persists as to whether the failure of memory following onset represents a kind of facultative failure to retrieve stored memories, as would be consistent with the theoretical construct of repression, or whether its mechanism lies in a defect in the initial encoding of new information. In the latter case, the episodic nature of the personal anterograde amnesia found in these cases might be explained by a temporary disruption of encoding as a consequence of high arousal precipitated by an emotive triggering event (35). While plausible, the theory does seem counterintuitive in that these episodic amnesias are commonly taken to be reversible. In addition, their reversal is known to be sometimes, if by no means invariably, enhanced by the use of positive suggestion as an aid to recall, by hypnosis, and by abreaction. (For a further discussion, see: "the treatment of psychogenic amnesias", below.)

POSTTRAUMATIC STRESS DISORDER

Situational amnesia need not occur in isolation. When a psychologically traumatic event leads to the posttraumatic stress syndrome then intrusive phenomena usually dominate the clinical picture in the form of forced recollections, dreams, or flashbacks (36). These are each likely to be distressing, thematically linked to the precipitating trauma, and prone to repetition. However, in many sufferers some aspects of the original trauma are subject instead to amnesia. This is a common but not invariable component of the syndrome, and when it occurs resembles the situational form of amnesia described above. (When marked affective changes are also present, continuing memory difficulties of the kind discussed below under "depressive dementia" can also be encountered in patients having PTSD.)

PSYCHOGENIC FUGUE

This has the status of a distinct syndrome in DSM-III-R. In psychogenic fugue an amnesia arises during, and can be subsequently limited to, a period in which there is evident behavioral change. These changes take the form of wandering in a superficially purposeful way, and during which the subject is unable to recall their past. As a consequence of this, the patient may assume a different identity. These episodes are usually brief, but if the initial amnesia for identity persists, the new identity may be consolidated and retained as in a highly remarkable and much quoted case that was first reported by Pratt (37).

Case History 3

A 45-year-old man was admitted to hospital for investigation of 'fits.' He said that 15 years previously he had been brought to a hospital unaware of his personal identity and of any event in his previous life. His amnesia had persisted, but he had been able to relearn general information quickly and had obtained a job as an engineering foreman. When informed of the whereabouts of his wife and family he had elected not to join them, his amnesia still persisting, and instead he had set up home with a new partner. His 'fits,' thought to be nonorganic, responded to superficial psychotherapy, though again with no change being observed in his amnesia. He did not meet his wife and children until his mother's final illness. Only at her deathbed did the memory of his former life return in full.

Although usually more mundane in their course, psychogenic fugues appear always to follow a precipitating trauma, with cases being more frequently reported in wartime settings. A history of prior head injury is not uncommon (38). Furthermore, they have been linked to acute depression of affect, with individual cases often being interpreted as a means of coping with active suicidal impulses as trenchantly observed by Stengel (39). It can be important to differentiate clinically between this form of perplexed wandering, and the consequences of epileptic automatism. Some points of contrast are summarized in Table 2. A further important diagnostic distinction must be made from

Table 2 Clinical Assessment of Fugue States

Psychogenic fugue	Postictal fugue
Identifiable emotional precipitant (may be preceded by fit or head injury)	Unlikely to be patient's first presentation of epilepsy
"Wandering" is socially appropriate	Perambulation accompanied by evident confusion
Recovery of orientation usually gradual	Recovery rapid
EEG usually normal	EEG abnormal

the consequences of a prolonged alcoholic blackout in someone with a significant prior drinking history. Unfortunately, alcoholism, head injury, secondary seizures, and depressive fugues tend to afflict a similar (largely male) population, emphasizing the need for great care in its diagnosis.

A NOTE ON "PSEUDODEMENTIA"

This term is often taken to apply to persisting symptoms of memory loss and intellectual impairment that mimic those attributed to cerebral dementias, but which are attributed to the presence of an independent psychiatric disorder. Depression, schizophrenia, hysteria, and personality disorders have been variously implicated, and, as was observed above, the psychogenic amnesias that result have not been well accommodated by the classification of DSM-III-R as yet. At the same time, the authors feel the term "pseudodementia" is a misnomer, and would urge its abandonment in neuropsychiatric discussion. It appears to have first occurred in the literature in an article by Madden et al. (40), in which a series of elderly patients who made unexpected clinical recoveries were reviewed. There "pseudodementia" was attributed to a variety of underlying disorders which would embrace affective and schizophrenic disorders in modern nomenclature. As, by definition, "dementia" was seen as a progressive disorder at that time, the neologism signaled a therapeutically significant distinction. In Kiloh's influential 1961 review of "pseudodementia," he was anxious also to underscore the therapeutic responsiveness of intellectual deficits seen in the course of "functional" illnesses, and in depression in particular (41). However, the idea of irreversibility is fortunately no longer accepted as central to the concept of dementia, making it far more appropriate to refer in such an instance not to pseudodementia, but instead to a depressive dementia in distinction to multi-infarct or primary degenerative dementia. Another source of resistance to such a move has been an equation between "dementia" and underlying neuropathology. A concept of depressive dementia, already advocated by Folstein and McHugh (42) is likely to gain increasing support as several lines of research continue to converge to suggest that changes intermediate between those found among "organically" demented patients and unaffected controls can be demonstrated in the CNS of elderly depressed patients. These include an increased latency of auditory and somatosensory evoked potentials (which appear to correlate with depressives' cognitive impairments rather than their affective symptoms) (43), and a decrease in brain tissue density on CT scanning (44).

In the hands of Kiloh (41) and Post (45), pseudodementia was described almost exclusively as an important if atypical form of depressive illness. Later champions of "pseudodementia" have claimed that it represents an independent syndrome, irrespective of the nature of the underlying "functional" disorder (46,47). However, like McAllister (48), we would dispute this assertion, believing that some of the features catalogued by Wells and others are more typical of depressive cases, while others are features of a syndrome produced by hysterical mechanisms. These are each described below.

DEPRESSIVE DEMENTIA

A measure of cognitive impairment is commonly found in patients with a significant degree of depression. However, in some patients failures in memory and concentration can dominate the clinical picture, which may not be one of overt depressive illness. The presence of a marked degree of cognitive impairment does not appear to be a reliable guide to the severity of the associated affective disturbance in such patients, although when depression takes this form, it tends to breed true from episode to episode in the same individual.

Case History 4
Mr. C.D. was a 50-year-old accountant who, following errors at work, had had some of his responsibilities removed from him by his employers. Mr. C.D. had nevertheless become increasingly anxious about his performance, constantly relying on notebooks for his work. He had been referred through a company psychiatrist anxious to exclude an organic cause for his patient's apparent decline. In his history, he had had subclinical episodes of compulsive washing in early adult life, and had in fact been forgetful and withdrawn for a period of weeks some years before. On examination he exhibited only mild depressive symptoms in the form of ahedonia, anergia, and loss of libido. He performed satisfactorily on brief clinical tests of cognitive function, despite his own protests to the contrary. However, when formally tested by a psychologist he cooperated with all tests, but was noted to perform badly on tests of recognition memory in a way that was inconsistent with his ability to orientate himself and with the rest of his test performance. His confidence and subjective satisfaction with his memory improved as his depressive symptoms remitted with appropriate treatment. A significant component of this was liaison with his employers to reduce the anxiety his performance at work had come to engender.

Symptoms suggestive of depression and intellectual decline commonly occur together among elderly patient populations, and the clinical differentiation between dementia and a primary depressive illness can still defeat the most experienced of clinicians. Apart from clinical examination of the cognitive state, there are several additional areas in which diagnostic clues can be sought in coming to a decision. A brief summary of some of these is provided in Table 3.

Further discussion of this differentiation may be obtained from Post (45), who emphasized the benefits of paying detailed attention to the history of onset in order to establish whether depressive symptoms preceded cognitive changes or vice versa. He emphasized also such qualitative features as the depressive's tendency to give "don't know" rather than inaccurate answers, and the frequent shallowness of the dementing patient's affect. Wells has pointed also to the potential usefulness of behavioral observations made during interview (e.g., discrepancies between spontaneous speech and response to questions); in unfamiliar situations (e.g., discrepancies between disorientation under questioning and in practice); and at home (where dementing

Table 3 Differentiation of Depressive Dementia from Organic (Alzheimer Type) Dementia

Depressive dementia	Degenerative dementia
History	
Family history of affective disorder	Family history of dementia
Past episodes of affective illness or resolving episodes of cognitive impairment	Recent history of subtle personality change
Rapid onset	Insidious onset
Associated features	
Biological and cognitive symptoms of depression	Symptoms of cortical involvement (i.e., dysphasias, dyspraxias, etc.)
Behavior	
Patient complains of memory (and other inadequacies)	Insight linked to denial and catastrophic reactions
Orienting skills largely intact	Visible problems with topographic memory
Mental state	
Affect depressed and real	Affect shallow even if depressed
Poor performance on cognitive tests through lack of participation (i.e., "don't know" responses)	Poor performance through incorrect responses which reflect objective difficulty of test
Course	
Resolving with treatment for affective symptoms	Exacerbated by CNS depressants

patients show more evidence of self neglect (49). Nonetheless, some caution should be expressed about Wells' descriptions, for instance, of exaggerated dependency among his "pseudodementia" patients, as a very high proportion of those in his published series had personality disorders rather than depression as their principal diagnosis (46). The "pseudodementia" they showed would be expected to have features in common with the next topic for discussion.

HYSTERICAL DEMENTIA

Although currently unfashionable, the term "hysterical" is retained here in a well-established role. This is to refer to conditions where the clinical features represent an imperfect imitation of the features of a (usually neurological) disorder, but which appear instead to correspond to an idea in the mind of the patient rather than to the known consequences of any local or systemic pathology. Indeed, because this component of imitation is evident in many cases of dementia, writers such as McAllister (48), while endorsing the view that the term "pseudodementia" is inappropriate for the dementia of depression, have recommended that it be applied solely to hysterical dementias instead. However, any attempt to artificially redesignate "pseudodementia" would only compound confusion: "hysterical dementia" has the merit of being largely self-explanatory.

Like other hysterical disorders, hysterical dementias differ from simple malingering in being removed from immediate conscious control, allowing them to be sustained in cases over long periods of time, albeit with periodic inconsistencies in performance. Although they most commonly take the form of a quite transparent imitation in patients of low intelligence (50), their features can be highly individual, and a significant cause of clinical confusion.

Case History 5
The patient, a married woman in her 40s, presented complaining of memory problems dating from the time of an alleged assault some four years before. She claimed to spend most of her time attempting to read while maintaining that she was mentally unable to absorb a word that she saw. Over many consultations and investigations she had insisted on being accompanied by her husband at all times. She had a long history of previously unexplained illness, and her amnesia had been accompanied at different times by complaints of pain, weakness and visual impairment. There was no significant history of depressive symptomatology. Her memory for past personal events was highly variable, alternating between vagueness and a tendency to make apparently unsubstantiated accusations of past assault. On routine psychological testing she kept the tester busy for 3 hours despite refusing many items. Her scores on tests of intellectual function and memory

showed extreme internal inconsistency, and her scores on tests of new learning were often worse than those of a severely demented person, and of a sort recorded previously only in patients with hysterical syndromes.

In summary, some of the points that would contrast a truly hysterical dementia from a depressive dementia are summarized in Table 4. It must be emphasized, however, that either type represents a pure form encountered relatively infrequently as such in practice. Mood changes often appear to bring hysterical mechanisms into play psychologically, making a varying mixture of features common. This was evident in Case History 2 reported above; the patient had a history of both affective and conversion symptoms, and the phenomenology of his cognitive difficulties embraced features typical of both depressive and hysterical dementias.

Table 4 Comparison of Two Modes of Persistent Psychogenic Amnesia

Hysterical dementia	Depressive dementia
Onset:	
(Both rapid and may follow emotional precipitants)	
Hysterical dementia more likely to follow a physical trauma	
Incidence:	
Rare; all adults	Common, especially elderly depressives
Past history:	
Conversion symptoms	Affective episodes
Course:	
Highly unpredictable	Remitting and recurring with affective disorder
Presentation:	
Lack of expressed concern, ready demonstrations of inability to remember	Protestations of memory loss (in excess of actual difficulties)
Associated findings:	
(often) conversion symptoms (e.g., dysphasias, anesthesias)	Other features of depression, *viz*, agitation, retardation, fatigue
Memory loss:	
Bizarre in pattern (e.g., global retrograde with loss of personal identity; e.g., continuous amnesia with defective immediate recall)	Patchy anterograde with some difficulty learning new material
Test performance:	
Highly variable, Might produce paradoxically bad responses	Particularly bad on tests requiring effort after active recall

HYSTERICAL AMNESIA

Very occasionally, chronic hysterical syndromes arise in which there are surprisingly consistent patterns of memory deficit that are nevertheless bizarre
in the extreme, and which occur in the apparent absence of other intellectual
difficulties. These include the rarer forms of hysterical amnesia described
by Janet (6), of which the extended amnesia for the patient's past life in his
"general" amnesia is probably the best known example. The atypical fugue
state described in Case History 3 may be seen as having ushered in a lasting
hysterical amnesia of this type, accounting for the extraordinary persistence
of the initial retrograde amnesia over many years. Another rare presentation
may be the phenomenon of so-called "continuous" amnesia, with apparent
inability to add to the stock of memory after a given time up to the present,
which appears to have occurred in an exaggeratedly pure form, and persisted
for decades, in the celebrated case of Grunthall and Storring. The following
report is adapted from that offered by Zangwill (51).

Case History 6
The patient, Br., was a 24-year-old foundry locksmith when he was suddenly rendered unconscious by a leak of coal gas. He was unconscious for
90 minutes and hospitalized for a week. Memory deficits were noted only
on his subsequent return to work, when they took the form of inability to
remember any events following the accident even as they occurred. The
span of his immediate memory was less than 5 seconds, and appears to
have varied over subsequent years, being, for instance, as little as 1 second
when rigorously tested at 5 years, but as great as 15 minutes from observations made by his wife some 10 years after the accident. A retrograde
amnesia of 4 days appears to have quickly remitted to one of a few hours
only. The patient remained severely disabled by this defect for the rest of
his adult life, but although he appeared to become less forthcoming in
spontaneous speech, no other intellectual deficits were reported despite
repeated investigation. He continued to maintain that his age was 24 under
questioning, and despite his inability to recall new memories since that
age, his behavior showed some acquired familiarity with changed surroundings, and recognition of new acquaintances.

According to Zangwill, the profile of Br.'s difficulties were so unusual as
to render it impossible to align them on the basis of similarity either with previous organic or psychogenic amnesias, although Zangwill makes no reference
to Janet in the discussion he offers of the case. Again, the association with
an initial physical insult had ensured a protracted medical controversy, one
which extended over 40 years, but a consensus finally emerged that any organic component to Br.'s predicament had given way to maintenance of the
symptoms through psychological mechanisms in the early years of the illness.

THE GANSER SYNDROME

This very rare syndrome is mentioned here as it is sometimes confused with hysterical dementia, while in fact it differs in having clouding of consciousness as a prominent feature, sometimes with hallucinosis present in addition (52). It has continued to be promoted as a hysterical complaint by those who choose to associate hysteria with the idea of "secondary gain" because Ganser's original report linked its occurence specifically with imprisonment (53), although subsequent reports have mainly come from other settings. It invites comparisons with dementing illnesses because of what has subsequently been dubbed the "Ganser symptom" (54). or "vorbeireden," when subjects respond to questions with answers that are consistently wrong, yet which approximate to the true answer sufficiently closely to betray a knowledge of the required response. The Ganser syndrome could represent a variety of psychogenic amnesia as subjects lack recall for their behavior during the circumscribed episode. However, it should be noted that the Ganser symptom, like the other features, is not specific to the Ganser syndrome, leading to considerable doubt as to its nosological validity. Whitlock concluded on the basis of his own observations that the syndrome did not represent a variety of hysteria but a form of transient psychosis, while admitting that none of the patients he reported actually matched Ganser's descriptions in all particulars (52). Ganser's original prison psychosis appears to have been more lasting, but like most subsequent reports the illness was initiated by physical trauma such as head injury or fever, yet sudden in its eventual remission (53). When Ganser states exhibiting clouding of consciousness and hallucinosis do, very rarely, occur, the role of psychogenesis would seem to be very variable.

HISTRIONIC PERSONALITY DISORDER

This diagnosis seems to have been treated with considerable circumspection in recent years, many of its classic features (exaggerated yet shallow emotionalism, attention-seeking, seductiveness) seeming to be an unreliable basis for diagnosis, if not simply pejorative (55). However, as DSM-III-R properly indicates, such patients also can have a highly characteristic style of description that is "excessively impressionistic and lacking in detail." This vagueness can be extremely unsettling for the physician expecting to elicit a factual history from such a patient, and would appear to reflect a distinct cognitive style in which the patient's memory for their past appears never to operate as efficiently as for other people of comparable intelligence. It was elaborated upon by Shapiro who, in his study on neurotic styles (56), contrasted it with the characteristically highly focused memory of the patient having a markedly obsessional personality. Shapiro felt that the hysteric's imprecision reflected a lack of focussing both in attending to events and in their recall, prompting a heavy reliance on global, emotional impressions. As a result, a person would be more susceptible to external suggestion, and would use repression as a characteristic defence against conflicting emotions leading to further imprecision of memory.

The topic of cognitive style is one which appears to deserve more detailed attention. Personality style is important also in the clinical assessment of other amnesias: the obsessional patient is more likely to complain about relatively small degrees of memory impairment than others for instance. As occurred in Case History 3, it is not uncommon for the complaints of a patient presenting with depressive dementia to be aggravated for this reason.

MULTIPLE PERSONALITY DISORDER

This phenomenon is discussed in DSM-III-R as a "dissociative" disorder in which a patient is likely to complain of inability to remember the full sequence of their personal history. There is an assumption that such gaps are accounted for by another personality having been adopted for the corresponding period, and who in turn might possess appropriate memories. It has been said to be the outcome of a bizarre pattern of psychological development, set in motion by highly traumatic experiences during formative years (57). While the authors have no wish to be numbered among the "extreme" sceptics recently referred to by Dell (58), they have had no personal experience of patients presenting in this way who did not reveal an underlying schizophreniform disorder in the course of psychiatric assessment.

THE TREATMENT OF PSYCHOGENIC AMNESIAS

Repeated reference has been made to the association of several of these conditions with physical trauma, and special attention should be paid to the possibility that the patient may consequently be suffering other physical and psychological impairments that require additional investigation. Moreover, where the forgetfulness is a manifestation of an independent psychiatric disorder, as in depressive dementia, then the treatment appropriate to the primary disorder should be the order of the day.

However, where the case is strongest that the patient's amnesia is situational or the product of hysterical mechanisms, then the timing as well as the form of "treatment" may need careful consideration in both acute and chronic cases. In amnesias of recent onset, a patient's response to simple measures can be gratifying in providing confirmatory evidence of the diagnosis, but it is important to respect the possible impact upon a patient of recovering memory for a situation that they had apparently been unable to tolerate at the onset of the amnesia. Exceptionally, this could mean a re-experiencing of suppressed suicidal impulses of the sort that may anticipate some fugue states, and so it is important to ensure that adequate support is available following active interventions designed to abort amnesic episodes.

The techniques adopted most commonly in this respect are those of structured cuing, hypnosis, and the amytal interview. Kennedy and Neville report attempts to assist recall with members of their series of patients exhiting brief amnesia, and recommended both suggestion with a vehicle (e.g., a placebo) or hypnosis according to the preference of the interviewer (30). Merskey has suggested that hypnosis itself is indeed a sophisticated placebo, and is sceptical of the authenticity of the ''suggested'' memories that hypnosis can elicit (59). (It is interesting to note that, through a combination of interviewing and these special techniques, Kennedy and Neville claimed credit for relief of amnesia in 70 of their 74 cases despite reporting organic pathology in 27 of the total). The amytal interview has been recommended as a more potent aid to recall in clinical use (60), although it also has been associated with the production of what Sargant and Slater termed a ''mixture of truth and fantasy'' (61). Conversely, it must be remembered that the success of these devices is highly variable in practice, especially once an amnesia is well established, and that failure to elicit information through their use does not necessarily imply that the amnesia is ''organic'' in origin.

When dealing with entrenched hysterical dementia or dysmnesia, where maintaining factors are likely to have assumed an importance they did not have at the onset of the syndrome, a more indirect, rehabilitative approach may need to be considered. Attempts aimed at direct restoration of lost memories are likely to be less effective therapeutically with the passage of time, although confrontation of the patient with the suspicion that they are deliberately malingering is important where these are honestly held. However, motives are more likely to have become a complicated mixture of the more and less conscious where chronic symptoms are involved, with the amount of face to be lost through the success of overtly psychological measures prone to increase with the passage of time, even when help is actively sought. Attempts to encourage the patient to improve their performance that are based on behavioral strategies and environmental adjustments can then offer the advantage that they are visibly neutral with respect to the question of etiology, and therefore that of whether, in the eyes of others, the patient had or had not been responsible for their plight. Such treatment should start from a position of accepting the patient's current limitations, attempt accurate assessment of their associated handicaps and disabilities, followed by negotiation of a structured program designed to minimize the handicaps associated with the patient's complaint.

SUMMARY

In the context of amnesia, the concept of 'psychogenesis' appears to beg as many questions as it has when applied elsewhere. While it appears to be impossible to maintain an absolute distinction between "psychogenic" and other origins of amnesia, there is a group of syndromes in which the occurence of significant memory difficulty has traditionally been explained without reference to neurological mechanisms, and these are discussed here.

They include situational amnesia, psychogenic fugue, hysterical dementia, and depressive dementia, as well as posttraumatic stress syndrome, the Ganser syndrome, multiple personality disorder, and histrionic personality disorder. In attempting to alleviate the diagnostic confusion which can surround the concept of "psychogenic amnesia," these syndromes are distinguished by references to variations in the character of the memory loss, the accompanying features with which this may be associated, and their chronicity. Attention is also drawn to the relevance of these latter two aspects for prognosis and treatment.

The failure of contemporary psychology to add to understanding of the pathogenesis of these disorders is noted, in the hope that future research might allow mechanisms linking memory disorders and their psychological precipitants to be explained by concepts other than "dissociation" and "repression." Though these were integral components to the theories of a century ago, they still bear on scientific discussion of amnesia only by virtue of a longstanding dissociation within the field of psychology.

ACKNOWLEDGMENT

The authors are grateful to Dr. Maria Ron for permission to use two of the case histories included here.

REFERENCES

1. American Psychiatric Association (1980). *Diagnostic and Statistical Manual of Mental Disorders*, 3rd ed. APA, Washington, D.C.
2. American Psychiatric Association (1987). *Diagnostic and Statistical Manual of Mental Disorders*, 3rd ed. revised. APA, Washington, D.C.
3. Trimble, M.R. (1982). Functional disease. *Br. Med. J.* 285:1768-1770.
4. Khan, A.U. (1986). Functional disorders of memory. In *Clinical Disorders of Memory*. Edited by A.U. Khan. Plenum, New York, pp. 199-218.
5. Lewis, A. (1972). 'Psychogenic': a word and its mutations. *Psychol. Med.* 2:209-215.
6. Janet, P. (1901). *The Mental State of Hystericals* (tr. Putnam). Macmillan, New York, p. 332.

7. Janet, P. (1889). *L'Automatisme Psychologique*. Paris, Alcan.
8. Dumas, R.A. (1977). EEG alpha-hynotizability correlations: a review. *Psychophysiology 14*:431-438.
9. McLeod-Morgan, C., and Lack, L. (1982). Hemispheric specificity: a physiological concomitant of hynotizability. *Psychophysiology 19*:687-690.
10. Nemiah, J. (1979). Dissociative amnesia: a clinical and theoretical reconsideration. In *Functional Disorders of Memory*. Edited by J.F. Kihlstrom and F.J. Evans. Lawrence Erlbaum, Hillsdale, NJ, pp. 303-324.
11. Hilgard, E. (1977). *Divided Consciousness*. Wiley, New York.
12. Feldman, M. (1977). Amnesia: a psychoanalytic viewpoint. In *Amnesia*, 2nd ed. Edited by C.W.M. Whitty and O.L. Zangwill. Butterworth, London, pp. 233-244.
13. Freud, S. (1905). Repression. In *The Complete Words* (*Standard Edition*), Vol. XIV. Hogarth, London, pp. 146-158.
14. Schilder, P. (1935). *The Image and Appearance of the Human Body*. Paul Kegan, London, p. 74.
15. Lloyd, G., and Lishman, W.A. (1975). Effect of depression on the speed of recall of pleasant and unpleasant experiences. *Psychol. Med. 5*:173-180.
16. Lishman, W.A. (1972). Selective factors in memory. Part 2: affective disorder. *Psychol. Med. 2*:248-253.
17. Lishman (1988). Possible mechanisms in psychogenic amnesia. In *Organic Psychiatry*, 2nd ed. Edited by W.A. Lishman. Blackwell, Oxford, p. 36.
18. Schacter, D.L. (1986). Amnesia and crime: how much do we really know? *Am. Psychol. 41*:286-295.
19. Parwatikar, S.D., Holcomb, W.R., and Menninger, K.A. (1985). The detection of malingered amnesia in accused murderers. *Bull. Am. Acad. Psychiatry Law 13*:97-103.
20. Bradford, J.W., and Smith, S.M. (1979). Amnesia and homicide: the Padola case and a study of thirty cases. *Bull. Am. Acad. Psychiatry Law 7*:219-231.
21. Fenton, G.W. (1984). Discussion II: Borderlands. In *What is Epilepsy?* Edited by M.R. Trimble and E.H. Reynolds. Churchill Livingstone, London, p. 332.
22. Taylor, P.J., and Kopelman, M.D. (1984). Amnesia for criminal offences. *Psychol. Med. 14*:581-588.
23. Scarf, M.B., Kathy Fletcher, A.C.P., and Graham, J.P. (1988). Comparative amnestic effects of benzodiazepine hypnotic agents. *J. Clin. Psychiatry 49*:134-137.
24. Maziere, B., Comar, D., and Maziere, M. (1986). Pharmacokinetic studies using PET. In *New Brain Imaging Techniques and Psychopharmacology*. Edited by M.R. Trimble. Oxford University Press, Oxford, pp. 63-76.
25. Fenton, G.W. (1972). Epilepsy and automatism. *Br. J. Hosp. Med. 7*:57-64.
26. Lishman, W.A. (1988). Physiogenesis and psychogenesis in the 'Post-concussional syndrome'. *Br. J. Psychiatry 153*:460-469.
27. Cronholm, B., and Ottoson, J.O. (1961). Memory functions in endogenous depression: before and after electroconvulsive therapy. *Arch. Gen. Psychiatry 5*:193-199.

28. Squire, L.R., and Slater, P.C. (1983). Electroconvulsive therapy and complaints of memory dysfunction: a three-year follow-up study. *Br. J. Psychiatry 142*:1-8.
29. Freeman, C.P.L., Weeks, D., and Kendell, R.E. (1980). ECT: II: Patients who complain. *Br. J. Psychiatry 137*:17-25.
30. Kennedy, A., and Neville, J. (1957). Sudden loss of memory. *Br. Med. J. 2*: 428-433.
31. Croft, P.B., Heathfield, K.W.G., and Swash, M. (1973). Differential diagnosis of transient amnesias. *Br. Med. J. 4*:593-596.
32. Lewis, A. (1961). Discussion on amnesic syndromes: the psychopathological aspect. *Proc. R. Soc. Med. 54*:955.
33. Zangwill, O.L. (1983). Disorders of memory. In *Handbook of Psychiatry*. Edited by M. Shepherd and O.L. Zangwill. Cambridge University Press, Cambridge, pp. 97-112.
34. Janet, P. (1907). *The Mental State of Hystericals* (translated by Corson). Macmillan, New York, pp. 76-90.
35. Kopelman, M. (1987). Amnesia: organic and psychogenic. *Br. J. Psychiatry 150*:428-442.
36. Horowitz, M.J., Wilner, N., Kaltreider, N., and Alvarez, W. (1980). Signs and symptoms of post-traumatic stress disorders. *Arch. Gen. Psychiat. 37*:85-92.
37. Pratt, R.T.C. (1977). Psychogenic loss of memory. In *Amnesia*, 2nd ed. Edited by C.W.M. Whitty and O.L. Zangwill. Butterworth, London, pp. 224-232.
38. Berrington, W.P., Liddell, D.W., and Foulds, G.A. (1956). A reevaluation of the fugue. *J. Ment. Sci. 102*:280-286.
39. Stengel, E. (1941). On the aetiology of the fugue states. *J. Ment. Sci. 87*:572-599.
40. Madden, J.J., Luhan, M.D., Kaplan, L.A., and Manfredi, H.M. (1952). Nondementing psychoses in older persons. *JAMA 150*:1567-1570.
41. Kiloh, I.G. (1979). Pseudo-dementia. *Acta. Psychiatr. Scand. 37*:336-361.
42. Folstein, M.F., and McHugh, P.R. (1978). Dementia syndrome of depression. In *Alzheimer's disease: Senile Dementia and Related Disorders*. Edited by R. Katzman, R.D. Terry, and K.L. Bick. Raven Press, New York, pp. 87-93.
43. Hendrickson, E., Levy, R., and Post, F. (1979). Averaged evoked responses in relation to cognition and affective state of elderly psychiatric patients. *Br. J. Psychiatry 134*:494-501.
44. Jacoby, R., Dolan, R.J., and Levy, R. (1983). Quantitative computed tomography in depressed elderly patients. *Br. J. Psychiatry 143*:124-127.
45. Post, F. (1975). Dementia, depression and pseudodementia. In: *Psychiatric Aspects of Neurological Disease*. Edited by D.F. Benson and D. Blumer. Grune & Stratton, New York, pp. 99-120.
46. Wells, C.F. (1979). Pseudodementia. *Am. J. Psychiatry 136*:895-900.
47. Caine, E.D. (1981). Pseudodementia. *Arch. Gen. Psychiatry 38*:1359-1364.
48. McAllister, T.W. (1983). Overview: pseudodementia. *Am. J. Psychiatry 140*: 528-533.
49. Wells, C.F. (1982). Pseudodementia and the recognition of organicity. In *Psychiatric Aspects of Neurological Disease,* Vol. II. Edited by D.F. Benson and D. Blumer. Grune & Stratton, New York, pp. 167-178.

50. Lishman, W.A. (1987). Hysterical pseudodementia. In *Organic Psychiatry*, 2nd ed. Blackwell, Oxford, pp. 407-409.
51. Zangwill, O.L. (1967). The Grunthal-Storring case of amnesic syndrome. *Br. J. Psychiatry 113*:113-128.
52. Whitlock, F.A. (1967). The Ganser syndrome. *Br. J. Psychiatry 113*:19-29.
53. Scott, P.D. (1965). The Ganser syndrome. *Br. J. Criminol. 5*:127-131.
54. Ganser, S. (1898). A peculiar hysterical state. (Tr. C.E. Schorer) In *Themes and Variations in European Psychiatry*. Edited by S.R. Hirsch and M. Shepherd. John Wright, Bristol, pp. 67-73.
55. Slavney, P.R. & McHugh, P. (1974). The hysterical personality: a controlled study. *Arch. Gen. Psychiat. 30*:325-329.
56. Shapiro, D. (Ed.). (1965). The hysterical style. In *Neurotic Styles*. Basic Books, New York, pp. 108-133.
57. Coons, P.M., Bowman, E.S., and Milstein, V. (1988). Multiple personality disorder: a clinical investigation of 50 cases. *J. Nerv. Ment. Dis. 176*:519-527.
58. Dell, P.F. (1988). Professional skepticism about multiple personality. *J. Nerv. Ment. Dis. 176*:528-531.
59. Merskey, H. (1971). An appraisal of hypnosis. *Postgrad. Med. J. 47*:572-580.
60. Perry, C.J., and Jacobs, D. (1982). Overview: clinical applications of the amytal interview in psychiatric emergency settings. *Am. J. Psychiatry 139*:552-559.
61. Sargant, W., and Slater, E. (1941). Amnesic syndromes in war. *Proc. Roy. Soc. Med. 34*:757-764.

Part V

TREATMENT

21

Treatment of Memory Disorders

Ronald C. Petersen and Takehiko Yanagihara
Mayo Clinic and Mayo Foundation
Rochester, Minnesota

Richard C. Mohs
Mount Sinai School of Medicine
New York, New York

Harvey S. Levin
University of Texas Medical Branch
Galveston, Texas

Felicia C. Goldstein
Emory University
Atlanta, Georgia

The treatment of memory disorders is a difficult, challenging, and controversial area. There can be no simple or uniform solution to the problem because, as indicated in earlier chapters in this volume, there are many types and causes of memory disorders. Despite this multitude of factors, certain anatomical structures and neurochemical systems appear to predominate in memory function, and investigators have used these features to design remediation strategies in an attempt to improve memory function.

This chapter outlines two basic classes of treatment approaches: pharmacologic and behavioral. Relatively few studies have addressed the pharmacologic treatment of pure memory disorders; namely amnesia. There is, however, a rather extensive literature on the treatment of dementia and, in particular, Alzheimer's disease. Consequently, much of the subsequent discussion of pharmacologic treatment of memory disorders will be in the context of research on dementia. It is important to realize, however, that often the primary measure of efficacy in these drug trials is an index of memory function; thus, when a drug is demonstrated to ameliorate a dementia, it also frequently enhances memory function.

The pharmacologic treatment of dementia is a very active area of research currently with many of the pharmaceutical companies investigating one or more compounds. Several excellent reviews have been written on the drug treatment of dementia (1-3). Most of these compounds are designed to affect one or more of the neurotransmitter systems in an attempt to augment memory function. The initial section of this chapter reviews this literature with an emphasis on memory function.

The second section of this chapter addresses the issue of cognitive rehabilitation of memory disorders. This is a controversial area, and there is no consensus on its efficacy (4-7). Most of these studies arose from head injury research, and consequently, there are many variables which affect the outcomes of these studies. In addition to the impairment of a specific cognitive function, other factors such as the interaction of multiple cognitive deficits, motivation of the subject, attentional issues, depression, and the severity of the injury, to name a few, contribute to the ultimate outcome. Recently, computer-assisted techniques for enhancing memory and cognitive function have been employed, and here again, the efficacy of this work is still being evaluated. Glisky et al. (8,9) have employed a novel approach based on the application of computer techniques to cognitive theory to assess a specific technique for enhancement of memory functions. These studies will be reviewed later but provide an interesting insight into possible new rehabilitation strategies. These issues will be addressed in the section on behavioral therapy.

PHARMACOLOGIC TREATMENT

CHOLINERGIC DRUGS

Several lines of research have converged to implicate the role of the cholinergic system in memory function. Research in patients with Alzheimer's disease has indicated that the loss of choline acetyltransferase (CAT) correlates with cognitive impairment which also relates to the degeneration of cholinergic axons and the subsequent loss of cell bodies in the nucleus basalis of Meynert (10-12). Cognitive impairment in patients with parkinsonian dementia has also been correlated with cholinergic cell loss (13). The second line of research concerns the well-known anatomical relation of cholinergic pathways in normal learning and memory functions (see Chap. 4). Mesulam has postulated that the cholinergic system may perform a modulatory function in regulating sensory-limbic connections (14). In this fashion, cholinergic drugs may enhance or impair memory functions. In a more direct fashion, cholinergic pathways exhibit a great deal of reciprocal innervation between the basal forebrain and other limbic and paralimbic regions. Mesulam and Van Hoesen demonstrated projections from the basal forebrain to the cortex, and since that time, selective loss of cholinergic cells has been found in the basal forebrain in patients with Alzheimer's disease (15,16). While it is recognized that cholinergic cell loss is not the only transmitter dysfunction in Alzheimer's disease, or even central to the cognitive impairment, it no doubt plays a role in learning and recall functions.

In addition to the anatomical rationale for the role of the cholinergic system in memory function, several clinical studies have implicated the cholinergic system in these functions as well. Investigators have shown that the administration of scopolamine can produce memory impairments in normal young individuals which are similar to those seen in normal aging and perhaps in Alzheimer's disease (17-20). Drachman and Leavitt (17,18) and Petersen (19,20) have shown with a variety of tasks that scopolamine can produce impairments in learning and memory similar to those seen in Alzheimer's disease. Petersen (19) in a dose response study of the effects of scopolamine on learning and memory in normal volunteers demonstrated that scopolamine has its primary effect on the acquisition of new information. Material acquired prior to the administration of the drug was relatively preserved. In a subsequent study, however, Petersen (20) showed that scopolamine also has the ability to produce state-dependent memory effects implying that it may affect retrieval processes as well.

More recently, Sunderland and colleagues (21,22) have shown on tests of attention and memory that patients with Alzheimer's disease are more sensitive to low doses of scopolamine than are elderly control subjects. This work nicely demonstrates the role of the cholinergic system in learning and memory functions in Alzheimer's disease and presumably in normal aging.

Based on these lines of evidence, many attempts have been made to enhance learning and memory functions through the augmentation of the cholinergic system. Three basic strategies exist for enhancing cholinergic activity: (a) providing dietary precursors such as lecithin or choline, (b) inhibiting acetylcholinesterase and thereby prolonging the activity of acetylcholine (ACh) at the receptor site, or (c) using direct cholinergic agonists.

PRECURSORS

Acetylcholine is produced in the cholinergic nerve terminal from choline and acetylcoenzyme A by the enzyme CAT. The rate-limiting step appears to involve the uptake of choline into the nerve terminal rather than the availability of choline or the enzyme CAT (23). Choline cannot be synthesized de novo and must be supplied by dietary sources. Consequently, one strategy to enhance cholinergic functioning has been to supply the dietary precursor of ACh, for instance, choline or phosphatidylcholine (lecithin). Most trials employing this strategy have been unsuccessful in enhancing memory function. While some studies have shown that ACh concentrations in the brain increase following supplementation with dietary choline (24,25), the trials in humans using only dietary precursors to treat dementia have been largely unsuccessful (26-30).

Several possible explanations for the lack of the effect of dietary precursors have been offered, but no consensus has been reached. There is some evidence that the effect of scopolamine can be attenuated by pretreatment with choline (31), but this does not appear to be a robust finding (32). One long-term trial of the administration of lecithin to Alzheimer patients showed some behavioral improvement but no significant effects on cognition (33). In general, the use of dietary precursors to enhance memory function in Alzheimer patients and normal elderly subjects has been unsuccessful.

CHOLINESTERASE INHIBITORS

The second strategy to enhance cholinergic functioning involves the use of acetylcholinesterase (AChE) inhibitors such as physostigmine or tacrine (tetrahydroaminoacridine, THA). This class of drugs has produced some positive results with respect to the enhancement of memory and cognition, but the effects have not been dramatic. The rationale for this class of compounds involves the inhibition of AChE, the degradative enzyme for ACh. By inhibiting AChE, one hopes to prolong the activity of ACh at the receptor site.

One problem with this class of compounds involves potential toxicity. Physostigmine is reasonably safe at low doses but can cause cardiac arrhythmias at higher doses (34,35). Tacrine (THA) appears to have some hepatic toxicity (36), while physostigmine has a short half-life (30 minutes) and only recently has become available in oral form.

Physostigmine has been studied most extensively, and some improvement has been shown in memory when the drug is administered intravenously or subcutaneously (37-40). There have been some studies which have also shown improvement with oral administration (41-45), but there have also been studies which have failed to show positive results by either route of administration (34,46-50). One possible explanation for the negative results concerns the length of administration of the physostigmine. Consequently, several investigators have pursued long-term oral treatment with physostigmine, and some of these studies have yielded positive results (51-53). Currently, a multicenter trial of sustained-release oral physostigmine in Alzheimer's dissease is underway.

It appears that most individuals have an optimum level of cholinergic functioning or a "cholinergic window" of activity. Consequently, many of the strategies which have shown positive results with AChE inhibitors have first obtained an optimum dose for the patients through preliminary dose titration studies. However, even when the optimal-dose-finding strategy has been employed, the results have been equivocal (49,54). Harrell and colleagues have been able to characterize responders and nonresponders on several indices of red blood cell and plasma choline levels as well as on neuropsychological tests (54). It also appears that the response to AChE inhibition correlates with central activity of the drug as assessed by AChE inhibition in the cerebrospinal fluid (44).

Relatively few studies have been done using the longer-acting, better-absorbed AChE inhibitor, tacrine (THA). Summers et al. and Davis and Mohs (55-57) generated a great deal of interest with a study published in 1986 claiming that most of his 17 Alzheimer patients responded to THA. This study has since been criticized (58), but nonetheless, large multicenter trials involving tacrine and tacrine plus lecithin are currently underway. The initial trial with tacrine was interrupted due to an increase in liver enzymes at the higher doses of the drug, but all of the abnormalities were reversible. Additionally, a study of an orally active hydroxylated metabolite of THA (HPO29) from Hoechst-Roussel is currently underway. This compound may provide a somewhat better safety to efficacy profile than THA itself (59).

In summary, several of the studies involving cholinesterase inhibitors have shown positive effects on memory; however, most of the changes have been modest. It is not clear if the bioavailability is the problem or if only certain patients respond to cholinergic manipulation. Finally, when patients do respond, the responses are modest and shortlived.

DIRECT AGONISTS

The third strategy in cholinergic treatment encompasses the use of direct cholinergic agonists. This class of agonists has similar toxicity to the AChE inhibitors and is limited in that respect. Arecoline is the single cholinergic agonist which has received the most intensive evaluation. Transient memory improvement has been found in subcutaneous administration of arecoline to young adults (60) and patients with Alzheimer's disease (37). Oxotremorine is another direct agonist which has received some study; however, it too is toxic at high doses, and one study had to be terminated because of the toxicity; no benefit was demonstrated (61). However, other cholinergic agonists such as RS-86 from Sandoz and pilocarpine are currently under investigation. Some results are positive with RS-86 (62), but others are more equivocal (34,63).

INTRAVENTRICULAR CHOLINERGIC AGONIST

Harbaugh and colleagues reported preliminary data regarding the intraventricular administration of the direct agonist, bethanechol in dementia (64). In this uncontrolled trial, there was a suggestion of improvement in the demented patients as reported by families when the agonist was administered via this route. This finding implied that cholinergic compounds could ameliorate some of the symptoms of dementia if the compounds could be effectively delivered to the central nervous system. This preliminary trial led to a more rigorous multicenter trial using this technique, and the results of this trial have been reported recently (65). In general, the results of the multicenter trial were not encouraging, and consequently, this approach is not being recommended for the treatment of dementia.

CENTRAL NERVOUS SYSTEM GRAFTING

Finally, there is some interest in the restoration of memory function through septohippocampal grafts, primarily in Alzheimer's disease (66). Research on the topic of central nervous system grafting was stimulated by the work of Madrazo and colleagues on adrenal-brain transplants in Parkinson's disease (67). More recent work on that procedure, however, has been less dramatic, and many centers are now reassessing the advisability of this approach in Parkinson's disease (68).

The rationale for grafting in the cholinergic system derives from early animal research which suggests improved cholinergic functioning. It is possible that a graft may elicit trophic factors for the host brain which then would perform a reparative function on the injured tissue (69,70). Nerve growth factor may serve a function in this role. The graft may also provide neurotransmitter at the site of action and enhance function in this fashion (71). Finally, the graft may actually replace the damaged tissue and become integrated into the host's neurocircuitry (71). The concept of neurografting is exciting and may prove beneficial in certain circumstances; however, a great number of issues including ethics, sources of material, site of grafting, and the mechanics of the procedure remain to be elucidated.

SUMMARY

The cholinergic system has a role in learning and memory functions, and the system appears to be impaired in various disease states (e.g., Alzheimer's disease). The majority of the attempts to enhance cholinergic function and secondarily memory and learning have been unsuccessful. A number of studies have shown modest improvements, but nothing is dramatic and the benefits are not sustained. There are several reasons that attempts at enhancing cholinergic function may fail.

1. Only certain people may benefit from enhancement of cholinergic functions.
2. Most people appear to have a "cholinergic window" which may be small and needs careful titration to determine its proper dose range.
3. Most cholinergic compounds have difficulties with bioavailability and short half-lives.
4. The toxicity of cholinergic compounds is significant and often curtails higher dose treatments.
5. Cholinergic neurons that project to the cortex are felt to be diminished. These nerve endings normally contain high levels of CAT and have presynaptic muscarinic, M_2 receptors that modulate the release of ACh.

Mash and colleagues have demonstrated that both CAT and the presynaptic M_2 receptors are decreased in patients with Alzheimer's disease (72). This decrease was also associated with an up-regulation of the numbers of postsynaptic M_1 muscarinic receptors on the target neurons. Thus, it has been proposed that the most efficacious type of cholinergic therapy should involve a selective M_1 agonist rather than the relatively nonspecific cholinergic agonists currently being used (73). Several pharmaceutical companies are currently developing selective M_1 agonists.

In spite of a lack of dramatic breakthrough, the rationale for using cholinergic compounds is strong and intense investigation continues.

ADRENERGIC DRUGS

While most of the attention on the pharmacologic manipulation of memory has involved the cholinergic system, other neurotransmitter systems are involved in memory deficits in young, old, and demented individuals. The noradrenergic system has received attention for its role in memory both in isolation and as a modulator of other pharmacologic systems. In all likelihood, the role of neurotransmitters in memory and cognitive function in general is quite complex and involves multiple interacting systems.

The anatomical focus of the noradrenergic system resides in the locus coeruleus. Some studies indicate that the number of cells in the locus coeruleus decreases with age with the implication that this cell loss may contribute to memory impairment. For example, in mice it has been shown that retention performance correlates well with locus coeruleus cell count, namely, those mice with poor retention performance generally had fewer cells in the locus coeruleus than mice performing well (74). In fact, in one study, the correlation between the locus coeruleus cell count and the behavioral measure of retention performance was 0.98 (74). In addition to the anatomical work, several investigators have reported reduced activity in the catecholamine system in the aged animal brain (75-77), and postmortem human studies have shown reduced levels of dopamine and norepinephrine related to age (78,79). There is also reasonably strong evidence that the noradrenergic system is involved in a variety of cognitive functions in normal subjects (80,81).

It is also possible that the noradrenergic system may work in a modulatory fashion on the cholinergic system, and consequently, manipulation of a single system may not be fruitful. There are several brain regions in which the noradrenergic and cholinergic systems may interact. For example, the locus coeruleus axons traverse the basal forebrain region (82,83), but it is not known if the locus coeruleus actually innervates this area. The cortex is another possible site of interaction since noradrenergic and cholinergic innervation patterns have been shown to overlap (84,85).

A variety of studies have reported various manipulations of the noradrenergic system with ultimate effects on memory function (81,86,87). Zornetzer reviewed his findings on the noradrenergic system in mice and concluded that age-related memory loss is not inevitable and that appropriate intervention strategies may delay the onset of memory difficulties in aging (74).

There is less information on memory enhancement with adrenergic agonists in man. McEntee and Mair reported a significant improvement in memory function in patients with Korsakoff's disease using the alpha-2 noradrenergic agonist, clonidine (88). These authors indicate that there is evidence for deficient central noradrenergic activity in Korsakoff's disease which correlates with the level of cognitive impairment. Levels of 3-methoxy-4-hydroxy-phenylglycol and homovanillic acid, the primary brain metabolites of norepinephrine and dopamine, respectively, are diminished in cerebrospinal fluid samples of these patients (89,90). In other human work, Bondareff and colleagues demonstrated a cell loss in the locus coeruleus in a subset of patients with Alzheimer type dementia (91). In one group of patients with Alzheimer's disease who were particularly young at the time of death and had a rather severe form of the disease, a loss of 80% of locus coeruleus neurons was found.

In a recent review of the role of catecholamines in the memory impairment found in normal aging, McEntee and Crook cite evidence for the involvement of catecholamines in aged humans and animals (92-96). They state that spatial memory is impaired in old monkeys which may relate to dysfunction in the dorsolateral prefrontal cortex, the site of catecholamine projections (97,98). McEntee and Crook contend that while the memory deficits associated with normal aging are likely to be multifactorial, involving at least the cholinergic and noradrenergic systems, norepinephrine may have a key modulatory function in memory and consequently may deserve special attention for the augmentation of memory function in normal aging. Thus far, however, manipulation of the noradrenergic system with clonidine has produced mixed results (99-102), and another study using a nonphysiologic precursor of norepinephrine, DL-threo-dihydroxyphenylserine in Korsakoff's disease produced an improvement in only one of several memory functions (103).

It appears that norepinephrine does have a role in memory function in humans, and it is likely to serve as a modulator. The enhancement of noradrenergic function in man may serve to increase attention and arousal and consequently augment memory through attentional mechanisms. This may constitute the cognitive counterpart of the modulatory role at the neurochemical level.

SEROTONERGIC DRUGS

There has been increasing evidence that the serotonergic system is affected in Alzheimer's disease (104). Not only is brain serotonin content and uptake reduced, but serotonergic cell density in the raphe nuclei is also reduced (105-110). Serotonergic receptors (S_1 and S_2) have been shown to be decreased in aging, and a recent report has indicated diminished serotonin binding in Alzheimer's disease which most likely represents a decrease in receptor number (111).

In an attempt to augment neuropsychological performance through manipulation of the serotonergic system, zimelidine, a relatively specific serotonin reuptake blocker was evaluated (112). Four patients with Alzheimer's disease were assessed in a double-blind, placebo-controlled crossover study. There were no significant effects of zimelidine on memory or reaction time when compared to placebo; thus, it appears from this small study that zimelidine is not effective in enhancing cognition.

PEPTIDES

VASOPRESSIN

A great deal of research has been conducted evaluating the effects of various neuropeptides on learning and memory. The rationale for much of this research comes from animal work on the effects of vasopressin on learning and memory performance. Evidence for the role of vasopressin is derived from research involving three different situations: neurohypophysectomy, learning and memory performance in the Brattleboro strain of rats with hereditary diabetes insipidus, and the administration of vasopressin antisera in assessing memory performance. De Wied and associates have shown that removal of the posterior pituitary in rats does not affect acquisition of avoidance behavior but does interfere with the maintenance of that performance (113). Administration of vasopressin to these animals restores the maintenance of this behavior. The administration of vasopressin to normal rats has also been shown to increase their resistance to extinction of avoidance behavior which is a sensitive index of retention on these tasks (114,115). Vasopressin can also protect against amnesia induced in mice by a variety of means including the administration of puromycin (116,117), CO_2 inhalation, and electroconvulsive shock (118). Although these animal data suggest that vasopressin might play a role in normal memory functioning and, conceivably, in memory disorders, there is no direct evidence for vasopressin abnormalities in brains of individuals who die with Alzheimer's disease or other dementing illnesses.

The Brattleboro strain of rats is homozygous for diabetes insipidus and consequently is genetically incapable of synthesizing vasopressin. These animals can initially learn passive avoidance behavior but have impaired retention of this type of behavior (119). Extinction of the learned behaviors is quite rapid (120,121). However, when these rats are administered various forms of vasopressin after learning the passive avoidance response, the behavior is retained implying that vasopressin has an effect on consolidation processes (122).

Additionally, the role of vasopressin in animal learning and memory function is also supported by investigations using intracerebroventricular injections of antisera to vasopressin. When the normal rats are administered antisera via this route, they behave in a fashion similar to that of the Brattleboro strain of rats. However, when vasopressin is given systemically, these changes in behavior are not appreciated implying the role of vasopressin in modifying these behaviors is central (123). These three lines of evidence in the animal literature point to the role of vasopressin in learning and memory function. While the precise mechanism of action of vasopressin on the central nervous system is unknown, its role in modulating certain neurotransmitter systems is well known. It has been speculated that vasopressin may facilitate memory by modulating noradrenergic transmission (124), but vasopressin also interacts with the cholinergic (125), serotonergic (126), and dopaminergic systems (127-129).

Animal studies have provided the rationale for a variety of clinical trials using vasopressin. In one study involving patients with apparently normal cognition, age 50-65, lysine vasopressin or a placebo was administered, and those who received vasopressin performed better on attention and memory tasks than those receiving placebo (130). In another study, small positive correlations were found between the level of circulating neurophysins in men between ages 50 and 65 and an index of long-term memory (131).

In a study on mood disturbances and cognitive impairment, Gold and Goodwin reported significant cognitive enhancement on verbal learning during treatment with 1-desamino-8-D-arginine vasopressin (DDAVP) (132). The performance returned to baseline six weeks after termination of the treatment with DDAVP.

Weingartner and colleagues studied six young cognitively unimpaired subjects and showed a significant increase in learning and memory performance when the subjects were given DDAVP for two to three weeks (133). In a subsequent study, two patients who were being treated with electroconvulsive therapy received DDAVP prior to the treatment, and their retrograde amnesia following electroconvulsive therapy was reduced.

Several small trials have been conducted using various vasopressin analogs in posttraumatic amnesia and amnesia associated with the excessive use of alcohol. One study involving three patients who had posttraumatic amnesia and one with alcohol-induced amnesia demonstrated some improvement in memory and mood following administration of vasopressin (134). In a double-blind single case study of a patient with Korsakoff's syndrome, improvement in learning and memory function was shown after two weeks of treatment with lysine vasopressin (135). However, another study on a single patient with Korsakoff's syndrome failed to show any response to lysine vasopressin (136). Similarly, another study on six severe posttraumatic amnesia patients using DDAVP failed to show any significant improvement in memory function; however, these patients were rather severely impaired (137).

More recently, several studies have been conducted investigating the role of vasopressin in the treatment of dementia. Weingartner and colleagues using DDAVP demonstrated some improvement in performance on a word association task but relatively little direct effect on memory (138). Another study involving 17 patients with Alzheimer's disease being treated for 10 days failed to show any significant changes on a variety of measures of learning and memory (139). However, some improvement was noted on reaction time measures implying an alternative mechanism of action.

In a trial of lysine vasopressin in 20 subjects with mild to moderate dementia, small but consistent improvements were seen on several memory tests (140). In this study, a selective reminding task and a reaction time task did not show differences although there was a trend on the reaction time task. There may have been a subtle improvement in mood in some of the patients.

Peabody and colleagues have performed several studies evaluating the effects of various vasopressin analogs on memory and learning functions (141). In general, this group has found their clinical trials with the vasopressin analogs to be unimpressive. In one study involving alcoholic patients and dementia patients, there was a trend toward a positive DDAVP effect on verbal learning; however, the magnitude was small (142). In a double-blind parallel group study, 17 demented patients with either suspected Alzheimer's disease or alcoholic dementia were given desglycinamide-9-arginine-vasopressin (DGAVP) for one week. The DGAVP group improved on a selective reminding task involving low imagery words but failed to exhibit any other appreciable behavioral effects. In all, the authors felt that this trial was negative but indicated that the compound should be studied further (141).

Data on the role of vasopressin on memory are controversial. It appears that the thesis that vasopressin modulates memory function directly is becoming less likely, but the notion that it modulates memory function secondarily through autonomic nervous system action is possible (143). Vasopressin's primary effect may be to modulate arousal mechanisms and thereby alter attentional functions which secondarily enhance memory processes. Support for this comes from Beckwith and colleagues (144) but not from Sahgal et al. (145). Sahgal's group reviewed the literature on vasopressin and memory and suggested that vasopressin may affect behavior by both peripheral and central actions. The peripheral action may serve as a reinforcement for behavior while the central role may actually modulate arousal level and secondarily affect learning and memory (146). The primary evidence for an arousal effect of vasopressin comes from its frequent biomodal effect on behavior implying that an appropriate level of arousal is necessary for optimal behavior. In a similar vein, LeMoal and colleagues have hypothesized that vasopressin induces peripheral autonomic responses which stimulate arousal and hence promote learning. They indicate that this hypothesis does not preclude other central mechanisms of vasopressin on memory (147).

ACTH

Other peptides related to vasopressin have also been postulated as having a role in learning and memory (148). ACTH has received a great deal of interest especially since the development of synthetic analogs which are devoid of the hormonal action of ACTH (149). One compound, ACTH 4-10, has been shown to affect acquisition and adaptive behavior yet it does not release steroids (150). The synthetic peptide, ORG 2766, has received the most attention, and while a few positive reports exist (151), most studies have failed to yield a consistent cognitive improvement (152-154). In general, ACTH does not appear to have a significant effect on cognition in dementia (3).

ACETYL-L-CARNITINE

Some attention has been given recently to acetyl-l-carnitine for the treatment of dementia and memory disorders. Acetyl-l-carnitine (l-β-acetyloxy γ-trimethylamino-butyric acid chloride) is the acetyl ester of l-carnitine, both of which occur naturally in the body. The structural formula of acetyl-l-carnitine is very similar to acetylcholine, and numerous studies have evaluated the similarities between these two compounds. Acetyl-l-carnitine has been shown to provide acetyl groups for acetylcholine synthesis, to activate choline acetyltransferase, to enhance the high-affinity uptake of choline, and exert a cholinomimetic effect on certain cholinergic receptors (155-158).

Acetyl-l-carnitine has been evaluated in several European studies on geriatric patients with compromised cognition due to degenerative or cerebrovascular diseases. Several open-label studies have been done in Europe investigating the role of acetyl-l-carnitine in Alzheimer's disease. One study on nine patients with Alzheimer's disease reported an improvement in attention and insight in most of the patients (159). Another study involving 25 patients with Alzheimer's disease showed an improvement in 12 patients in the areas of memory and behavior and the remaining 13 patients either had an equivocal response or no significant change in function (160). A third study involving 12 patients claimed to show a significant improvement, and perhaps equally as important, a decline in neuropsychological function when the medication was discontinued (161). A final study on 15 patients with dementia again showed an improvement in two-thirds of the patients with no change in the remainder (162).

More recently, 8 double-blind placebo-controlled studies have been conducted on over 300 patients with various stages and degrees of cognitive impairment. Agnoli and colleagues, in particular, noted improvement on acquisition, delayed recall, and a memory index after three months of treatment with acetyl-*l*-carnitine when compared with a placebo group (163). Other studies have indicated a positive effect on mental function (164), spatial and temporal judgment, and in a large study involving 212 patients treated over 3 months, an improvement in clinical global impression of performance (165). Bonavita and colleagues studied 40 patients classified as senile who received 3 g of acetyl-*l*-carnitine or placebo for 40 days and demonstrated small but significant changes from baseline on several measures of cognitive function in the treated group (166). Additional studies involving groups of patients as large as 50 being treated for 6 months have also shown a positive effect of the compound on cognition (167,168). Finally, Mantero and colleagues showed an improvement in patients with moderately severe Alzheimer's disease on the Mini-Mental State Examination after three and six months of treatment with acetyl-*l*-carnitine (169).

The compilation of this research has been sufficiently encouraging to lead to a national multicenter trial of acetyl-*l*-carnitine in Alzheimer's disease. Since this compound is a naturally occurring substance, it is felt to be virtually free of side effects and, in that sense, constitutes an interesting compound to evaluate for memory and dementia in elderly patients.

SOMATOSTATIN

Somatostatin is a hypothalamic tetradecapeptide which inhibits growth hormone release and is found in substantial quantity in the rat's cerebral cortex and hippocampus (170,171). There is also a suggestion that somatostatin in the hippocampus may be intrinsic and confined to local interneurons (172). Somatostatin may play a role in Alzheimer's disease as indicated by the following findings: (a) cerebrospinal fluid levels of somatostatin have been shown to be reduced in patients with Alzheimer's disease (173-177); (b) somatostatinlike immunoreactivity in the cortex has been shown to be reduced in Alzheimer's disease and this appears to correlate with glucose hypometabolism (178-182); (c) a reduction in somatostatin correlates with senile plaque counts; (d) neuronal tangles have been identified in somatostatinergic neurons (181); and (e) a recent study on cerebrospinal fluid somatostatin levels and neuropeptide Y suggests that somatostatin levels are decreased while neuropeptide Y levels are unchanged in Alzheimer's disease (183). These findings suggest that the administration of somatostatin in patients with Alzheimer's disease and memory disorders may be beneficial.

One small study involving the intravenous administration of a somatostatin analog failed to show an improvement in memory function in patients with Alzheimer's disease (184). Since part of the lack of effectiveness of in-travenous somatostatin may be due to the ineffective delivery of the compound to the brain, intrathecal administration has been suggested. However, a recent trial of intracranial, intrathecal somatostatin administration to monkeys resulted in marked neurotoxicity (185). Consequently, while the hypothesis regarding the role of somatostatin in memory function and in Alzheimer's disease remains interesting, considerable further research needs to be done before the compound can be given to patients with Alzheimer's disease.

NOOTROPICS

A class of drugs described as nootropics has been investigated in memory disorders since the mid-1970s. Giurgea referred to this class of drugs as compounds which act in a relatively specific fashion on cognitive function yet have relatively few side effects (1,186,187). The term does not imply any specific mechanism of action, and in general, no specific pharmacologic profile has been derived for the members of this class. The basic features of the nootropics are that they are meant to enhance learning and memory, facilitate information processing, antagonize processes which impair cognitive function, and in general lack cognitive or other systemic side effects. The prototypical drug in this class is piracetam. Other members of this group include pramiracetam, oxiracetam, and aniracetam.

Piracetam has been the most extensively studied compound in this group and is a γ-aminobutyric acid (GABA) analog with varied effects on the brain and performance (186). It is thought that piracetam has a nonspecific enhancing effect on neuronal function and perhaps augments certain neurochemical systems (e.g., the cholinergic system) (188,189).

Nootropics produce few side effects and consequently are felt to be safe when given to brain injured or elderly individuals (190). Several animal studies have shown that piracetam augments performance on a variety of tasks (188,190-193), but its use in humans has yielded variable results. Several studies have investigated piracetam in dyslexic children with generally mildly positive results in improving reading ability (194), learning and recall (195), reading and writing ability (196), and reading speed (197). However, each study also failed to show improvement in other cognitive measures, and there was no consistent pattern of performance across studies.

Since piracetam may have an effect on the cholinergic system, several animal studies have been undertaken assessing performance involving piracetam and cholinergic manipulations (188,198). These studies have been suggestive and consequently have led to several clinical trials. An initial study by Smith and colleagues demonstrated positive findings using piracetam plus lecithin (199), but Growdon and colleagues failed to show any benefit from piracetam or piracetam plus lecithin in any of their patients with Alzheimer's disease (200). One study designed to assess the effects of piracetam on post-electroconvulsive amnesia demonstrated an improvement in memory function following electroconvulsive therapy in a piracetam-treated group (201). In this study, a group of patients with a variety of clinical diagnoses who were to undergo ECT received piracetam prior to the electroconvulsive therapy, and this group performed somewhat better after ECT than the untreated group.

Another nootropic which has received attention largely from Italian investigators is oxiracetam. Oxiracetam is more potent electrophysiologically than piracetam and may display a broader spectrum of activity (202). The mechanism of action of oxiracetam is unknown, but changes in cholinergic activity have been reported (203). For example, it has been shown that oxiracetam can prevent the decrease in brain ACh levels induced by scopolamine and electroconvulsive shock and can alter the decrease in brain ACh levels following the intracerebroventricular administration of hemicholinium (204,205).

One double-blind placebo-controlled study involving 43 patients with organic brain syndrome which included dementia of the Alzheimer type, multi-infarct dementia, and affective disorders showed improved cognition following treatment with oxiracetam 800 mg twice daily for 8 weeks. Several other psychological parameters improved as well (206). However, another study on oxiracetam involving a group of 106 middle-aged patients suffering from mild to moderate organic brain syndrome secondary to prolonged exposure to organic solvents found no differences in neuropsychological test performance following treatment (207).

When oxiracetam was used on a group of patients with a variety of disorders including memory deficits, intellectual dysfunction, and affective disturbances, improvement was seen in short-term memory and a variety of subjective symptoms after one week of treatment with oxiracetam when compared with placebo (208). However, by four weeks, the differences on a general geriatric assessment scale were not significant.

In a multicenter double-blind placebo-controlled trial to evaluate the efficacy of oxiracetam when given for 24 weeks to patients with probable or possible Alzheimer's disease, some improvement was seen on a psychiatric and somatic complaint scale as well as on certain scales of the Luria-Nebraska Neuropsychological Battery. The 16 patients on oxiracetam, as a group, showed improvement over time while the 14 patients on placebo remained unchanged or tended to deteriorate. No differences were seen between the two groups in side effects (209).

Less work has been done on the other nootropics in the piracetam class. An electrophysiological study of aniracetam showed some increase in alertness in 10 geriatric patients (210) and preliminary findings from Dajas showed memory improvement using this compound (211). Sourander showed some improvement in immediate and delayed recall in a placebo-controlled double-blind study involving aniracetam in 44 patients with Alzheimer type dementia, but failed to show an overall clinical effect (212).

In general, the nootropics have been rather extensively investigated, but the overall result is not encouraging. The mechanism of action of these compounds is unknown and most of the studies have used heterogeneous groups of patients. Additionally, the outcome variables have varied considerably among the studies and consequently it is difficult to determine the efficacy of this group of agents.

VASODILATORS

It was formerly believed that atherosclerosis was a major cause of dementia in the elderly. Some of the reasoning behind this belief involved the coexistence of atherosclerosis and dementia in the elderly. Because atherosclerosis reduced blood flow to the brain, it was presumed that this ultimately led to neuronal deterioration and dementia. As knowledge of the pathophysiology of dementing illnesses has evolved, this explanation for cognitive impairment in the elderly has been replaced with other theories on the etiology of the disorder.

Nevertheless, several drug studies were spawned and designed to assess the effects of vasodilators on cognition. Generally, these drugs have been cerebral vasodilators, and while initially they were thought to exert their effects through vasodilation, it is now felt that these drugs may also have other, perhaps metabolic, antidepressant, or anxiolytic actions (213). Yesavage and colleagues reviewed this extensive literature of well over 100 studies and concluded that drugs with mixed vasodilating and metabolic effects have generally produced more positive effects than have drugs which were primarily vasodilators (214). However, the overall effectiveness of this class of drugs has been felt to be marginal.

One of the most popular drugs in this category is dihydroergotoxine mesylate (Hydergine). This compound has been widely studied, and typically, it has been compared with placebo or placebo and papaverine. Many studies have been done using dihydroergotoxine mesylate, and often, behavioral variables show a statistically significant improvement compared with placebo (215-226). The variables which showed some improvement include alertness, orientation, confusion, memory, depression, anxiety, motivation, agitation, and overall impression of change; however, dihydroergotoxine mesylate fairs less well when cognitive measures are used (227). Most of the studies which showed some improvement did not use objective tests of cognitive function, but, nevertheless, some showed continuous improvement in behavioral variables for extended periods up to 12 weeks. It may be that dihydroergotoxine mesylate is of benefit to some patients with dementia. It is not clear if this represents a group of patients with a vascular component to their dementia or whether this is a nonspecific alerting effect which may benefit a variety of dementias.

Papaverine is another compound in this class which has been investigated and has been shown to have an effect on cerebral blood flow (228-231). Some studies have shown improved cognition, but in comparison with studies using dihydroergotoxine mesylate, the latter compound has been found to be slightly superior (215,216).

Cyclandelate is another vasodilator which has been investigated rather extensively with mixed results. In the better control studies, little, if any, positive effect has been realized from the treatment with cyclandelate (214). More recent uncontrolled studies suggest that cyclandelate may be worth pursuing further in multi-infarct dementia (232,233). An interim analysis in one open-study indicated improvement in cognitive functions, orientation, and verbal communication as assessed by the Blessed Dementia Scale and Parkside Behavioral Scale (225). In an uncontrolled trial of cyclandelate in 10 patients with multi-infarct dementia and 10 patients with alcohol-related amnesia, some subscales of the Wechsler Memory Scale showed improvement with cyclandelate for 6 weeks of treatment (233). Finally, in a comparison between cyclandelate and flunarizine in vascular dementia, cyclandelate appeared superior on several memory parameters (234).

There have been several methodological problems with many of the studies investigating vasodilators. One problem concerns the definition of the patient population. Most of the studies have been done on patients presumed to have multi-infarct dementia, yet a precise definition of this concept is not available. Attempts have been made at lending some objectivity to this concept, but controversy remains (235-237). Additionally, many of the trials have been uncontrolled and have used behavioral scales rather than cognitive measures to assess the effects of the compounds. These scales have made the assessment of cognitive effects of these drugs difficult, and a concern over a placebo effect in uncontrolled trials is a significant factor. Finally, the mechanism of action of many of these compounds has been elusive. Some appear to work as vasodilators while others appear to have various metabolic actions. In general, there has been no compelling evidence that these compounds exert any significant positive effects on memory.

CALCIUM CHANNEL ANTAGONISTS

Calcium channel antagonists have recently been studied for their possible role in the treatment of primary degenerative dementia. The primary drug of interest in this group is nimodipine which is a 1,4 dihydropyridine and is lipid soluble, thus enabling it to cross the blood-brain barrier more effectively.

It has been shown to be a potent cerebrovasodilator. The drug has recently been marketed in the United States for prevention of cerebral vasospasm following subarachnoid hemorrhage (238-242). Nimodipine appears to enhance cerebral blood flow following ischemic stroke (243-246), and numerous animal studies have shown that nimodipine increases cerebral blood flow following experimental ischemic strokes (247-253). In two studies involving lightly anesthetized rats, regional cerebral blood flow was increased after nimodipine administration in several regions known to be involved in dementia (e.g., hippocampus, cerebral cortex, and thalamus) (254,255). However, this factor is not thought to be its primary mechanism of action in treating primary degenerative dementia. The entry of calcium into the neuron may constitute the final common pathway resulting in cell death following ischemia (245), and it is possible that this factor may play a role in dementia.

In aging, many changes occur within the central nervous system including a variety of neurotransmitter changes, receptor alterations, cell loss, as well as an alteration in calcium metabolism. Calcium-activated potassium currents have been found to be prolonged in hippocampal neurons in the aging brain, and this may relate to memory deficits occurring in normal aging (256). Furthermore, certain alterations in calcium homeostatsis in aged individuals may be toxic to neurons (257,258). Consequently, it has been suggested that calcium channel antagonists may improve learning and memory function in aged individuals by decreasing the neuronal influx of calcium and thereby reducing calcium-activated currents or minimizing calcium toxicity in the aged brain. A recent study by Deyo and colleagues studied this question by investigating the effect of nimodipine on associative learning in aging rabbits (259). These investigators demonstrated an accelerated acquisition of a conditioned eye-blink response in both young and aging rabbits without causing an increase in nonspecific responding. Based on this work, these authors felt that nimodipine may be effective in treating age-related learning and memory deficits. As a result of these animal studies and pilot work involving elderly humans, a multicenter trial of nimodipine in primary degenerative dementia is currently underway.

ADDITIONAL THERAPIES

A variety of other classes of pharmacologic agents have been proposed for the treatment of memory disorders and/or dementia. Many of these compounds have been evaluated in only limited clinical trials, and consequently, no definite conclusions can be drawn.

L-DEPRENYL

Deprenyl or selegiline has recently been released for treatment of Parkinson's disease. A great deal of interest has been generated based on studies that appear to indicate that deprenyl may retard the progression of the disorder (260,261). Deprenyl is a selective monoamine oxidase-B inhibitor at low doses and thereby prolongs the action of dopamine. Also, it may have a role in reducing the formation of a potentially toxic compound in the brain of patients with Parkinson's disease.

Deprenyl has been evaluated in a group of 17 patients with Alzheimer's disease at both 10 and 40 mg/day. Half of the patients improved clinically with increased activity and social interaction particularly at the lower dose. There were, however, only minimal changes in cognitive function in these patients as indicated by a variety of neuropsychological measures (262). Patients received the medication for four to five weeks at each dose, and consequently, longer effects of the drug were not assessed. If the outcome of the studies on Parkinson's disease is applicable to Alzheimer's disease, longer treatment intervals may be necessary to assess any positive protective effects of deprenyl on memory function in dementia.

PHOSPHATIDYLSERINE

A recent multicenter trial of phosphatidylserine suggests that this compound may improve performance on selected cognitive variables in dementia (263). Phosphatidylserine is a naturally occurring phospholipid that may stabilize neuronal membranes as well as exert other metabolic effects. In this double-blind randomized placebo-controlled trial, 70 patients received phosphatidylserine and 70 patients received a placebo for a period of three months. Improvement in performance was found in the treated group on some cognitive measures, but considering the large number of outcome measures used, this was not felt to be particularly significant. In another trial, Delwaide and colleagues evaluated 42 hospitalized demented patients and documented a trend toward improvement in the phosphatidylserine-treated patients (264). Further work is underway on this compound.

GABA

The role of gamma-aminobutyric acid (GABA) in memory function has been investigated in several animal studies. Drugs that enhance GABA activity generally impair memory performance, while drugs that decrease GABA activity enhance memory function (265). Most of the memory work on the GABA system has involved the evaluation of the effect of benzodiazepines on memory. Benzodiazepines impair new learning but produce less of an effect on retrieval of previously acquired information (266-270). Lawlor and colleagues have reviewed this aspect of memory function elsehwere in this volume. The benzodiazepine receptor antagonist, RO-15-1788, appears to block benzodiazepine-induced amnesia (271).

Some evidence suggests GABA interneurons may receive cholinergic input from the basal forebrain (46) and the GABA neurons may be abnormal in Alzheimer's disease (272-274). Consequently, a trial of a GABA agonist was undertaken in a group of six patients with Alzheimer's disease of mild to moderate severe degree. However, no significant cognitive effects were found in any of these patients following treatment, and consequently, Mohr and colleagues felt that GABA probably does not play a major role in the cognitive impairment in Alzheimer's disease (275).

OPIOIDS

Animal studies have suggested that opioids can have a facilitative effect on memory (276). Most of the studies have involved the effects of the opiate antagonist, naloxone, but the results are dependent upon the dose, route of administration, and particular task used to test the memory function. This complex relationship has been reviewed by Wolkowitz et al. (277). Additionally, the effects of opioids on learning and memory function may also reflect the secondary involvement of other neuropharmacologic systems such as the catecholaminergic system (278).

Several human studies have found a deleterious effect of naloxone on memory function in normal individuals (268,279,280). One small open trial found a beneficial effect of naloxone in treatment of patients with senile dementia of the Alzheimer type (281), but a larger trial involving 12 patients with Alzheimer's disease revealed no positive effect (282). Similarly, a trial involving the opiate antagonist, naltrexone, produced only a slight enhancement in one cognitive measure following acute treatment (283). Finally, a multicenter trial of naloxone in patients with Alzheimer's disease has been reported recently, and no significant findings resulted from this study (284). It does not appear that opioid antagonists are generally useful in enhancing memory function in normal persons or in patients with dementia of the Alzheimer type.

NERVE GROWTH FACTOR

Nerve growth factor (NGF) is a protein considered to be neurotrophic. In peripheral sympathetic neurons, NGF is synthesized by target tissues and acts on receptors located on the projecting neurons. Nerve growth factor is then internalized and transported in a retrograde fashion to the cell bodies of the neurons where it stimulates the synthesis of proteins essential for survival and influences transmitter-specific properties of the neuron (285). Nerve growth factor is the most well understood of a large group of compounds that are involved in neuronal growth and maintenance.

Nerve growth factor levels are high in the hippocampus, cortex, septum, and nucleus basalis region which are known target areas for cholinergic projections (286). This suggests that NGF is produced by target cells of cholinergic neurons of the basal forebrain. In addition, when NGF is injected into the target areas of forebrain cholinergic neurons, it is taken up by these neurons and transported in a retrograde fashion to cholinergic nerve cell bodies in the basal forebrain (287,288). Hefti and Weiner (285) note that the stimulation of NGF receptors on cholinergic neurons mediates trophic influences on these cells, and NGF has been shown to elevate levels of choline acetyltransferase (289-291).

These and other data indicate that NGF is present in the brain and can affect cholinergic neurons in the basal forebrain by acting on specific receptors on the cells. It appears that NGF can affect survival, fiber growth, and expression of certain enzymes in cholinergic neurons.

Based on this evidence, enthusiasm has grown for the role of NGF in the treatment of Alzheimer's disease and memory disorders, and a workshop was organized at the National Institute on Aging to discuss the potential use of NGF in Alzheimer's disease. The workshop recognized the potential value of NGF but also cautioned premature use of NGF pending the availability of a reliable source of NGF, a method for determining the activity of NGF, appropriate toxicity studies in animals and humans, and trials in non-human primates (292). These issues are currently being addressed by investigators in this field.

EXCITATORY AMINO ACID ANTAGONISTS

Glutamate and aspartate are excitatory amino acids that have been implicated in a variety of clinical disorders including epilepsy, movement disorders, and dementia (293). Adequate clinical trials have not been done on excitatory amino acid agonists and antagonists, but there is increasing evidence for the role of these amino acids in cognitive changes with aging (294). It appears that excess accumulation of glutamate or aspartate can cause neuronal death in the absence of anoxia, and this finding has lead to speculation about the role of excitatory amino acids in cell death of other etiologies, e.g., degenerative brain diseases. The status of glutamate in Alzheimer's disease is controversial with some evidence for alterations in binding (293) and some evidence for no change (295). There is evidence for the depletion of glutamate in the hippocampal perforant pathway of patients with Alzheimer's disease when compared to nondemented control subjects (296). The excitatory amino acid antagonist, MK801, has been shown to have some positive effects in a form of attentional deficit disorder (297), but its possible role in other cognitive disorders has not been explored adequately (298).

ACE INHIBITORS

Recently, the effects of several antihypertensive drugs on cognition have been investigated. Most notably, the angiotensin-converting enzyme (ACE) inhibitor, captopril, has been associated with better work performance and life satisfaction when compared with propranolol and methyldopa (299). Memory effects of ACE inhibitors have also been noted (300). While the mechanism by which these changes may take place is unclear, it appears that the ACE inhibitors may increase cerebral blood flow while decreasing systemic blood pressure (301,302). Captopril is currently being investigated for any possible effects it may have on cognition.

CHELATION THERAPY

The role of aluminum in Alzheimer's disease remains controversial (303-305). An increase in aluminum content has been found in neurofibrillary tangles in the brains of patients with Alzheimer's disease, but its role as being primary or secondary in the disorder is unclear (303-305). Chelation therapy has been proposed by some as a form of treatment for Alzheimer's disease, but no clinical trials have been conducted. This remains a controversial area, and there is little evidence to recommend this as a form of treatment for Alzheimer's disease (306).

BEHAVIORAL TREATMENTS

ASSESSMENT CONSIDERATIONS

The widespread nature of memory disorders after closed head injury (CHI) emphasizes the importance of adequately evaluating patients' impairments and abilities in order to maximize the potential for rehabilitation. Assessment should include measures covering modalities such as verbal, visual, and spatial memory. The observation that one modality is relatively spared is critical for treatment since patients can be taught in a manner that exploits the preserved ability, e.g., the use of visual cues to learn the stages of transferring from a wheelchair when visual as opposed to verbal functions are intact (307). Testing should also evaluate differences between recall and recognition within a particular modality. In recall, patients demonstrate memory in the absence of specific cues whereas in recognition, cues are provided such as the beginning letters of a target word or the target word paired with distractors. The ability to recognize but not to recall information indicates that storage of material has occurred and that the use of cuing techniques may aid performance. However, when cuing does not facilitate memory functioning, this may suggest that the emphasis should be placed on ensuring that encoding takes place. Finally, the evaluation needs to encompass measures of immediate versus delayed memory since inclusion of the former condition alone may give a spuriously high estimate of performance.

The relevance of laboratory tasks such as recalling words or designs to performance in naturalistic situations raises a number of issues. First, to what extent do standardized tests capture components necessary to perform daily activities such as remembering acquaintances, telephone numbers, or appointments? Second, how can laboratory tests be better designed to offer more concrete suggestions for rehabilitation of memory in the environment? At present, our techniques are sensitive to grading of cerebral damage such as the severity of closed head injury, and they allow us to monitor recovery. However, the tasks often seem removed from the types of abilities needed for successful everyday functioning. In response to these criticisms, Wilson, Cockburn, and Baddeley developed the Rivermead Behavioral Memory Test (RBMT) in order to examine ecologically valid aspects of memory and to guide therapists in the identification of treatment needs (308). The RBMT assesses a number of areas relevant to everyday situations such as remembering a name, an appointment, faces, a route, and a hidden belonging. Wilson reports that performance of patients on the RBMT correlates with opinions of occupational therapists concerning patients' memory abilities (309). The sensitivity of the RBMT to better predict and to characterize memory problems beyond traditional laboratory tests remains to be examined.

In addition to the specific evaluation of memory functions, assessment needs to identify aspects that potentially contribute to memory problems. For example, depression may produce an "apparent" memory disturbance (e.g., the patient who performs poorly due to a lack of effort) or may prolong an underlying disturbance (e.g., the patient who is uninterested in applying techniques to improve impaired memory performance). Depression is a common affective feature in survivors of CHI and appears across the spectrum of severity. Fordyce et al. observed an intensification of emotional distress in patients tested six months or later after injury as compared to cases assessed earlier (310). Dikmen and Reitan reported a relationship between items on a personality inventory measuring somatic preoccupation, depression, and anxiety and the presence of cognitive deficits, suggesting the interrelationship of affective and cognitive dimensions (311). Evaluation of vegetative signs of depression (e.g., sleep and appetite disturbances) and reports of family members can be useful in the diagnosis of an affective component.

The amount of insight and awareness of a memory problem is also an important feature of evaluation. A failure to appreciate deficits may produce an impaired capacity for benefitting from treatment efforts (312). Studies have indicated that survivors rate their memory performance similar to controls without brain damage and that there are weaker correlations between patients' reports of their memory abilities and objective data as opposed to their relatives' ratings (313,314). Poor insight regarding memory functioning may reflect the inability to remember occurrences of forgetting (314), the denial of problems due to anxiety and avoidance, or an organically induced syndrome. Damage to the frontal lobes, for example, may produce alterations in behavior consisting of indifference and lack of initiative (315). Levin and colleagues found that disturbances encompassing self-appraisal (e.g., exaggerated self-opinion, overrating ability or underrating change as compared with relative and clinician opinions) and planning (poor formulation of future goals) were common in patients sustaining severe injuries (316). The relationship of frontal lobe lesions in the CHI population to deficits in awareness of sequelae remains to be examined. Assessment of the patient's appreciation of a memory problem can be compared to actual test performance and relatives' observations to determine the likelihood that techniques will be employed.

Finally, the neuropsychological evaluation needs to consider additional cognitive sequelae that may produce an "apparent" memory disturbance such as impaired language or perceptual abilities. For example, a patient may perform poorly on a test of reproductive memory for designs as a result of impaired visuomotor functions (e.g., drawing) or may recall few words on a verbal memory procedure due to aphasia. Clearly, assessment should be as broad-based as possible to adequately characterize the underlying reasons for the obtained pattern of performance.

REMEDIATION CONSIDERATIONS

It was previously noted that some CHI survivors are unaware or deny that they have memory problems and thus may be unwilling to actively participate in treatment. Another subset of patients may have misconceived notions concerning how memory operates and the benefits of mnemonic aids. For example, they may view memory as a "muscle" that needs to be exercised and the employment of techniques as weakening their recovery process. Moreover, certain patients may feel embarrassed to utilize aids that set them apart from individuals without brain damage. As a result of these issues that can thwart remediation attempts, several programs have emphasized the importance of incorporating awareness training and education into the direct treatment of memory disturbances (312,317).

There is evidence suggesting that amnesic patients are capable of learning and retaining skills that could potentially be adapted for job-related tasks. The work of Schacter and Glisky (318-320) on teaching domain-specific knowledge (i.e., knowledge relevant to a particular task) has demonstrated that memory-disordered patients, including those with head injuries, can acquire the vocabulary and techniques necessary to operate a computer. These investigators have employed the "method of vanishing cues" to help patients learn technical jargon. In this technique, a specific computer term (e.g, SAVE) is initially paired with a definition, and the number of target letters is gradually increased (e.g., S _ _ _; SA _ _; SAV _) until patients can identify the correct vocabulary term. On subsequent trials, fewer letters are provided until ultimately the definition itself elicits the correct term. Schacter and Glisky (318) compared this training technique with a rote rehearsal procedure that simply presented the terms and the definitions in a repeated fashion. Relative to a group that received rote rehearsal, patients in the vanishing cue condition demonstrated greater retention of the target terms after a six-week interval.

In a second phase of training, Schacter and Glisky examined the ability of patients to utilize their knowledge to interact with a computer, that is, to learn basic operating terms and to write simple programs. Training consisted of graded steps involving the acquisition of relevant vocabulary and implementation of these terms on the computer. Again, patients with severe memory deficits were able to effectively interact with the computer.

Schacter, Glisky, and McGlynn also designed a strategy to increase awareness of a memory deficit in a patient who developed amnesia following a ruptured anterior communicating artery aneurysm (317). The patient was asked to predict his recall performance for words and actions, was then presented with tasks measuring these abilities, and was subsequently given feedback concerning actual versus predicted performance. Feedback took place over numerous sessions. Compared with baseline findings, the patient now reported that he had memory difficulties and that these problems could interfere with his ability to return to work. However, the patient still overestimated his performance on extraexperimental memory tasks despite reminders that he had trouble on laboratory tests. As Schacter and colleagues noted, the generalization of awareness training to situations in the environment is an important part of rehabilitation. These preliminary results are encouraging in terms of the potential for restoring adaptive functioning in CHI patients.

Group sessions and diaries are used at the Transitional Learning Community in Galveston, Texas. Survivors of severe CHI meet daily to discuss the impact of their injuries on functioning, to dispel myths, for example, concerning whether memory is made weaker by mnemonic techniques, and to develop realistic expectations regarding recovery. Trainees are also required to keep a notebook in which they describe the activities performed in each therapy. This technique helps patients keep track of their schedules and reminds them of previous tasks. Finally, videotaping the patient's examples of forgetting (e.g., of names) can also be employed to increase awareness.

Apart from willingness to utilize mnemonic strategies, the ability and likelihood of survivors to employ these techniques must be considered. Internal/external mnemonics illustrate some of the factors that play a part in choosing techniques. Internal strategies encompass skills such as mental retracing (e.g., reconstructing one's actions in order to find lost keys), face-name association (visualizing hills growing out of a person's beard to remember the name of "Mr. Hills"), and story elaboration (forming an intricate scenario linking to-be-remembered words). External strategies, on the other hand, include environmental aids such as schedule books, diaries, and a watch-alarm that buzzes at set times to remind one of activities, e.g., to take medications (321).

One issue concerning the choice of an overall strategy involves whether these techniques are natural for patients to employ. In general, internal techniques suggested in the literature such as visual imagery, semantic elaboration, and ridiculous stories/bizarre images are not widely adopted by people without brain damage (322-328). In a survey of memory techniques used by college students, Harris reported that external aids such as calendars and notebooks were more often relied on than internal strategies (329). This finding suggests that internal strategies may not have been employed premorbidly by patients and thus will be more difficult to train and to achieve generalization. A second issue concerns the level of cognitive ability required by particular mnemonic aids. Crovitz et al. described the difficulty of their patients in acquiring the skills needed to remember words by forming bizarre interacting images (323). For example, one CHI patient with frontal lobe damage used concrete rather than bizarre images. Another consideration involves the load placed on memory in utilizing these aids. Techniques such as story elaboration (e.g., remembering *key, door,* and *kitchen* by forming the sentence "He put the *key* into the *door* and walked into the *kitchen.*") are often intricate and appear more difficult to remember than the three words. External strategies, in contrast, tend to take the burden away from memory since the patient is not asked to store or retrieve information. Finally, a particular remediation approach should normalize as much as possible the utilization of certain techniques. For example, the tendency of individuals without brain damage to employ aids such as schedule books may enhance their attractiveness and increase the likelihood of being used.

Currently, there is no compelling evidence that any one particular strategy significantly enhances the memory performance or adaptive functioning of survivors of CHI. This state of the art may reflect the numerous features that go into planning a remediation program (e.g., awareness, cognitive level of patients, potential resistance), thus making a simplified training approach difficult. Additionally, few techniques have attempted to capitalize on preserved capabilities of patients, that is, aspects of functioning that can be utilized during rehabilitation.

CONCLUSION

The field of memory remediation is in its infancy. As reviewed here, a great deal of work has been carried out on the pharmacological treatment of memory disorders, yet no single therapy has emerged as being uniformly successful.

This is not unexpected considering the various types of memory disorders outlined in earlier chapters.

The anatomical substrate of memory has been reasonably well delineated, and to a somewhat lesser extent, the pharmacological foundation of memory has also been described. Based on these principles, certain treatment strategies have been proposed largely involving manipulation of pharmacological systems. The cholinergic system has received the most attention, and while dramatic changes are not apparent from these studies, this still remains a viable approach for memory remediation. Most investigators feel that a manipulation of a single neurotransmitter system will not be adequate to treat memory disorders, and ultimately we may need a pharmacological "cocktail" to address these questions. Further, the "cocktail" may vary depending upon the nature of the memory deficit. Newer strategies involving nerve growth factor and neural grafting are intriguing, but definitive answers are not available.

Finally, behavioral tactics hold promise in some situations. Research is just beginning in this area, and it is too early to determine its efficacy. Complete remediation may not be likely, but partial improvement would make significant differences in many aspects of these patients' lives.

The field of memory research remains a fascinating enterprise and in many respects is central to work on all aspects of cognition. The solutions will not be simple, but any advances will be enthusiastically received.

REFERENCES

1. Crook, T. (1988). Pharmacotherapy of cognitive deficits in Alzheimer's disease and age-associated memory impairment. *Psychopharmacol. Bull. 24*:31-38.
2. Mohs, R.C., and Davis, K.L. (1987). The experimental pharmacology of Alzheimer's disease and related dementias. In *Psychopharmacology: The Third Generation of Progress.* Edited by H.Y. Meltzer. Raven Press, New York, pp. 921-928.
3. Whalley, L.J. (1989). Drug treatments of dementia. *Br. J. Psychiatry 155*:595-611.
4. Berrol, S. (1990). Issues in cognitive rehabilitation. *Arch. Neurol. 47*:219-220.
5. Volpe, B.T., and McDowell, F.H. (1990). The efficacy of cognitive rehabilitation in patients with traumatic brain injury. *Arch. Neurol. 47*:220-222.
6. Levin, H.S. (1990). Cognitive rehabilitation: Unproved but promising. *Arch. Neurol. 47*:223-224.
7. Hachinski, V. (1990). Cognitive rehabilitation. *Arch. Neurol. 47*:224.
8. Glisky, E.L., Schacter, D.L., and Tulving, E. (1986). Computer learning by memory-impaired patients: Acquisition and retention of complex knowledge. *Neuropsychologia 24*:313-328.
9. Glisky, E.L., Schacter, D.L., and Tulving, E. (1986). Learning and retention of computer-related vocabulary in memory-impaired patients: Method of vanishing cues. *J. Clin. Exp. Neuropsychol. 8*:292-312.

10. Perry, E.K. (1987). Cortical neurotransmitter chemistry in Alzheimer's disease. In *Psychopharmacology: The Third Generation of Progress*. Edited by H.Y. Meltzer. Raven Press, New York, pp. 887-896.

11. Bowen, D.M., and Davison, A.N. (1986). Biochemical studies of nerve cells and energy metabolism in Alzheimer's disease. *Br. Med. Bull.* 42:75-80.

12. Perry, E.K., Tomlinson, B.E., Blessed, G., Bergmann, K., Gibson, P.H., and Perry, R.H. (1978). Correlation of cholinergic abnormalities with senile plaques and mental test scores in senile dementia. *Br. Med. J.* 2:1457-1459.

13. Perry, E.K., Curtis, M., Dick, D.J., Candy, J.M., Atack, J.R., Bloxham, C.A., Blessed, G., Fairbarin, A., Tomlinson, B.E., and Perry, R.H. (1985). Cholinergic correlates of cognitive impairment in Parkinson's disease: Comparisons with Alzheimer's disease. *J. Neurol. Neurosurg. Psychiatry* 48:413-421.

14. Mesulam, M.M. (1986). The cholinergic connection in Alzheimer's disease. *NIPS 1*:107-109.

15. Mesulam, M.M., and Van Hoesen, G.W. (1976). Acetylcholinesterase-rich projections from the basal forebrain of the rhesus monkey to neocortex. *Brain Res.* 109:152-157.

16. Whitehouse, P.J., Price, D.L., Clark, A.W., Coyle, J.T., and DeLong, M.R. (1981). Alzheimer disease: Evidence for selective loss of cholinergic neurons in the nucleus basalis. *Ann. Neurol. 10*:122-126.

17. Drachman, D.A., and Leavitt, J. (1974). Human memory and the cholinergic system. A relationship to aging? *Arch. Neurol. 30*:113-121.

18. Drachman, D.A. (1977). Memory and cognitive function in man: Does the cholinergic system have a specific role? *Neurology 27*:783-790.

19. Petersen, R.C. (1977). Scopolamine induced learning failures in man. *Psychopharmacology 52*:283-289.

20. Petersen, R.C. (1979). Scopolamine state-dependent memory processes in man. *Psychopharmacology 64*:309-314.

21. Sunderland, T., Tariot, P.N., Mueller, E.A., Murphy, D.L., Weingartner, H., and Cohen, R.M. (1985). Cognitive and behavioral sensitivity to scopolamine in Alzheimer patients and controls. *Psychopharm. Bull. 21*:676-679.

22. Sunderland, T., Tariot, P.N., Cohen, R.M., Weingartner, H., Mueller, E.A. 3d, and Murphy. D.L. (1987). Anticholinergic sensitivity in patients with dementia of the Alzheimer type and age-matched controls. A dose-response study. *Arch. Gen. Psychiatry 44*:418-426.

23. Simon, J.R., and Kuhar, M.G. (1975). Impulse-flow regulation of high affinity choline uptake in brain cholinergic nerve terminals. *Nature 255*:162-163.

24. Brunello, N., Cheney, D.L., and Costa, E. (1982). Increase in exogenous choline fails to elevate the content or turnover rate of cortical, striatal, or hippocampal acetylcholine. *J. Neurochem. 38*:1160-1163.

25. Haubrich, D.R., Wang, P.F., Clody, D.E., and Wedeking, P.W. (1975). Increase in rat brain acetylcholine induced by choline or deanol. *Life Sci. 17*:975-980.

26. Bartus, R.T., Dean, R.L. 3d, Beer, B., and Lippa, A.S. (1982). The cholinergic hypothesis of geriatric memory dysfunction. *Science 217*:408-414.

27. Fovall, P., Dysken, M.W., Lazarus, L.W., Davis, J.M., Kahn, R.L., Jope, R., Finkel, S., and Rattan, P. (1980). Choline bitartrate treatment of Alzheimer-type dementias. *Comm. Psychopharmacol. 4*:141-145.

28. Mohs, R.C., Davis, K.L., Tinklenberg, J.R., and Hollister, L.E. (1980). Choline chloride effects on memory in the elderly. *Neurobiol. Aging 1*:21-25.
29. Mohs, R.C., Davis, K.L., Tinklenberg, J.R., Hollister, L.E., Yesavage, J.A., and Kopell, B.S. (1979). Choline chloride treatment of memory deficits in the elderly. *Am. J. Psychiatry 136*:1275-1277.
30. Thal, L.J., Rosen, W., Sharpless, N.S., and Crystal, H. (1981). Choline chloride fails to improve cognition in Alzheimer's disease. *Neurobiol. Aging 2*:205-208.
31. Mohs, R.C., Davis, K.L., and Levy, M.I. (1981). Partial reversal of anticholinergic amnesia by choline chloride. *Life Sci. 29*:1317-1323.
32. Mohs, R.C., and Davis, K.L. (1985). Interaction of choline and scopolamine in human memory. *Life Sci. 37*:193-197.
33. Levy, R., Little, A., Chuaqui, P., and Reith, M. (1983). Early results from double-blind, placebo controlled trial of high dose phosphatidylcholine in Alzheimer's disease. *Lancet 1*:987-988.
34. Caine, E.D. (1980). Cholinomimetic treatment fails to improve memory disorders. *N. Engl. J. Med. 303*:585-586.
35. Dysken, M.W., and Janowsky, D.S. (1985). Dose-related physostigmine-induced ventricular arrhythmia: Case report. J. Clin. Psychiatry 46:446-447.
36. Summers, W.K., Kaufman, K.R., Altman, F., Jr., and Fischer, J.M. (1980). THA—A review of the literature and its use in treatment of five overdose patients. *Clin. Toxicol. 16*:269-281.
37. Christie, J.E., Shering, A., Ferguson, J., and Glen, A.I. (1981). Physostigmine and arecoline: Effects of intravenous infusions in Alzheimer presenile dementia. *Br. J. Psychiatry 138*:46-50.
38. Blackwood, D.H., and Christie, J.E. (1986). The effects of physostigmine on memory and auditory P300 in Alzheimer-type dementia. *Biol. Psychiatry 21*:557-560.
39. Davis, K.L., Mohs, R.C., Tinklenberg, J.R., Pfefferbaum, A., Hollister, E., and Koppell, B.S. (1978). Physostigmine: Improvement of long-term memory processes in normal humans. *Science 201*:272-274.
40. Peters, B.H., and Levin, H.S. (1979). Effects of physostigmine and lecithin on memory in Alzheimer disease. *Ann. Neurol. 6*:219-221.
41. Beller, S.A., Overall, J.E., and Swann, A.C. (1985). Efficacy of oral physostigmine in primary degenerative dementia. A double-blind study of response to different dose level. *Psychopharmacology 87*:147-151.
42. Jenike, M.A., Albert, M.S., Heller, H., Gunther, J., and Goff, D. (1990). Oral physostigmine treatment for patients with presenile and senile dementia of the Alzheimer's type: A double-blind, placebo-controlled trial. *Clin. Psychiatry 51*:3-7.
43. Mohs, R.C., Davis, B.M., Johns, C.A., Mathe, A.A., Greenwald, B.S., Horvath, T.B., and Davis, K.L. (1985). Oral physostigmine treatment of patients with Alzheimer's disease. *Am. J. Psychiatry 142*:28-33.
44. Thal, L.J., Fuld, P.A., Masur, D.M., and Sharpless, N.S. (1983). Oral physostigmine and lecithin improve memory in Alzheimer disease. *Ann. Neurol. 13*:491-496.
45. Muramoto, O., Sugishita, M., and Ando, K. (1984). Cholinergic system and constructional praxis: A further study of physostigmine in Alzheimer's disease. *J. Neurol. Neurosurg. Psychiatry 47*:485-491.

46. Coyle, J.T., Price, D.L., and DeLong, M.R. (1983). Alzheimer's disease: A disorder of cortical cholinergic innervation. *Science 219*:1184-1190.

47. Wettstein, A. (1983). No effect from double-blind trial of physostigmine and lecithin in Alzheimer disease. *Ann. Neurol. 13*:210-212.

48. Jotkowitz, S. (1983). Physostigmine and Alzheimer's disease. Lack of clinical efficacy of chronic oral physostigmine in Alzheimer's disease. *Ann. Neurol. 14*:690-691.

49. Stern, Y., Sano, M., and Mayeux, R. (1987). Effects of oral physostigmine in Alzheimer's disease. *Ann. Neurol. 22*:306-310.

50. Jenike, M.A., Albert,M.S., Heller, H., Gunther, J., and Goff, D. (1990). Oral physostigmine treatment for patients with presenile and senile dementia of the Alzheimer's type: A double-blind placebo-controlled trial. *J. Clin. Psychiatry 51*:3-7.

51. Beller, S.A., Overall, J.E., Rhoades, H.M., and Swann, A.C. (1988). Long-term outpatient treatment of senile dementia with oral physostigmine. *J. Clin. Psychiatry 49*:400-404.

52. Stern, Y., Sano, M., and Mayeux, R. (1988). Long-term administration of oral physostigmine in Alzheimer's disease. *Neurology 38*:1837-1841.

53. Thal, L.J., Masur, D.M., Blau, A.D., Fuld, P.A., and Klauber, M.R. (1989). Chronic oral physostigmine without lecithin improves memory in Alzheimer's disease. *Geriatr. Soc. 37*:42-48.

54. Harrell, L.E., Jope, R.S., Falgout, J., Callaway, R., Avery, C., Spiers, M., Leli, D., Morere, D., and Halsey, J.H. (1990). Biological and neuropsychological characterization of physostigmine responders and nonresponders in Alzheimer's disease. *Geriatr. Soc. 38*:113-122.

55. Summers, W.K., Majovski, L.V., Marsh, G.M., Tachiki, K., and Kling, A. (1986). Oral tetrahydroaminoacridine in long-term treatment of senile dementia, Alzheimer type. *N. Engl. J. Med. 315*:1241-1245.

56. Davis, K.L., and Mohs, R. C. (1986). Cholinergic drugs in Alzheimer's disease. *N. Engl. J. Med. 315*:1286-1287.

57. Summers, W.K., Viesselman, J.O., Marsh, G.M., and Candelora, K. (1981). Use of THA in treatment of Alzheimer-like dementia: Pilot study in twelve patients. *Biol. Psychiatry 16*:145-153.

58. Pirozzolo, F.J., Baskin, D.S., Swihart, A.A., and Appel, S.H. (1987). Oral tetrahydroaminoacridine in the treatment of senile dementia, Alzheimer's type. *N. Engl. J. Med. 316*:1603-1605.

59. Richter, R.W., Murphy, M.F., Allen, R., Nash, R.J., Dobsen, C., Demkovich, J.J., and Hardiman, S. (1990). Clinical pharmacology study of HP029 (1,2,3,4-tetrahydro-9-aminoacridin-1-OL maleate) in Alzheimer's disease. *Neurology 40*:229.

60. Sitaram, N., Weingartner, H., and Gillin, J.C. (1978). Human serial learning: Enhancement with arecholine and choline impairment with scopolamine. *Science 201*:274-276.

61. Davis, K.L., Hollander, E., Davidson, M., Davis, B.M., Mohs, R.C., and Horvath, T.B. (1987). Induction of depression with oxotremorine in patients with Alzheimer's disease. *Am. J. Psychiatry 144*:468-471.

62. Wettstein, A., and Spiegel, R. (1984). Clinical trials with the cholinergic drug RS-86 in Alzheimer's disease (AD) and senile dementia of the Alzheimer type (SDAT). *Psychopharmacology 84*:572-573.

63. Bruno, G., Mohr, E., Gillespie, M., Fedio, P., and Chase, T.N. (1986). Muscarinic agonist therapy of Alzheimer's disease. A clinical trial of RS-86. *Arch. Neurol. 43*:659-661.

64. Harbaugh, R.E., Roberts, D.W., Coombs, D.W., Saunders, R.L., and Reeder, T.M. (1984). Preliminary report: Intracranial cholinergic drug infusion in patients with Alzheimer's disease. *Neurosurgery 15*:514-518.

65. Harbaugh, R.E., Reeder, T.M., Senter, H.J., Knopman, D.S., et al. (1989). Intracerebroventricular bethanechol chloride infusion in Alzheimer's disease. Results of a collaborative double-blind study. *J. Neurosurg. 71*:481-486.

66. Bond, N.W., Walton, J., and Pruss, J. (1989). Restoration of memory following septo-hippocampal grafts: A possible treatment for Alzheimer's disease. *Biol. Psychol. 28*:67-87.

67. Madrazo, I., Drucker-Colin, R., Diaz, V., Martinez-Mata, J., Torres, C., and Becerril, J.J. (1987). Open microsurgical autograft of adrenal medulla to the right caudate nucleus in two patients with intractable Parkinson's disease. *N. Engl. J. Med. 316*:831-834.

68. Ahlskog, J.E., Kelly, P.J., vanHeerden, J.A., Stoddard, S.L., Tyce, G.M., Windebank, A.J., Bailey, P.A., Bell, G.N., Blexrud, M.D., and Carmichael, S.W. (1990). Adrenal medullary transplantation into the brain for treatment of Parkinson's disease: Clinical outcome and neurochemical studies. *Mayo Clin. Proc. 65*:305-328.

69. Gage, F.H., and Bjorklund, A. (1987). Trophic and growth-regulating mechanisms in the central nervous system monitored by intracerebral neural transplants. *CIBA Found. Symp. 126*:143-159.

70. Kesslak, J.P., Nieto-Sampedro, M., Globus, J., and Cotman, C.W. (1986). Transplants of purified astrocytes promote behavioral recovery after frontal cortex ablation. *Exp. Neurol. 92*:377-390.

71. Gash, D.M., Collier, R.J., and Sladek, J.R. (1985). Neural transplantation: A review of recent developments and potential applications to the aged brain. *Neurobiol. Aging 6*:131-150.

72. Mash, D.C., Flynn, D.D., and Potter, L.T. (1985). Loss of M2 muscarine receptors in the cerebral cortex in Alzheimer's disease and experimental cholinergic denervation. *Science 228*:1115-1117.

73. Goyal, R.K. (1989). Muscarinic receptor subtypes: Physiology and clinical implications. *N. Engl. J. Med. 321*:1022-1029.

74. Zornetzer, S.F. (1986). The noradrenergic locus coeruleus and senescent memory dysfunction. In *Treatment Development Strategies for Alzheimer's Disease*. Edited by T. Crook, R.T. Bartus, S. Ferris, S. Gershon. Mark Powley Associates, Inc., Madison, CT, pp. 337-360.

75. Algeri, S., Bonati, M., Brunello, N., and Ponzio, F. (1978). Biochemical changes in central catecholaminergic neurons in the senescent rat. In *Neuro-Psychopharmacology. Proceedings of the 10th Congress of the Collegium International Neuro-Psychopharmacologicum, Quebec, July 4-9, 1976: Vol. II. Workshop 6.*

Models in geriatric neuro-psychopharmacology. Edited by P. Deniker, C. Radouco-Thomas, A. Villeneuve, D. Baronet-LaCroix, F. Garcin. Pergamon Press, Oxford.

76. Finch, C.E. (1973). Catecholamine metabolism in the brains of ageing male mice. *Brain Res. 52*:261-276.

77. Finch, C.E. (1976). The regulation of physiological changes during mammalian aging. *Rev. Biol. 51*:49-83.

78. Adolfsson, R., Gottfries, C.G., Roos, B.E., and Winbald, B. (1979). Post mortem distribution of dopamine and homovanillic acid in human brain, variations related to age and a review of the literature. *J. Neural Trans. 45*:81-105.

79. Carlsson, A., and Winblad, B. (1976). Influence of age and time interval between death and autopsy on dopamine and 3-methoxytyramine levels in human basal ganglia. *J. Neural Trans. 38*:271-276.

80. Mason, S.T. (1981). Noradrenaline in the brain: Progress in theories of behavioral function. *Prog. Neurobiol. 16*:263-303.

81. Zornetzer, S.F., Abraham, W.C., and Appleton, R. (1978). Locus coeruleus and labile memory. *Pharm. Biochem. Behav. 9*:227-234.

82. Fallon, J.H., Koziell, D.A., and Moore, R.Y. (1978). Catecholamine innervation of the basal forebrain: II. Amygdala, suprarhinal cortex and entorhinal cortex. *J. Comp. Neurol. 180*:509-532.

83. Fallon, J.H., and Moore, R.Y. (1978). Catecholamine innervation of the basal forebrain: III. Olfactory bulb, anterior olfactory nuclei, olfactory tubercle and piriform cortex. *J. Comp. Neurol. 180*:533-544.

84. Morrison, J.H., Grzanna, R., Molliver, M.E., and Coyle, J.T. (1978). The distribution and orientation of noradrenergic fibers in neocortex of the rat: An immunofluorescence study. *J. Comp. Neurol. 181*:17-40.

85. Jacobowitz, D.M., and Palkovitse, M. (1974). Topographic atlas of catecholamine and acetylcholinesterase-containing neurons in the rat brain: I. Forebrain (telencephalon, diencephalon). *J. Comp. Neurol. 157*:13-28.

86. Zornetzer, S.F., and Gold, M.S. (1976). The locus coeruleus: Its possible role in memory consolidation. *Physiol. Behav. 16*:331-336.

87. Stein, L., Belluzzi, J.D., and Wise, C.D. (1975). Memory enhancement by central administration of norepinephine. *Brain Res. 84*:329-335.

88. McEntee, W.J., and Mair, R.G. (1980). Memory enhancement in Korsakoff's psychosis by clonidine: Further evidence for a noradrenergic deficit. *Ann. Neurol. 7*:466-470.

89. McEntee, W.J., Mair, R.G., and Langlais, P.J. (1984). Neurochemical pathology in Korsakoff's psychosis: Implications for other cognitive disorders. *Neurology 34*:648-652.

90. Mair, R.G., McEntee, W.J., and Zatorre, R.J. (1985). Monoamine activity correlates with psychometric deficits in Korsakoff's disease. *Behav. Brain Res. 15*:247-254.

91. Bondareff, W., Mountjoy, C.Q., and Roth, M. (1982). Loss of neurons of origin of the adrenergic projection to cerebral cortex (nucleus locus coeruleus) in senile dementia. *Neurology 32*:164-168.

92. McEntee, W.J., and Crook, T.H. (1990). Age-associated memory impairment: A Role for catecholamines. *Neurology 40*:526-530.

93. Finch, C.E. (1978). Age-related changes in brain catecholamines: A synopsis of findings in C57BL/6J mice and other rodent models. *Adv. Exp. Med. Biol.* *113*:15-39.
94. Goldman-Rakic, P.S., and Brown, R.M. (1981). Regional changes of monoamines in cerebral cortex and subcortical structures of aging rhesus monkeys. *Neuroscience 6*:177-187.
95. Winblad, B., Hardy, J., Backman, L., and Nilsson, L.G. (1985). Memory function and brain biochemistry in normal aging and in senile dementia. *Ann. N.Y. Acad. Sci. 444*:255-268.
96. Reis, D.J., Ross, R.A., and Joh, T.H. (1977). Changes in the activity and amounts of enzymes synthesizing catecholamines and acetylcholine in brain, adrenal medulla, and sympathetic ganglia of aged rat and mouse. *Brain Res. 136*:465-474.
97. Arnsten, A.F., and Goldman-Rakic, P.S. (1985). Alpha 2-adrenergic mechanisms in prefrontal cortex associated with cognitive decline in aged nonhuman primates. *Science 230*:1273-1276.
98. Brozoski, T.J., Brown, R.M., Rosvold, H.E., and Goldman, P.S. (1979). Cognitive deficit caused by regional depletion of dopamine in prefrontal cortex of rhesus monkey. *Science 205*:929-932.
99. Mohr, E., Schlegel, J., Fabbrini, G., Williams, J., Mouradian, M.M., Mann, U.M., Claus, J.J., Fedio, P., and Chase, T.N. (1989). Clonidine treatment of Alzheimer's disease. *Arch. Neurol. 46*:376-378.
100. Brodie, D.A., LeWitt, P., Berchou, V., Berchou, R., Bagne, C., Siegel, B., and Near, E. (1989). Cognitive effects from long-term clonidine therapy in Alzheimer's disease and in normal elders. *Neurology 39*:254.
101. Frith, C.D., Dowdy, J., Ferrier, I.N., and Crow, T.J. (1985). Selective impairment of paired associate learning after administration of a centrally-acting adrenergic agonist (clonidine). *Psychopharmacology 87*:490-493.
102. Mair, R.G., and McEntee, W.J. (1986). Cognitive enhancement in Korsakoff's psychosis by clonidine: A comparison with L-Dopa and ephedrine. *Psychopharmacology 88*:374-380.
103. Langlais, P.J., Mair, R.G., Whalen, P.J., McCourt, W., and McEntee, W.J. (1988). Memory effect of DL-threo-3,4-dihydroxyphenylserine (DOPS) in human Korsakoff's disease. *Psychopharmacology 95*:250-254.
104. Azmitia, E.C. (1978). Chemical pathways in the brain. In *Handbook of Psychopharmacology.* Edited by L. Iverson, S.D. Iverson, S.H. Snyder. Plenum Press, New York.
105. Arai, H., Kosaka, K., and Iizuka, R. (1984). Changes of biogenic amines and their metabolites in postmortem brains from patients with Alzheimer-type dementia. *J. Neurochem. 43*:388-393.
106. Carlsson, A., Adolfsson, R., Aquilonius, S.M., Gottfries, C.G., Oreland, L., Svennerholm, L., and Winblad, B. (1980). Biogenic amines in human brain in normal aging, senile dementia, and chronic alcoholism. *Adv. Biochem. Psycho. Pharmacol. 23*:295-304.
107. Sparks, D.L., Markesbery, W.R., and Slevin, J.T. (1986). Alzheimer's disease: Monoamines and spiperone binding reduced in nucleus basalis. *Ann. Neurol. 19*:602-604.

108. Sparks, D.L., and Slevin, J.T. (1985). Determination of tyrosine, tryptophan and their metabolic derivatives by liquid chromatography-electrochemical detection: Application to post mortem samples from patients with Parkinson's and Alzheimer's diseases. *Life Sci. 36*:449-457.

109. Mann, D.M.A., and Yates, P.O. (1983). Serotonin nerve cells in Alzheimer's disease. *J. Neurol. Neurosurg. Psychiatry 46*:96.

110. Yamamoto, T., and Hirano, A. (1985). Nucleus raphe dorsalis in Alzheimer's disease: Neurofibrillary tangles and loss of large neurons. *Ann. Neurol. 17*:573-577.

111. Sparks, D.L. (1989). Aging and Alzheimer's disease. Altered cortical serotonergic binding. *Arch. Neurol. 46*:138-140.

112. Cutler, N.R., Haxby, J., Kay, A.D., Narang, P.K., et al. (1985). Evaluation of zimeldine in Alzheimer's disease. Cognitive and biochemical measures. *Arch. Neurol. 42*:744-748.

113. de Wied, D. (1965). The influence of the posterior and intermediate lobe of the pituitary and pituitary peptides on the maintenance of a conditioned avoidance response in rats. *J. Neuropharmacol. 4*:157.

114. de Wied, D. (1971). Long term effect of vasopressin on the maintenance of a conditioned avoidance response in rats. *Nature 232*:58-60.

115. de Wied, D., and Bohus, B. (1966). Long term and short term effects on retention of a conditioned avoidance response in rats by treatment with long acting pitressin and a-MSH. *Nature 212*:1484-1486.

116. Lande, S., Flexner, J.B., and Flexner, L.B. (1972). Effect of corticotropin and desglycinamide 9-lysine vasopressin on suppression of memory by puromycin. *Proc. Natl. Acad. Sci. (USA) 69*:558-560.

117. Walter, R., Hoffman, P.L., Flexner, J.B., and Flexner, L.B. (1975). Neurohypophyseal hormones, analogs and fragments: Their effect on puromycin-induced amnesia. *Proc. Natl. Acad. Sci. (USA) 72*:4180-4184.

118. Rigter, H., van Riezen, H., and de Wied, D. (1974). The effects of ACTH- and vasopressin-analogues on CO_2-induced retrograde amnesia in rats. *Physiol. Behav. 13*:381.

119. Brito, G.N., Thomas, G.J., Gingold, S.I., and Gash, D.M. (1981).Behavioral characteristics of vasopressin-deficient rats (Brattleboro strain). *Brain Res. Bull. 6*:71-75.

120. Bohus, B., van Wimersma Greidanus, T.J.B., and de Wied, D. (1975). Behavioral and endocrine responses of rats with hereditary hypothalamic diabetes insipidus (Brattleboro strain). *Physiol. Behav. 14*:609-615.

121. de Wied, D., Bohus, B., and van Wimersma Greidanus, T.J.B. (1975). Memory deficit in rats with hereditary diabetes insipidus. *Brain Res. 85*:152-156.

122. de Wied, D., and Versteeg, D.H. (1979). Neurohypophyseal principles and memory. *Fed. Proc. 38*:2348-2354.

123. van Wimersma Greidanus, T.J.B., Bohus, B., and de Wied, D. (1975). CNS sites of action of ACTH, MSH, and vasopressin in relation to avoidance behavior. *Anatomical Neuroendocrinology*. Edited by W.S. Stumpf and L.D. Grant. Basel, Karger, pp. 284-290.

124. Kovacs, G.L., Bohus, B., and Versteeg, D.H.G. (1979). Facilitation of memory consolidation by vasopressin: Mediation by terminals of the dorsal noradrenergic bundle. *Brain Res. 172*:73-85.

125. Castro de Souza, E.M., Rocha, E., and Silva, M. Jr. (1977). The release of vasopressin by nicotine: Further studies on its site of action. *J. Physiol. 265*: 297-311.

126. Ramaekers, F., Rigter, H., and Leonard, B.E. (1977). Parallel changes in behavior and hippocampal serotonin metabolism in rats following treatment with desglycinamide lysine vasopressin. *Brain Res. 120*:485-492.

127. Tanaka, M., de Kloet, E.R., de Wied, D., and Versteeg, D.H.G. (1977). Arginine vasopressin affects catecholamine metabolism in specific brain nuclei. *Life Sci. 20*:1799-1808.

128. Versteeg, D.H.G., Tanaka, M., and de Kloet, E.R. (1978). Catecholamine concentration and turnover in discrete regions of the brain of the homozygous Brattleboro rat deficient in vasopressin. *Endocrinology 103*:1654-1661.

129. Kovacs, G.L., Bohus, B., Versteeg, D.H.G., de Kloet, E.R., and de Wied, D. (1979). Effect of oxytocin and vasopressin on memory consolidation: Sites of action and catecholaminergic correlates after local microinjection into limbic midbrain structures. *Brain Res. 175*:303-314.

130. Legros, J.J., Gilot, P., Seron, X., Claessens, J., Adam, A., Moeglen, J.M., Audibert, A., and Berchier, P. (1978). Influence of vasopressin on learning and memory. *Lancet 1*:41-42.

131. Legros, J.J., Gilot, P., Schmitz, S., Bruwier, M., et al. (1980). Neurohypophyseal peptides and cognitive function: A clinical approach. In *Progress in Psychoneuroendocrinology*. Edited by F. Brambilla, G. Racagni, D. de Wied. Elsevier-North Holland, Biomedical Press, pp. 325-338.

132. Gold, P.W., and Goodwin, F.K. (1978). Vasopressin in affective illness. *Lancet 1*:1233-1236.

133. Weingartner, H.P., Gold, P.W., Ballenger, J.C., Smallberg, S.A., Summers, R., Rubinow, D.R., Post, R.M., and Goodwin, F.K. (1981). Effects of vasopressin on human memory functions. *Science 211*:601-603.

134. Oliveros, J.C., Jandali, M.K., Timsit-Berthier, M., Remy, R., Benghezal, A., Audibert, A., and Moeglen, J.M. (1978). Vasopressin in amnesia. *Lancet 1*: 42.

135. LeBoeuf, A., Lodge, J., and Eames, P.G. (1978). Vasopressin and memory in Korsakoff syndrome. *Lancet 2*:1370.

136. Blake, D.R., Dodd, M.J., and Evans, J.G. (1978). Vasopressin in amnesia. *Lancet 1*:608.

137. Jenkins, J.S., Mather, H.M., Coughlan, A.K., and Jenkins, D.G. (1979). Desmopressin in post-traumatic amnesia. *Lancet 2*:1245-1246.

138. Weingartner, H., Kaye, W., Gold, P., Smallberg, S., Petersen, R., Gillin, J.C., and Ebert, M. (1981). Vasopressin treatment of cognitive dysfunction in progressive dementia. *Life Sci. 29*:2721-2726.

139. Chase, T.N., Durso, R., Fedio, P., and Tamminga, C.A. (1982). Vasopressin treatment of cognitive deficits in Alzheimer's disease. In *Alzheimer's Disease: A report of progress in research*. Edited by S. Corkin, K.L. Davis, J.H. Growden, E. Usdin, R.J. Wurtman. Raven Press, New York, pp. 457-462.

140. Ferris, S.H., Reisberg, B., Brook, T., Friedman, E., Schneck, M.K., Mir, P., Sherman, K.A., Corwin, J., Gershon, S., and Bartus, R.T. (1981). Treating dementia with neuropeptides and piracetam. In *Alzheimer's Disease: A Report*

of Progress in Research. Edited by S. Corkin, K.L. Davis, J.H. Growden, E. Usdin, R.J. Wurtman. Raven Press, New York, pp. 475-482.

141. Peabody, C.A., Thiemann, S., Pigache, R., Miller, T.P., Berger, P.A., Yesavage, J., and Tinklenberg, J.R. (1985). Desglycinamide-9-arginine-8-vasopressin (DGAVP, Oragnon 5667) in patients with dementia. *Neurobiol. Aging 6*: 95-100.

142. Tinklenberg, J.R., Peabody, C.A., and Berger, P.A. (1981). Vasopressin effects of cognitive and affect in the elderly. In *Neuropeptide and Hormone Modulation of Brain Function and Homeostasis.* Edited by J.M. Ordy, J.R. Sladek, B. Reisberg. Raven Press, New York.

143. Gash, D.M., and Thomas, G.J. (1983). What is the importance of vasopressin in memory processes. *Trends Neurosci. 6*:197-198.

144. Beckwith, B.E., Couk, D.I., and Till, T.S. (1983). Vasopressin analog influences the performance of males on a reaction time tasks. *Peptides 4*:707-709.

145. Sahgal, A., Wright, C., and Ferrier, I.N. (1986). Desamino-D-arg8-vasopressin (DDAVP), unlike ethanol, has no effect on a boring visual vigilance task in humans. *Psychopharmacology 90*:58-63.

146. Sahgal, A. (1984). A critique of the vasopressin-memory hypothesis. *Psychopharmacology 83*:215-228.

147. Le Moal, M., Dantzer, R., Mormede, P., Baduel, A., et al. (1984). Behavioral effects of peripheral administration of arginine vasopressin: A review of our search for a mode of action and a hypothesis. *Psychoneuroendocrinology 9*:319-341.

148. Quarton, G.C., Clark, L.K., Cobb, S., et al. (1955). Mental disturbance associated with ACTH and cortisone: A review of explanatory hypotheses. *Medicine 34*:13-50.

149. de Wied, D. (1969). Effects of peptide hormones on behavior. *Frontiers Neuroendocrinol.* 97-140.

150. Pigache, R.M. (1983). The human psychopharmacology of peptides related to ACTH and alpha MSH. In *Clinical Pharmacology in Psychiatry.* Edited by L. Gram et al. Macmillan, London.

151. Kragh-Sorensen, P., Olsen, R.B., Lund, S., et al. (1986). Neuropeptides: ACTH-peptides in dementia. *Prog. Neuropharm. Biol. Psychiatry 10*:479-492.

152. Branconnier, R., Cole, J., and Gardos, G. (1979). ACTH 4-10 in the amelioration of neuropsychological symptomatology associated with senile organic brain syndrome. *Psychopharmacology 61*:161-165.

153. Ferris, S.H., Sathananthan, G., Gershon, S., et al. (1976). Cognitive effects of ACTH 4-10 in the elderly. *Pharmacol. Biochem. Behav. 5*:73-78.

154. Soininen, H., Koskinen, T., Helkola, E., et al. (1985). Treatment of Alzheimer's disease with a synthetic ACTH 4-9 analog. *Neurology 35*:1348-1351.

155. Dolezal, V., and Tucek, S. (1981). Utilization of citrate, acetylcarnitine, acetate, pyruvate, and glucose for the synthesis of acetylcholine in rat brain slices. *Neurochemistry 36*:1323-1330.

156. Angelucci, L., and Ramacci, M. (1986). Neuropharmacological potentials in the senescent rat. In *Developments in Psychiatry*, Vol. 7. Edited by C. Chagass, R. Josiassen, W. Bridger, K. Weiss, D. Stoff, G. Simpson. Elsevier, Amsterdam.

157. Angelucci, L., Ramacci, M., Taglialatela, G., et al. (1988). Nerve growth factor binding in aged rat central nervous system: Effect of acetyl-l-carnitine. *J. Neurosci. Res. 20*:491-496.

158. Fariello, R., Ferraro, T., Golden, G., and DeMattei, M. (1988). Systemic acetyl-l-carnitine elevates nigral levels of glutathione and GABA. *Life Sci. 43*:289-292.

159. Pierelli, F., Pozzessere, G., Rizzo, P.A., Calvani, M., and Lazzari, R. (1981). Uso della L-acetil-carnitina nella malattia di Alzheimer: Studio clinico ed electrofisiologico. *Rivista Italiana EEG Neurofisiologica Clin 1*:45-46.

160. Bergamasco, B., Tarenzi, L., Leotta, D., Scarzella, L., Iannuccelli, M., and Bianco, C. (1985). Activity of acetyl-l-carnitine in primary degenerative dementia. IVth World Congress of Biological Psychiatry, Philadelphia, September 8-13.

161. Loeb, C., Iannucceli, M., Traverso, F., and Albano, C. (1985). Evaluation of the activity of acetyl-l-carnitine in the senile dementia Alzheimer type. IVth World Congress of Biological Psychiatry, Philadelphia, September 8-13.

162. Testa, G., Giaretta, D., Pellegrini, A., Chemello, R., Freddo, L., and Angelini, C. (1982). A preliminary trial with acetylcarnitine in dementia. *Riv. Neurol. 52*:185-197.

163. Agnoli, A., Manna, V., Martucci, N., and Cassabgi, F. (1985). Effects of acetyl-l-carnitine after acute administration on brain bioelectrical activity mapping in different aged healthy volunteers. IVth World Congress of Biological Psychiatry, Philadelphia, September 8-13.

164. Bergonzi, P., Diodata, S., Ferri, R., Gigli, G.L., Mazza, S., Mennuni, G., and Pola, P. (1982). The effect of L-acetyl carnitine on mental deterioration in the elderly: Neuropsychological assessment and computerized EEG analysis. Symposium "The Aging of the Brain," Mantova, March 26-29.

165. Hiersemenzel, R., Dietrich, B., and Herrmann, W.M. (1988). Therapeutic and EEG-effects of acetyl-l-carnitine in elderly outpatients with mild to moderate cognitive decline. Results of two double-blind placebo-controlled studies. In *Senile Dementia*. Edited by A. Agnoli, J. Cahn, N. Lassen, R. Mayeux. John Libbey Eurotext, Paris, pp. 427-432.

166. Bonavita, E. (1986). Study of the efficacy and tolerability of L-acetylcarnitine therapy in the senile brain. *Int. J. Clin. Pharmacol. Ther. Toxicol. 24*:511-516.

167. Mantero, M., Grosso, V., Barbero, M., Giannini, R., Tommasina, C., and Iannuccelli, M. (1986). A double blind study of acetyl-l-carnitine vs placebo in patients with pathological brain aging. Congress on "Hypothalamic Dysfunction in Neuropsychiatric Disorders." Rome, Italy, April 9-12.

168. Bassi, S., Ferrarese, C., Finoia, M.G., Frattola, L., Iannuccelli, M., Meregalli, S., and Piolti, R. (1988). L-acetyl-carnitine in Alzheimer disease (AD) and senile dementia Alzheimer type (SDAT). In *Senile Dementia*. Edited by A. Agnoli, J. Cahn, N. Lassen, R. Mayeux. John Libbey Eurotext, Paris, pp. 461-466.

169. Mantero, M.A., Barbero, M., Giannini, R., Grosso, V.G., Tomasina, C., and Iannuccelli, M. (1989). Acetyl-l-carnitine as a therapeutic agent for mental

deterioration in geriatric patients (double-blind controlled versus placebo study). *Clin. New Trends Clin. Neuropharmacol. 3*:17-24.

170. Brownstein, M., Arimura, A., Sato, H., Schally, A.V., and Kizer, J.S. (1975). The regional distribution of somatostatin in the rat brain. *Endocrinology 96*: 1456-1461.

171. Kobayashi, R.M., Brown, M., and Vale, W. (1977). Regional distribution of neurotensin and somatostatin in rat brain. *Brain Res. 126*:584-588.

172. Petrusz, P., Sar, M., Grossman, G.H., and Kizer, J.S. (1977). Synaptic terminals with somatostatin-like immunoreactivity in the rat brain. *Brain Res. 137*:181-187.

173. Wood, P.L., Etienne, P., Lal, S., Gauthier, S., Cajal, S., and Nair, N.P.V. (1982). Reduced lumbar CSF somatostatin levels in Alzheimer's disease. *Life Sci. 31*:2073-2079.

174. Francis, P.T., Bowen, D.M., Neary, D., Palo, J., Wikstrom, J., and Olney, J. (1984). Somatostatin-like immunoreactivity in lumbar cerebrospinal fluid from neurohistologically examined demented patients. *Neurobiol. Aging 5*: 183-186.

175. Serby, M., Richardson, S.B., Twente, S., Siekierski, J., Corwin, J., and Rotrosen, J. (1984). CSF somatostatin in Alzheimer's disease. *Neurobiol. Aging 5*:187-189.

176. Beal, M.F., Growdon, J.H., Mazurek, M.F., and Martin, J.B. (1986). CSF somatostatin-like immunoreactivity in dementia. *Neurology 36*:294-297.

177. Raskind, M.A., Peskind, E.R., Lampe, T.H., Risse, S.C., Taborsky, G.J. Jr., and Dorsa, D. (1986). Cerebrospinal fluid vasopressin, oxytocin, somatostatin, and beta-endorphin in Alzheimer's disease. *Arch. Gen. Psychiatry 43*:382-388.

178. Rossor, M.N., Emson, P.C., Mountjoy, C.Q., Roth, M., and Iversen, L.L. (1980). Reduced amounts of immunoreactive somatostatin in the temporal cortex in senile dementia of the Alzheimer type. *Neurosci. Lett. 20*:373-377.

179. Davies, P., Katzman, R., and Terry, R.D. (1980). Reduced somatostatin-like immunoreactivity in cerebral cortex from cases of Alzheimer disease and Alzheimer senile dementia. *Nature 288*:279-280.

180. Quirion, R., Martel, J.C., Robitaille, Y., Etienne, P., Wood, P., Nair, N.P., and Gauthier, S. (1986). Neurotransmitter and receptor deficits in senile dementia of the Alzheimer type. *Can. J. Neurol. Sci. 13*:503-510.

181. Gauthier, S., Leblanc, R., Robitaille, Y., Quirion, R., et al. (1986). Transmitter replacement therapy in Alzheimer's disease using intracerebroventricular infusions of receptor agonists. *Can. J. Neurol. Sci. 13*:394-402.

182. Beal, M.F., Mazurek, M.F., Svendsen, C.N., Bird, E.D., and Martin, J.B. (1986). Widespread reduction of somatostatin-like immunoreactivity in the cerebral cortex in Alzheimer's disease. *Ann. Neurol. 20*:489-495.

183. Atack, J.R., Beal, M.F., May, C., Kaye, J.A., Mazurek, M.F., Kay, A.D., and Rapoport, S.I. (1988). Cerebrospinal fluid somatostatin and neuropeptide Y. Concentrations in aging and in dementia of the Alzheimer type with and without extrapyramidal signs. *Arch. Neurol. 45*:269-274.

184. Cutler, N.R., Haxby, J.V., May, C., Burg, C., Narag, P.K., and Reines, S.A. (1985). L-363,586, a somatostatin analog: An assessment of memory function in Alzheimer's disease. *Neurology 35*:265.

185. Leblanc, R., Gauthier, S., Gauvin, M., Quirion, R., Palmour, R., and Masson, H. (1988). Neurobehavioral effects of intrathecal somatostatinergic treatment in subhuman primates. *Neurology 38*:1887-1890.

186. Giurgea, C. (1976). Piracetam: Nootropic pharmacology of neurointegrative activity. *Curr. Dev. Psychopharmacol. 3*:221-273.

187. Nicholson, C.D. (1989). Nootropics and metabolically active compounds in Alzheimer's disease. *Biochem. Soc. Trans. 17*:83-85.

188. Bartus, R.T., Dean, R.L., 3d, Sherman, K.A., Friedman, E., and Beer, B. (1981). Profound effects of combining choline and piracetam on memory enhancement and cholinergic function in aged rats. *Neurobiol. Aging 2*:105-111.

189. Wurtman, R.J., Magil, S.G., and Reinstein, D.K. (1981). Priacetam diminishes hippocampal acetylcholine levels in rats. *Life Sci. 28*:1091-1093.

190. Giurgea, C.E. (1981). *Fundamentals to a Pharmacology of the Mind*. Charles C Thomas, Springfield, IL.

191. Sara, S.J., and David-Remacle, M. (1974). Recovery from electroconvulsive shock-induced amnesia by exposure to the training environment: Pharmacological enhancement by piracetam. *Psychopharmacologia 36*:59-66.

192. Sara, S.J., and Lefevre, D. (1972). Hypoxia-induced amnesia in one-trail learning and pharmacological protection by piracetam. *Psychopharmacologia 25*: 32-40.

193. Giurgea, C., and Mouravieff-Lesuisse, F. (1972). Multi-trial learning facilitation in the rat by piracetam. *J. Pharmacol. 3*:17-30.

194. Wilsher, C.R., Bennett, D., Chase, C.H., Conners, C.K., et al. (1987). Piracetam and dyslexia: Effects on reading tests. *J. Clin. Psychopharmacol. 7*: 230-237.

195. Helfgott, E., Rudel, R.G., and Kairam, R. (1986). The effect of piracetam on short- and long-term verbal retrieval in dyslexic boys. *Int. J. Psychophysiol. 4*:53-61.

196. Tallal, P., Chase, C., Russell, G., and Schmitt, R.L. (1986). Evaluation of the efficacy of piracetam in treating information processing, reading and writing disorders in dyslexic children. *Int. J. Psychophysiol. 4*:41-52.

197. DiIanni, M., Wilsher, C.R., Blank, M.S., Conners, C.K., Chase, C.H., et al. (1985). The effects of piracetam in children with dyslexia. *J. Clin. Psychopharmacol. 5*:272-278.

198. Platel, A., Jalfre, M., Pawelec, C., Roux, S., and Porsolt, R.D. (1984). Habituation of exploratory activity in mice: Effects of combinations of piracetam and choline on memory processes. *Pharmacol. Biochem. Behav. 21*:209-212.

199. Smith, R.C., Vroulis, G., Johnson, R., and Morgan, R. (1984). Comparison of therapeutic response to long-term treatment with lecithin versus piracetam plus lecithin in patients with Alzheimer's disease. *Psychopharmacol. Bull. 20*: 542-545.

200. Growdon, J.H., Corkin, S., Huff, F.J., and Rosen, T.J. (1986). Piracetam combined with lecithin in the treatment of Alzheimer's disease. *Neurobiol. Aging 7*:269-276.

201. Ezzat, D.H., Ibraheem, M.M., and Makhawy, B. (1985). The effect of piracetam on ECT-induced memory disturbances. *Br. J. Psychiatry 147*:720-721.

202. Olpe, H.R., Jones, R.S.G., and Haas, H.L. (1984). Comparative extracellular- and intracellular-electrophysiological investigations on the action of oxirace-tam and piracetam on hippocampal slices. *Clin. Neuropharmacol. S417*:774-775.

203. Spignoli, G., Pedata, F., Giovannelli, L., Banfi, S., Moroni, F., and Pepeu, G. (1986). Effect of oxiracetam and piracetam on central cholinergic mech-anisms and active avoidance acquisition. *Clin. Neuropharmacol. 9*:S39-S47.

204. Spignoli, G., and Pepeu, G. (1987). Interactions between oxiracetam, anir-acetam and scopolamine on behavior and brain acetylcholine. *Pharmacol. Biochem. Behav. 27*:491-495.

205. Pepeu, G., and Spignoli, G. (1990). Neurochemical actions of "nootropic drugs." *Adv. Neurol. 51*:247-252.

206. Moglia, A., Sinforiani, E., Zandrini, C., Gualtieri, S., Corsico, R., and Arrigo, A. (1986). Activity of oxiracetam in patients with organic brain syndrome: A neuropsychological study. *Clin. Neuropharmacol. 9*:S73-S78.

207. Hjorther, A., Browne, E., Jakobsen, K., Viskum, P., and Gynthelberg, F. (1987). Organic brain syndrome treated with oxiracetam. A double-blind ran-domized controlled trial. *Acta Neurol. Scand. 75*:271-276.

208. Saletu, B., Linzmayer, L., Grunberger, J., and Pietschmann, H. (1985). Dou-ble-blind, placebo-controlled, clinical, psychometric and neurophysiological investigations with oxiracetam in the organic brain syndrome of late life. *Neu-ropsychobiology 13*:44-52.

209. Smirne, S., Truci, G., Pieri, E., Monza, G.C., Piccolo, I., deFilippi, F., Mar-chetti, C., and Motta, A. (1987). Efficacy and tolerability of oxiracetam in Alzheimer's disease—A double blind, six month study. *Clin. Neurol. Neuro-surg. 89*(2):19.

210. Saletu, B., Grunberger, J., and Linzmayer, L. (1980). Quantitative EEG and psychometric analyses in assessing CNS activity of Ro 13-5057—A cerebral insufficiency improver. *Methods Find. Exp. Clin. Pharmacol. 2*:269-285.

211. Dajas, F., Romero, S., Florens, M., Lorenzo, J. et al. (1983). Neuropsycho-logical and psychiatric assessment of the effects of aniracetam (RO 13-5057) on age related brain deficits. Preliminary results. Presented at the 6th Int Neuro-psychological Soc (INS) Eur. Conf., Lisbon, June 14-17, 1983. The INS Bulle-tin, p. 12.

212. Sourander, L.B., Portin, R., Molsa, P., Lahdes, A., and Rinne, U.K. (1987). Senile dementia of the Alzheimer type treated with aniracetam: A new noo-trophic agent. *Psychopharmacology 91*:90-95.

213. Reisberg, B., Ferris, S.H., and Gershon, S. (1981). An overview of pharma-cologic treatment of cognitive decline in the aged. *Am. J. Psychiatry 138*:593-600.

214. Yesavage, J.A., Tinklenberg, J.R., Hollister, L.E., and Berger, P.A. (1979). Vasodilators in senile dementia. *Arch. Gen. Psychiatry 36*:220-223.

215. Bazo, A.J. (1973). An ergot alkaloid prepatation (Hydergine) versus papa-verine in treating common complaints of the aged: Double-blind study. *J. Am. Geriatr. Soc. 21*:63-71.

216. Rosen, H.J. (1975). Mental decline in the elderly: Pharmacotherapy (ergot alkaloids versus papaverine). *J. Am. Geriatr. Soc. 23*:169-174.

217. Rehman, S.A. (1973). Two trials comparing "Hydergine" with placebo in the treatment of patients suffering from cerebrovascular insufficiency. *Curr. Med. Res. Opin. 1*:456-462.

218. McConnachie, R.W. (1973). A clinical trial comparing "Hydergine" with placebo in the treatment of cerebrovascular insufficiency in elderly patients. *Curr. Med. Res. Opin. 1*:463-468.

219. Thibault, A. (1974). A double-blind evaluation of "Hydergine" and placebo in the treatment of patients with organic brain syndrome and cerebral arteriosclerosis in a nursing home. *Curr. Med. Res. Opin. 2*:482-487.

220. Banen, D.M. (1972). An ergot preparation (Hydergine) for relief of symptoms of cerebrovascular insufficiency. *J. Am. Geriatr. Soc. 20*:22-24.

221. Rao, D.B., and Norris, J.R. (1972). A double-blind investigation of hydergine in the treatment of cerebrovascular insufficiency in the elderly. *Johns Hopkins Med. J. 130*:317-324.

222. Jennings, W.G. (1972). An ergot alkaloid preparation (hydergine) versus placebo for treatment of symptoms of cerebrovascular insufficiency: Double-blind study. *J. Am. Geriatr. Soc. 20*:407-412.

223. Triboletti, F., and Ferri, H. (1969). Hydergine for treatment of symptoms of cerebrovascular insufficiency. *Curr. Ther. Res. 11*:609-620.

224. Ditch, M., Kelly, F.J., and Resnick, O. (1971). An ergot preparation (hydergine) in the treatment of cerebrovascular disorders in the geriatric patient: Double-blind study. *J. Am. Geriatr. Soc. 19*:208-217.

225. Gerin, J. (1969). Symptomatic treatment of cerebrovascular insufficiency with hydergine. *Curr. Ther. Res. 11*:539-546.

226. Roubicek, J., Geiger, C., and Abt, K. (1972). An ergot alkaloid preparation (hydergine) in geriatric therapy. *J. Am. Geriatr. Soc. 20*:222-229.

227. Kugler, J., Oswald, W.D., Herzfeld, U., Seus, R., Pingel, J., and Welzel, D. (1978). Longterm treatment of cerebrovascular changes in the elderly. *Dtsch. Med. Wochenschr. 103*:456-462.

228. Stern, F.H. (1970). Management of chronic brain syndrome secondary to cerebral arteriosclerosis with special reference to papaverine hydrochloride. *J. Am. Geriatr. Soc. 18*:507-512.

229. Ritter, R.M., Nail, H.R., Tatum, P., and Blazi, M. (1971). The effect of papaverine on patients with cerebral arteriosclerosis. *Clin. Med. 78*:18-22.

230. McQuillan, L.M., Lopec, C.A., and Vibal, J.R. (1974). Evaluation of EEG and clinical changes associated with pavabid therapy in chronic brain syndrome. *Curr. Ther. Res. 16*:49-58.

231. Branconnier, R.J., and Cole, J.O. (1977). Effects of chronic papaverine administration on mild senile organic brain syndrome. *J. Am. Geriatr. Soc. 25*: 458-462.

232. Blakemore, C.B. (1987). Cyclandelate in the treatment of multi-infarct dementia. Interim findings from a multicentre study in general practice. *Drugs 33*:110-113.

233. Ananth, J. (1987). Specific effects of cyclandelate on memory. *Drugs 33*:97-102.

234. Albizzati, M.G., Bassi, S., Calloni, E., Sbacchi, M., Piolti, R., and Frattola, L. (1987). Cyclandelate versus flunarizine. A double-blind study in a selected group of patients with dementia. *Drugs 33*:90-96.

235. Hachinski, V.C., Iliff, L.D., Zilhka, E., Boulay, G.H.D., McAllister, V.L., Marshall, J., Russell, R. W., and Symon, L. (1975). Cerebral blood flow in dementia. *Arch. Neurol. 32*:632-637.

236. Hachinski, V.C., Lassen, N.A., and Marshall, J. (1974). Multi-infarct dementia. A cause of mental deterioration in the elderly. *Lancet 2*:207-210.

237. Scheinberg, P. (1988). Dementia due to vascular disease—a multifactorial disorder. *Stroke 19*:1291-1299.

238. Philippon, J., Grob, R., Dagreou, F., Guggiari, M., Rivierez, M., and Viars, P. (1986). Prevention of vasospasm in subarachnoid haemorrhage. A controlled study of nimodipine. *Acta Neurochir. 82*:110-114.

239. Wilkins, R.H. (1986). Attempts at prevention of treatment of intracranial arterial spasm: An update. *Neurosurgery 18*:808-825.

240. Pickard, J.D., Murray, G.D., Illingworth, R., Shaw, M.D.M., et al. (1989). Effect of oral nimodipine on cerebral infarction and outcome after subarachnoid haemorrhage: British aneurysm nimodipine trial. *Br. Med. J. 298*:636-642.

241. Petruk, K.C., West, M., Mohr, G., Weir, B.K.A., et al. (1988). Nimodipine treatment in poor-grade aneurysm patients. Results of a multicenter double-blind placebo-controlled trial. *J. Neurosurg. 68*:505-517.

242. Allen, G.S., Ahn, H.S., Preziosi, T.J., Battye, R., Boone, S.C., et al. (1983). Cerebral arterial spasm—a controlled trial of nimodipine in patients with subarachnoid hemorrhage. *N. Engl. J. Med. 308*:619-624.

243. Forsman, M., Aarseth, H.P., Nordby, H.K., Skulberg, A., and Steen, P.A. (1989). Effects of nimodipine on cerebral blood flow and cerebrospinal fluid pressure after cardiac arrest: Correlation with neurologic outcome. *Anesth. Analg. 68*:436-443.

244. Gelmers, J.H. (1985). Calcium-channel blockers: Effects on cerebral blood flow and potential uses for acute stroke. *Am. J. Cardiol. 55*:144B-148B.

245. Gelmers, H.J. (1987). Effect of calcium antagonist on the cerebral circulation. *Am. J. Cardiol. 59*:173B-176B.

246. Scriabine, A., and van den Kerckhoff, W. (1988). Pharmacology of nimodipine. *Ann. N.Y. Acad. Sci. 522*:698-706.

247. Harper, A.M., Craigen, L., and Kazda, S. (1981). Effect of the calcium antagonist, nimodipine, on cerebral blood flow and metabolism in the primate. *J. Cereb. Blood Flow Metab. 1*:349-356.

248. Steen, P.A., Newberg, L.A., Milde, J.H., and Michenfelder, J.D. (1983). Nimodipine improves cerebral blood flow and neurologic recovery after complete cerebral ischemia in the dog. *J. Cereb. Blood Flow Metab. 3*:38-43.

249. Haws, C.W., Gourley, J.K., and Heistad, D.D. (1983). Effects of nimodpine on cerebral blood flow. *J. Pharmacol. Exp. Ther. 225*:24-28.

250. Steen, P.A., Newberg, L.A., Milde, J.H., and Michenfelder, J.D. (1984). Cerebral blood flow and neurologic outcome when nimodipine is given after complete cerebral ischemia in the dog. *J. Cereb. Blood Flow Metab. 4*:82-87.

251. McCalden, T.A., Nath, R.G., and Thiele, K. (1984). The effects of a calcium antagonist (nimodipine) on basal cerebral blood flow and reactivity to various agonists. *Stroke 15*:527-530.

252. Grabowski, M., and Johansson, B.B. (1985). Nifedipine and nimodipine: Effect on blood pressure and regional cerebral blood flow in conscious normotensive and hypertensive rats. *J. Cardiovasc. Pharmacol. 7*:1127-1133.

253. Milde, L.N., Milde, J.H., and Michenfelder, J.D. (1986). Delayed treatment with nimodipine improves cerebral blood flow after complete cerebral ischemia in the dog. *J. Cereb. Blood Flow Metab. 6*:332-337.

254. Mohamed, A.A., Mendelow, A.D., Teasdale, G.M., Harper, A.M., and McCulloch, J. (1985). Effect of the calcium antagonist nimodipine on local cerebral blood flow and metabolic coupling. *J. Cereb. Blood Flow Metab. 5*:26-33.

255. Mohamed, A.A., McCulloch, J., Mendelow, A.D., Teasdale, G.M., and Harper, A.M. (1984). Effect of the calcium antagonist nimodipine on local cerebral blood flow: Relationship to arterial blood pressure. *J. Cereb. Blood Flow Metab. 4*:206-211.

256. Landfield, P.W., and Pitler, T.A. (1984). Prolonged Ca 2 + -dependent after hyperpolarizations in hippocampal neurons of aged rats. *Science 226*:1089-1092.

257. Gibson, G.E., and Peterson, C. (1987). Calcium and the aging nervous system. *Neurobiol. Aging 8*:329-343.

258. Siesjo, B.K. (1981). Cell damage in the brain: A speculative synthesis. *J. Cereb. Blood Flow Metab. 1*:155-185.

259. Deyo, R.A., Straube, K.T., and Disterhoft, J.F. (1989). Nimodipine facilitates associative learning in aging rabbits. *Science 243*:809-811.

260. Tetrud, J.W., and Langston, J.W. (1989). The effect of deprenyl (selegiline) on the natural history of Parkinson's disease. *Science 245*:519-522.

261. The Parkinson's Study Group. (1989). Effect of deprenyl on the progression of disability in early Parkinson's disease. *N. Engl. J. Med. 321*:1364-1371.

262. Tariot, P.N., Cohen, R.M., Sunderland, T., Newhouse, P.A., et al. (1987). L-Deprenyl in Alzheimer's disease. Preliminary evidence for behavioral change with monoamine oxidase B inhibition. *Arch. Gen. Psychiatry 44*:427-433.

263. Amaducci, L. (1988). Phosphatidylserine in the treatment of Alzheimer's disease: Results of a multicenter study. *Psychopharmacol. Bull. 24*:130-134.

264. Delwaide, P.J., Gyselynck-Mambourg, A.M., Hurlet, A., and Ylieff, M. (1986). Double-blind randomized controlled study of phosphatidylserine in senile demented patients. *Acta Neurol. Scand. 73*:136-140.

265. Katz, R.J., and Liebler, L. (1978). GABA involvement in memory consolidation: Evidence from posttrial amino-oxyacetic acid. *Psychopharmacology 56*: 191-193.

266. Ghoneim, M.M., and Mewaldt, S.P. (1977). Studies on human memory: The interactions of diazepam, scopolamine, and physostigmine. *Psychopharmacology 52*:1-6.

267. Ghoneim, M.M., and Mewaldt, S.P. (1990). Benzodiazepines and human memory: A review. *Anesthesiology 72*:926-938.

268. Wolkowitz, O.M., and Tinklenberg, J.R. (1985). Naloxone's effect on cognitive functioning in drug-free and diazepam-treated normal humans. *Psychopharmacology 85*:221-223.

269. Wolkowitz, O.M., Weingartner, H., Thompson, K., Pickar, D., Paul, S.M., and Hommer, D.W. (1985). Diazepam-induced amnesia: A neuropharmaco-

logical model for the "organic amnestic syndrome." *Am. J. Psychiatry 144*: 25-29.

270. Petersen, R.C., and Ghoneim, M.M. (1980). Diazepam and human memory: Influence on acquisition, retrieval, and state-dependent learning. *Prog. Neuro. Psychopharmacol. 4*:81-89.

271. O'Boyle, C., Lambe, R., Darragh, A., Taffe, W., Brick, I., and Kenny, M. (1983). RO-15-1788 antagonizes the effects of diazepam in man without affecting its bioavailability. *Br. J. Anaesth. 55*:349-356.

272. Perry, E.K., Gibson, P.H., Blessed, G., Perry, R.H., and Tomlinson, B.E. (1977). Neurotransmitter enzyme abnormalities in senile dementia. Choline acetyltransferase and glutamic acid decarboxylase activities in necropsy brain tissue. *J. Neurol. Sci. 34*:247-265.

273. Davies, P. (1979). Neurotransmitter-related enzymes in senile dementia of the Alzheimer type. *Brain Res. 171*:319-327.

274. Rosor, M.N., Garrett, N.J., Johnson, A.L., Mountjoy, C.O., Roth, M., and Iversen, L.L. (1982). A post-mortem study of the cholinergic and GABA systems in senile dementia. *Brain 105*:313-330.

275. Mohr, E., Bruno, G., Foster, N., Gillespie, M., et al. (1986). GABA-agonist therapy for Alzheimer's disease. *Clin. Neuropharmacol. 9*:257-263.

276. Kovacs, G.L., and DeWied, D. (1981). Endorphin influences on learning and memory. In *Endogenous Peptides and Learning and Memory Processes.* Edited by J.L. Martinez Jr., R.A. Jensen, R.B. Messing, H. Rigter, J.L. McGaugh. Academic Press, New York, pp. 231-247.

277. Wolkowitz, O.M., Tinklenberg, J.R., and Weingartner, H. (1985). A psychopharmacological perspective of cognitive functions. II. Specific pharmacologic agents. *Neuropsychobiology 14*:133-156.

278. Izquierdo, I., and Graudenz, M. (1980). Memory facilitation by naloxone is due to release of dopaminergic and beta-adrenergic systems from tonic inhibition. *Psychopharmacology 67*:265-268.

279. File, S.E., and Silverstone, T. (1981). Naloxone changes self-ratings but not performance in normal subjects. *Psychopharmacology 74*:353-354.

280. Volavka, J., Dornbush, R., Mallya, A., and Cho, D. (1979). Naloxone fails to affect short-term memory in man. *Psychiatry Res. 1*:89-92.

281. Reisberg, B., Ferris, S.H., Anand, R., Mir, P., Geibel, V., de Leon, M.J., and Roberts, E. (1983). Effects of naloxone in senile dementia: A double-blind trial. *N. Engl. J. Med. 308*:721-722.

282. Tariot, P.N., Sunderland, T., Weingartner, H., Murphy, D.L., Cohen, M.R., and Cohen, R.M. (1986). Naloxone and Alzheimer's disease. Cognitive and behavioral effects of a range of doses. *Arch. Gen. Psychiatry 43*:727-732.

283. Pomara, N., Roberts, R., Rhiew, H.B., Stanley, M., and Gershon, S. (1985). Multiple, single-dose naltrexone administrations fail to effect overall cognitive functioning and plasma cortisol in individuals with probable Alzheimer's disease. *Neurobiol. Aging 6*:233-236.

284. Henderson, V.W., Roberts, E., Wimer, C., Bardolph, E.L., Chui, H.C., Damasio, A.R., et al. (1989). Multicenter trial of naloxone in Alzheimer's disease. *Ann. Neurol. 25*:404-406.

285. Hefti, F., and Weiner, W.J. (1986). Nerve growth factor and Alzheimer's disease. *Ann. Neurol. 20*:275-281.

286. Korsching, S., Auburger, G., Heumann, R., Scott, J., and Thoenen, H. (1985). Levels of nerve growth factor and its mRNA in the central nervous system of the rat correlate with cholinergic innervation. *EMBO 4*:1389-1393.

287. Schwab, M.E., Otten, U., Agid, Y., and Thoenen, H. (1979). Nerve growth factor (NGF) in the rat CNS: Absence of specific retrograde axonal transport and tyrosine hydroxylase induction in locus coeruleus and substantia nigra. *Brain Res. 168*:473-483.

288. Seiler, M., and Schwab, M.E. (1984). Specific retrograde transport of nerve growth factor (NGF) from neocortex to nucleus basalis in the rat. *Brain Res. 300*:33-39.

289. Gnahn, H., Hefti, F., Heumann, R., Schwab, M.E., and Thoenen, H. (1983). NGF-mediated increase of choline acetyltransferase (ChAT) in the neonatal rat forebrain; Evidence for a physiological role of NGF in the brain? *Brain Res. 285*:45-52.

290. Mobley, W.C., Rutkowski, J.L., Tennekoon, G.I., Buchanan, K., Johnston, M.V., et al. (1986). Choline acetyltransferase activity in striatum of neonatal rats increased by nerve growth factor. *Science 229*:284-287.

291. Mobley, W.C., Rutkowski, J.L., Tennekoon, G.I., Buchanan, K., and Johnston, M.V. (1986). Nerve growth factor increases choline acetyltransferase activity in developing basal forebrain neurons. *Brain Res. 387*:53-62.

292. Phelps, C.H., Gage, F.H., Growdon, J.H., Hefti, F., Harbaugh, R., Johnston, M.V., Khachaturian, Z.S., Mobley, W.C., Price, D.L., Raskind, M., et al. (1989). Potential use of nerve growth factor to treat Alzheimer's disease. *Neurobiol. Aging 10*:205-207.

293. Greenamyre, J.T., Penney, J.B., Young, A.B., D'Amato, C.J., Hicks, S.P., and Shoulson, I. (1985). Alteration in l-glutamate binding in Alzheimer's and Huntington's diseases. *Science 227*:1496.

294. Greenamyre, J.T. (1986). The role of glutamate in neurotransmission in neurologic disease. *Arch. Neurol. 43*:1058.

295. Perry, T.L., Yong, V.W., Bergeron, C., Hansen, S., and Jones, K. (1987). Amino acids, glutathione, and glutathione transferase activity in the brains of patients with Alzheimer's disease. *Ann. Neurol. 21*:331.

296. Hyman B.T., Van Hoesen G.W., Damasio A.R. (1987). Alzheimer's disease: Glutamate depletion in the hippocampal perforant pathway zone. *Ann. Neurol. 22*:37-40.

297. Reimherr, F.W., Wood, D.R., and Wender, P.H. (1986). The use of MK-801, a novel sympathomimetic, in adults with attention deficit disorder, residual type. *Psychopharmacol. Bull. 22*:237.

298. Meldrum, B. (1985). Possible therapeutic applications of antagonists of excitatory amino acid neurotransmitters. *Clin. Sci. 68*:113-122.

299. Croog, S.H., Levine, S., Tests, M., et al. (1986). The effects of antihypertensive therapy on the quality of life. *N. Engl. J. Med. 314*:1657-1664.

300. Lichter, I., Richardson, P., and Wyke, M. (1986). Differential effects of atenolol and enalapril on memory during treatment for essential hypertension. *Br. J. Clin. Pharmacol. 21*:641-645.

301. Britton, K., Granowska, M., Nimmon, C.C., et al. (1985). Cerebral blood flow in hypertensive patients with cerebrovascular disease: Technique for measurements and effects of captopril. *Nucl. Med. Comm.* 6:251-261.
302. Rajagopalan, B., Raine, A.E.G., Cooper, R., et al. (1984). Changes in the cerebral blood flow in patients with severe congestive heart failure before and after captopril treatment. *Am. J. Med.* 76:86-90.
303. Crapper, D., Krishnan, S., and Dalton, A. (1973). Brain aluminum distribution in Alzheimer's disease and experimental neurofibrillary degeneration. *Science 180*:511-512.
304. DeBoni, V., and Crapper McLachlan, D. (1981). Biochemical aspect of SDAT and aluminum as a neurotoxic agent. In *Strategies for the Development of an Effective Treatment for Senile Dementia*. Edited by T. Crook, S. Gershon. Mark Powley Association, Connecticut.
305. Markesbery, W., Ehmann, W., Hossain, T., et al. (1981). Instrumental neutron activation analysis of brain aluminum in Alzheimer's disease and aging. *Ann. Neurol.* 10:511-516.
306. Cardelli, M., Russell, M., Gabne, C., and Pomara, N. (1985). Chelation therapy, unproved modality in the treatment of Alzheimer-type dementia. *J. Am. Geriatr. Soc. 33*:548-551.
307. Wilson, B. (1984). Memory therapy in practice. In *Clinical Management of Memory Problems*. Edited by B.A. Wilson and N. Moffat. Aspen Systems Corporation, Rockville, MD, pp. 89-111.
308. Wilson, B., Cockburn, J., and Baddeley, A. (1985). *The Rivermead Behavioral Memory Test*. Thames Valley Test Company, England.
309. Wilson, B. (1987). *Rehabilitation of Memory*. Guilford Press, New York.
310. Fordyce, D.J., Roueche, J.R., and Prigatano, G.P. (1983). Enhanced emotional reactions in chronic head trauma patients. *J. Neurol. Neurosurg. Psychiatry 46*:620-624.
311. Dikmen, S., and Reitan, R.M. (1977). Emotional sequelae of head injury. *Ann. Neurol. 2*:492-494.
312. Prigatano, G.P. (1987). Personality and psychosocial consequences after brain injury. In *Neuropsychological Rehabilitation*. Edited by M.J. Meier, A.L. Benton, and L. Diller. Churchill Livingstone, New York, pp. 355-378.
313. Sunderland, A., Harris, J.E., and Baddeley, A.D. (1983). Do laboratory tests predict everyday memory? A neuropsychological study. *J. Verb. Learn. Verb. Behav. 22*:341-357.
314. Sunderland, A., Harris, J.E., and Gleave, J. (1984). Memory failures in everyday life following severe head injury. *J. Clin. Neuropsychol. 6*:127-142.
315. Stuss, D.T., and Benson, D.F. (1986). *The Frontal Lobes*. Raven Press, New York.
316. Levin, H.S., High, W.M., Jr., Goethe, K.E., Sisson, R.A., et al. (1987). The neurobehavioral rating scale: Assessment of the behavioural sequelae of head injury by the clinician. *J. Neurol. Neurosurg. Psychiatry 50*:183-193.
317. Schacter, D.L., Glisky, E.L., and McGlynn, S.M. (1990). Impact of memory disorder on everyday life: Awareness of deficits and return to work. In *The Neuropsychology of Everyday Life. Volume I. Theories and Basic Competencies*. Edited by D. Tupper and K. Cicerone. Martinus Nijhoff, Boston.

318. Schacter, D.L., and Glisky, E.L. (1986). Memory remediation: Restoration, alleviation, and the acquisition of domain-specific knowledge. In *Clinical Neuropsychology of Intervention*. Edited by B. Uzzell and Y. Gross. Martinus Nijhoff, Boston, pp. 257-282.

319. Glisky, E.L., and Schacter, D.L. (1988). Long-term retention of computer learning by patients with memory disorders. *Neuropsychologia 26*:173-178.

320. Glisky, E.L., and Schacter, D.L. (1989). Extending the limits of complex learning in organic amnesia: Computer training in a vocational domain. *Neuropsychologia 27*:107-120.

321. Harris, J. (1984). Methods of improving memory. In *Clinical Management of Memory Problems*. Edited by B.A. Wilson and N. Moffat. Aspen Systems Corporation, Rockville, Maryland, pp. 46-62.

322. Crovitz, H.F. (1979). Memory retraining in brain-damaged patients: The airplane list. *Cortex 15*:131-134.

323. Crovitz, H.F., Harvey, M.T., and Horn, R.W. (1979). Problems in the acquisition of imagery mnemonics: Three brain-damaged cases. *Cortex 15*:225-234.

324. Gianutsos, R., and Gianutsos, J. (1979). Rehabilitating the verbal recall of brain-injured patients by mnemonic training: An experimental demonstration using single-case methodology. *J. Clin. Neuropsychol. 1*:117-136.

325. Glasgow, R.E., Zeiss, R.A., Barrera, M. Jr., and Lewinsohn, P.M. (1977). Case studies on remediating memory deficits in brain-damaged individuals. *J. Clin. Psychol. 33*:1049-1054.

326. Jones, M.K. (1974). Imagery as a mnemonic aid after left temporal lobectomy: Contrast between material-specific and generalized memory disorders. *Neuropsychologia 12*:21-30.

327. Lewinsohn, P.M., Danaher, B.G., and Kikel, S. (1977). Visual imagery as a mnemoic aid for brain-injured persons. *J. Consult. Clin. Psychol. 45*:717-723.

328. Wilson, B. (1982). Success and failure in memory training following a cerebral vascular accident. *Cortex 18*:581-594.

329. Harris, J.E. (1980). Memory aids people use: Two interview studies. *Mem Cognit. 8*:31-38.

Index

Acetylcholine, 63, 459, 468
Acetylcholinesterase, 63, 80,
    459-461
Acetyl-1-carnitine, 468, 469
ACh (*see* Acetylcholine)
AChE (*see* Acetylcholinesterase)
Acquired immunodeficiency
    syndrome, 399-400
ACTH (*see* Adrenocorticotropic
    hormone)
Acute confusional state, 200, 206,
    214, 287, 401 (*see also*
    Delirium)
ADH (*see* Antidiuretic hormone)
Adrenal-brain transplant, 462
Adrenergic drugs, 453, 464
Adrenocorticotropic hormone,
    103, 468
Aging, 347-363
Agnosia, 382
AIDS (*see* Acquired immunode-
    ficiency syndrome)
Alcohol, 104, 105, 401
Alcoholic blackout, 401, 441
Alcoholics, 236, 239, 241, 244-246
Aluminum, 478
Alzheimer's disease, 12, 13, 15, 28,
    35, 48, 86, 88, 98, 100-102,
    117-119, 121, 122, 148, 170,
    173-175, 178, 181, 182,

[Alzheimer's disease]
    186, 239, 242, 243, 269,
    374, 375, 377, 380-385,
    399, 404, 457, 459, 460,
    462, 463, 465, 467-471,
    475-478
Amnesia (*see also* Amnesic
    syndrome)
anterograde, 11, 23, 24, 26, 28,
    29, 32, 33, 37, 41, 45-47,
    49, 50, 102, 166, 171, 173,
    203, 204, 209-211, 230-234,
    236, 244, 245, 247, 261,
    279, 283, 300, 301, 313,
    314, 330, 331, 334, 336,
    377, 383, 398, 401-403,
    405, 434, 439
continuous, 438, 446
diencephalic, 28-31, 37-41, 203,
    206
functional, 429, 430
general, 438, 446
global, 438
hysterical, 446
localized, 438
postictal, 314
posttraumatic, 12, 256, 259,
    261-266, 435
psychogenic (*see* Psychogenic
    amnesia)

[Amnesia]
  retrograde, 12, 24, 26, 47, 48,
    50, 166, 203, 204, 206, 209-
    211, 234-238, 244, 247,
    259, 263-265, 279, 283,
    303, 305, 313, 315, 377,
    383, 398, 399, 403, 405,
    435, 437, 446
  selective, 438
  situational, 438, 439
  source, 357, 358, 362
  temporal lobe, 24-28
Amnesic syndrome, 165-168
Amphetamine, 105
Amygdala, 24-28, 34-37, 39, 41,
    42, 45-48, 53, 65, 67, 68,
    72, 78, 80, 83, 171, 207,
    214, 288, 300, 301, 304,
    306, 307, 322, 331, 334,
    335, 370, 371, 381, 398
Aneurysm
  anterior communicating artery,
    172, 211-213, 481
  basilar artery, 213
Angiotensin-converting enzyme
    inhibitor, 477
Aniracetam, 470-472
Anticonvulsants, 312, 402
Antidiuretic hormone, 103
Antihypertensive drugs, 402
Aphasia, 335, 383
Apraxia, 382
Arecholine, 461
Artery
  anterior cerebral, 45, 206, 211
  anterior choroidal, 198, 203
  anterior communicating, 45, 211
  basilar communicating, 201, 202
  Heubner's recurrent, 211, 212
  hippocampal, 198
  inferior temporal, 198
  interpeduncular profundus (see
    paramedian thalamic)

[Artery]
  paramedian mesencephalic, 204
  paramedian thalamic, 202, 203
  polar (see tuberothalamic)
  posterior cerebral, 198-200
  posterior choroidal, 198
  premamillary (see tuberothalamic)
  thalamoperforating (see para-
    median thalamic)
  tuberothalamic, 202, 203
Aspartate, 477
Aura, 313, 315
Automatic processing, 16, 267,
    270, 271
Automatism, 313, 434, 440
AVLT (see Rey auditory-verbal
    learning test)

Basal forebrain, 28, 46, 48, 64,
    65, 174, 212, 245, 371, 381,
    398, 458, 475
Basal ganglia, 182, 206, 238, 369-
    373
Benzodiazepines, 99, 101-103, 401,
    434, 475
Bethanechol, 461
Binswanger disease, 186, 208
Block-tapping test, 331
Boston naming test, 175, 177, 179,
    181, 242, 243
Bradyphrenia, 374
Brain stem, 63, 182, 243
Brain tumors, 283, 413-420 (see
    also Craniopharyngioma,
    gliomas, meningioma, pitui-
    tary adenoma)
  frontoseptal, 417
  thalamic, 416, 417
  in third ventricle, 414-416

Calcium channel antagonist, 473,
    474

California verbal learning test, 157-160, 167, 242
Captopril, 477, 478
Carbamazepine, 312, 313, 402
CCK (see Cholecystokinin)
Cerebellum, 182, 243, 379, 380
ChAT (see Choline acetyltransferase)
Chelation, 478
Cholecystokinin, 103
Choline, 459, 460
Choline acetyltransferase, 63, 65, 67, 75, 78, 80, 83, 86, 101, 174, 371, 378, 458, 459, 462, 463, 468, 477
Cholinergic system, 245, 371, 381, 466
Cingulectomy, 423
Classical conditioning, 51
Clonidine, 464
Closed head injury, 12, 13, 143, 171, 255-273, 434, 435, 478-482
  impaired consciousness in, 256, 258, 267
  ocular responses in, 256, 258, 267
Commissure, anterior, 68
Commissurotomy, 423
Computerized memory assessment, 161-163
Confabulation, 229, 230
Controlled word association task, 168
Conversion syndrome, 445
Corpus callosotomy, 423
Corpus callosum, 200, 417, 418
Cortex (see also Gyrus)
  anterior insula, 26
  entorhinal, 24, 28, 32, 36, 41, 42, 44, 45, 53, 174, 381
  orbitofrontal, 26, 41, 370, 398
  paraolfactory, 378

[Cortex]
  perirhinal, 36
  piriform, 370
  prefrontal, 28, 45, 362, 370, 371, 419
  prepiriform, 24
  retrosplenial, 210
Craniopharyngioma, 414, 415 (see also Brain tumors)
Creutzfeldt-Jakob disease, 173, 399
CVLT (see California verbal learning test)
Cyclandelate, 473

Deja vu, 307, 308
Delayed nonmatching-to-sample task, 33, 34, 36, 37, 39, 40, 46, 51
Delayed recognition span test, 167, 169, 175, 179
Delayed word recall test, 148
Delirium, 206, 287, 401 (see also Acute confusional state)
Dementia (see also Dementia syndrome)
  alcoholic, 242, 243
  in amyotrophic lateral sclerosis, 399
  cortical, 373, 380-382
  depressive, 437, 438, 440, 442-445
  frontal lobe type (see Dementia of frontal lobe type)
  hysterical, 438, 444, 445, 449
  in lacunar state, 186, 208, 421
  multi-infarct, 185-187, 208, 473
  subcortical, 182, 373, 374, 377, 378, 399, 404
Dementia of frontal lobe type, 178-180, 384
Dementia syndrome, 173-187

Denman neuropsychology memory
    scale, 154
Deprenyl, 474, 475
Depression, 17, 123, 235, 347,
    361, 441, 479
Diagonal band of Broca, 66-68
Diencephalon, 24, 50, 63, 112,
    143, 168, 289
Dihydroergotoxine mesylate, 472,
    473
Dissociation, 431
Divided attention, 352, 355
DL-threo-dihydroxyphenylserine,
    464
Dopamine, 182, 375, 378
Dopaminergic system, 466
    mesencephalic, 371
    mesocorticolimbic, 369-371, 378
Down's syndrome, 28
Drilled word span test, 144, 145

Effort-demanding processing, 16,
    17, 99, 103, 120, 269-271,
    375
Electric stimulation
    cerebral cortex, 305, 306
    hippocampus, 305
    temporal lobe, 305, 307, 404,
        405
Electroconvulsive therapy, 235,
    263, 303, 404-406, 436,
    471
Embedded figures test, 168, 242
Encephalitis
    herpes simplex, 12, 13, 26, 35,
        48, 166, 167, 170, 398
    limbic, 400
Encephalopathy, 400-402
Endorphins, 103
Epilepsy, 308-312 (see also Seizure)
    generalized, 308
    nontemporal lobe, 309
    temporal lobe, 308-311, 314

Epileptiform discharges
    generalized, 306
    in temporal lobe, 306, 307
Excitatory amino acids, 477

Flunarizine, 473
Fornicotomy, 422, 423
Fornix, 29, 34-37, 44, 65, 206,
    207, 211, 371, 415-418
Fugue
    postictal, 441
    psychogenic, 437-441

GABA (see Gamma aminobutyric
    acid)
Galveston orientation and amnesia
    test, 262, 263
Gamma aminobutyric acid, 102,
    470, 475, 476
Ganser syndrome, 437, 438, 447
Glasgow coma scale, 256-258, 267
Gliomas, 413-419 (see also Brain
    tumors)
Global ischemia, 213, 214
Globus pallidus, 68
Glutamate, 477
Gyrus (see also Cortex)
    cingulate, 26, 72, 78, 80, 207,
        210, 212, 370, 371, 381,
        398, 419
    fusiform, 199
    lingual, 198
    parahippocampal, 24, 26, 28,
        36, 41, 42, 53, 78, 80, 83
        198, 214, 322, 331, 337

Habenula, 78, 371
Hallervorden-Spatz disease, 379
Hidden objects test, 145
Hippocampal formation (see
    Hippocampus)
Hippocampectomy, 37, 51, 331-334

Hippocampus, 25-37, 40-42, 44-48,
     53, 65, 66, 80, 83, 84, 99,
     102, 119, 171, 172, 198,
     199, 288, 300, 301, 306,
     307, 322, 331, 335-337,
     362, 370, 381, 383, 398,
     400, 418, 419, 469, 474,
     476, 477
  CA1 region of, 26, 28, 42, 214,
     302, 304, 334
  CA2 region of, 26, 42, 44, 304
  CA3 region of, 26, 42, 304
  CA4 region of, 41
Histrionic personality disorder,
     437, 438, 447, 448
Homovanillic acid, 464
Huntington's disease, 117, 118,
     173, 174, 184, 238, 239,
     373, 376, 377, 404
Hydrocephalus, 420-422
  noncommunicating, 422
  normal pressure, 420-422
Hypnosis, 431, 439, 449
Hypothalamus, 68, 78, 168, 211,
     212, 371
Hypoxia (*see* Global ischemia)
Hysterical dysmnesia, 438, 449

Infarct (*see* Thromboembolism)
Intracerebral hemorrhage, 209, 210
  in cerebral cortex, 210
  in thalamus, 209

Korsakoff's syndrome, 12, 13,
     28-30, 37, 41, 44, 45, 99,
     115, 120, 139, 167, 170,
     264, 269, 272, 420, 422,
     430, 434, 464, 466, 467
  alcoholic, 166-169, 227-247
  after aneurysm surgery, 211-213
  in brain tumors, 413-418
  confabulation in, 229

[Korsakoff's syndrome]
  etiology of, 245
  in global ischemia, 213
  in herpes simplex encephalitis,
     398
  neurological bases of, 243-245
  personality in, 228
  problem solving in, 227, 237,
     239, 242, 246
  in subarachnoid hemorrhage,
     211-213
  in thromboembolism, 206
  visuoperceptual processing in,
     227, 242, 243, 246

Lecithin, 459-461, 471
Leukoaraiosis, 209
Lewy body disease, 378
Limbic system, 370, 371
Locus coeruleus, 373, 463, 464
Long-term potentiation, 302-304

Malingering, 433
Mammillary bodies, 28-31, 36, 37,
     40, 41, 44, 168, 244, 398,
     415, 418
Mammillothalamic tract, 29, 39,
     40, 203, 204, 206, 209, 289,
     415, 416, 418
Mattis dementia rating scale, 175,
     176, 183
Medial forebrain bundle, 370
Melanocyte-stimulating hormone,
     103
Memory
  anterograde (*see* Amnesia,
     anterograde)
  autobiographical, 236, 243, 384
  declarative, 16, 18, 50, 52, 238,
     263, 374, 383
  episodic, 15, 18, 50, 52, 99, 100,
     102, 103, 112, 114-118, 120,
     121, 123, 124, 141, 206,

[Memory]
    230, 231, 237, 326, 327,
    349, 357, 362, 383, 398,
    399
  explicit, 11, 15, 18, 112, 116-118,
    122, 124, 239, 356, 359,
    362, 383
  genuine, 146
  global, 267, 269
  immediate, 156, 166
  implicit, 11, 15, 18, 112, 116-
    118, 122, 124, 167, 239,
    356, 357, 359, 362
  incidental, 15
  intentional, 15
  long-term, 14, 18, 33, 49, 113,
    167, 266, 285, 323, 348,
    352-358, 398, 405
  material-specific, 267, 269, 322,
    324, 331
  nonverbal, 160, 310, 311, 329-
    333 (*see also* Memory, visual)
  primary, 11, 14, 17, 112-114,
    117, 118, 123, 139, 140,
    166, 173, 350, 351, 383
  procedural, 16, 18, 50, 51, 117,
    238, 263, 349
  prospective, 350, 358
  recent, 14
  remote, 14, 124, 141, 142, 170,
    171
  retrograde (*see* Amnesia, retro-
    grade)
  secondary, 14, 18, 112, 113,
    117, 118, 123, 139, 166,
    167, 170, 173, 174, 350,
    352-358, 383
  semantic, 15, 18, 50, 101, 112,
    114-118, 120-122, 124, 206,
    231, 237, 326, 327, 349,
    357, 359, 398

[Memory]
  short-term, 11, 13, 17, 24, 49,
    51, 113, 166, 230, 266, 283,
    305, 323, 348, 350-352
  state-dependent, 375, 459
  verbal, 156, 160, 308, 310, 311,
    324-331
  visual, 156, 308, 330 (*see also*
    Memory, nonverbal)
  working, 14, 114, 118, 119, 123,
    162, 328, 348, 351, 352,
    362, 374, 403
Memory testing, 153-163
Meningioma, 414, 419, 420 (*see
    also* Brain tumors)
Metacognitive process, 16, 18
Metamemory, 323, 334, 360 (*see
    also* Metacognitive process)
3-Methoxy-4-hydroxyl-phenylglycol, 464
Migraine, 214, 283, 287, 289
Mini-mental state exam, 142, 176-
    180, 183, 187
Mnemonic aids, 480-482
MSH (*see* Melanocyte-stimulating
    hormone)
Multiple personality disorder, 437,
    438, 448
Multiple sclerosis, 402-404
Multiple system atrophy, 379

Naloxone, 476
National adult reading test, 242
Nerve growth factor, 462, 476, 477
Neuropeptide, 103, 104, 465-467,
    469
Neuropeptide Y, 469
Neuropsychological testing, 165-187
NGF (*see* Nerve growth factor)
Nimodipine, 473
N-methyl-D-aspartate, 376, 477
NMDA (*see* *N*-methyl-D-aspartate)

Noneffortful processing (*see* Automatic processing)
Nootropics, 102, 470-472
Noradrenergic system, 373, 463
Norepinephrine, 245, 464
Nucleus
  accumbens, 64, 212, 370, 371
  anterior thalamic (*see* Thalamus, anterior nucleus of)
  basalis of Meynert, 28, 67, 70, 101, 211, 371, 380, 381, 458
  caudate, 64, 378, 417
  dorsomedialis of thalamus (*see* Thalamus, dorsomedial nucleus of)
  lateral dorsal thalamic (*see* Thalamus, lateral dorsal nucleus of)
  parataenial of thalamus (*see* Thalamus, parataenial nucleus of)
  raphe, 373
  septal, 66, 68, 78, 211, 212, 370, 398, 476

Olfactory bulb, 65, 67
Olfactory tubercle, 64
Olivopontocerebellar atrophy, 379, 380
Opioids, 476
Oxiracetam, 470, 471
Oxotremorine, 461
Oxytocin, 103

Papaverine, 472, 473
Paragraph recall, 149
Parasubiculum, 84
Parkinsonism, 374-376, 421
Parkinsonism-ALS-dementia complex of Guam, 376
Parkinson's disease, 100, 173, 181, 183, 239, 371, 374, 462, 474, 475

[Parkinson's disease]
  with Alzheimer's disease, 376
  familial, 375
  idiopathic, 374, 375
Peptide (*see* Neuropeptide)
Perseveration, 243, 383
Personality disorder, 441
Phenobarbital, 402
Phenytoin, 312, 313, 402
Phosphatidylserine, 475
Physostigmine, 86, 101-103, 460
Pick's disease, 173, 174, 178, 180, 384
Piracetam, 470, 471
Pituitary adenoma, 415 (*see also* Brain tumors)
Postconcussion syndrome, 256, 435
Postencephalitis (*see* Encephalitis, herpes simplex)
Postictal fugue (*see* Fugue)
Posttraumatic stress disorder, 429, 437-440
Pramiracetam, 470
Presubiculum, 44
Primidone, 312
Priming effect, 11, 16, 33, 51, 52, 116, 117, 120, 122, 124, 167, 182, 238, 239
Proactive interference, 118, 167, 231, 242
Processing resources, 353, 355, 362
Progressive aphasia syndrome, 384, 385
Progressive subcortical gliosis, 178, 180
Progressive supranuclear palsy, 173, 174, 182, 377, 378
Prosopagnosia, 381, 382
Pseudodementia, 100, 441, 442, 444

Psychogenesis, 430-437
Psychogenic amnesia, 288, 429-450
Psychogenic fugue (*see* Fugue)
Putamen, 64

Receptor
   dopamine, 378
   glutamate, 376
   N-methyl-D-aspartate, 302, 303, 376, 477
Reduplicative paramnesia, 210, 382
Remediation method of vanishing cues, 480
Repression, 431, 439
Rey auditory verbal learning test, 146, 147, 157-161, 167
Rey-Osterrieth complex figure, 149, 311
Rivermead behavioral memory test, 154, 358, 479

Schizophrenia, 430, 441
Scopolamine, 86, 100, 459, 460
Seizure, 283, 287 (*see also* Epilepsy)
   absence, 314
   complex partial, 313-315, 321, 419
   grand mal, 314, 315
   partial, 285, 304
   temporal lobe, 308-311, 314
      dominant, 311
      nondominant, 311
Selective reminding memory test, 146, 157, 159, 267
Selegiline (*see* Deprenyl)
Septohippocampal graft, 462
Septum pellucidum, 417
Serotonergic system, 373, 466
Short test of mental status, 142

Shy-Drager syndrome, 379
Sodium amytal test, 334-338
Somatostatin, 381, 469
Spike discharges (*see* Epileptiform discharges)
Splenium, 200, 210
Spreading depression, 214
Status epilepticus, 303, 309, 314
Stimulants, 105
Stria terminalis, 68
Striatonigral degeneration, 379
Subarachnoid hemorrhage, 210-213
Subiculum, 26, 42, 44, 53, 84, 174, 214, 381
Substantia innominata, 67, 370, 371
Superior colliculus, 78

Tacrine (*see* Tetrahydroaminoacridine)
Temporal lobectomy, 12, 139, 166, 300, 301, 321-339
   dominant, 322, 324-329
   nondominant, 322, 329-331
Tetrahydroaminoacridine, 101, 460, 461
THA (*see* Tetrahydroaminoacridine)
Thalamus
   anterior nucleus of, 39, 44, 203, 209, 214, 415, 416
   centrum medianum of, 203, 417
   dorsomedial nucleus of, 29-31, 39-41, 44-46, 168, 203-207, 244, 289, 371, 416, 418
   lateral dorsal nucleus of, 45, 52
   parataenial nucleus of, 30
Three words and three shapes test, 143
Thromboembolism, 198-209, 283, 286, 287, 290

[Thromboembolism]
in anterior cerebral artery, 206
in anterior choroidal artery,
203, 207
in internal carotid artery, 207
in middle cerebral artery, 206
in paramedian thalamic artery,
203, 204
in posterior cerebral artery,
198-201
in tuberothalamic artery, 203
Trail making test, 175, 179, 185
Transient global amnesia, 214,
215, 279-298, 314, 419, 420,
422
antecedent events in, 281
associated medical conditions
in, 283
cerebral blood flow in, 215
clinical feature of, 282
differential diagnosis in, 287,
288
electroencephalography in, 284,
285
incidence of, 280
mechanism of, 289, 290
neuroanatomy of, 288, 289
neuropsychological assessment
of, 283
prognosis of, 285, 286
Transitional learning community,
481

Uncus, 25, 331, 335

Valproic acid, 312, 313, 402
Vasodilator, 472
Vasopressin, 103, 104, 465-468
Ventral pallidum, 371
Ventral striatum, 369-372, 378
Ventral tegmental area, 370, 371
Visual search test, 242, 243
Visual spatial learning test, 160

Wechsler adult intelligence scale,
37, 154, 166, 172, 178, 184,
228, 308, 322, 325
Wechsler adult intelligence scale-
revised, 154, 175, 242, 243
Wechsler memory scale, 37, 139,
149, 150, 166, 167, 171,
175, 176, 179, 180, 183-185,
228, 308-311, 324
Wechsler memory scale-revised,
150, 154-156, 161, 162, 167,
228, 233, 234, 242
Wernicke-Korsakoff syndrome,
228, 236, 243-246
Wernicke's encephalopathy, 228,
236, 243, 244, 246
Wisconsin card sorting test, 168,
237, 239, 242, 243
Wilson's disease, 378, 379

Zimelidine, 465

about the editors

TAKEHIKO YANAGIHARA is a Professor of Neurology at the Mayo Medical School and a Consultant in Neurology at the Mayo Clinic, Rochester, Minnesota. He is a member of the American Neurological Association, American Academy of Neurology, American Association of Neuropathologists, and American Society for Neurochemistry. Dr. Yanagihara received the M.D. degree (1960) from the Osaka University School of Medicine, Osaka, Japan.

RONALD C. PETERSEN is an Assistant Professor of Neurology at the Mayo Medical School and a Consultant in Neurology at the Mayo Clinic, Rochester, Minnesota. He is a member of the American Academy of Neurology, Behavioral Neurology Society, and International Neuropsychology Society. Dr. Petersen received the Ph.D. degree (1972) in experimental psychology from the University of Minnesota, Minneapolis, Minnesota, and M.D. degree (1980) from the Mayo Medical School, Rochester, Minnesota. He also completed a fellowship in behavioral neurology at Beth Israel Hospital, Harvard Medical School, Boston, Massachusetts.